PUBLIC HEALTH IN THE 21$^{ST}$ CENTURY

# PREGNANCY AND ALCOHOL CONSUMPTION

# PUBLIC HEALTH IN THE 21ST CENTURY

Additional books in this series can be found on Nova's website under the Series tab.

Additional E-books in this series can be found on Nova's website under the E-books tab.

PUBLIC HEALTH IN THE 21ST CENTURY

# PREGNANCY AND ALCOHOL CONSUMPTION

JOSHUA D. HOFFMAN
EDITOR

Nova Science Publishers, Inc.
*New York*

LIBRARY OF CONGRESS CATALOGING-IN-PUBLICATION DATA
Pregnancy and alcohol consumption / editor, Joshua D. Hoffman.
p. ; cm.
Includes bibliographical references and index.
ISBN 978-1-61761-122-3 (hardcover)
1. Fetal alcohol syndrome. I. Hoffman, Joshua D.
[DNLM: 1. Pregnancy Complications--etiology. 2. Alcohol
Drinking--adverse effects. 3. Ethanol--toxicity. 4. Fetus--drug effects.
5. Maternal-Fetal Exchange--drug effects. WQ 240]
RG629.F45P74 2010
618.3'268--dc22
2010027157

*Published by Nova Science Publishers, Inc. † New York*

# CONTENTS


**Preface** **vii**

**Chapter 1** The Biochemistry of Prenatal Alcohol Exposure **1**
*Ernst van Faassen and Onni Niemelä*

**Chapter 2** Mechanisms of Fetal Toxicity to Alcohol with Special Consideration to Fetal Zinc Deficiency **67**
*P. Coyle, B. L. Summers-Pearce, C. J. Cowley, and A. M. Rofe*

**Chapter 3** Alcohol Use Pre- and Late-Pregnancy: Epidemiology and Comments from Postpartum Surveys **105**
*Diana Cheng, Laurie Kettinger, Douglas D'Agati, Paula J. Lockhart and Lee Hurt*

**Chapter 4** Medaka (Oryzias latipes) as a Model to Study Fetal Alcohol Spectrum Disorder **129**
*Yuhui Hu, Minghui Wu, Ikhlas A. Khan, and Asok K. Dasmahapatra*

**Chapter 5** Research on Interventions to Prevent Alcohol Consumption during Pregnancy **155**
*Katrina Kully-Martens, Katy Wyper and Carmen Rasmussen*

**Chapter 6** Fetal Alcohol Exposure and Risk to the Premature Newborn **175**
*Theresa W. Gauthier, Sowmya S. Mohan and Lou Ann S. Brown*

**Chapter 7** Alcohol-Pregnancy and Placental Hypoxia Versus Fetal Development **195**
*Cleofina Bosco and Eugenia Díaz*

**Chapter 8** The Timing of Alcohol Consumption during Pregnancy and Fetal Alcohol-Induced Brain Damage **225**
*Susan E. Maier and Wei-Jung A. Chen*

**Chapter 9** The French Paradox: Forbidding Alcohol during Pregnancy, but Making an Exception for Wine! **245**
*Agnès Dumas, Stéphanie Toutain and Laurence Simmat-Durand*

| | | |
|---|---|---|
| **Chapter 10** | Medicolegal Considerations Concerning Fetal Alcohol Spectrum Disorders<br>*Christos I. Evaggelakos, Stavroula A. Papadodima and Chara A. Spiliopoulou* | **263** |
| **Chapter 11** | Fetal Alcohol Syndrome in Urban Schools<br>*Giorgie Petković and Ingeborg Barišić* | **281** |
| **Chapter 12** | Life as an Adult with Foetal Alcohol Syndrome<br>*Stéphanie Toutain* | **299** |
| **Chapter 13** | Factors Associated with Alcohol Abuse among Women of Child-Bearing Age<br>*Sanna J. Thompson and Jina Jun* | **315** |
| **Chapter 14** | Alcohol and Time to Pregnancy<br>*Audra L. Gollenberg, Maureen A. Cooney and Courtney D. Lynch* | **331** |
| **Chapter 15** | Biological Markers of Exposure of Foetus to Alcohol during Pregnancy<br>*S. Lamy and F. Thibaut* | **347** |
| **Chapter 16** | Alcohol and Pregnancy: History, Current Situation in France and Descriptive Study of the Development of Addictive Behaviors during Pregnancy -<br>*M. Tanguy and S. Fanello* | **359** |
| **Index** | | **365** |

# PREFACE

Prenatal alcohol exposure has been directly implicated in a wide range of deficits that adversely influence the development of affected individuals. Fetal Alcohol Spectrum Disorder (FASD) is an umbrella term referring to a continuum of effects that occur in individuals who were prenatally exposed to alcohol. FASD is a permanent birth defect, and a leading cause of mental retardation and developmental delay. This book gathers the latest research in the study of pregnancy and alcohol consumption from authors around the globe, including the biochemistry of prenatal alcohol exposure; research on interventions to prevent alcohol consumption during pregnancy; medico-legal considerations concerning fetal alcohol spectrum disorders; life as an adult with fetal alcohol syndrome; and biological markers of exposure of the fetus to alcohol during pregnancy.

Chapter 1 – In this contribution the authors review the biochemical pathways of ethanol and its metabolites in humans in the context of pregnancy. Special emphasis is devoted to the implications for fetal and neonatal development. The review covers primary direct effects of ethanol as well as downstream effector pathways involving modulation of receptor and hormonal signaling, and the enzymatic status of the offspring. Special attention is given to the implications of maternal alcohol consumption for the nutritional status of compounds with recognized relevance for pregnancies, such as folate, unsaturated fatty acids and zinc. The field of ethanol induced developmental disorders is enormous and still growing rapidly. Since pre-2000 material has been well covered by excellent review publications already, our manuscript concentrates on the more recent exciting developments in the field, like the interference of ethanol with neurosteroid and neuropeptide signaling. Accordingly, the references are biased heavily towards publications from the last decade. The emphasis is firmly on the biochemical pathways behind the manifestations of maternal alcohol in the neural development, physiological regulation and the immune competence of the fetus and the neonate. Extensive attention is given to the relatively new concept of *in utero* programming of fetal development. The epidemiological, social, or economic aspects of alcohol consumption during pregnancy are not covered by this review, as they are reviewed in other chapters of this volume. The chapter concludes with a summary discussion of the implications of ethanol exposure for fetal and neonatal health.

Chapter 2 – Alcohol use in pregnancy is associated with a wide range of adverse pregnancy outcomes and whilst the likelihood of these increases with heavy drinking patterns, morbidity to the fetus may nevertheless result from an acute episode of alcohol consumption (i.e. "binge-drinking"). Increased maternal age, genetic susceptibility to alcohol, low socio-economic status, tobacco smoking and illicit drug use have all been reported to contribute to increased risk from alcohol exposure in pregnancy. Fundamental to understanding the risks associated with alcohol consumption in pregnancy and to providing an insight into factors that may contribute to comorbidity, is a basic understanding of how alcohol causes fetotoxicity. In this chapter we will review the potential mechanisms causing alcohol-mediated damage to the fetus, including altered retinoic acid metabolism, excess prostaglandins, oxidative stress and alterations in placental structure and function, with a particular focus on the accumulating evidence that fetal zinc deficiency may underpin many of events that interrupt developmental processes. This chapter also includes new findings in regard to zinc homeostasis, including the roles of the metal binding protein metallothionein and zinc transporters, and the regulation of these by inflammatory mediators.

Chapter 3 – *Background:* Avoidance of maternal alcohol consumption during pregnancy is the only way to prevent the harmful effects of alcohol on the fetus known as fetal alcohol spectrum disorder (FASD).

*Objective:* To assess the prevalence of pre- and late-pregnancy alcohol consumption among women and to determine maternal opinions about prenatal alcohol use.

*Methods:* Data were obtained from a stratified random sample of 12,611 Maryland mothers who delivered live born infants during the years 2001-2008 and completed the Maryland Pregnancy Risk Assessment Monitoring System (PRAMS) survey. Univariable and bivariable analyses were conducted using Proc Surveyfreq in SAS v9.2. Multivariable logistic regression analysis, using Proc Surveylogistic in SAS, was used to control for potential confounding factors. Maternal quotes about alcohol use were taken verbatim from mothers who wrote comments either next to the survey questions or on the last blank page of the survey.

*Results:* Nearly 8% of Maryland mothers reported any alcohol consumption during the last three months of pregnancy. Alcohol consumption occurred most frequently among mothers who were white non-Hispanic, 35+ years of age, college graduates, and married. Less than 1% of mothers reported binge drinking during the last three months of pregnancy. Binge drinking occurred most frequently among mothers who were under 20 years of age and unmarried. During the three months before pregnancy, 51% of women reported consuming alcohol and 16% reported binge drinking. Alcohol use and binge drinking increased significantly between 2001 and 2008.

Many mothers voiced their opinions about the adverse consequences of alcohol use during pregnancy. Some urged mothers not to drink, others wanted to help mothers stop drinking, a few thought women were selfish to continue drinking during pregnancy and several thought this was a form of child abuse. It was clear that many mothers were not assessed for alcohol use during their prenatal visits and some went so far as to say that their physicians sent mixed messages about alcohol use. Among mothers who reported alcohol use during pregnancy, most wanted to minimize its use by conveying that the amount consumed was small or for a special occasion. Some confirmed that they drank during early pregnancy before the pregnancy was confirmed.

*Conclusion:* Pre and late-pregnancy alcohol use was common among women—especially those who are usually at low risk for adverse pregnancy outcomes such as college graduates. Screening all women for alcohol use before and during pregnancy will improve identification of women who need help or treatment for alcohol use reduction. This will facilitate the achievement of an alcohol-free pregnancy—theoretically the only sure way to prevent FASD.

Chapter 4 – Alcohol abuse during pregnancy produces permanent brain damage in the fetus and is associated with the development of a life-long behavioral, social, and cognitive disorder known as fetal alcohol spectrum disorder (FASD). Fetal alcohol syndrome (FAS) is the most clinically recognizable form of FASD and is characterized by a set of facial dysmorphogenesis, mental dysfunction, growth retardation, cardiovascular and limb defects. Human studies of FAS are very limited because of ethical constraints. However, several non-human vertebrate and invertebrate animal models are currently used, and our major understanding about FASD is mainly based on the studies on these animals. We have used Japanese medaka (*Oryzias latipes*) as a non-mammalian vertebrate model to elucidate the mechanism(s) of FASD. We have demonstrated that fertilized medaka embryos exposed to ethanol developed several phenotypic features in cardiovascular, craniofacial, and skeletal systems which are comparable to the FASD features observed in human. Moreover, the effects at the cellular level have shown that ethanol is able to reduce total protein, RNA, and DNA contents of the embryos in a dose- and time-dependent manner. The alcohol metabolizing enzyme mRNA expression such as alcohol dehydrogenase (ADH5 and ADH8) and aldehyde dehydrogenase ( Aldh1A2 and Aldh9A) mRNAs also showed a developmental stage-specific reduction after alcohol treatment. Our studies indicate that medaka embryogenesis might be used as an alternative non-mammalian model for investigating the molecular mechanisms involved in FASD.

Chapter 5 – Prenatal alcohol exposure (PAE) has been directly implicated in a wide range of deficits that adversely influence the development of affected individuals. Fetal Alcohol Spectrum Disorder (FASD) is an umbrella term referring to a continuum of effects that occur in individuals who were prenatally exposed to alcohol (Chudley, Conry, Cook, Loock, Rosales, and LeBlanc, 2005). FASD is a permanent birth defect, and a leading cause of mental retardation and developmental delay in North America (Chudley et al., 2005; Canadian Paediatric Society, 2002). In the United States and Canada, approximately 1 of every 100 children is affected with FASD (AADAC, 2004; Health Canada, 2006;, May and Gossage, 2001; Sampson et al., 1997).

Individuals affected by FASD may require lifetime support and extensive services related to health, social services, education and training, addictions, justice, and family supports due to various neuropsychological, physical, and behavioral sequelae, which are often costly and difficult to treat (Government of Alberta, 2005; Health Canada, 2006). The annual cost of FASD in Canada for individuals aged 0 to 53 is estimated at $5.3 billion, with an annual cost per individual of nearly $22,000 (Stade et al., 2009). Further, U.S. estimates place the lifetime cost of a child with FASD at $2 million (Lupton, Burd, and Harwood, 2004). These costs reflect, among other factors, the increased use of the above-mentioned services, as well as externalizing behaviors and lost personal or caregiver productivity. The overwhelmingly negative effects that PAE has on affected individuals and their families, combined with enormous societal costs and the fact that FASD is, in theory, entirely preventable, make research on the efficacy of FASD prevention programs vital. In this chapter we will review research on selective and indicated FASD prevention strategies. The strategies reviewed include screening methods, brief interventions with and without motivational features, and longer-term prevention programs including enhanced case management.

Chapter 6 – Despite its well publicized risks, maternal alcohol use during pregnancy remains a common exposure for the developing neonate. Maternal alcohol use during pregnancy significantly increases the risk of premature delivery, and as such a large number of both term and premature newborns are exposed to this toxic substance in utero. Clinical evidence suggests that fetal alcohol exposure increases the risk of sepsis in both premature and term newborns, but the risks of alcohol exposure on the various morbidities suffered by premature newborns remain under investigation. Alcohol-induced alterations in antioxidant redox defenses occur in both the mother and the developing neonate during pregnancy, placing the premature newborn at particular risk for exaggerated oxidant-induced morbidities. These alcohol-induced redox alterations, particularly in the glutathione system, adversely affect the developing lung and its resident inflammatory cell the alveolar macrophage. This chapter will review the need for detection of the alcohol-exposed newborn, including the premature newborn and explore current biomarkers of fetal alcohol exposure such as fatty acid ethyl esters. Alterations of the glutathione redox system affecting the alcohol-exposed fetal lung are examined using animal models of fetal ethanol exposure. The ethanol-induced oxidant injury to the resident alveolar macrophage of the developing lung deranges immune functioning and increases the risk of pulmonary infection. However, availability of the antioxidant glutathione holds promise as a therapeutic intervention for the at-risk premature lung. Continued investigations of in utero alcohol's effects on the risk of adverse outcomes to all vulnerable organs of the developing newborn will allow for a better understanding of in utero alcohol's effects on this high-risk patient population.

Chapter 7 – Sustained alcohol abuse by pregnant women is clearly on the rise, so their effects on pregnancy outcomes are important public health issues. Alcohol is one of the commonest teratogenic agents and its uncontrolled consumption by pregnant women can give rise to an irreversible condition in the child called Fetal Alcohol Syndrome (FAS). This syndrome is characterized by intrauterine growth restriction (IUGR), craniofacial malformations, physical and mental retardation and cardiac septal defects. However, FAS represents only a part of the spectrum of fetal alcohol effects on pregnancy. Another syndrome expressing a lesser degree of deformities associated to FAS, some times unnoticeable except by close examination, is the Fetal Alcohol Effect (FAE), which only characteristic is a variable degree of mental retardation.

It must be emphasized that all children of mothers who abuse consume of alcohol during pregnancy do not necessarily develop FAS/FAE. This fact suggests that there may be others factors involved, besides the degree of exposure to alcohol, which predisposed the fetus to FAS/FAE syndrome. The potential source of individual variability includes differences in the pattern, frequency and duration of the period of drinking, differences in maternal, fetal and placental metabolism of ethanol/acetaldehyde, as well as genetic factors.

In addition, studies in animal models suggest that acetaldehyde, the primary hepatic oxidative metabolite of ethanol, reaches the fetus either by placental production or placental transference. Acetaldehyde may contribute to alter placental function, which in turn could affect fetal growth and development. The most likely hypothesis regarding the decrease of fetal growth is thought to be via hypoxia and increased oxidative stress, which interfere with cellular processes that require oxygen in order to function adequately, e.g. placental transport.

This review summarizes recent findings on placental hypoxia, oxidative stress and fetal development that may play a role in the impairment of the normal transference of essential fetal metabolites that could be related with FAS/FAE syndrome.

Chapter 8 – One of the most challenging goals in fetal alcohol research is to identify the risk factors and mechanisms that influence the outcomes of alcohol exposure during pregnancy since not every woman who drinks alcohol during pregnancy will deliver an offspring with fetal alcohol spectrum disorder or fetal alcohol syndrome. Various key risk factors have been studied that can account for some of the variability in the severity of fetal alcohol-induced damage observed among the affected offspring, and the timing of alcohol exposure during gestation relative to specific developmental events appears to play a significant role affecting the variability in offspring deficits. Although the clinical research on this risk factor is sparse due to the difficulty in partitioning timing, duration and amount of alcohol consumed during pregnancy, considerable pre-clinical research shows a distinct pattern of offspring deficits when the timing of alcohol exposure is well-controlled in laboratory settings. This review outlines the effects of timing of alcohol exposure during gestation in various animal model systems and draws parallels between the effects observed in laboratory settings with those from clinical outcomes.

Chapter 9 – France was the second country in the world to adopt a radical position with regard to the consumption of alcohol during pregnancy, with a campaign recommending "zero alcohol during pregnancy", and compulsory labelling of all containers of alcoholic beverages (even Champagne). This position is surprising in view of the fact that no updated prevalence data is available nationally whether on consumption by pregnant women or on the numbers of infants affected by neonate alcohol syndrome. In addition, until recently, advice to pregnant women allowed one to two glasses of wine a day, good for the heart, and the consumption of beer was even recommended to facilitate breast feeding. Generally speaking, pressure from lobbies to have red wine recognised as a foodstuff and not as alcohol, or the famous "French paradox" reputed to prove that life expectancy increases with regular moderate consumption of red wine, seemed to leave very little chance for the message to be adopted in France.

After the issue was avoided for some twenty years, giving as pretext this French paradox, it suddenly came into the limelight in the media in 2004, the state fearing legal action against it (by women giving birth to children with foetal alcohol syndrome and considering they had not been informed of the risk) and this led to legislation that made the warning labels on alcoholic beverages compulsory in 2004.

Although no risk threshold has been defined in the international medical literature, this radical position was justified by what was viewed as the simplicity of the message, despite the fact that it is quite inadequate in a country where total abstinence is still far from standard. Even if surveys on knowledge about the dangers of alcohol during pregnancy reflect better levels of information in the general population, health professionals as individuals and women generally feel they are not really concerned, and view the danger as being related drinking strong alcohols or concerning alcoholics.

This chapter, in addition to a review of the literature, of the French debate and of the surveys available, sets out to provide original results from the prevalence surveys at present underway.

Chapter 10 – Prenatal, intrauterine exposure to alcohol can cause life-long physical, neurological, and psychological impairments, totally named FASD (Fetal Alcohol Spectrum Disorders). The neurological and psychological impairments, including learning disabilities, impulsivity, hyperactivity, social ineptness, and poor judgment, can increase susceptibility to victimization and involvement in the criminal justice system (CJS) , and consequently, their disabilities must be considered at all stages in the legal process. Whether people with FASD appear in court as complainant, witness or accused, their testimony should be taken under great consideration and doubt. Even in case of illegal or criminal behaviour, this category of people requires special treatment. They must be punished with increased lenity and incarceration is not always an ideal solution for them. In principles, people with FASD should be helped to understand the court rules and their legal rights, which is sometimes very difficult for them to achieve. Of course, FASD should be officially diagnosed by experts, such as general practitioners, psychiatrists and medical examiners. Judges and lawyers need to be advised and informed by these kinds of professionals on the impacts FASD have induced on every individual patient, assessing how decisive this syndrome is for his/her behavior.

Chapter 11 – Learning disabilities are frequent and important cause of poor school performance. One of the most frequent causes of mental and learning problems in children is fetal alcohol syndrome (FAS). The syndrome is caused by maternal alcohol consumption during pregnancy which causes facial anomalies, growth retardation and neurological manifestations in children. One of the hallmarks of FAS is an impaired neurological function with attention deficiency, speech, reasoning, and learning disabilities. Dyscalculia is the most frequent learning problem present in these children. Later-life complications include poor academic performance, low income, and unemployment, which lead to other undesirable social consequences.

Estimated FAS prevalence is highly variable, and ranges from 3.1 to 74.2 per 1000 schoolchildren. A high variability of FAS prevalence is attributed to the differences between races, ethnic groups, socioeconomic status, educational level, and alcohol consumption habits. Most studies performed so far, have focused on rural high-risk populations of low socioeconomic status. However, recent studies have revealed important changes in lifestyle and alcohol consumption habits among women. These studies have suggested that urban, employed women with higher income and higher educational level represent another high-risk population when it comes to drinking during pregnancy. However, FAS studies in urban schoolchildren populations are rare.

In this work we have reviewed drinking habits reported in women, together with risk factors and pregnancy drinking habits. These habits pose a risk factor for the development of FAS in children. We have also reviewed clinical characteristics and estimated FAS prevalence of FAS in general schoolchildren population, with a special emphasis put on urban population.

FAS is one of the most common congenital but preventable causes of neurological deficits in children. Epidemiologic studies have contributed to the degree of awareness on this problem among healthcare professionals, and have improved the primary prevention in terms of reducing alcohol intake among women of the childbearing age. It is necessary to further increase the awareness of school personnel in order to enhance secondary prevention of later-life complications by adequate scholastic interventions carried out among these children. These interventions should help the children with their scholastic curriculum so as to become productive members of society.

Chapter 12 – For more than fifty years, it was supposed that Maria had inherited the slight mental handicap of her mother and her half sister. In reality, she is a victim of her mother's alcoholism and was born with foetal alcohol syndrome (FAS). Besides the physical handicaps (dysmorphy, deformations), this syndrome provokes deficiencies of the central nervous system, mild to moderate mental retardation, social and professional difficulties as well as dysfunctional families (Danel, Karila and Mezerete, 2007). FAS children are clearly handicapped by their syndrome and their future is further jeopardized by the absence of suitable care programmes for them. The follow-up of a cohort of American children (Streissguth and al., 1991) shows that 43 % of the children exposed to alcohol in utero were later excluded from the school system, 70 % interrupted their education, 60 % spent some time in prison and 30% in psychiatric hospitals, 65% presented sexual deviances and 80% faced endemic problems with finding and keeping a job or a secure place to live. The relation of cause and effect between FAS and social problems thus seems rather undeniable. At its most serious, the syndrome results in the association of characteristics which tend to become less conspicuous with age: small heads, slanty eyes, thin superior lips, smooth-grooved upper lips, some abnormal internal organs, a slower growth ante and postnatal and some confusion in their neurological development (small intelligence quotients). If the physical characteristics of this syndrome tend to become less obvious with age, the abnormalities of the central nervous system remain irreversible. At its least severe form, the syndrome becomes "foetal alcohol spectrum disorders" (FASD). In this case, facial dysmorphy is not necessarily visible. Maria's story, from birth to adulthood (she is now 58) is that of a typical FAS victim. It is extremely useful in throwing light on the difficulties FAS victims face in our society.

Chapter 13 – It is estimated that of the 15.1 million alcohol-abusing or alcohol-dependent individuals in the United States, nearly one-third (5,277,000) are women. Drinking behavior differs with age, life role, and marital status among women. In general, the incidence of alcohol dependence is greater among women of child-bearing age and the development of consequences associated with alcohol use may be accelerated. Women are more sensitive to alcohol, become addicted quicker, develop alcohol-related problems sooner, and die at a younger age than men with similar drinking problems. Equal proportions of black and white women drink heavily; however, African American women report fewer alcohol-related personal and social problems than white women, but a greater proportion of black women experience alcohol-related health problems.

Chapter 14 – Secular trends showing a decrease in fertility across countries and an increase in the use and demand of infertility treatment in recent years have heightened the search for preventable contributors to impaired fecundity. There has been particular interest in the association between common exposures, such as alcohol intake, and reduced fecundability, given its global accessibility across socioeconomic gradients and thus, potential impact on markers of fecundity. An important marker of fecundity is time to pregnancy (TTP), measured as the at-risk time (in months or cycles) it takes a couple to achieve pregnancy. Sparse literature is available on the association between alcohol use and TTP and the existing studies have found conflicting results, largely from methodologic limitations and variability in study design. For example, some studies were based on large samples (>5,000) of participants, but collected alcohol information on only one partner, others used retrospective capture of both alcohol use and TTP information, a method which can be fraught with inaccuracies and bias. Several of the studies have observed a decreased fecundity for those consuming any alcohol as compared to unexposed individuals, yet still others have suggested a protective effect from certain types of alcoholic beverages. Moreover, other work has suggested that heavy drinking may contribute to the development of ovulatory disorders and thus, a difficulty in conceiving. It is important when reviewing the current state of the literature to take into consideration the different methodologies used in studying this association. Overall, the field requires more large, prospective cohort studies to elucidate the association between alcohol use by type and frequency and markers of fecundity using a couple-based approach before we can definitively inform couples regarding the risks and benefits of preconception alcohol use.

Chapter 15 – The potential consequences of the increasing use of alcohol by pregnant women are a major public health concern. According to different studies, 20 to 89 % of women may drink alcohol during their pregnancy. Current research suggests that the consumption of seven or more standard drinks of alcohol (one standard drink = 13.6 grams of absolute alcohol) per week during pregnancy places the baby at risk of serious, lifelong developmental and cognitive disabilities. Maternal alcohol use during pregnancy may lead to fetal alcohol spectrum disorder (FASD). FASD is characterized by typical facial features, growth retardation, intellectual dysfunction and behavioral problems. The FASD is the first cause of developmental abnormalities known. Psychological and educational interventions may help women to reduce their alcohol intake during pregnancy. The National Institute of Drug Abuse (USA) reported that 75% of the infants exposed to alcohol or substance during pregnancy present medical problems as compared to only 27% of the nonexposed infants. The modalities of alcohol and substance use have changed during the last years and there is increasing evidence for polyconsumption (e.g. among cannabis users, 52.3% smoke tobacco and 32.4% use alcohol several times per week). The toxic effects of these substances during pregnancy may be increased by their combination. Alcohol and substance use prevalence (tobacco, cannabis, cocaine…) during pregnancy remains under estimated. Most of the published studies were based on the mother's interview. In most cases, the mother underreport the amount of alcohol used. Further studies measuring alcohol use in the mother's blood, hair or in the newborn's meconium are needed. In addition, a serious challenge in diagnosing FASD is the need for markers of alcohol use during pregnancy. Detecting patterns of maternal drinking that place fetuses at risk for fetal alcohol spectrum disorders (FASDs) is critical to diagnosis, treatment, and prevention but is challenging because information on antenatal drinking collected during pregnancy is often insufficient or lacking. Serum Gamma-glutamyltransferase (GGT), carbohydrate-deficient transferrin (CDT), and mean corpuscular volume of erythrocytes (MCV) appear to be the most efficient laboratory markers for detecting excessive alcohol consumption. Ethyl glucuronide (EtG) and ethyl sulfate (EtS) are also biomarkers of excessive alcohol use. They can be measured in the mother’s blood, newborn’s blood or meconium. Recently, fatty acid ethyl esters (FAEEs) measurements in meconium emerged as reliable, direct biological markers for establishing gestational ethanol exposure. We will review the available markers of alcohol use during pregnancy. Until now, when examining the association between prenatal alcohol exposure and fetal effects, epidemiological studies have ignored the timing and intensity of the exposure. New epidemiological study combining biological, pharmacological and mothers’ interview approaches should permit a better evaluation of the consequences for the newborn and child exposed to alcohol during pregnancy as a function of intensity and timing of alcohol exposure.

Chapter 16 - Alcohol consumption in France, a country with a strong wine tradition, is widely associated with conviviality, friendship and loyalty. However, excessive alcohol consumption is associated with well known adverse effects. During pregnancy, the problem is more severe. Binge drinking - a growing practice in France – and chronic consumption can cause disability to the unborn.

These damages are described as Foetal Alcohol Syndrome (FAS), Foetal Alcohol Effects (FAE) and Foetal Alcohol Spectrum Disorder (FASD). They can be avoided by informing women and encouraging abstinence from alcohol during pregnancy. Moreover, mothers who have an alcohol problem may find support and assistance. In France, mainly since 2002, public health policies have improved public information, prevention and management of disorders related to alcohol consumption during pregnancy. These measures need to be supported by careful training of all professionals providing health care to pregnant women.

In: Pregnancy and Alcohol Consumption
Editor: Joshua D. Hoffman, pp. 1-65

ISBN 978-1-61761-122-3


*Chapter 1*

# THE BIOCHEMISTRY OF PRENATAL ALCOHOL EXPOSURE

***Ernst van Faassen[1]* and Onni Niemelä[2]•***

1. Debye Institute, Utrecht University,
Utrecht, The Netherlands
2. EP Central Hospital,
Seinäjoki and University of Tampere,
Finland

## ABSTRACT

In this contribution we review the biochemical pathways of ethanol and its metabolites in humans in the context of pregnancy. Special emphasis is devoted to the implications for fetal and neonatal development. The review covers primary direct effects of ethanol as well as downstream effector pathways involving modulation of receptor and hormonal signaling, and the enzymatic status of the offspring. Special attention is given to the implications of maternal alcohol consumption for the nutritional status of compounds with recognized relevance for pregnancies, such as folate, unsaturated fatty acids and zinc. The field of ethanol induced developmental disorders is enormous and still growing rapidly. Since pre-2000 material has been well covered by excellent review publications already, our manuscript concentrates on the more recent exciting developments in the field, like the interference of ethanol with neurosteroid and neuropeptide signaling. Accordingly, the references are biased heavily towards publications from the last decade. The emphasis is firmly on the biochemical pathways behind the manifestations of maternal alcohol in the neural development, physiological regulation and the immune competence of the fetus and the neonate. Extensive attention is given to the relatively new concept of *in utero* programming of fetal development. The epidemiological, social, or economic aspects of alcohol consumption during pregnancy are not covered by this review, as they are reviewed in other chapters of this volume. The

* E-Mail: faassen@phys.uu.nl.
• E-Mail: onni.niemela@epshp.fi.

chapter concludes with a summary discussion of the implications of ethanol exposure for fetal and neonatal health.

## ACRONYMS

| | |
|---|---|
| 3α,5α-THP | allopregnanolone, a neurosteroid |
| 4-MP | 4-methylpyrazole, inhibitor of ADH |
| 5-HT | 5-hydroxytryptamine (serotonin), a neurotransmitter |
| 8-iso$PGF_{2\alpha}$ | 8-isoprostaglandin $F_{2\alpha}$, a marker for membrane lipid peroxidation |
| αLN | α-linolenic acid, ALA (C18 : 3ω-3) |
| AA | acetaldehyde |
| ACTH | adrenocorticotropin hormone |
| ADH | alcohol dehydrogenase |
| ADNF | activity dependent neurotrophic factor |
| ADNP | activity-dependent neuroprotective protein |
| AIF | apoptosis inducing factor |
| ALDH | aldehyde dehydrogenase |
| AVP | arginine vasopressin, also vasopressin, antidiuretic hormone |
| BAC | blood alcohol concentration |
| BBB | blood-brain barrier |
| cAMP | cyclic adenosine monophosphate |
| CDT | carbohydrate deficient transferrin |
| cGMP | cyclic guanosine monophosphate |
| CNS | central nervous system |
| CRH | corticotrophin releasing hormone |
| CYP2E1 | Cytochrome P450 II E1 enzyme |
| Cys | cysteine |
| CySS | cystine, disulfide of cysteine |
| DA | dopamine, a catecholamine neurotransmitter and neurohormone |
| dG | deoxyguanosine |
| DHA | docosahexaenoic fatty acid (C22 : 6ω-3) |
| DHN-GSH | 1,4 dihydroxynonene-glutathione |
| DNA | deoxyribonucleic acid |
| DPA | docosapentaenoic fatty acid (C22 : 5ω-3) |
| DPI | diphenyleneiodonium, a NOX inhibitor |
| EPA | eicosapentaenoic fatty acid (C20 : 5ω-3) |
| EtOH | ethanol, alcohol |
| EtONO | ethyl nitrite, O-nitrosated ethanol |
| FAEE | fatty acid ethyl esters, from non-oxidative EtOH metabolism |
| FAE | fetal alcohol effects |
| FAS | fetal alcohol syndrome |
| FSH | follicle stimulating hormone (FSH) |
| GABA | gamma-aminobutyric acid, inhibitory neurotransmitter |
| GAD | glutamate decarboxylase, synthesizes GABA |
| GGT | gamma-glutamyltransferase |
| GSH | glutathione |

| | |
|---|---|
| GSNO | S-nitrosoglutathione |
| GSSG | glutathione disulfide |
| hCG | human chorionic gonadotropin (hCG), a glycoprotein hormone |
| HNE | 4-hydroxynonenal, oxidation product of polyunsaturated ω-6 lipids |
| HPA | hypothalamic – pituitary – adrenal axis |
| ICAM-1 | inter-cellular adhesion molecule-1 (CD54) |
| IgA | immunoglobulin A, transferred by lactation |
| IgG | immunoglobulin G, the only maternal Ig that crosses the placental barrier |
| IGF-1 | insulin-like growth factor-1 |
| IL-6, IL-10 | interleukins, a class of cytokines |
| L1 | a membrane glycoprotein cell adhesion molecule |
| LA | linoleic acid (C18 : 2ω-6) |
| LCPUFA | long-chain polyunsaturated fatty acids |
| LH | luteinizing hormone from anterior pituitary, triggers ovulation |
| MDA | malondialdehyde |
| MEOS | microsomal alcohol-oxidizing system |
| MGE | medial ganglionic eminence, a transitory fetal brain structure |
| MPT | mitochondrial permeability transition |
| MT | metallothionein, cysteine rich protein binding a broad spectrum of metal ions |
| NAA | N-acetyl aspartate/creatine |
| nCAM | neural cell adhesion molecule |
| NMDA | N-methyl-D-aspartate (synthetic activator of NMDA-R) |
| NMDA-R | glutaminergic NMDA receptor of the CNS |
| NO | nitric oxide radical, activator of guanylate cyclase |
| NOS | nitric oxide synthase (eNOS, nNOS, iNOS) |
| NOX | a class of NADPH oxidases for transmembrane electron transport |
| PdG | 1,N(2)-propano-2'-deoxyguanosine |
| PDI | psychomotor development index |
| PI-3 | phosphatidylinositol 3'kinase |
| PNS | peripheral nervous system |
| PREGS | pregnenolone sulfate (a neurosteroid) |
| PS | phosphatidylserine |
| PUFA | polyunsaturated fatty acid |
| RNA | ribonucleic acid |
| $rT_3$ | 3,3',5'-triiodothyronine, a non-hormone metabolite of $T_4$ |
| sGC | soluble guanylate cyclase, produces cGMP |
| SOD | superoxide dismutase |
| $T_3$ , $T_4$ | 3,5,3-triiodothyronine, thyroxine (thyroid hormones) |
| TGFβ | Transforming Growth Factor-β |
| TLR | Toll like receptor |
| TNF-α | tumor necrosis factor-α |
| TSH | thyroid-stimulating hormone |
| VCAM-1 | vascular cell adhesion molecule-1 (CD106) |
| VIP | vasoactive intestinal peptide |

## INTRODUCTION

In recent years, industrialized nations have seen an increasing prevalence of alcohol consumption among women. Epidemiological studies have shown that 90% of women drink alcohol regularly, and approximately 3 % exceed the limit of heavy drinking. In women, alcohol related problems concerning pregnancy add another dimension to the problem of excessive alcohol consumption *per se*.

Consequently, the detrimental health effects have continued to grow. While there may be significant racial, genetic and interindividual variation in the susceptibility to fetotoxic effects towards ethanol [licona09], epidemiological data has shown that alcohol use exceeding 3-5 daily drinks is associated with a 30-50% risk of delivering a child with fetal alcohol effects. The incidence of fetal alcohol syndrome (FAS) has been estimated to vary between 1.7 and 5.9 per 1000 live births, depending on the ethnic group and the criteria used to define the phenotype. In comparison with other complications of fetal development, alcohol related fetal complications are quite unusual in that they are completely avoidable. In reality, fetal alcohol induced damage is a widespread phenomenon with a wide clinical spectrum ranging from mild fetal alcohol effects (FAE) to fully developed FAS. Conspicuous manifestations are dysfunction of the central nervous system, characteristic congenital anomalies and growth retardation [sokol03, sulik05].

Disturbing as the cases of manifest FAS are, they represent only the tip of a much larger iceberg of detrimental effects of alcohol on the children that are prenatally exposed to alcohol by their mothers. The invisible part of the iceberg may attract less attention and prominence, but the sheer size and diversity of the submerged portion necessitates a careful study as well. Rapid advances in recent years have identified a surprising range of effects on a subtler scale than fully developed FAS. The damaging effect of alcohol on fetal development has been well documented in the scientific literature. But recently, the emphasis has shifted more to the new concept of prenatal programming. Many *in vivo* studies have revealed the phenomenon of prenatal programming whereby gestational stimuli predispose the fetus to abnormal development at later stages [matthews02, myatt06, koeners07, weinberg08, kapoor08, hellemans10]. These later stages may extend far beyond the neonatal period, into puberty and adult stages. At time of birth, the alcohol related damage may not yet be manifest, but is carried along in a preprogrammed fashion until its manifestation at a far later time.

The purpose of the present contribution is to update research on the primary mechanisms and biochemical pathways underlying the toxic effects of ethanol during pregnancy. A proper mapping of such pathways is necessary for the planning and execution of intervention programs to prevent the devastating consequences of maternal alcohol use on child development. The epidemiological, social and behavioural aspects of alcohol consumption have been covered by other contributions to this volume, and will not be considered further in this chapter. Instead, we will focus on the molecular mechanisms behind the manifestations of prenatal alcohol exposure.

## ALCOHOL METABOLISM IN HUMANS

After alcohol (ethanol, EtOH) is consumed, it may enter the blood compartment by absorption in the stomach and intestines. This absorption is affected by several factors, such as the quantity and type of food in the gastrointestinal tract. The ensuing blood alcohol levels are determined by competition between the rate of absorption and oxidation of alcohol by metabolic pathways. The rate of absorption is determined by the time needed for the transfer of the stomach content into the intestines. This transfer is slow after consumption of food with a high fat content. Accordingly, after a heavy meal containing fat, protein and carbohydrates, alcohol absorption is threefold slower than on an empty stomach. Alcohol is subsequently detoxified through successive oxidations by a chain of dehydrogenases (cf scheme 1).

**Scheme 1: The oxidation cascade of EtOH, and the main enzymatic mediators**

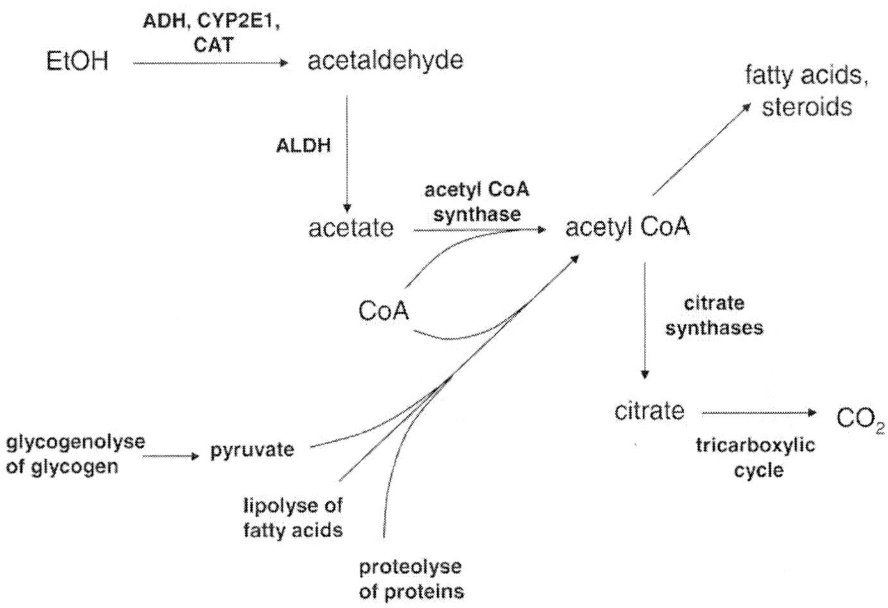


*Two initial enzymatic steps oxidize EtOH to acetate. This intermediate species is enzymatically coupled with coenzyme-A (CoA) to form acetyl-CoA, the substrate for the tricarboxylic acid (TCA) cycle of aerobic respiration. In the course of TCA cycling, the acetate is ultimately broken down to $CO_2$ and exhaled.*

The first step is catalyzed by three independent pathways: (1) alcohol dehydrogenases (ADH); (2) microsomal cytochrome P450IIE1 (CYP2E1); (3) catalase. The relative importance between these pathways depends crucially on the developmental stage. All the three pathways have been extensively discussed in an abundant quantity of literature for decades. In this chapter, we restrict ourselves to a few basic properties.

*(1) The ADH pathway*: Mammalian alcohol dehydrogenases are cytosolic dimeric enzymes with considerable polymorphism and genetic variations between ethnic populations. Six mammalian classes of ADH have been identified so far, five of which have been identified in humans [jornvall00]. ADH isoforms are found in almost every adult mammalian tissue type [reviews: green07, jelski08]. These isoforms have significantly variable capacity to oxidize EtOH: ADH-I has highest efficiency for EtOH, while ADH-IV has tenfold lower activity [duester98]. ADH-V has not been well characterized ([jornvall00] and references therein), and appears not significant for EtOH metabolism in adults. However, small quantities of mRNA for ADH-V were detected in human fetal liver [estonius96]. Since the other isoforms were not yet expressed at this stage, it was proposed that ADH-V may actually be the dominant isoform in fetal tissues at this stage of development [estonius96]. The third class ADH-III is somewhat of a misnomer, since this isoform does not show reactivity towards EtOH (cf table 1). Instead, it plays an important physiological role in lungs through the oxidation of formaldehyde [sanghani03] and reduction of the endogenous bronchodilator S-nitrosoglutathione (GSNO) [duester98, thompson09]. In conclusion, ADH-I has highest relevance in the context of EtOH clearance. In human adults, hepatic ADH-I is the dominant pathway for EtOH oxidation, and the quantity of hepatic ADH-I appears the rate limiting factor of the alcohol oxidation chain *in vivo.* In healthy adult Caucasians, the liver metabolizes ca 120 mg of EtOH per hour and kg body weight. In healthy adults, this ADH pathway is the dominant mechanism for oxidation of EtOH. Minor expression of ADH was found ubiquitously in all other types of adult mammalian tissue, like the gastrointestinal tissues, lung, kidney, smooth and skeletal muscle as well as brain.

The human ADH dimer has total weight of 80,000 D. Each subunit has one active site, and two essential Zn atoms. One zinc atom stabilizes the protein structure and has no catalytic activity, whereas the other is positioned in the catalytic cleft. The zinc binding is rather weak, since the enzymatic activity of ADH may be reversibly suppressed by removal of Zn with metal chelators like EDTA or 1,10-phenanthroline bipyridine. Like most mammalian ADH's, human ADH has low specificity and accepts a broad spectrum of substrates including aliphatic, cyclic and aromatic alcohols, retinol, diols, $\omega$-hydroxylated fatty acids, 2-enoic acids as well as their respective aldehydes. ADH has also been implied in the oxidation of cardiac glycosides administered therapeutically to treat congestive heart failure and cardiac arrhythmias. Given this low specificity of ADH, EtOH may act as a potential competitor for any of these physiological substrates. Competition of EtOH with retinol as substrates for ADH-IV activity has been firmly established, and will be discussed in more detail below.

The above remarks apply to tissues from adults, but the expression of ADH is markedly dependent on developmental stage: ADH activity is very low in human fetal tissues, and increases to normal adult level only after ca 5 years. At 10 – 16 weeks of gestation, human fetuses have not yet developed the capacity to oxidize ethanol [pikkarainen71]. The entire range of ADH isoforms is detected only several weeks post partum (for review cf. eg. [agarwal90]). This makes fetuses and young children particularly sensitive to EtOH. At partum, human liver has very low ADH activity and amounts to less than 10% of adult activity [pikkarainen71]. Similarly, ADH-I could not be detected in second trimester fetal brain [estonius96]. Therefore, it has been questioned whether ADH-I is the dominant pathway for fetal alcohol clearance.

(2) *The CYP2E1 pathway*. In adults, under chronic alcohol consumption, the rates of alcohol elimination can increase significantly by activation of a new microsomal alcohol-

oxidizing system (MEOS) [lieber04]. This MEOS is based on the second pathway catalyzed by CYP2E1, with deleterious effects on the cellular redox status [koop06]. In comparison with ADH-I, CYP2E1 has low affinity for EtOH (high binding constant $K_m \sim 10$ mM) [lu08]. Accordingly, at moderate alcohol doses, hepatic CYP2E1 plays a relatively minor role in ethanol clearance. In adults, CYP2E1 is expressed in a variety of tissues, including liver, brain and placenta. Different ethnic groups express a variation of isoforms [gemma07]. It has been found that CYP2E1 is expressed already at early stages of human fetal development: Significant enzymatic activity of CYP2E1 was detected in microsomal fractions of human fetal brain and liver already after ca 50 days of gestational age [brzezinski99]. At this time point fetal organogenesis and cellular differentiation are well under way. It was shown that chronic maternal EtOH consumption affects not only maternal CYP2E1 expression: In rats and guinea pigs, fetal CYP2E1 activity in liver mitochondrial and microsomal fractions was enhanced in alcohol consuming dams [hewitt10, lu08].

It should be noted that CYP2E1 fulfils other roles that might be connected to EtOH toxicity. It has been found that CYP2E1 may release significant quantities of superoxide in normally oxygenated tissues [lu08]. Microsomes from chronic EtOH consuming rats release 2 – 3 fold higher quantities of superoxide and $H_2O_2$. Inhibition of microsomal CYP2E1 activity by anti-CYP2E1 IgG suppressed not only the NADPH oxidase activity but also lipid peroxidation, one of the indicators of ROS release. Another mechanism for serious toxicity comes from the effect of CYP2E1 on polyunsaturated fatty acids. In adults enhanced expression of hepatic CYP2E1 may result from dietary patterns with high lipid content. It seems plausible that the same will occur in fetuses of pregnancies with such diets. A large body of data by the Cederbaum group [wu05, wu06, lu08] has implied CYP2E1 in the oxidation of polyunsaturated fatty acids such as arachidonic or linoleic acid (LA), lipids with a characteristic polyunsaturated ω-6 chain. The oxidation leads to 4-hydroxynonenal (HNE), which has been recognized as highly toxic inducer of neuronal cell death if applied at higher levels > 5 μM [dianzani03, moneypenny05]. Due to its reactivity, HNE is toxic via several mechanisms. In the literature, prominence is given to the genotoxic reaction of HNE with deoxyguanosine moieties on DNA [brooks05, minko09]. More details on this pathway will be given in the section on DNA. HNE may also react and form stable adducts with lysine, cysteine, and histidine residues on proteins [henderson99, yan06]. Mammalian tissues apparently do not possess significant capacity to clear HNE, and this metabolite is only slowly cleared from the lipid compartment. Several pathways have been identified so far [alary03]. First, glutathione-S-transferases conjugate HNE with glutathione (GSH) to 1,4 dihydroxynonene-glutathione (DHN-GSH), a more watersoluble adduct that is cleared from the circulation. A second pathway involves ω-hydroxylation by cytochrome P450 4A. Some reactivity towards HNE has also been reported for aldose reductase, ADH and ALDH [gardner03]. It has been demonstrated that human fetal tissues are more prone to HNE accumulation since fetal liver tissues at second trimester have fivefold lower capacity to detoxify HNE than adult liver [gardner03]. More details on the formation of HNE from PUFA will be given in the section on lipid metabolism (see below).

*(3) The catalase pathway.* Given the susceptibility of CNS tissue to EtOH toxicity, it is significant that only small quantities of ADH are found in adult and fetal brain. In this compartment EtOH clearance was dominated by catalase instead [hamby97].

Similarly, catalase activity and expression in fetal rat brain homogenates was far higher than that in adult rat brain (4.5 and 2.5 times, respectively) [hamby97]. Applying selective inhibitors for ADH, CYP and catalase, these authors demonstrated that the oxidation of EtOH to AA in fetal and adult rat brain homogenates is dominated by catalase activity. It was confirmed that the catalase activity of human fetal brain also varies considerably with time as gestation proceeds: Just like in rats, human fetal brain has catalase activity during the first two trimesters that is ca 50% higher than in the final period [de86]. We note that this catalase kinetics seems peculiar for fetal brain and is not shared with other fetal tissues like liver and kidney, where catalase activity remained fairly constant throughout gestation [de86]. Human placenta also has considerable catalase activity which varies through early gestation. Placental catalase was concentrated in the peroxisomes of the stromal macrophages and cytotrophoblast cells. The placental catalase activity increased ca threefold between weeks 6 and 17 of gestation, with the greatest increase between 12 and 17 weeks [watson98].

This still leaves the question as to the dominant pathway for EtOH detoxification during the embryonic stage, in particular during the very early gestational period prior to expression of ADH-1 and CYP2E1. Experiments in early mouse embryos have demonstrated that the appearance of retinoic acid at E7.5 is concomitant with mRNA levels of ADH-IV. This class IV isoform is mainly responsible for the retinol dehydrogenase activity in mammals. This enzymatic activity is essential for early embryonic retinoid signaling [duester98]. We note that ADH-IV is rather insensitive to ethanol ($K_m \sim 10$ mM [han98]). Therefore, retinoid signaling will be disrupted if local EtOH levels exceed ca 10 mM (cf table 1). Such levels are easily reached in parental alcohol consumption.

**Table 1. Ethanol inhibits the oxidation of retinol to retinaldehyde by human ADH isoforms in vitro**

| ADH class | isoform | $K_m$ (retinol) (μM) | $k_{cat}$ ($min^{-1}$) | $K_i$ (EtOH) (mM) | Inhibition (%) at [EtOH] = 5 mM | Inhibition (%) at [EtOH] = 20 mM | Inhibition (%) at [EtOH] = 50 mM |
|---|---|---|---|---|---|---|---|
| I | αα | 36 | 11.0 | 3.8 | 51 | 81 | 91 |
| | $\beta_1\beta_1$ | 30 | 1.2 | 0.04 | 99 | 99.7 | 99.9 |
| | $\beta_2\beta_2$ | 96 | 17.0 | 0.3 | 94 | 98 | 99 |
| | $\gamma_1\gamma_1$ | 74 | 7.2 | 0.4 | 91 | 98 | 99 |
| II | ππ | 7.3 | 3.3 | 6.9 | 23 | 55 | 78 |
| III | χχ | ---- | ---- | ---- | ---- | ---- | ---- |
| IV | μμ | 27 | 120 | 11 | 25 | 57 | 76 |
| V † | | unknown | unknown | unknown | | | |

† small quantities of mRNA for ADH-V were found in human fetal liver [estonius96], but this isoform has not yet been characterized and its kinetic constants appear unknown.

ADH-III is the only isoform that does not show significant oxidation of retinol [thompson09]. It is noted that modest mM concentrations of EtOH already strongly inhibit the retinol processing by ADH. (table adapted from [han98] and references therein). The isoform ADH-IV has by far the highest conversion rate for retinol, but even here conversion is significantly inhibited at modest EtOH. $K_m$ is the Michaelis constant for retinol binding to ADH. $k_{cat}$ is the catalytic turnover rate for retinol oxidation. $K_i$ is the competitive inhibition constant for inhibition by EtOH. These constants were fitting parameters with estimated accuracy of ca 10 %. The rightmost three columns give calculated inhibition factors at various relevant EtOH concentrations.

Alternatively, human ADH-V has been proposed as the dominant type of fetal ADH since low quantities of mRNA levels of ADH-V were found in human fetal liver [estonius96], while mRNA of the other isoforms remained undetected. In addition, fetal brain and organ tissues show considerable catalase activity already before the twelfth week of gestation [de86]. Combined, these data show unambiguously that fetal tissues have several competent pathways operational for EtOH oxidation, even at early stages prior to induction of hepatic ADH-1. In fetal tissues, and particularly the susceptible fetal CNS tissue, the microsomal and catalase pathways seem dominant mechanisms for detoxification of EtOH. However, the slow rate of fetal alcohol clearance indicates that the combined capacity of these pathways is still very modest and remains an order of magnitude below that found in the adult circulation [brien83]. The hepatic ADH activity starts to increase towards adult values only *post partum* (for rats, cf eg fig 2 below).

The above noted the considerable variations in rates of EtOH uptake and detoxification between individuals. This results in considerable variations in the endogenous EtOH levels induced by ingestion of a given quantity of EtOH. There is far less variation in the effects of a given blood alcohol level on human behaviour.

Given this broad spectrum, we note that ethanol may act as a competitive inhibitor for the other, non-alcoholic, substrates of ADH. Competition with retinol in particular has been investigated. The class of ADH-IV provides the major retinol dehydrogenase activity in mammals, and the level of ADH-IV has been identified as the rate limiting step in the oxidation of retinol (vitamin A) to retinaldehyde, the precursor for retinoic acid. Secondary retinol dehydrogenase activity is in human ADH-I and ADH-II (ADH-III is not active even at supraphysiological levels of 100 μm retinol) [han98]. We note that the production of retinaldehyde is essential for embryonic and fetal development, since retinoic acid binds and activates retinoic nuclear receptors [clagett02]. Such receptors belong to the nuclear hormone receptor superfamily and regulate embryonic morphogenesis and organogenesis [chambon96, maden00, germain06]. The relevance of retinoic signaling for embryonic development has been reviewed in [perrotta03].

The viewpoint that ethanol may outcompete retinol was confirmed by *in vitro* experiments on human ADH isoforms [han98]. The critical EtOH levels for interference with retinol processing may be estimated from the substrate binding constants. The ADH isoforms have typical binding constants $K_m \sim 10 - 70$ μM for retinol, but thousandfold higher inhibition constants $K_i \sim 0.3 - 7.0$ mM for EtOH (cf table 1) [han98, yin02]. Therefore, significant interference with production of retinaldehyde is expected at EtOH levels found after moderate alcohol consumption already. We note that vitamin A deficiencies were the first dietary causes of congenital malformations to be recognized.

The second step of scheme 1 involves the oxidation of AA to acetate. This step is mainly catalyzed by aldehyde dehydrogenases (ALDH). Three isoforms have been identified (reviewed in [crabb04]): First, cytosolic ALDH1 with intermediate affinity for AA (intermediate binding constant $K_m \sim 30$ μM). Second, mitochondrial ALDH2 with high affinity for AA (low $K_m \sim 1$ μM). Third, ALDH3 with low affinity for AA (high $K_m \sim 10$ mM ) for AA. ALDH3 is expressed primarily in the digestive tract, cornea and various tumours [seitz06]. The differences in affinity for AA indicate that the rate of AA clearance of a given tissue will depend on the local AA concentration. Given that human plasma levels of AA will remain below 5 μm (see above), only mitochondrial ALDH2 is expected to be relevant for AA clearance. Accordingly, the ALDH2 isoform is most widely considered in the context of alcohol detoxification. It has been experimentally confirmed that AA levels in blood of ALDH2 - knockout mutant mice reach far higher levels ([AA] up to 200 μM) after bolus injection of EtOH [kiyoshi09]. In accordance, blood acetate levels remained considerably lower in these mutants than in wild type (1.3 mM vs 2.1 mM).

The third step of scheme 1 involve the conversion of acetate to acetyl coenzyme A (acetyl CoA) by acetyl CoA synthase. This enzyme is expressed in the cytosol and mitochondria of liver, kidney, skeletal muscle and cardiac muscle. Like other acetyl carrying compounds, acetyl CoA mainly functions as substrate for citrate production by citrate synthases as the initial step of the mitochondrial tricarboxylic cycle to generate ATP. Competing reaction pathways may convert acetyl CoA to fatty acids, steroids or ketone bodies.

Absorption and metabolism of alcohol has a marked gender difference: Due to women's smaller average body weight, a given quantity of alcohol leads to higher BAC in women than in men. Factors that contribute to sex differences in absorption, distribution and metabolism include mean body mass, total body water, liver size, and basal levels of alcohol metabolizing enzymes in the digestive tract and liver of women and men. In addition, the levels of sex hormones estrogen and testosterone can also affect the absorption and metabolism of alcohol. The gender differences in alcohol metabolism were reviewed in [thomasson95]. As the details of gender differences fall outside of the scope of this review, they will not be considered further.

## Dramatis Personae: The Main Metabolites of Ethanol

Subsequent to the consumption of EtOH, a wide range of downstream metabolites may be detected in tissues or body fluids. These metabolites have their own pharmacological characteristics, tissue distribution and time dependence of clearance. Many metabolites are scrutinized for teratogenic, carcinogenic or toxicologic hazards. Some are surprisingly long lived and may be used as biomarkers for alcohol consumption [niemela07, littner07]. The most prominent metabolites are listed below.

*Acetaldehyde (AA):* The main source of this metabolite is hepatic ADH-I, but smaller contributions come from ADH activity in other tissues as well (including placenta [karl88, gemma07]). In adults, AA is oxidized to acetate by ALDH at a much faster rate than it is released by the ADH activity in the liver. The *in vivo* lifetime of a bolus dose of AA in blood is only a few minutes [quertemont05]. Accordingly, even after intoxicating alcohol consumption, peripheral venous acetaldehyde levels remain below ca 1 μM in caucasian males, and 3 μM in caucasian females. Only straightforward inhibition of aldehyde dehydrogenase allows venous acetaldehyde levels to rise to ca 40 – 60 μM. AA readily crosses the blood-brain barrier (BBB), and its presence is readily detected in the cerebrospinal compartment [quertemont05]. However, the enzymatic activity of ALDH in the brain microvasculature keeps AA concentrations in the cerebrospinal fluid and brain tissues significantly below that of peripheral blood ([quertemont05] and references therein). Although the dominant fraction of AA is removed by ALDH, a small subfraction is lost via competing pathways that give rise to further downstream metabolites. In fact, AA can react with a wide range of compounds due to its general reactivity towards nucleophilic moieties.

Relevant examples are amines in general, lysine or cystine protein residues, or peptide N-terminals. In accordance, a broad spectrum of adducts of AA have been found in various tissues of alcoholic humans. A special section has been devoted to the discussion of such secondary AA adducts (*vide infra).* To conclude this section, it should be noted that endogenous oxidation of EtOH is not the sole source of AA. Many foodstuffs contain AA as a result of fermentation processes during preparation (eg beer, fruit juices, yoghurt). The aldehyde content of food and especially fermented (eg alcoholic) drinks like sherry may also contribute significantly to systemic AA levels. The above concerns the role of ALDH in adults. Much less is known about expression and distribution of ALDH during gestation. In Wistar fetuses, cytosolic and mitochondrial ALDHs were detectable after 15 days of gestation. Mitochondrial ALDH activity increased until day 21 [cao89]. Therefore, a certain degree of protection against endogenous or maternal AA seems operational in rat fetuses during the third trimester.

It has been confirmed that AA crosses the BBB, and that placental transmission of maternal AA to the fetus is feasible [karl88].

*Acetate:* Basal acetate concentrations in venous plasma of fasting humans are 50 – 60 μM [tollinger79]. This basal value rises to ca 100 μM after consumption of a standard breakfast. Such basal acetate levels do not arise from the oxidation cascade of EtOH, but from basal lipolysis or from decomposition of endogenous acetyl-CoA by enzymes like acetyl-CoA hydrolase or hepatic acetyl-CoA synthetase (both enzymes catalyze the forward as well as the backward reaction). It should be noted that most mammalian tissues may act as net producers as well net consumers of acetate, depending on endogenous acetyl-CoA levels. Following a bolus injection of acetate, the timescale for relaxation back to basal levels is about an hour in humans. Acetate levels in arterial plasma are consistently higher than in venous plasma. Plasma acetate levels are significantly enhanced in acidosis and liver diseases. After ingestion of a modest quantity of 0.5 g/kg EtOH (ca 2 standard drinks), plasma acetate levels in adults rise by an order of magnitude to 0.5 – 0.7 mM. This effect may be reinforced by coadministration of fructose. The subsequent relaxation back to basal levels is rather slow on a timescale of 5 – 7 hrs [sarkola02]. The major metabolic pathway for removal of excess acetate is the reaction with coenzyme-A (Co-A) to give acetyl-CoA, the substrate for the tricarboxylic acid cycle of aerobic respiration. This reaction is catalyzed by acetyl-CoA hydrolases and synthetases and seems distributed over many different tissues [sarkola02]. Via downstream reaction steps in the tricarboxylic acid cycle, the acetate is ultimately converted to $CO_2$. Like EtOH and AA, acetate readily crosses the blood-brain barrier [deelchand09].

*Ethyl nitrite (EtONO): in vitro* experiments have demonstrated the formation of ethyl nitrite in acid solutions containing ethanol and nitrite. EtONO is the ethanolic member of the alkyl nitrites. As a class, such O-nitrosated species have potent vasodilating activities *in vivo* (reviewed in ch17 of [faassen07]). Accordingly, such compounds are under investigation as potential nitric oxide donors. EtONO is a gas at room temperature and pressure, and admixtures of EtONO in inhaled breath (up to 0.125 %) has been used to improve the postductal arterial oxygenation in hypoxaemic infants [moya02, discussed in abman02, auten07]. The beneficial effect of inhalation of ethyl nitrite were attributed to S-nitrosation of thiol moieties by EtONO [auten07, gago08]. Interestingly, detectable quantities of EtONO are endogenously formed if EtOH enters the blood circulation: The *in vivo* formation of up to 0.5 μM levels of EtONO has been demonstrated in blood of rats after intraperitoneal injection of ethanol [deng04]. In whole liver tissues, EtONO reached ca 0.2 μM. We note that these levels exceed those reported for basal levels of S-nitrosothiols ([S-NO] ~ 10 – 20 nM in heart and brain, ~ 1.4 nM in blood plasma cf eg chapter 9 of ref [faassen07]). The pathways of endogenous EtONO formation are still controversial. Nitrosating species like $N_2O_3$ or peroxynitrite have been shown to produce EtONO by O-nitrosation of ethanol *in vitro*. However, it is highly unlikely that this reaction be relevant under *in vivo* conditions. In mammalian tissues, peroxynitrite is far more likely to be scavenged by ubiquitous $CO_2$ ~ 25 mM in the rapid bimolecular reaction described by Lymar and Hurst [Lymar95] (reaction rate $k = 3 \cdot 10^4 \ (Ms)^{-1}$). Also, nitrosating species like $N_2O_3$ have an abundance of alternative targets for nitrosation *in vivo* (for a general discussion cf eg chapters 1 and 9 of ref [faassen07]). A plausible alternative pathway has been proposed for the stomach, where the acidic gastric conditions promote the O-nitrosation of ethanol by protonized dietary nitrite [gago08, takahama08]. It is likely that many observations of ethanol-induced vasodilation are in fact mediated by EtONO: NO release from ethyl nitrite has been reported *in vivo* [cederqvist94], and EtONO has proven capacity to transfer its NO moiety to thiols in a facile trans-nitrosation reaction [gago08]. Accordingly, inhalable EtONO is a facile and rapid method to increase cardiopulmonary levels of S-nitrosothiols.

*5-Hydroxytryptophol (HTOL):* the long lifetime of this metabolite makes that HTOL remains elevated for 10 – 20 hrs after the clearance of ethanol from the body. It may be detected in body fluids like urine or plasma, and has been used as diagnostic marker for recent alcohol consumption [beck03]. HTOL appears as a reaction product of serotonin, but the reaction pathway remains controversial. Serotonin is predominantly produced by the enterochromaffin cells in the gut, and far smaller quantities by the serotonergic neurons of the central nervous system. Significant quantities of serotonin are stored by the blood platelets. Due to the localized character of serotonin production and storage, the physiogical significance of HTOL formation remains unclear. Reports of physiological effects or toxicity seem not reported for this metabolite.

*Fatty acid ethyl esters (FAEE):* FAEE comprises a class of ethyl esters that result from conjugation of EtOH to endogenous free fatty acids. The dominant fractions are ethyl palmytoleate, ethyl oleate, ethyl linoleate and ethyl arachidonate. Basal levels of FAEE are nonzero even in abstainers, and significantly raised in plasma of alcohol consumers for a timespan of ca 10 – 15 hrs after alcohol intake. FAEE is mostly produced in liver tissue. Circulating mononuclear cells also have proven capacity to metabolize EtOH to FAEE [alhomsi06]. Significant levels of FAEE are found in liver, pancreas and adipose tissues. Circulating plasma FAEE levels may reach up to 10 μM in heavy drinkers [laposata02]. FAEE is toxic *in vitro* and *in vivo* (the older literature is reviewed in [laposata02]). As FAEE is rapidly metabolized by the microsomal fraction of the placenta, maternal FAEE is prevented from crossing into the fetus [chan04]. Nevertheless, some FAEE is found in the meconium of alcohol consuming pregnancies [bearer05]. This meconial FAEE has been attributed to EtOH metabolism by the fetus itself [chan04]. It seems to be a general property that FAEE promote apoptosis and necrosis *in vitro* in isolated human mononuclear cells [alhomsi08], and in cultured rhombencephalic neurons [antonio08]. It was proposed that FAEE might be toxic for white blood cells and contribute to the observed damping of the immune system in chronic alcohol consumers [alhomsi06, alhomsi08].

*Phosphatidylethanol (PEth):* This metabolite is attributed to activity of phospholipase D and has a long *in vivo* half life ~ 4 days in the blood circulation of alcoholics. This metabolite is very specific as it only forms in the presence of ethanol. Accordingly, PEth cannot be detected in blood of non-drinkers. In blood of alcohol consumers, PEth is found mainly in the red blood cells. Typical PEth concentrations in blood are up to 8 μM for heavy habitual drinkers. The diagnostic sensitivity of PEth was found to be very high and exceeded that of established ethanol markers like carbohydrate deficient transferrin (CDT) or gamma-glutamyltransferase (GGT) [aradottir06]. Given its long lifetime, this PEth seems an unreactive endproduct of ethanol. Apparently, no reports of toxicity of PEth seem to have appeared in the scientific literature.

## Pharmacology of Ethanol in Pregnancy

The kinetics of alcohol consumption in humans is one of the best documented pharmacological processes (for a recent review cf [spanagel09] and references therein). A crucial parameter is the maximal blood alcohol content (BAC) after consumption of alcohol. Given that a standard drink contributes 17.75 ml of EtOH, the consumption of five standard drinks in rapid succession will lead to blood alcohol levels of ca 1.1 – 1.3 ‰ in males, and 1.3 – 1.6 ‰ in females of average adult weight (60 – 70 kg). Women reach significantly higher levels due to their larger body fat content. EtOH is very miscible with water and tends to concentrate in the polar aqueous compartment. In women, this aqueous compartment is relatively smaller, and a given dose results in higher EtOH concentration. A BAC of 1 ‰ (1 promille) corresponds to

$$1‰ \sim [\text{EtOH}] = 0.94 \text{ g / l blood} \sim 21.7 \text{ mM}$$

At 1 ‰ physical and mental coordination are significantly impaired. At 2 ‰ the motor area of the brain is depressed (difficulty with walking, standing, talking), and judgment distorted. At 3 ‰ confusion and stupor results. At 4 ‰ coma is likely, with a mortality rate of ca 50 %. At 5 ‰, survival is unlikely unless immediate medical assistance is provided.

Given the above, the blood alcohol levels in pregnant women are not likely to exceed an upper limit of ca 2.5 ‰ (EtOH concentrations up to ca 50 mM). Excessive values of [EtOH] ~ 200 mM, though often used in *in vitro* studies of tissues and cell cultures, are therefore wholly unrealistic for human physiology. These order of magnitude estimates should be kept in mind when considering the implications of *in vitro* results to the human physiology. For our purposes, the relevant physiological alcohol concentrations are in the range from modest (ca 25 mM) to high (ca 50 mM).

Normal EtOH clearance in human adults is mainly due to metabolism (ca 87 %), with minor quantities being cleared by urinary excretion (ca 10 %) or by exhalation (ca 3 %). A very small fraction is excreted in sweat or tears. The metabolic pathway in adults is dominated by hepatic ADH-I activity, whereas other ADH isoforms and CYP2E1 give minor contributions to the oxidation of EtOH to AA (scheme 1). Minor quantities of EtOH are metabolized via other, non-oxidative pathways: Conjugation of EtOH to free fatty acids constitutes a minor non-oxidative metabolic pathway, leading to fatty acid ethyl esters (FAEE). These metabolites are toxic and stimulate apoptosis *in vitro* and *in vivo* [laposata02, bearer05, alhomsi08].

Given obvious ethical objections, clearance studies in pregnant humans are rare. A typical clearance rate of alcohol from the blood in moderate drinkers is between 15 ± 5 mg/dl/h (ca 3 mM/h). Markedly higher rates of over 20 mg/dl/h (ca 4 mM/h) may be found in habitual drinkers, who have developed ethanol tolerance. At present, it is still unknown what parameter acts as limiting factor for EtOH clearance in adults. Two plausible theories have been proposed. The first assumes that ADH-I content is the main limiting factor. An alternative hypothesis assumes that reoxidation of NADH to $NAD^+$ is the rate limiting step in hepatic oxidation of EtOH to AA. Strong support for the NADH viewpoint comes from the observation that the clearance rate in humans and rodents may be enhanced significantly by concomitant consumption of sugars like glucose or fructose, or by intravenous administration of amino acids [lisander06]. It has been proposed that these agents promote a rapid reoxidation of reduced coenzyme NADH back to $NAD^+$, and thereby accelerate the metabolic state and the activity of the hepatic mitochondrial respiration.

With lower body and liver mass, adult women have slightly lower metabolic clearance. Their metabolic rate seems unaffected by pregnancy [brien83]. In an older study [brien83] of young healthy pregnancies, EtOH clearance of a modest quantity of alcohol (1.5 standard drink) was indeed similar to that in non-pregnant women. In rats, it was explicitly confirmed that hepatic ADH-I activity was unaffected by pregnancy [badger05]. However, these rat models did show massive fourfold increase in maternal hepatic ALDH2 activity, and sixfold reduction of hepatic CYP2E1 activity [badger05].

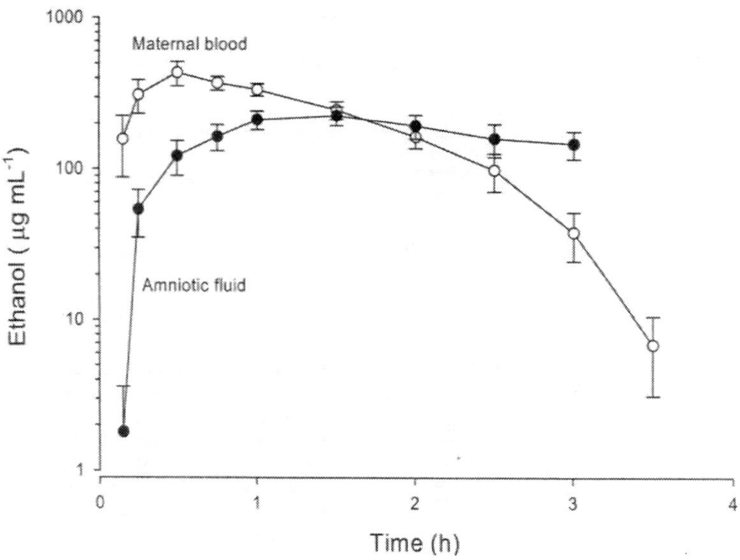


Figure 1. kinetics of EtOH clearance from maternal blood and amniotic fluid of six young healthy pregnant women (from [nava04] with permission). The oral alcohol dose of ca 300 mg / kg body weight corresponds to ca 1.5 standard drinks. The experiment shows EtOH clearance at 16 – 18 weeks of gestation.

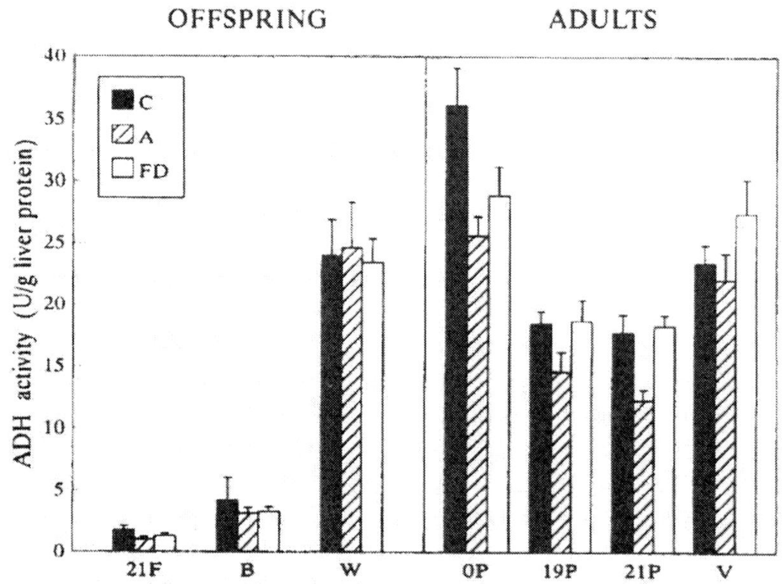


Figure 2: Effect of chronic alcohol consumption on the hepatic ADH activity of rats and offspring. Offspring: 21 days of fetal age (21F), birth (B) and weaned pups (W). Adults: pregnant (0P, 19P, 21P days of pregnancy) and virgin (V) rats. The three groups are control (C), alcohol (A), and fibre diet (FD). From [traves95] with permission.

Given that CYP2E1 contributes significantly to EtOH clearance in habitual alcohol users only, this suggests that maternal EtOH clearance might be impaired in alcoholic pregnancies. In normal pregnancies, EtOH clearance is dominated by hepatic ADH-I, which remains unaffected. At the same time, hepatic AA clearance seems higher during pregnancy.

In view of the above, the usual kinetics and amplitudes of EtOH clearance should be representative for pregnant clearance as well. However, it is interesting to consider the level of fetal exposure at a given maternal BAC. Again, for ethical reasons, few human data exist. Interestingly, the peak EtOH level of the amniotic fluid (0.2 mM) was only slightly below that of maternal blood (0.4 mM). It seems highly significant, however, that the EtOH clearance from the amniotic fluid was very much slower than that from the maternal circulation (figure 1) [nava04, brien83]. Therefore, amniotic levels remained significantly higher than maternal blood levels ca 2 hrs after intake.

This suggests that steady state EtOH levels in amniotic fluid of chronic drinkers may even exceed (!) the steady state EtOH levels in maternal blood. This situation was subsequently confirmed with pregnant rats with chronic alcohol intake [traves95]. The steady state EtOH concentrations in maternal blood, fetal blood and amniotic fluid were determined at various timepoints during gestation. While maternal blood had [EtOH] = 0.4 – 0.5 mg / ml, the amniotic fluid had far higher steady state levels (1.1 mg / ml at day 19, 0.8 mg / ml at day 21). In accordance, the steady state fetal blood levels were far higher (0.8 – 0.9 mg / ml) than maternal levels. These data demonstrate succinctly that fetal tissues experience significantly higher and enduring alcohol exposure than the consuming mother. This observation reflects the fact that fetal liver has far lower capacity for EtOH clearance than adult liver (cf fig 2). This is mainly due to low expression of ADH-I in fetal liver. Interestingly, hepatic ADH activity of the offspring was not lowered by maternal EtOH (figure 2). However, chronic EtOH consumption significantly reduced hepatic ADH activity in the pregnant mother rats.

## Effects of Ethanol on Lactation

The negative effects of maternal alcohol consumption on offspring continue post-partum through noticeable changes in lactation. The existing literature was reviewed recently by [giglia06]. Although the American Academy of Pediatricians considers alcohol consumption 'compatible with breastfeeding', it was noted that EtOH consumption higher than 0.5 g/kg maternal weight reduced the volume of milk consumed by the infant. At higher EtOH levels a significant decrease of the milk ejection reflex was noted. This reflex promotes expulsion from the mammal alveoli into the collecting ducts to the nipple, and is under hormonal control of oxytocin (secreted by the posterior pituary gland) (cf eg. [neville01]). The reflex assists in the emptying of the breast by the suckling infant. EtOH was found to inhibit the release of oxytocin and to disrupt the hormonal milieu of lactating women [mennella01, mennella05, pueta08]. After EtOH consumption, plasma oxytocin levels were lower by ca 25 %, whereas plasma prolactin levels were 30 % higher [mennella05]. Although increased prolactin suggests higher milk production by the mammal glands, the let-down of milk to the suckling infant is actually controlled by oxytocin. Studies have confirmed that this leads to reduced milk intake by the infant ([mennella05] and references therein). On a longer timescale, infant weight, growth, and other developmental parameters are compromised.

EtOH enters breast milk by passive diffusion from the maternal blood circulation. Accordingly, EtOH reaches the milk within ca 30 min after ingestion, and will attain concentrations similar to that in the mother. For ethical reasons, the effect of EtOH on the suckling infant can only be estimated from a hypothetical calculation: At a maternal 1.2 ‰ blood concentration, a reasonable quantity of 200 ml breast milk should contain a total EtOH dose of ca 250 mg. In a small infant this would probably induce a blood alcohol level of ca 0.1 ‰ ([EtOH] ~ 2.2 mM). In the suckling, this quantity would be circulating far longer than in an adult due to the immature liver and very low ADH expression in neonates (see above). A large epidemiological study has revealed a strong inverse relationship between chronic exposure to EtOH via breast milk and the Psychomotor Development Index (PDI) ([giglia06] and references therein). Sleeping patterns of sucklings consuming EtOH tainted milk are also significantly affected, with shortened periods of active sleep [mennella01].

There is no scientific experimental support for the widely circulating folklore that women should consume alcohol, in particular beer, to enhance breast milk volume and improve breastfeeding. The acute rise in maternal prolactin levels after EtOH consumption is well documented and might seem beneficial for lactation at first glance. However, lactational performance is determined by maternal oxytocin, rather than prolactin. Human and rodent studies have clearly established that maternal EtOH reduces in volume and duration of lactation [mennella05], and requiring larger effort from the suckling. Recent experiments with lactating rats have shown that EtOH decreased daily weight gain of the pups significantly, and changed the composition of the milk [azara08]. The milk from EtOH consuming mothers was higher in protein (+20 %), lower in carbohydrate (-20 %), with lipid content unchanged. Their pups had lower concentrations of essential minerals like $Ca^{2+}$, P and $Cl^-$ in the neuronal tissues [azara08]. Maternal EtOH also brings enhanced risk of folate deficiency in the offspring. This essential B-group vitamin plays several critical roles in fetal and neonatal development [lucock03]. Older literature has indicated that maternal EtOH does not significantly impede maternal-fetal folate transfer through the placenta [lin91]. However, it is generally known that pregnancy carries significant risk of maternal folate deficiency, and dietary folate supplementation is generally recommended for pregnant women. The risk of systemic folate deficiency is considerably increased by alcohol consumption, since EtOH in the circulation enhances urinary excretion of folate from humans (see below), including pregnant women. The risk continues *post partum*. It has been noted that milk from EtOH consuming mothers also has lower folate levels [murillo03]. We note that lactation provides the only source of folate to the suckling during the first months of life. Therefore, maternal EtOH consumption exacerbates the risk of folate deficiency in the offspring during gestational and neonatal periods. After birth, three cumulative effects of EtOH compound the risk of folate deficiency in the neonate: First, lactation quantity and duration are reduced [mennella05]. Second, the milk *per se* has lower folate content. Third, EtOH exposure *in utero* reduces the intestinal capacity of the weanling to absorb the dietary folate from maternal milk [murillo03].

## Effects of Ethanol on the Developing Nervous System

The development and ripening of fetal brain is a very complex process and quite sensitive to environmental, i.e. mainly maternal factors. The main stages of normal fetal brain development are reviewed in e.g. [joseph00]. This normal development is compromised by maternal EtOH consumption via a broad spectrum of mechanisms.

EtOH has a wide spectrum of acute effects on the human CNS. The pleasant sensations form the main motivation of alcohol consumption of adults and, together with social motives, the main stimulus for development of dependency. These acute effects are manifold, and are described extensively in other chapters of this volume. On a molecular level, the administration of EtOH acutely affects the normal signal transduction in the CNS, depending on the type of neurotransmitter involved (cf eg pollard08]). An overview of the main mammalian neurotransmitters is given in table 2. In the context of EtOH toxicity, two receptor types have attracted particular attention. Both belong to the central nervous system (CNS): The inhibitory GABAergic receptors, and the excitatory glutaminergic NMDA receptors (NMDA-R). EtOH tends to stimulate the inhibitory GABAergic system. The net effect is damping of CNS activity. In the glutaminergic system, EtOH has downregulating effect on the NMDA-R. Again, the net effect is damping of CNS acitivity. Interestingly, EtOH-like effects appear *in vivo* in human volunteers treated with either the NMDA antagonist ketamine, or with the $GABA_A$ agonist thiopental [dickerson10]. Accordingly, it appears that these acute effects on CNS signaling are elicited by EtOH *per se*, rather than by some downstream metabolite.

Recent advances in MRI have allowed non-invasive assessment of certain chemicals in human tissues. Just like the neurotransmitter glutamate, N-acetyl aspartate/creatine (NAA) and creatine (Cr) are found throughout mammalian brain in very high concentrations ([NAA] ~ 9 - 11 mM; [Cr] ~ 6-8 mM [christiansen93]). NAA contributes significantly to the osmotic fluid balance of the CNS, and is needed for synthesis of the neuronal dipeptide N-acetylaspartylglutamate [moffett06]. The ratio of NAA to creatine (*NAA/Cr*) can be non-invasively measured by proton-Magnetic Resonance spectroscopy, and is widely used as a reliable marker of neuronal integrity and function. It has been found that NAA/Cr was significantly enhanced in children that had been prenatally exposed to alcohol [cortese06]. In these children, the caudate nucleus, a brain region crucial for learning and memory, was found to be markedly less developed than in controls. Clearly, in these children the normal status of the aspartate cascade is significantly and irreversibly disturbed.

**Table 2. The mammalian neurotransmitters and their postsynaptic receptors**

| transmitter | acronym | receptor type | main action |
|---|---|---|---|
| Acetylcholine | Ach | nicotinic receptor ($Na^+$ / $K^+$ channel); muscarinic 7-helix receptor | excitatory |
| Dopamine | | dopamine 7-helix receptor | excitatory |
| γ-butyric acid | GABA | $Cl^-$ channel; 7-helix β-type GABA receptor | inhibitory† |
| Glycine | Gly | $Cl^-$ channel | inhibitory |
| Glutamate | Glu | $Na^+$ / $K^+$ channel, $Na^+/K^+$ / $Ca^{2+}$ channel; NMDA-R channel‡ | excitatory, dominant neuronal transmitter |
| Aspartate | Asp | NMDA-R channel‡ | excitatory |
| Serotonin (5-hydroxytryptamine) | 5-HT | 5-HT3 channel; 7-helix serotonin receptor | excitatory |
| Norepinephrine | NE | 7-helix adrenergic receptor | excitatory |
| Nitric oxide | NO | soluble Guanylate cyclase | excitatory burst of cGMP |
| Carbon monoxide | CO | heme bound $K^+$ channel | reversible liganding of heme |
| oxytocin | | metabotropic oxytocin receptor | promotes lactation |

†inhibitory in adult, but excitatory at early stages of development[benari07]. See text.

‡The NMDA receptor has a complicated activation mechanism involving both ligand (glutamate or aspartate) binding and modulation of the membrane potential. Its name is somewhat misleading since NMDA itself is not a physiological neurotransmitter but a synthetic chemical not naturally found in mammals. Note that not all synapses rely on signal transduction via release of neurotransmitters: Excitatory action of 'electrical' synapses involves direct coupling of the presynaptic and postsynaptic cytosolic compartments via gap junctions. Glycine and GABA are usually considered inhibitory. However, this depends on the intracellular chlorine levels. Prior to induction of the chlorine pumps, the GABAergic action in immature neuronal cells is excitatory rather than inhibitory (see text). Nitric oxide (NO) and carbon monoxide (CO) are gaseous neurotransmitters. Neuronal signal transmission via such gaseous transmitters is rare but significant in hippocampus and cerebellum, as well as the Auerbach plexus (plexus myentericus) of the intestinal tract. In addition, over 50 different neuroactive peptides are known so far. Most act as modulators of the action of a conventional small-molecule transmitter, but some peptide transmitters act as primary transmitter per se. Presynaptic $Zn^{2+}$ release is also considered as a neurotransmitter by some [hirano08]. Some aspects of $Zn^{2+}$-homeostasis in the context of pregnancy are discussed in the text. The central nervous system has many neurotransmitters, whereas the peripheral nervous system relies on just Ach and NE.

Many studies have documented that EtOH disturbs the molecular mechanisms of NMDA-R activation acutely [feyder10]. As mentioned above, administration of the NMDA antagonist ketamine elicits effects in human volunteers quite reminiscent of those of EtOH [dickerson10]. The NMDA-R channel belongs to the ionotropic glutamate receptors of the CNS. The activity of this channel is modulated by a broad spectrum of endogenous ligands like glycine, Zn, polyamines and a variety of neurosteroids [ron04]. In addition, its activity is modulated by (de)phosphorylation of the tyrosine residue of the NR2 subunit (the conductivity of this channel is enhanced in phosphorylated state). Experimental evidence suggests that acute EtOH promotes dephosphorylation of the tyrosine [ferrani03, ron04]. Such dephosphorylation is a plausible mechanism for the observed inhibitory affect of EtOH on the NMDA receptors. It has been noted, however, that the state of phosphorylation is modulated locally by the presence of specific proteins that are selectively expressed in different regions of the human brain. Examples are the scaffolding protein RACK1, which localizes close to NMDA-R in the hippocampus [yaka03]. Another example is the DARPP-32 protein that is preferentially expressed in the dopaminergic neurons of the neostriatum. DARPP-32 also mediates the downregulation of neostriatal NMDA-R conductivity by dephosphorylation [maldve02]. Clearly, the molecular mechanisms behind EtOH effects represent quite complex cascades and combined action of several agents. Apparently, the acute effect of EtOH on the phosphorylation of the NMDA receptor presents the basic pathway. This basic pathway functions throughout the CNS, but with significant regional variations in coupling strength [ron04]. It should be noted that these acute effects on GABAergic receptor signaling are elicited by EtOH *per se*, rather than by some downstream metabolite.

The process of neurulation, i.e. the formation of the neural tube, appears to be a particularly sensitive to maternal EtOH. In humans, neurulation occurs during the third week of gestation. In mice, maternal alcohol consumption during embryonic neurulation (E7 – E18 in mice) significantly reduced serotonin innervation in the embryos [zhou05]. Fewer serotonic 5-HT fibers were found in the hypothalamus and septal nucleus, with both organs having reduced size. Prenatal EtOH has long term effects on the 5-HT-mediated reponses of the hypothalamic-pituitary-adrenal axis in adult rats [hofmann07].

There are numerous reports of effects of EtOH on the developing nervous system. Prominent anatomical deficiencies are decreased brain mass [chen03, zhou05], with corresponding decreased mass of subregions like hippocampus, hypothalamus, septal nucleus, deformation of the corpus callosum etc ([chen03, handmaker06, bookstein06, bookstein07] and references therein). The observed effects span the whole range of processes in neural development: On a cellular level EtOH affects neuronal proliferation, differentiation and migration.

EtOH has a marked proapoptotic effect on neurons via a combination of different pathways, and a special section below is dedicated to this important phenomenon. On a systemic level, it affects the development of the synaptic network, the natural apoptotic selection of the neural network, and the myelination of the axons. The physiological changes to neonatal brain have been reviewed in other chapters of this volume, and we here restrict ourselves to effects on a molecular level. Moreover, we restrict ourselves to cases where the prime effector was identified as EtOH itself, rather than one of its downstream metabolites.

First we consider a number of pathways involving the migration and proper positioning of neural cells during brain development. This process is a very complex and synchronized sequence of proliferation, differentiation, migration, adhesion and systemic integration (for reviews cf [rakic90, guan03, huang07]). Even prior to finishing migration, neurons project neurites that actively seek their targets under guidance of dedicated molecules like netrins, semaphorins, or ephrins. These compounds are evolutionary conserved and crucial for axonal integration in late embryonic, fetal and early neonatal development [uziel06, salinas08]. EtOH interferes with normal migration and systemic integrations of neurons via several pathways. To start with, it disrupts the signaling pathways of Transforming Growth Factor-β (TGFβ). This growth factor can affect cellular migration by modulating the expression of cell adhesion proteins (CAP) that promote the migration and subsequent adhesion of several non-neural cells types, like osteoclasts, immune and endothelial cells. It was recently found that low concentrations of TGFβ1 ligand promote migration of rat neural cells as well [siegenthaler04, powrozek09]. TGFβ upregulates the neural cell adhesion molecule (nCAM) in immature neurons and neuroblastomal cells [miller02] and thereby promotes neuronal migration. This assists cortical development by promoting the migration of young neurons from the proliferative population towards the target. Prenatal EtOH exposure *in vivo* reduces both TGFβ receptor expression and level of TGFβ1 ligand [Siegenthaler04] in the cortex. This inhibits the neural migration promoted by TGFβ1, and is likely to impair the final positioning of the cortical neurons. EtOH also inhibits ripening and normal migration of callosal cells to such an extent that callosal cells end up in an abnormal position [livy08]. Aberrant migratory neural profiles may result not only from inhibitory effects of EtOH: Recently, a mouse model demonstrated that EtOH actually promotes (!) premature tangential migration of primordial GABAergic interneurons from the medial ganglionic eminence (MGE) into the cortex [cuzon08] and leads to aberrant cell distributions. Interestingly the $GABA_A$ receptor has been found to have a direct effect on the neuronal migration in the developing neocortex [heck06]. This receptor is known as a direct target of EtOH (see below).

A more recent hypothesis proposes that EtOH compromises fetal brain development via an indirect pathway, namely by reducing maternal levels of thyroid hormones. Placental transfer of maternal thyroid hormones modulates neuronal migration at early stages of gestation, i.e. before fetal thyroid function has developed. The hypothesis is based on observations that maternal thyroid hormones affect the organization of the cytoskeleton of fetal brain cells, and also promote neuronal migration, ripening, and integration. In addition, maternal thyroid hormones promote expression of the crucial guidance molecule laminin on astrocyte membranes. This interesting mechanism has been reviewed in [farwell05]. The effect of EtOH on fetal thyroid levels is discussed in more detail in the section on hormonal status (see below).

The natural migratory ripening of neurons may also be affected at subsequent embedding stages of the migratory cascade:

EtOH has been reported to interact with the beneficial role of neuroprotective proteins, like activity-dependent neuroprotective protein (ADNP) and activity dependent neurotrophic factor (ADNF) (reviewed in [sari06, gozes07, mandel08]). Both proteins are expressed in astroglial cells already during fetal development and essential for proper brain development. Both proteins participate in the signaling cascade controlled by vasoactive intestinal peptide (VIP). VIP plays an important role in the proliferation and differentiation of many cell types, and is prominently expressed in hematopoietic stem cells and megakaryocytes from the bone marrow [nam09]. However, VIP also is a major neuropeptide in the brain and has large effect on the growth and development of fetal brain. Studies of neuronal cells from mice and rats have demonstrated that VIP regulates embryonic growth by controlling the release of ADNP and ADNF [sari06].

The biochemical pathways underlying these actions of VIP are still under investigation, but certain details have emerged form *in vitro* studies on cultured neuronal cells. The octapeptide NAP-fragment of ADNP stimulates neurite outgrowth *in vitro* by promoting tyrosine phosphorylation of Fyn kinase and the scaffold protein Cas [chen08]. *In vitro* experiments have shown that modest levels of EtOH ($IC_{50}$ ~ 17 mM) inhibit the activation of Fyn kinase and Cas by the NAP fragment.

In their effect on the Fyn kinase pathway, EtOH and ADNP appear to antagonize each other: On the one hand, the beneficial effects of ADNP on neurite outgrowth were suppressed by EtOH *in vitro* in cultured rat cerebral granule neurons [chen08]. On the other hand, suppletion of ADNP and ADNF is neuroprotective against EtOH [zhou04, zhou08, sari06] *in vitro* and *in vivo*. Other neuroprotective proteins, like SALLRSIPA or NAPVSIPQ, similarly rescue the retardation of brain growth by EtOH [zhou04]. These small polypeptides appear to act via their function as agonist of ADNF and ADNP, respectively [zhou08].

Low doses of EtOH disable the neural cell adhesion molecule L1. This 200 kD transmembrane adhesion protein is deeply involved in axon guidance, neuronal targeting, axonal fasciculation and synaptic plasticity in the fetal brain. L1 also promotes activation of extracellular receptor kinases [yeaney09]. Mutations of L1 lead to morphological abnormalities, reminiscent of fetal alcohol syndrome, such as hypoplasia of the corpus callosum, cerebellar dysplasia, and hydrocephalus. Proper expression and functioning of L1 is neuroprotective against alcohol induced cell death [gubitosi07]. It is known that modest EtOH concentrations as reached after two standard drinks, already inhibit L1-mediated cell-cell adhesion significantly, and L1-mediated neurite outgrowth [bearer99]. Recent *in vitro* experiments have investigated the molecular mechanism of the interaction between EtOH and L1. EtOH did not affect the expression of L1, but promoted significant phosphorylation of a tyrosine moiety on L1 [yeaney09]. In addition, recent experiments have identified a binding site for EtOH on the extracellular domain of L1. It was noted that this binding site is located in a sensitive domain, that is, in proximity to sites where mutations induce severe neurological disorders [arevalo08].

The above examples illustrate the negative effect of EtOH on proper neuronal migration in the developing brain. However, many other effects on parts of the CNS have been reported. In most regions of the adult vertebrate brain, two antagonistic types of neurons can be distinguished: a majority of excitatory principal neurons, and a minority of inhibitory interneurons. The inhibitory interneurons dampen and regulate the excitatory activity of the principal network to a controlled level of activity required for functional balance of the CNS. Various neuronal cells use their characteristic transmitter for signal transduction. In the inhibitory interneurons γ-aminobutyric acid (GABA) plays a prominent role, and GABA is usually viewed as the main inhibitory neurotransmitter in vertebrates. However, recent research has shown that GABA plays a more differentiated role in the developing brain. It has been recently discovered that during early stages of brain development GABA has excitatory rather than inhibitory action [benari07] and that it plays an essential role in morphological maturation of cortical neurons. This excitatory activity promotes neuronal growth and systemic neuronal integration [liu06]. In rats, this transition from excitatory action at early, and inhibitory action at mature stages of development occurs postnatally 5-7 days after birth. It may also occur transiently during delivery under influence of the surge in maternal oxytocin [tyzio06]. This hormone acts as a neurotransmitter in the brain, facilitates delivery and lactation, and affects social recognition, bonding, and maternal behaviour. In humans, the timepoint of transition seems not known, but is likely to be soon after birth as well. The molecular mechanism for the transition from excitatory to inhibitory action is complex [benari07, liu06] and may be understood from the action of GABA: Activation of the ionotropic $GABA_A$ receptor creates an influx of chloride into the cell. In mature cells, this hyperpolarizes the membrane and raises the threshold for activation (inhibition). In contrast, immature neurons have not yet expressed the KCC2 chloride transporter and carry a higher cytosolic chloride concentration than mature cells. Accordingly, GABA receptor activation acts depolarizing in the immature cell (excitation). Other fundamental differences between immature and mature stages have been found: In the mature CNS, GABA is synthesized by glutamate decarboxylases (GAD). This class of enzymes catalyzes the decarboxylation of glutamic acid to GABA and $CO_2$. Several isoforms are known and labelled according to their molecular weight in kD. Two isoforms appear in mature neuronal cells (GAD65, GAD67), and two additional embryonic isoforms were identified in the developing brain (GAD25 and GAD44 respectively). In very early stages of development GAD enzymes are not yet induced and GABA originates from putrescein [cancedda07, benari07]. This second pathway for GABA was found to be significant far into the postnatal stage [sequerra07]. The role of GABA innervation in the development and ripening of the CNS has been reviewed in [huang07]. In the context of maternal alcohol consumption it seems highly significant that EtOH has multiple direct effects on GABAergic signaling. Presynaptically, it enhances the release of GABA [carta04, hayward04]. Postsynaptically, EtOH sensitizes the $GABA_A$ receptor to GABA and increases its activity. The effects combine so that GABAergic signaling is significantly enhanced by acute EtOH. The physical relevance of this enhancement is illustrated by recent experiments with thiopental in human volunteers. This $GABA_A$ receptor agonist acutely produced effects reminiscent of EtOH [dickerson10]. It should be noted that these acute effects on GABAergic receptor signaling are elicited by EtOH *per se*, rather than by some downstream metabolite.

Under chronic EtOH administration, changes in the GABAergic parameters of certain regions of the CNS are apparent: The steady-state tissue GABA concentrations in the central amygdala of adult rats were more than twofold higher than in EtOH naive rats (50 nM vs 20 nM) [breese06]. The EtOH induced increase in GABA has regional specifity and is not apparent in all brain regions [breese06, criswell08]. We already noted that the $GABA_A$ receptor has a direct effect on the neuronal migration in the developing neocortex [heck06]. In accordance, it was recently shown that chronic *in utero* exposure to EtOH reduces the number of cortical neurons in macaques [miller06] and the density of GABAergic cells in the cortex of guinea pigs [bailey04]. In both cases, the most dramatic reductions were found in cortical layers II – III, i.e. the somatosensory regions. In the course of development, the cortex develops from the telencephalon, i.e. the most anterior part of the neural tube. This region is known to be particularly sensitive to chronic as well as acute EtOH exposure at certain time windows [isayama09]. In a recent report, it was noted that acute exposure to high, supraphysiological (100 mM) EtOH levels, promotes expression of $GABA_B$ receptors and protein kinase A-α (PKA) in cultivated cortical and hippocampal neural cells from rat fetuses [naseer10]. This effect could be largely abolished by cotreatment with ascorbate.

The above shows that EtOH has profound effect on the inhibitory GABAergic signaling in the developing brain. Despite intense research efforts over the last decade, the basic mechanisms behind the alterations in $GABA_A$ receptor function are still controversial. The hypotheses range from changes in membrane receptor expression, receptor phosphorylation, subcellular localization, changes in receptor subunit composition, and indirect effects via neurosteroids. The experimental support for these various propositions has been reviewed in [kumar04, breese06].

Besides the GABAergic system, EtOH has many other effects on neural signal transduction and development. Systemic EtOH increases the levels of neuroactive steroids in the brain and alters its functional response. Such neurosteroids have strong modulatory influence on postsynaptic activation by interacting with many receptors (like $GABA_A$). Given the important role of neurosteroids in pregnancy, a special section has been dedicated to this mechanism (see below).

It has been recognized that EtOH affects the activity of other neurotransmitters as well (the older literature on brain ligand-gated ion channels is reviewed in [costa00]). Many anesthetics or anticonvulsants have actions reminiscent of EtOH in various signaling pathways [ikonomidou01], and similarly promote neuronal apoptosis (for EtOH induced neuronal apoptosis see below). During the human brain growth spurt, the developing brain seems particularly vulnerable to irreversible damage by the presence of EtOH or anesthetics. In humans, this spurt spans the time interval from $6^{th}$ month of gestation.

Glycinergic signaling pathways are also affected by maternal alcohol consumption [eggers04]. Glycinergic transmission is involved in control of the respiratory network, and it was noted that pre- and postnatal EtOH exposure significantly reduces respirational ventilation in rats [dubois06, dubois08]. The neonates developed polycythaemia to compensate for the low basal level of ventilation. Moreover, the hypoxic response was blunted due to central glycinergic tonic inhibition, making the newborn more susceptible to hypoxia.

The serotonergic system in neonates is affected as well. Subsequent to prenatal EtOH exposure, rat fetuses and weanlings had decreased plasma concentrations of serotonin (5-HT) and its metabolites. Such animals showed physiological and behavioural abnormalities consistent with 5-HT deficiency, as well as abnormal expression and function of $5\text{-}HT_{1A}$ receptors [hellemans10]. The brains of these neonates also showed significantly blunted development of the serotonergic neurons [sliwowska08]. The physiological and behavioural manifestations of irreversible prenatal EtOH damage is reviewed in [hellemans10]. It was already noted that this detrimental effect of EtOH on serotonergic neurons may be rescued by interventions involving the downstream signaling pathways of vasoactive intestinal protein (VIP) [zhou08] (see above).

Dopaminergic systems may also be affected: Low doses of EtOH significantly increase the electrophysiological activity of the mesolimbic dopamine (DA) network in rats. Conversely, chronically drinking rats show a decrease in dopaminergic neuronal activity when EtOH is withdrawn. Subsequent *in vivo* studies [foddai04] have shown that AA administration elicits similar responses in the dopaminergic system. It suggests that the observed effects of EtOH on DA activity is mediated by the metabolite AA, rather than EtOH itself.

Recent *in vivo* experiments have revealed a new mechanism how maternal EtOH may affect the fetal CNS. The neural proteins complexin I and complexin II regulate the calcium dependence of neurotransmitter release from the presynaptic terminals. Their physiological relevance for cognition and memory formation has been confirmed. It was found that maternal EtOH significantly reduced the expression of these proteins in various regions of the neonatal brain, and impaired learning [zink09].

The above concentrates on the mechanisms through which EtOH affects the normal brain development in the fetal and neonatal stages. On top of this, we note that EtOH is definitely detrimental to existing brain structures. Phrased otherwise: Impaired development may be further aggravated by subsequent damage to existing structures of the immature CNS. The mechanisms for such neurodegeneration have been recently reviewed in [crews09].

## Ethanol and Neuronal Apoptosis

The mechanism behind the proapoptotic action of EtOH on neurons is still controversial. In the literature, multiple hypotheses have been forwarded. The first mechanism notes that EtOH dampens the activity of the phosphatidylinositol 3'kinase (PI-3) in rat neurons [antonio08]. This promotes apoptosis, since PI-3/Akt signaling pathway is a key regulator of cellular proliferation and survival (reviewed in [terragni08]). The downstream effects are complicated, manifold and poorly understood; Akt phosphorylation inhibits proapoptotic action of downstream kinases like GSK-3, and members of the Bcl-2 family like Bad [terragni08] or Bax [young03, nowoslawski05]. The damping of PI-3 also reduces the expression of pro-survival genes concomitantly. This proapoptotic pathway affects fetal tissues other than the CNS: Enhanced Bax expression has been confirmed *in vivo* in hepatic apoptosis in rat fetuses exposed to maternal EtOH *in utero* [perez06]. The second mechanism proposes that neuronal apoptosis is promoted by EtOH induced release of reactive oxygen species (ROS). The effects of ROS mediated oxidative stress on tissues are discussed in the section on the redox state of tissues (see below). A third hypothesis is based on the observation that EtOH neutralizes the antiapoptotic action of docosahexaenoic acid (DHA) [akbar06]. This role of DHA will be discussed further below. A fourth proposal has noted that EtOH suppresses cAMP production and activates transforming growth factor-β1 in cultured hypothalamic β-EP neurons from rats [chen06]. Fifth, we recall the endogenous formation of fatty acid ethyl esters (FAEE) when EtOH reacts with endogenous free fatty acids in the plasma membrane. Basal levels of FAEE are nonzero even in abstainers, and significantly raised in plasma of alcohol consumers for a timespan of ca 10 – 15 hrs after alcohol intake. FAEE are toxic and known to promote apoptosis *in vitro* and *in vivo* [laposata02, bearer05, alhomsi08].

The first mechanism involving IP-3 deserves more comment as it appears to be specific for ethanol signaling in neurons. Interestingly, an *in vitro* study of cultured pig pulmonary artery endothelial cells (PAEC's) observed the opposite effect: In PAEC, modest but chronic levels of EtOH enhanced endothelial NO production and eNOS protein levels through PI-3 mediated upregulation of eNOS transcription [polikandriotis05]. In this endothelial cell type, therefore, modest ethanol seems to act anti-apoptotically. We correlate this observation with clinical observations that low to modest doses of EtOH enhance the endothelial release of NO in humans (reviewed in [puddey01, deng07]).

In this context, it should be noted that neuronal apoptosis should not be regarded as a negative phenomenon *per se.* Rather, neuronal apoptosis is a key process in two important stages of normal brain development. In early stages of this development, an excessive quantity of neurons is produced, and requires controlled annihiliation of roughly half the neuronal cells produced. This controlled pruning is achieved in two apoptotic waves. The first removes the proliferating precursors and young postmitotic neuroblasts. The second wave removes a significant fraction of the postmitotic neurons (reviewed in [okouchi07]). This controlled and beneficial developmental apoptosis should be distinguished from neurodegenerative apoptosis of later stages in life (eg Alzheimer, Parkinson, dementia), and also from excessive apoptosis as induced by harmful external factors like EtOH, toxins, prolonged hypoxia, or similar agents that harm the normal development of the fetal brain.

## Effects of Ethanol on Levels and Function of Neurosteroids

Neuroactive steroids, or neurosteroids, modulate neuronal excitability by their interaction with neurotransmitter-gated ion channels. The neurosteroids are endogenously synthesized *de novo* in the central and peripheral nervous systems from cholesterol or steroidal precursors. Alternatively, they appear as metabolites of adrenal or gonadal steroids, especially testosterone or progesteron. The progesterone metabolite allopregnanolone (3α,5α-THP) has recently attracted attention due to its physiological role in alcohol dependent humans [morrow01, purdy05, porcu08, morrow09]. This neurosteroid is a positive modulator of the $GABA_A$ receptor and also promotes neurogenesis [grobin03, gago04, wang05]. It has been noted long ago that neonatal rats show reduced behavioural response to the neurosteroid pregnenolone sulfate (PREGS) after *in utero* exposure to maternal EtOH. Like other neurosteroids, PREGS is known to modulate the sensitivity of the $GABA_A$ receptor and the glutaminergic NMDA receptor. Accordingly, it is known as a GABA antagonist. These modulating effects of PREGS are blunted in fetuses after maternal EtOH [costa00b]. In addition, neurosteroid levels in brain may be affected: It was recently found that prenatal EtOH exposure enhances PREGS levels in the fetal and neonatal brain, but not other tissues. The enhancement was attributed to endogenous accumulation in the fetus, since the levels of these neurosteroids had remained normal in placenta and maternal blood [caldeira04]. Under acute EtOH, the neurosteroid 3α,5α-THP was also found enhanced in plasma, cerebral cortex and hippocampal tissue of adult rats [caldeira04]. Some effects of 3α,5α-reduced neurosteroids (like 3α,5α-THP or 3α,5α-PROG) are reminiscent of symptoms of acute EtOH administration. The acute effects of EtOH on neurosteroid levels can be surprisingly large: *In vivo* 3α,5α-THP levels in rat cerebral cortex were acutely enhanced fourfold ca 1 hr after injection of EtOH [morrow01]. 3α,5α-THP has a significant concentration dependent effect on the developing brain: At low concentrations (1 – 100 nM), 3α,5α-THP induced regression of hippocampal neuron neurites, and promoted the proliferation of hippocampal neuroprogenitor cells from rats and human neural stem cells from the cerebral cortex [wang05]. At high concentrations (> 1 μM) proliferation was strongly inhibited. It should be noted that maternal as well as fetal levels of 3α,5α-THP vary significantly during gestation: In fertile nonpregnant women, serum levels in the middle of the menstrual cycle are ca 4 nM. Serum levels are massively increased during pregnancy and reach ca 160 nM during the third trimester [luisi00]. In the fetus, progesterone and 3α,5α-THP are synthesized in the central nervous system throughout gestation. The production was located primarily in the pluripotent progenitor cells [gago04]. Highest 3α,5α-THP levels are found in late gestation. It is highly likely that fetal neurosteroid levels are influenced by maternal factors, and that this will affect the development as well as activity of the fetal central nervous system. It is known that small neurosteroids like 3α,5α-THP readily pass the placental and blood-brain barriers [wang05], so that maternal neurosteroids can reach the fetal brain.

## Effects of Ethanol on Lipid Metabolism and Membrane Composition

EtOH exposure has manifold effects on the lipids of the central nervous system. These effects were recently reviewed by Cazzaniga et al [cazzaniga09]. Prominent effects are changes in the overall unsaturated : saturated fatty acid ratio, and the asymmetric distribution of lipids in the cytosolic and apical blade of the plasma membrane. It has been noted that neural cell lipids are particularly sensitive to the presence of EtOH [cazzaniga09, monte09]. Prenatal EtOH exposure in rats alters the phospholipid composition of membranes in rat brain and hippocampus [wen04]. In addition, it inhibits the antiapoptotic action of docosahexaenoic acid (DHA) which is known to promote accumulation of phosphatidylserine (PS) in neuronal cells *in vitro* and *in vivo* (reviewed in [kim08]). PS has played a prominent role in research on neuronal apoptosis since PS presentation in the apical membrane leaflet was recognized as a marker for decreased aminophospholipid translocase activity and upregulation of calcium-dependent scramblases. The ensuing loss of asymmetry between the inner and outer membrane leaflet is often found in apoptotic cells (reviewed in [fadok98, elmore07]). In neuronal cells, accumulation of PS has an antiapoptotic effect, and may be stimulated by certain polyunsaturated fatty acids (PUFA) like DHA or, to a lesser extent, docosapentaenoic acid (DPA) [kim03]. In fetal and neonatal stages, PUFA and their metabolites affect both early immune development and immune maturation (reviewed in [harbige03, calder06, seyfarth08]). Neuronal membranes are particularly enriched in such PUFA, and DHA has been recognized as essential for normal neuronal development [carlson99, schuchardt10]. Some of the benefits of PUFA in neuronal membranes have been attributed to their promotion of PS accumulation [kim08] by upregulation of cellular PS synthesis. Accordingly, supplementation of PUFA has a clear antiapoptotic effect on neuronal cells *in vitro* and *in vivo* ([florent06], [kim08]). This protective mechanism of DHA is readily inhibited by modest levels of EtOH (25 mM) [akbar06, kim08]. We note that such EtOH levels are readily exceeded in fetal blood and amniotic fluid of alcohol consuming mothers.

The beneficial character of dietary polyunsaturated fatty acids (PUFA) has become a kind of mantra of the food and health industry. Less publicized is the toxic character of some of the oxidation products of PUFA as may arise in normal lipid metabolism. Recent scientific literature has documented the link between PUFA and the formation of 4-hydroxynonenal (HNE), one of the oxidation products of polyunsaturated ω-6 fatty acids like arachidonic, linoleic or docosadienoic acid. Work of the Cederbaum group (reviewed in [lu08]) has shown that microsomal and mitochondrial CYP2E1 is a highly relevant pathway for this reaction. Many studies *in vitro* and *in vivo* document the dangerous combination of arachidonic acids with CYP2E1. Inhibition of CYP2E1 with selective inhibitors or a high dose of nitric oxide abolishes the harmful effects of arachidonic acid, presumably by suppressing the release of

HNE [lu08]. By its high affinity for heme, nitric oxide is a well known inhibitor of various mammalian cytochrome P450 enzymes, and its inhibition of CYP2E1 has been explicitly confirmed. The mechanism involves reversible nitrosylation of the heme moiety, i.e binding of nitric oxide to the iron atom as an axial nitrosyl ligand perpendicular to the plane of heme. The NO levels required for this inhibition are unlikely to be reached under basal conditions (endogenous NO levels in mammals remain in the nanomolar range, cf eg [faassen07]). This is not surprising, given that unimpeded activity of cytochrome P450 in the smooth endoplasmatic reticulum is essential for life. Accordingly, the suppression of endogenous NO by NOS inhibitors like L-NAME will not significantly upregulate activity of CYP2E1. This has been verified *in vitro* [wu06]. In this context it should be mentioned that many cytochrome P450 isoforms have a significant capacity to reduce the nitrite anion ($NO_2^-$) to free NO radicals under conditions of hypoxia (for a review cf [faassen09]). Although not directly proven, it seems highly probable that CYP2E1 shares this capacity. The phenomenon of hypoxic reduction of nitrite has confirmed physiological relevance in the context of ischemia and hypoxia in mammals [faassen09, lundberg09].

It has been mentioned before that enhanced CYP2E1 expression is found in liver and brain of people on diets with high alcohol or high lipid content. Ominously, it has been recently reported [raza06] that HNE itself promotes further CYP2E1 expression in PC12 cells *in vitro* (this rat cell line is a widely used model for neuronal differentiation). Although the physiological relevance of this finding remains uncertain for humans, it demonstrates the existence in principle of a positive feedback loop for release of this harmful compound. The release of HNE has been implicated in a variety of diseases, apoptosis and neurodegenerative disorders like Alzheimer (the entire August 2003 issue of Molecular Aspects of Medicine, vol 24, is dedicated to the physiological roles of HNE). While low (1-5 μM) levels of HNE are considered beneficial, high levels (> 10μM) are definitely harmful and proapoptotic. In cultured rat fetal cortical neurons, formation of HNE correlates directly with EtOH induced apoptosis and oxidative stress [maffi08]. The genotoxic reaction of HNE with deoxyguanosine moieties in DNA has already been discussed above.

Interestingly, *in utero* alcohol exposure has promoted apoptosis in rat fetal brain [ramachandran01]. The rats received a high EtOH dosis reminiscent of 'binge drinking'. The mechanism was mediated by EtOH induced formation of HNE in the brain. This study also presented evidence that maternal alcohol intake induces the mitochondrial permeability transition (MPT) in fetal brain tissue, accompanied by mitochondrial swelling and the release of cytochrome c and apoptosis-inducing factor (AIF) from the mitochondria. We note that the MPT is a major cause of cell death. Similar observations of MPT, release of mitochondrial cytochrome c and caspase activation have been made in cultured rat hepatocytes exposed to 50 mM EtOH [higuchi01].

Another class of adducts from polyunsaturated fatty acids are the so called long-chain polyunsaturated fatty acids (LCPUFA). LCPUFA are synthesized from PUFA by repeated enzymatic desaturation and chain extension (repeated cycles of desaturase and elongase activity). For example, ω-6 linoleic acid may be extended to arachidonic acid by three successive enzymatic steps. ω-3 α-linolenic acid (αLN) may be extended to DHA by no less than six enzymatic steps. These conversions involve desaturase and elongase enzymes in the endoplasmatic reticulum of hepatocytes (cf eg [schuchardt10]). In humans, the efficiency of chain extension is low and sex specific: women have higher expression of the elongase and desaturase enzymes involved in the chain extension of αLN to DHA [kitson10].

Adults mostly rely on dietary sources to satisfy their LCPUFA requirements. It has been noted that alcoholics have lower concentrations of LCPUFA in their blood. The placenta lacks desaturase activity [hanebutt08], and fetal enzyme activity *in utero* is very low anyway. Therefore, the fetus is wholly dependent on placental transfer of maternal LCPUFA. Like other fatty acids, LCPUFA can readily cross the placental barrier (reviewed in hanebutt08]). The transfer appears to be actively supported, since *in vitro* and *in vivo* studies have shown that the fetal circulation is significantly enriched in LCPUFA when compared to maternal blood, whereas levels of saturated and mono-unsaturated fatty acids were comparable (cf table 3). Of various LCPUFA, DHA was transferred particularly well. After birth, dietary intake from maternal milk takes over. Maternal milk has a lipid composition with a high proportion of ω-3 LCPUFA, and this contribution is believed to improve neonatal immunity. It is known that ω-3 LCPUFA like DHA and eicosapentaenoic acid (EPA) are essential modulators of the human inflammatory and immune responses [chapkin09]. The details of this phenomenon are discussed below in the special section concerning immunity. Therefore, the fetus seems supplied by three sources of fatty acids: First, a very modest endogenous capacity for *de novo* synthesis. Second, a passive gradient-driven transport through the placental barrier. Third, a selective driven placental transport system for the physiologically important class of LCPUFA. Gestational alcohol exposure has been shown to enhance the levels of DHA and arachidonic acid of umbilical cord serum in humans [denkins00, beblo05]. The DHA content of umbilical plasma was 3.9 % of total lipid in EtOH exposed pregnancies. This is significantly higher than 3.0 % found in controls [denkins00]. EtOH exposed pregnancies had higher ω-3 /ω-6 ratio in cord blood. Higher fetal plasma levels do not imply that tissue levels are enhanced also. On the contrary, studies in rats have shown that serum levels of DHA were enhanced at gestational age 20, but tissue levels in brain were lower than in controls [denkins00]. Given the manifold relevance of LCPUFA in brain development and immunity, these effects of maternal alcohol consumptions give reason for worry.

EtOH also has detrimental effect on sphingolipids, a lipid class with special relevance for neural tissues. The fundamental structural unit common to all sphingolipids is the ceramide structure consisting of a fatty acid chain attached to the headgroup of sphingosine via an amide linkage. Besides a structural function in the cellular membrane, ceramides contribute to cellular signaling for the regulation of proliferation, differentiation, and apoptosis. Ceramides readily cross the BBB and exposure to ceramide induces neurodegeneration in vitro and in vivo. Ceramides and EtOH induce similar responses in cultured neuronal cells, and exposure to supraphysiological (100 mM) EtOH has caused accumulation of ceramides and triglycerides in cultured neurons [saito05]. Whether this link has relevance for the in vivo situation awaits confirmation, but seems plausible given that ceramide accumulation has been implicated in alcohol induced degeneration of liver and brain tissue [monte09]. Recent in vivo experiments on mice have shown that the sphingolipid metabolism in neonates may be profoundly affected by a single maternal alcohol binge around gestational day 15 [dasgupta07]. Highly significant increases in sphingosine were found throughout the brain regions already at modest binge doses (eg doubling of fetal sphingosine 15 days post partum after single maternal dose of 1.5 g EtOH/kg). Although sphingosine is metabolized to ceramide, no abnormalities in monoglycosylceramide were found in the neonatal brain. Neither were any abnormalities found in the sphingolipid content of offspring brain throughout the time window during which myelination takes place (from mid gestation to 30 days post partum in mice, from mid gestation to 2 yrs post partum in neonates) [kinney05].

Therefore, the physiological implications of this interesting finding remain unclear. The authors note that sphingosine per se has proven cytotoxicity in cultured cells [saito05].

**Table 3. fatty acid concentrations (in mg/dl) in maternal and umbilical cord plasma at partum**

| | Maternal plasma | Cord plasma |
|---|---|---|
| Saturated fatty acids | 47 ± 2 | 47 ± 2 |
| Mono-unsaturated FA | 15 ± 3 | 13 ± 2 |
| Arachidonic acid | 7.7 ± 1.9 | 16 ± 2 |
| Total ω-6 LCPUFA | 12 ± 2 | 23 ± 3 |
| DHA | 2.9± 1.0 | 4.8 ± 1.7 |
| Total ω-3 LCPUFA | 3.7± 1.2 | 5.4± 3 |

Data from [berghaus98]. Note that the fetal circulation is significantly enriched in LCPUFA when compared to maternal blood, whereas levels of saturated and mono-unsaturated fatty acids are similar in maternal and cord plasma.

It was mentioned above that fatty acid ethyl esters (FAEE) are metabolic adducts of EtOH. This class of esters results from non-oxidizing metabolic pathways of EtOH clearance. Such esters have proven toxicity in vitro and in vivo [laposata02], and induce apoptosis and necrosis in isolated human mononuclear cells in vitro [alhomsi08]. It suggests that FAEE might be toxic for white blood cells and contribute to the damping of the immune system in chronic alcohol consumers [alhomsi08]. FAEE have been detected in the meconium of neonates. Careful perfusion studies on human placental cotyledons [chan04] have shown that the human placenta has significant intrinsic capacity to degrade FAEE. This capacity is located in the microsomal compartment. At physiological levels of a few μM, maternal FAEE are not transferred to the fetus because of this placental degradation. These results imply that the meconial FAEE is produced from EtOH by the fetus itself [chan04].

There are indications that prenatal EtOH have irreversible effects on the cellular structures that stabilize the plasma membrane of hepatocytes. After maternal EtOH, hepatocytes from newborn rats contained enhanced quantities of tubulin and cytokeratin, but had markedly reduced capacity to assemble functional microtubules [azorin04]. It suggests that the properties of the postnatal hepatic cytoskeleton has been irreversibly altered by prenatal EtOH. It appears likely that cytoskeletal deficiency affects other cell types as well. We note that proper control of cytoskeletal organization of astrocytes and neurons is essential for neuronal migration, outgrowth and systemic integration [farwell05].

## EFFECTS OF ETHANOL ON PURINE METABOLISM

Purines are heterocyclic aromatic compounds containing a characteristic moiety of a pyrimidine ring joined to an imidazole ring. Two of the four deoxyribonucleotides as well as the corresponding ribonucleotides are purines, making that ca 50 % of all DNA and RNA are purines. (Hypo)xanthine, uric acid, adenosine and isoguanine are other small purines with immense relevance for human physiology. More complex purine based biomolecules are ATP, GTP, cyclic AMP and GMP, NADH, and coenzyme A (CoA). Certain purines act as neurotransmitters on purinergic receptors, and adenosine activates adenosine receptors. Given their physiological relevance, nature has developed an elaborate metabolic machinery for processing of purines. EtOH interferes with this machinery in many places. First and foremost, EtOH enhances adenine nucleotide degradation and increases lactic acid production, which readily leads to hyperuricemia [yamamoto05]. EtOH also increases the plasma concentrations and urinary excretion of hypoxanthine and xanthine via the acceleration of adenine nucleotide degradation and possible inhibition of xanthine dehydrogenase activity. There may also be additional beverage-specific effects. For example, in beer consumers, purines already present in the beverage itself contribute to the increase in plasma uric acid. Recent surveys among apparently healthy abstainers and moderate drinkers have indicated distinct gender-dependent impacts of increased body weight and alcohol drinking on serum uric acid [alatalo09]. While both obesity and alcohol consumption may induce oxidative stress and alterations in uric acid metabolism, it appears that moderate alcohol consumption is associated with elevated uric acid concentrations among men only, not in women [gao07]. Similarly, a greater intake of added sugars or sugar-sweetened drinks raised plasma uric acid concentrations in men but not in women. In women with type I diabetes, the initial increase in oxidative stress coincides with a reduction in plasma levels of uric acid [pitocco08]. Interestingly, serum uric acid seems to increase in menopause. Its concentration is influenced by nitric oxide (NO) and peroxynitrite production, and uric acid seems to play an important role in human antioxidant defence systems through its ability to scavenge free radicals. It also prevents the degradation of extracellular superoxide dismutase (SOD) [kurra09]. However, excessive concentrations of uric acid in circulation may also have pro-oxidant properties.

## Effects of Ethanol on Redox State of Tissues

Decades of research have firmly established that reactive oxygen species (ROS) play important roles in the mechanism through which EtOH induces apoptosis and teratogenesis in humans (cf eg [wu03]). Although the mechanisms remain controversial, indirect evidence for ROS involvement comes from clear experimental evidence that a wide range of antioxidants protects against ethanol teratogenicity. This situation arises in healthy alcohol consuming humans, as well as in children that were prenatally exposed to maternal EtOH (reviewed in [cohen03]). Fetal oxidant stress due to maternal EtOH is firmly documented ([henderson99] and references therein). Therefore, it is not surprising that oxidant stress is a symptom of many maternal complications during pregnancy as well [orhan03]. For example, in preeclampsia, many tissue markers attest to enhanced oxidant stress [kaur08, gupta09] and oxygen radical levels were found significantly enhanced in preeclamptic placentas [sikkema01]. Healthy nonpregnant adults also show an acute increase of urinary isoprostanes with peak levels ca 6 hrs after consumption of a single dose of EtOH [maegher99]. Such isoprostanes are oxidative markers of free radical attack on arachidonic acid. We note that human fetuses do not yet have well developed enzymatic defense against reactive oxygen species (ROS). For example, the superoxide dismutase activity in fetal brain and organ tissues is very low at early stages of gestation and only gradually rises as gestation proceeds. For example, SOD activity in liver at gestational age 12 – 15 weeks is ca threefold lower than at *partum* [de86].

The effects of EtOH induced oxidative stress extend *post partum:* It is known that *in utero* exposure to EtOH correlates with increased oxidant stress in the offspring post partum [gauthier10]. Low molecular weight thiols like cysteine (Cys) or glutathione (GSH) act as physiological redoxbuffers in tissues [moriarty04]. Adequate fetal levels of GSH are necessary for normal embryonic development: Insufficiency of fetal GSH induced release of toxic HNE and enhanced hydroxyurea teratogenicity in the mouse embryo during organogenesis, even in absence of EtOH [yan06]. Thus, the importance of proper GSH homeostasis for fetal development has been firmly established. Interestingly, intra- and extracellular compartments are stabilized at different redox potentials: The intracellular compartment is buffered by the GSH/GSSG redox couple at a potential in the range from -230 mV to -260 mV. Therefore, this intracellular compartment is stabilized in rather reduced state with GSH being the favored form. In contrast, the extracellular compartment is mainly stabilized by the Cys/CySS redox couple at a far higher potential, and the disulfide CySS is the favored form [moriarty04]. Interestingly, due to enzymatic activity, the cyteine and glutathione redox potentials in human plasma are set at different values: The Cys/Cyss couple is set at -80 ±9 mV. This level is considerably more oxidized than the GSH/GSSG couple with -137 ± 9 mV in plasma [moriarty04]. It should be noted that plasma Cys and Cyss levels are quite variable and respond on the timescale of an hour to dietary intake of food, in particular proteins. In correspondence, the redox potential of the Cys/Cyss couple shows a mild diurnal variation in humans [blanco07]. Deviations from the normal average thiol/disulfide ratio is often used as biomarker for oxidant stress tissues or plasma [Iyer09]. Adult alcoholics routinely show a significantly lowered ratio [yeh07]. It was recently confirmed [gauthier10] that pregnancy *per se* already lowers the maternal GSH/GSSG ratio somewhat (less negative redox potential). It suggests that maternal physiology is already exposed to enhanced oxidative stress during normal, non-alcoholic pregnancy. The plasma GSH redox potential has been reported at -120 ± 4 mV nonpregnant; -111 ± 30 mV non-alcoholic pregnancy; -93 ± 6 mV EtOH consuming pregnancy [blanco07, gauthier10]. These numbers apply to tissues other than components from the CNS. In the brain, GSH homeostasis is quite different in that extracellular GSH is kept at very low concentrations (below μM). Addition of extracellular GSH in the micromolar range is actually toxic for neurons due to the reaction of GSH with redox sites on the NMDA receptor. This reduced state activates the receptor and potentiates excitotoxicity [regan99]. Phrased otherwise, in the CNS, the extracellular compartment appears to be kept at deeply oxidized state [moriarty04].

The above observations suggest that the plasma GSH status of pregnant women reflects enhanced oxidative stress when EtOH is consumed. It should be noted, however, that other oxidative markers, like urinary 8-isoprostaglandin $F_{2\alpha}$ (8-iso$PGF_{2\alpha}$) or vasoactive prostaglandin metabolites, did not show significant differences between pregnant drinkers and non-drinkers [signore08] (with EtOH > 48 grams / day, the alcohol consumption in these two studies was comparable).

The symptoms of enhanced oxidant stress indicate that ethanol has shifted the normal equilibrium between production and scavenging of ROS. Possibly, ROS production was enhanced, or scavenging reduced, or both effects occurred simultaneously. Therefore, levels of catalase, superoxide dismutase (SOD) [de86], enolase enzymes, ADH and ALDH in neonatal tissues have been assessed. In rats, it was found that chronic maternal EtOH consumption prior to conception also significantly lowers the hepatic SOD activity, and decreases expression of ADH and ALDH in liver and brain of the offspring [ledig90]. In this case, these changes occurred without the offspring ever having been exposed to EtOH during gestation. The preconceptive EtOH consumption of the mother caused subsequent disturbances in the emotional reactivity and motoric activity of the weanlings.

As usual, brain tissues have been found to be very sensitive to such oxidative stress. EtOH induced marked oxidative stress in cultured murine neural crest cells [chen00], rat cortical neurons [ramachandran03] and mouse cerebellum [heaton06]. In cultured fetal rat cortical neurons, modest extracellular EtOH induces acute release of ROS and lowering of intracellular GSH, with concomitant increase of apoptotic markers [rathinam06]. Interestingly, fetal rat cortical neurons do show a marked heterogeneity in intracellular GSH content [maffi08]. The intracellular GSH content correlates inversely with EtOH induced apoptosis: The neurons with low GSH appear more vulnerable to EtOH induced apoptosis than GSH-rich neurons. These neurons with low GSH also contained a markedly higher quantity of adducts of HNE [maffi08], the characteristic oxidation product of polyunsaturated ω-6 fatty acids (see above). In accordance, marked increases in HNE-protein adducts have been observed in tissues of GSH depleted mouse embryos [yan06].

Despite intense research, the sources of such oxidative stress remain controversial. Experiments with mice have shown that EtOH induced ROS was significantly reduced in homogenized cerebellum of *bax* knock-out mutants [heaton06]. This mutant was also protected against EtOH induced loss of Purkinje cells. The *bax* gene has potent pro-apoptotic function *in vitro* and *in vivo*. The mechanism why *bax* knock-out inhibits release of ROS remains unknown. Alternatively, the NOX family of NADPH oxidases was proposed as source of the EtOH induced ROS generation [bedard07, dong10]. These authors used the NOX inhibitor diphenyleneiodonium (DPI) to identify the contribution of NOX to oxidative stress in mouse embryos 6 hrs after a high dose of EtOH was injected into the mother. The experiment was done on gestational day 9. They found that EtOH caused significant increases in mRNA expression of various NOX regulatory subunits, and also in the enzymatic activity of XOR. Maternal EtOH also induced oxidative DNA damage to the embryo, as quantified with 8-OH deoxyguanosine. It also enhanced the expression and activity of caspase-3, a marker for apoptosis. Co-treatment with DPI abolished these changes [dong10], suggesting that fetal NOX contribute significantly to EtOH induced oxidative stress.

Nevertheless, one should keep in mind that other potential sources of ROS are the mitochondrial respiratory chain, cytochrome P450 enzymes like CYP2E1 (see above), and xanthine oxidase. All these enzymes share the common property that their normal enzymatic activity depends on ambient oxygen levels: All start to function as nitrite reductases if local oxygen levels fall below certain thresholds. This phenomenon has considerable relevance for local NO levels in hypoxic tissues, and was reviewed in [faassen09].

## PROTEIN ADDUCTS OF ACETALDEHYDE AND LIPID PEROXIDATION PRODUCTS

All pathways of ethanol metabolism result in the production of acetaldehyde (AA), which under normal conditions is rapidly oxidized further (cf scheme 1). However, because of the electrophilic nature of the carbonyl carbon, AA readily reacts with a variety of nucleophilic groups to generate protein adducts. It binds primarily to reactive lysine residues, some aromatic amino acids and to cysteine [freeman05]. At physiological temperature and pH, AA reacts with ε-amino groups of internal lysine residues and the α-amino group on the N-terminal amino acid of unblocked proteins, forming unstable Schiff base adducts. Under appropriate reducing conditions proteins with abundant amounts of reactive lysine residues may generate stable N-ethyl lysine adducts at physiologically relevant concentrations of AA (<200 μM). In the absence of reducing agents, stable cyclic imidazolidinone structures are also formed between AA and the free alpha-amino group of the aminoterminal valine of haemoglobin. Such adducts may be stabilized by bond rearrangement to form the cyclic 2-methyl-imidazolidin-4-one derivative and accumulate in vivo in the blood of alcoholics. Alternatively, N-terminal cysteine residues are also nucleophilic, and potential targets for reaction with AA. The reaction product is a thiazolidine derivative. However, though feasible in principle, this pathway does not generate significant quantities of the thiohemiacetal adduct [freeman05].

Several lines of evidence from experimental animal models and from human alcoholics have indicated that ethanol metabolism per se and associated oxidative stress lead to the generation of various types of aldehydic products, which are capable of binding to proteins. Conditions of oxidative stress and enhanced lipid peroxidation generate increased levels of malondialdehyde (MDA), which can also react with amino groups of proteins and form protein adducts [Niemelä01; Freeman05]. In addition, lysine, cysteine, and histidine residues may react with HNE to appear to form stable HNE adducts. Earlier studies have shown that fetal tissues are prone to form and accumulate HNE [henderson99, ramachandran01]. In fetuses, the toxicity of HNE is compounded by the fact that human fetal liver has far lower capacity to detoxify HNE than adult liver [gardner03], presumably due to lower expression of glutathione S-transferases at this early stage of development. HNE affects fetal development in several ways: At low nM concentrations it arrests proliferation of hematopoietic stem cells *in vitro* [moneypenny05]. At μM levels it redirects differentiation pathways in such cells and at still higher levels it induces apoptosis [henderson99, moneypenny05]. Additionally, *in vitro* and *in vivo,* acetaldehyde and malondialdehyde may form toxic hybrid products that have been designated as MAA adducts. Depending on the stoichiometry, several classes of such MAA may be distinguished. For example, the so called MAA 2:1 adducts consist of 2 equivalents of MDA with 1 equivalent of AA. Alternatively, the MAA 1:1 adducts arise from the reaction of 1 equivalent of malondialdehyde with 1 equivalent of AA [tuma02]. The physiological relevance of these pathways is corroborated by the observation of enhanced amounts of aldehyde-derived protein adducts and their deposition in tissues under conditions of oxidative stress. Such conditions may arise from several factors, for example excess body iron, high fat diet [tsukamoto95] or by the lack of biological protective mechanisms (eg folate deficiency) [halsted02].

Certain target proteins seem particularly susceptible to aldehyde-derived modifications *in vivo* [Niemelä01]. *In vitro* studies have shown that erythrocyte membrane proteins and haemoglobin readily bind acetaldehyde. In accordance, *in vivo* studies have reported elevated concentrations of hemoglobin-acetaldehyde adducts in blood of chronic alcoholics. Formation of AA adducts does not require sustained EtOH consumption over a long period: hemoglobin-acetaldehyde adducts had accumulated in the erythrocytes of non-alcoholic volunteers even after single bout of heavy drinking. Experiments on both acute ethanol intake and on hospitalised chronic alcoholics further indicated that AA-adducts in erythrocytes remain elevated long after blood ethanol has been eliminated. AA-adducts were also found in erythrocytes from women who continued to drink during pregnancy and subsequently gave birth to children with fetal alcohol effects [Niemelä91, Stoler98].

Adduct formation has also been described to occur with major serum proteins which are synthesised in the liver. As a consequence, the physicochemical properties of proteins may be altered leading to disturbed cellular functions and aggravation of ethanol toxicity. The interference with protein function has been previously well characterized for microtubule function and for a variety of lysine dependent-enzymes. Acetaldehyde binding to tubulin alters the capacity of tubulin to polymerize thereby impairing protein secretion. *In vitro* addition of AA to enzymes with lysine residues in functionally critical locations leads to decreased catalytic activities. The generation of protein adducts may also play a role in the hematological derangements in peripheral blood cells, which are most typically present in erythrocytes of alcoholics (reviewed in [niemelä04]). In tissues, adduct deposition has been found from liver microsomes and from hepatocytes with zone 3 predominance. Interestingly, the areas of fatty deposition and cytochrome P450 induction are also sites of AA adduct generation [niemelä01]. Following ethanol administration, the occurrence of protein adducts in the gut, heart and skeletal muscle of experimental animals has also been demonstrated.

Although the formation of adducts in a wide range of tissues has now been firmly established, pathogenic significance of the adduct formation is still being discussed. It is known that human fetal tissues contain significant basal quantities of lipid peroxidation products as quantified by malondialdehyde formation [de86], even with abstaining mothers. Fetal brain contains 2-3-fold higher levels than other tissues like liver or kidney. The quantity of lipid peroxidation products is particularly high during the first trimester, and falls gradually towards *partum*. Several lines of recent evidence have supported a link between acetaldehyde action and alcohol-induced cardiac dysfunction and myopathy [niemelä01, freeman05]. It has also been found that aldehyde-derived protein adducts may stimulate immunological responses from the acquired immune system directed against the specific protein modifications. For example, immunoglobulins with anti-AA-adduct, anti-MDA, or anti-MAA adduct specificity have all been detected. The antibodies representing several immunoglobulin isotypes are found in plasma from human and rodent alcohol consumers. While the titers towards the AA-derived antigens seem to be predominantly of IgA isotype, IgG antibodies are typical for the lipid peroxidation derived antigens [vidali08]. Anti-AA-adduct IgA titers are elevated in 60-70% of patients with alcoholic liver disease and correlate well with the severity of the disease. In moderate and heavy drinkers without apparent liver disease, the titers of anti-AA adduct antibodies also show a correlation with the actual amounts of recent alcohol ingestion [latvala05] The generation such immune responses also involves release of IL-6, IL-10 [latvala05] and circulating TNF-$\alpha$ [vidali08], and may thereby fuel tissue damage in response to excessive ethanol intake. On the other hand, the antibody responses may also contribute to exclusion and neutralization of antigens resulting from the exposure of cellular structures to AA as released from ethanol oxidation.

## DNA Adducts of Acetaldehyde

Recent studies have emphasized a mutagenic and carcinogenic potential for AA, which is due to its ability to cause sister chromatid exchanges and chromosomal aberrations in human cells. [brooks05] Under physiological conditions AA is also capable of reacting with nucleic acids although the reaction products are mainly unstable and reversible in nature. There may also be different types of DNA adducts with different mutagenic potential. N(2)-ethyl-2`-deoxyguanosine is a typical adduct of the reaction of AA with DNA. Its *in vivo* formation has been demonstrated in hepatic DNA obtained from ethanol-treated rodents and from leukocytes of human heavy drinkers. Another type of AA adduct, 1,N(2)-propano-2`-deoxyguanosine (PdG), is generated in vivo in the presence of histones and other basic molecules. The PdG adduct appear to carry a higher genotoxic and mutagenic potential and can exist either as a ring-closed or a ring-open form. The ring-closed form is considered mutagenic, whereas the aldehyde form may be responsible for secondary lesions, such as DNA-protein cross-links and DNA interstrand crosslinks. Nucleoside adducts may also be formed by co-operative reaction of AA and ethanol, since the exocyclic amino groups of ribonucleosides and deoxyribonucleosides can react rapidly at ambient temperature with acetaldehyde and alcohol to yield mixed acetals. Deoxyguanosine (dG) is a preferred target for modification by EtOH metabolites[minko09]. Two prominent dG adducts with acetaldehyde have been identified: First, $N^2$-ethyl-2'-deoxyguanosine moieties on DNA from hepatic tissues or white blood cells from human alcoholics. Toxicity of these adducts is unclear for the moment. Second, the close homolog PdG that was mentioned before. PdG has proven genotoxic and mutagenic capacity in mammals. It appears either with a closed ring structure or as an aldehyde with open ring [brooks05]. In addition, dG moieties may also react with a variety of lipid peroxidation products, such as α,β-unsaturated aldehydes (eg acrolein or crotonaldehyde) or 4-hydroxynonenal (4-HNE). Enzymatic repair of such dG lesions is possible in principle, but difficult in practice since the repair involves a complex cascade of events [minko09]. It has been proposed that genetic variations in the coding of the repair enzymes contribute to observed variations in the susceptibility to EtOH induced carcinogenesis in humans [brooks05].

## Direct Physiological Effects of Acetaldehyde

In view of its high reactivity, acetaldehyde is incriminated in a variety of direct physiological effects and adverse consequences of alcohol consumption (reviewed in [quertemont06]). EtOH is converted in equimolar amounts to AA mainly in the liver. Accordingly, the liver is a major target for AA toxicity. Some of the AA is exported from the liver into the blood circulation, and other tissues may thus be affected as well. Prominent physiological manifestations of acetaldehyde accumulation in adults are increased skin temperature, facial flushing, increased heart and perspiration rates, bronchoconstriction, lowered blood pressure, as well as the symptoms of hangover (nausea, headache). These manifestations are readily enforced by administration of ALDH inhibitors like disulfiram. While the pharmacological effects of AA appear mainly mediated through the release of vasoactive compounds, wide-spectrum adduct formation with proteins or other cellular components seems the plausible mechanism for the manifest organ toxicity of AA.

Though well documented in adults, far less is known about the physiological effects of AA on fetuses or neonates. Earlier studies have indicated that rather high free concentrations of acetaldehyde may occur in fetal circulation following perfusion with rather low concentrations of $^{14}C$ ethanol. The human placenta may oxidize maternal EtOH to AA that is released into the fetal perfusate [karl88]. These investigators also demonstrated direct acetaldehyde transfer from the maternal to the fetal side. However, it is known that not all children who are exposed prenatally to the same amount of alcohol will be affected. Several lines of epidemiological evidence have supported the view that the different forms of the genes coding for alcohol-metabolizing enzymes determine the teratogenic potential of alcohol ingestion [Warren05]. Similar frequencies of high acetaldehyde levels among alcoholics and the rates of alcohol-related birth defects have also supported the role of acetaldehyde as a key factor in creating an abnormal outcome in child development [hard01].

Recent results showed that AA may act as a modulator of the production of corticotrophin releasing hormone (CRH, also called corticotrophin releasing factor) by the hypothalamus: Recent *in vitro* experiments on rat hypothalamic explants have shown that suppletion of 1 – 3 μM AA acutely increased hypothalamic CRH release by a massive factor 4 - 5 [cannizzaro10]. Note that such levels of AA are easily reached in the plasma of humans after moderate consumption of alcohol. Further downstream, CRH controls the release of adrenocorticotropin hormone (ACTH) by the anterior pituitary gland. This activation cascade might give a plausible explanation of one of the most prominent hormonal effects of ethanol, namely the activation of the hypothalamic-pituitary-adrenal (HPA) axis [cannizzaro10].

## Interference with Hormonal Status

EtOH consumption may affect the maternal hormone status in manifold ways [gabriel98, gill00, stevens05]. In this section we restrict ourselves to effects that appear likely to affect the outcome of pregnancy. First, we recall that EtOH upsets maternal prolactin/oxytocin balance and reduces milk production. The details were discussed before in the section dedicated to lactation (see above).

In adult mammals, ethanol markedly stimulates the HPA axis, i.e. the major controller of the neuroendocrine system, in particular the neuroendocrine response to stress. It leads to enhanced levels of cortisol and corticosterone, two prominent glucocorticoid hormones. This effect was observed in many adult mammalian species, including human [hellemans10]. However, maternal alcohol affects the development of the fetal HPA axis as well [haley06, weinberg08, hellemans10] and may results in a hyperresponsive juvenile HPA and enhanced plasma levels of ACTH. In fact, the development of the fetal HPA appears very susceptible to programming by a range of maternal factors during gestation [matthews02, kapoor06]. EtOH is one of these factors, as maternal EtOH or its downstream metabolites are known to affect the neuroendrocine functions of the fetus long after birth [zhang05]. The mechanism by which EtOH stimulates the HPA remains controversial. One hypothesis proposes that the effect is mediated by catecholamines, the adrenal stress hormones like epinephrine and norepinephrine (formerly (nor)adrenaline) or dopamine. Repeated EtOH exposure has been shown to enhance plasma levels of catecholamines and the expression of enzymes for catecholamine synthesis in the adrenal medulla of the rat [patterson05]. In accordance, epinephrine was recently shown to amplify the sensitization of mouse liver by EtOH [montfort08]. The catecholamine hypothesis is further supported by observations that stimulation elicits a stronger release of ACTH and corticosterone in the offspring of rats and mice that had consumed EtOH during pregnancy [zhang05]. We note that catecholamines induce release of ACTH. However, several alternative mechanisms have been proposed: Work of the Weinberg group has demonstrated that the effects of ethanol on the HPA axis are strongly affected by the levels of sex hormones like estrogen and testosterone [lan09a, lan09b]. In addition, a recent study with rats [choi08] noted that the EtOH induced hyperresponsiveness seems localized in the C1 adrenergic neurons of the ventrolateral medulla. This area plays an important function in transmission of stress signals to the hypothalamus. EtOH has other effects on the HPA in adult humans as well: enhanced levels of CRH and glucocorticoids are well known manifestations. These compounds cross into the fetal circulation via the placenta and may affect fetal and neonatal development. After all, glucocorticoids are key regulators of organogenesis and maturation (eg lung development).

The mechanism behind the stimulation of HPA by EtOH remained controversial so far, but recent publications suggest that the metabolite AA act as a modulator of CRH production by the hypothalamus: In the brain, CRH is secreted by the parvocellular cells in the hypothalamus, and transported by the portal circulation to anterior pituitary lobe where it stimulates the corticotropes to release ACTH and β-endorphin. Recent *in vitro* experiments on rat hypothalamic explants have shown that 30 mM EtOH acutely increased hypothalamic CRH release sevenfold [cannizzaro10]. A 4 – 5 fold increase of CRH was also observed after suppletion of 1 – 3 μM AA. Note that such levels of AA are quite realistic, since they simulate AA levels in the plasma of humans after moderate consumption of alcohol. The CRH enhancement was attributed to the EtOH metabolite AA rather than EtOH itself, since the outflow of CRH could be blocked by coincubation of the catalase inhibitor 3AT. Interestingly, significant quantities of CRH are also synthesized in the endometrium and placenta, where it fulfils many crucial functions from blastocyst implantation [makrigiannakis04] to control of the duration of the pregnancy. Levels of placental CRH rise significantly just prior to partum, and seem to have high relevance for proper parturition [lye01]. Fetal CRH actively controls the corticotropin axis long before *partum:* CRH has been detected in hypothalamic as well as extrahypothalamic tissues of primates throughout the third trimester (125 – 185 days of gestation in baboons) [dotzler04]. It has long been known that placental CRH production may be modulated by steroids.

Next to CRH, maternal glucocorticoids are also closely scrutinized for their potential for programming of the fetal HPA [kapoor06]. This problem has high clinical relevance, since synthetic glucocorticoids are widely applied to treat pregnant women with enhanced risk of preterm delivery and to promote maturation of the lungs of premature infants [kapoor08]. Long term effects of perinatal glucocorticoid treatment on pituitary morphology and ACTH status have been confirmed in rats [john06]. Finally, it has been proposed that EtOH stimulates the HPA by a mechanism involving nitric oxide (NO) [lee08]. NO is released as an excitatory neurotransmitter by some motor neurons of the parasympathetic branch of the

ANS. Moreover, NO has indirect effects in the CNS by inhibiting the function of neuronal monoamine transporters [kiss01]. In this way the monoaminergic system can be activated by the NO status of glutaminergic system, without having glutamate receptors or receiving synaptic excitatory signals from the glutaminergic system. NO was found to stimulate the HPA, and the sensitivity to this NO stimulus is enhanced by prenatal EtOH exposure [lee08]. Given these various possibilities, the dominant mechanism behind the observed sensitization of the HPA by EtOH remains to be established.

It has been long known that developmental delays due to prenatal alcohol exposure may be alleviated by thyroid hormone treatment [gottesfeld90]. The mechanism behind this effect has not been elucidated, but proper thyroid regulation of the cytoskeleton of fetal neuronal cells has been proposed as a possible explanation ([farwell05] and references therein). The effect of maternal EtOH seems partially mediated by the thyroid status of the mother: Pregnant EtOH consuming rats have significantly lower plasma levels of thyroid hormones like 3,5,3-triiodothyronine ($T_3$), thyroxine ($T_4$) and thyroid-stimulating hormone (TSH) [wilcoxon04]. The thyroid status of the offspring was unchanged during the neonatal period, but significant changes were found later in life: In adulthood, the offspring showed a combination of elevated TSH, and reduced $T_3$. Although the implications for human physiology are not clear yet, these observations clearly illustrate the phenomenon of prenatal thyroid programming by maternal EtOH. In this context it should be noted that the fetus relies on maternal thyroid hormones at early stages of gestation, i.e. prior the onset of fetal thyroid function at ca 18-20 weeks of gestation [morreale04]. Functional studies have shown that maternal thyroid hormones are essential for early fetal brain development [zoeller00, morreale04]. In normal pregnancies, the thyroid levels in fetal CNS show a well regulated timedependence (fig 3). We note that this figure shows a time window where the fetus is still fully dependent on maternal thyroid hormones that have crossed the placental barrier. Even after onset of fetal thyroid function, the mother continues to contribute significantly to fetal $T_4$ levels rught until *partum.*

An interesting structural class of human hormones are heterodimeric glycoproteins like luteinizing hormone (LH), thyroid stimulating hormone (TSH), follicle stimulating hormone (FSH), and human chorionic gonadotropin (hCG). In each case, the functional unit consists of one α-unit and one β-unit. LH, TSH, FSH and hCG share the same α-unit with a 92 aminoacid sequence, and are distinguished only by differences in the β-unit. LH is essential for reproduction in males (testical Leydig cells and production of testosterone) as well as females (controlling the menstrual cycle, inducing ovulation, and development of the corpus luteum). Acute EtOH is known to inhibit the NMDA-stimulated release of LH-releasing hormone (LHRH) [hiney99]. Chronic prenatal EtOH leads to additional effects on the LH axis: It was found that a single acute *in utero* exposure to EtOH during LHRH neuron formation reduces the number of LHRH-positive cells in the hypothalamus of young rats during the gestational and early postnatal stage [gavin94]. The impairment seemed temporary, as LHRH-positive cell numbers returned to normal at 60 days after birth. Interestingly, it was reported that the depressing effect of EtOH on LH levels may be abolished by *in vivo* administration of leptin [hiney99]. An *in vitro* study of rat hypothalamus has proposed that the inhibition of LHRH is mediated by activation of the endocannabinoid system [fernandez04]. EtOH also interferes with normal thyroid signaling: Pregnant EtOH consuming rats have significantly lower plasma levels of TSH, $T_3$ and $T_4$ [wilcoxon04]. The thyroid status of the offspring was unchanged during the neonatal period, but significant changes were found later in life: In adulthood, the offspring showed a combination of elevated TSH, and reduced $T_3$. Although the implications for human physiology are not clear yet, these observations clearly illustrate that thyroid signaling is prone to prenatal programming by maternal EtOH.

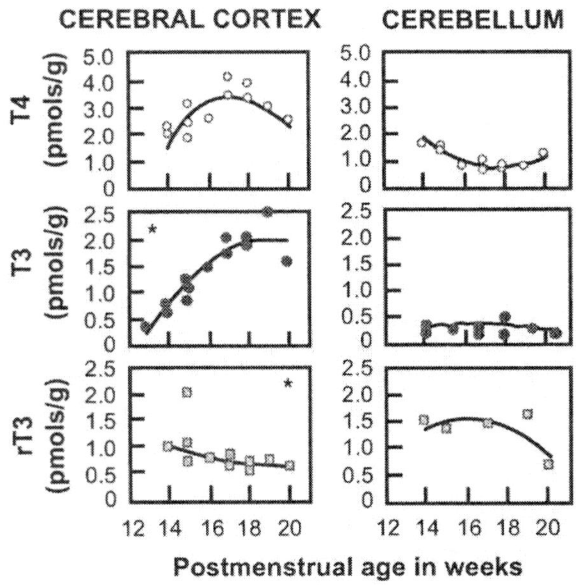


Figure 3. Changes in thyroid hormones $T_3$ and $T_4$ in human fetal CNS as function of time up to midgestation (for unborns, postmenstrual age equals gestational age). In this time window the mother is the only source of thyroid hormone for the fetus. $rT_3$ is 3,3',5'-triiodothyronine, a non-hormone metabolite of $T_4$. From [morreale04] with permission.

Chronic EtOH is known to depress levels of leptin in the circulation of mammals and humans [hiney99]. This 16 kD protein hormone regulates energy uptake and expenditure, but is also involved in the regulation of placental amino acid transporters [jansson03]. We note that intrauterine growth retardation is associated with deficiencies in levels of amino acids and leptin on the maternal as well as the fetal side [jones07].

Testosterone levels during fetal and neonatal stages are key regulators for sexual behaviour in adult life. Fetal testosterone regulation is prone to disruption by maternal EtOH: The characteristic fetal surges in testosterone levels of male rat fetuses was disrupted *in vivo* by maternal EtOH consumption ([ward03] and references therein). The important role of sex hormones like estrogen and testosterone on the activity of the HPA axis has already been mentioned before, and it was noted that the HPA response is amplified by EtOH [lan09a, lan09b].

EtOH also enhances the placental status of thromboxane (a vasoconstricting eicosanoid) [siler00] and prostaglandin E (PGE) [randall96] on the fetal side.

Studies of alcohol consumers have shown that chronic EtOH lowers production of vasopressin (AVP) from the posterior pituitary. AVP is also called antidiuretic hormone, since it promotes water reabsorption during renal filtration, and contracts arterioles. AVP deficiency implies reduced capacity for renal reabsorption and excess production of urine and dehydration, common symptoms in alcohol abusers. Interestingly, prenatal EtOH gives predisposition for lower AVP in adult rats [bird06]. Both the pituitary release and storage of AVP were permanently impaired by this example of prenatal programming. The underlying mechanism has not been elucidated.

The above list is by no means exhaustive, but illustrates that prenatal EtOH has a plethora of pathways to affect the maternal and fetal hormonal state. Some of these pathways involved prenatal programming. In most cases it is not yet clear whether EtOH *per se* or some downstream metabolite is implicated. We conclude this section with an example where the agent is clearly identified: AA has considerable reactivity to certain classes of hormones. For example, all amine moieties contain a characteristic lone pair of electrons on the very electronegative nitrogen atom. This lone pair makes all amines more or less nucleophile, and therefore prone to modification by AA. The reactivity of AA towards peptide α-amino groups has already been mentioned above in the section on protein adducts. Amine hormones also have this lone pair and are known to form such adducts with AA. The formation of such adducts has been confirmed *in vivo* [murrey10]. This pathway will certainly interfere with normal physiological signaling of these hormones, but this field seems not yet well investigated in the literature.

## Ethanol and Zn Status during Pregnancy

There is a remarkable similarity between the congenital abnormalities observed in FAS and those produced by maternal Zn deficiency. In the early eighties it was recognized that alcoholic mothers had significantly lower plasma levels of Zn than non-alcoholic mothers [flynn81]. Even more ominously, they noted a direct inverse relationship between maternal plasma Zn and incidence of fetal alcohol syndrome. Experimental studies in mammals and humans have shown that Zn-deficiency during pregnancy correlates with growth retardation and organ abnormalities like malformations of heart, lung, brain, and urinary tract. Extreme examples are the severe Zn deficiencies associated with acrodermatitis enteropathica. This rare human autosomal genetic disorder has catastrophic poor prognosis for outcome unless treated with large oral Zn supplements in the final trimesters (embryonic Zn requirements seem very low until the onset of cellular differentiation and organogenesis, ca 4 wks after fertilization).

Zinc is an essential nutrient. Although it does not participate in redox reactions directly, it is essential for the folding structure of many proteins and over 300 known enzymatic reactions [tapiero03]. It has special relevance for cell growth, but abnormal Zn status is known to affect cellular differentiation and survival. Zinc deficiency induces growth retardation, as well as severe deficiencies in the immune system. Moreover, Zn binds several signaling molecules and modulates their activity. Well known examples are the tyrosine phosphatases. Zn *per se* also plays a role as intracellular signaling molecule (reviewed in [hirota08]).

The whole body Zn content of healthy pregnant women is ca 7 % higher than that of non-pregnant women. In accordance, Zn absorption is increased by ca 30 % in late human pregnancy (for review cf [king00]). This additional Zn is deposited in the fetus (60 – 70 %) or the greatly enlarged uterus. Moreover, urinary loss of Zn during gestation is nearly double that during preconception [fung97]. In most cases, the enhanced demand for Zn is satisfied from dietary sources. However, the combination of high dietary calcium and phytate may inhibit the uptake of Zn from ingested food.

Maternal Zn status has particular relevance for alcohol consuming mothers. First, alcohol consumption reduces placental transport of Zn [ghishan82, carey00] and enhances urinary Zn losses. Given that Zn demand is enhanced during pregnancy anyway, maternal EtOH consumption significantly enhances the risk of Zn deficiency. Moreover, birthweight studies in rats showed that the combination of Zn deficiency with maternal alcohol consumption was more potent than either Zn deficiency or alcohol alone [keppen85].

It has been explicitly confirmed that maternal EtOH consumption alters the Zn distribution not only in the mother, but in the offspring as well. Recently, a rat model showed that neonates of chronic EtOH consuming Wistars have enhanced (!) Zn levels in kidney, spleen and testes, but significantly lower hepatic levels [murillo10].

Apart from dietary factors, maternal Zn status may also be compromised by the induction of metallothionein (MT) (tapiero03] and references therein). This cysteine rich intracellular protein has high affinity for a wide range of divalent metals. Mammalian MT binds four $Zn^{2+}$ in its α domain, and additional three $Zn^{2+}$ in the β domain. The binding and release of $Zn^{2+}$ ions by MT is integral part of the intercellular Zn signaling. Such Zn signaling is important both between and within neurons, and in regulation of the tumour suppressor protein p53. A broad spectrum of stimuli, including EtOH, is known to initiate MT synthesis. Divalent metal ions like $Cu^{2+}$, $Zn^{2+}$ or $Cd^{2+}$ stimulate MT expression primarily in the liver. However, adrenocorticosteroids as well as cytokines like TNF-α, IL-1 and IL-6 may act as endogenous inducers of hepatic MT, and cause sequestration of the metal ions in maternal liver. Animal pregnancy models have confirmed that many developmental toxins elevate maternal MT, with concomitant decrease of maternal plasma Zn and embryonic Zn uptake [keen93]. Experiments with MT-knockout mutant mice gave strong support to this concept that ethanol affects maternal and fetal Zn status through induction of maternal MT [carey00]. Later studies on mice showed that dietary Zn supplementation prevented the cognitive and memory impairments as caused by intraperitoneal alcohol injections on gestational day 8 (a model for incidental maternal binge drinking) [summers08].

## ETHANOL AND PLACENTAL FUNCTION DURING PREGNANCY

Good placental function is crucial for fetal development, and many reports document that maternal EtOH consumption has wide range of adverse effects on placental development and function. A recent overview over the clinical studies in humans can be found in [burd07]. Although the adverse effects are quite clear and undisputed, the underlying mechanisms are often controversial. For example, high EtOH consumers have a sixfold higher risk of placental abruption than modest drinkers (29 % risk vs 5 %, [leunen03]). But no obvious clinical cause for this phenomenon could be established. High consumers carry fourfold higher risk of stillbirth than abstainers (4 % vs 1 % [burd07]). In these cases, the general term of 'fetoplacental dysfunction' was recognized as the decisive factor, but, again, the underlying mechanism remained obscure.

Clearly, proper supply of oxygen and nutrients are important, as well as transfer of certain parts of the maternal immunity (in particular immunoglobulin G (IgG), the most prominent plasma immunoglobulin and the only maternal isotype that crosses the placental barrier into the fetus). The placenta is also essential for controlled transfer of maternal hormones to the fetus, in particular in early stages of gestation where the fetal hormonal system is not yet functional. A good example is the total reliance of the fetus on maternal thyroid hormones up to midgestation (cf fig 3). The transplacental transfer appears to be a tightly regulated process since fetal levels are maintained at far lower levels than maternal concentrations [morreale04].

The placental barrier does not protect the fetus from maternal EtOH or some of its metabolites: EtOH does readily cross from maternal to fetal side, as does AA [karl88]. In addition, the human placenta may oxidize maternal EtOH to AA that is released into the fetal perfusate [karl88]. The accumulation and slow clearance of amniotic EtOH and AA has already been mentioned above. In contrast, term placental tissue has adequate capacity to metabolize maternal FAEE, thereby preventing crossing of maternal FAEE into the fetus [chan04].

Several pathways have so far been discovered where maternal EtOH affects placental function. First and foremost, EtOH induces acute placental vasoconstriction in a dose-dependent manner. This vasoconstriction increases fetal-placental vascular resistance and the placental perfusion pressure on the fetal side ([burd07] and references therein). A broad spectrum of effects of EtOH on placental transport of essential nutrient like biotin, amino acids, or vitamin $B_6$ has been collected and reviewed in [burd07].

EtOH affects the placental hormonal status as well: EtOH increased the release of vasoconstricting thromboxane from human placenta and enhanced the thromboxane levels on the fetal side [siler00]. In contrast, the vasodilator prostacyclin was unchanged. Production of prostaglandin E (PGE) was similarly enhanced by perfusion of term human placentas with 25 mM EtOH [randall96]. In addition, EtOH interferes selectively with placental handling of unsaturated fatty acids [chan04, haggarty02]. In particular, the transfer of docosahexaenoic acid (DHA) through human term placentas was threefold slower in presence of ca 45 mM (2 mg/ml) EtOH. Transfer of linoleic acid and α-linolenic acid (αLN) were inhibited as well, but by smaller amounts. Overall, EtOH shows strongest inhibition of placental transfer of ω-3 type PUFA. It has been remarked before that dietary deficiency of ω-3 type PUFA such as DHA during critical gestational time windows may cause irreversible damage to the fetus. Many studies have documented disturbed development of the CNS and cognitive abilities *post partum* (cf preceding section on lipid metabolism).

Not surprisingly, gene expression profilings have revealed a manifold spectrum of effects of EtOH on the expression of placental proteins: Placental CYP2E1 expression was enhanced in EtOH consuming pregnancies [gemma07]. In rats, a recent microarray screening of placental gene expression has revealed at least 22 genes with significant (more than fivefold) changes in expression under moderate chronic EtOH consumption [rosenberg09]. These genes involved the whole spectrum of developmental processes (CNS development, organ morphogenesis, immune response, skeletal, vascular and cartilage development).

It has already been noted that EtOH consumption induces oxidative stress and promotes release of ROS, and superoxide in particular. Placental superoxide is thought to disrupt placental function, and was confirmed experimentally in human preeclamptic placentas [sikkema01].

## ETHANOL AND FOLATE STATUS DURING PREGNANCY

EtOH induces a rapid and significant transient reduction in circulating folate levels in humans. This vitamin is essential for cellular proliferation, and biosynthesis of purines, pyrimidines, and some essential amino acids. Folate deficiency disturbs hepatic methionine metabolism and aggravates EtOH induced liver injury *in vivo* [halsted02]. Folate cannot be synthesized by mammals *de novo,* but is obtained by modification of formylated of methylated tetrahydrofolate precursors extracted from dietary sources. The relevance of maternal folate status for embryonic and fetal development is well documented, and folate requirements are significantly enhanced during pregnancy. It protects against fetal neural tube defects although the mechanism is still unknown (for review cf [blom06]). The efficacy of folate is attested by recommendations of dietary folate supplements during or when planning a pregnancy. Folate also is beneficial for proper NO production by NOS enzymes, in particular in preventing enzymatic uncoupling and release of superoxide radicals [stroes00, huisman00]. The strong effect of EtOH on plasma folate is attributed to disruption by EtOH of folate reabsorption in the renal proximal tubule. Proper recycling of folate is essential for conservation of folate stores. In accordance, EtOH consumption acutely enhances urinary excretion of folate in humans ([gowder09] and references therein). Epidemiologic studies have confirmed the precarious folate status of alcohol consumers, in particular drinking mothers. Recent experiments in cultured human proximal tubular cells have suggested that the effects of EtOH on folate reabsorption are mediated by an endothelin signaling pathway and protein kinase-C [gowder09, hamid09].

## ETHANOL AND SKELETAL DEVELOPMENT

Human studies have shown that maternal EtOH consumption hampers the general growth and skeletal development of the fetus. Skeletal ossification as well as growth rates are affected. By the eighth week of gestation, cartilaginous prototypes of all the major skeletal components have been formed and endochondral ossification starts. The process of ossification appears impaired at lower doses of EtOH [simpson05]. Different bones were found to vary in their susceptibility to EtOH effects, with a markedly higher sensitivity of those bones that develop largely *in utero* [snow07]. The observed effects of EtOH appear irreversible and do not show rapid normalization after birth. The mechanism has not been established in detail, but appears to function via interference of EtOH with normal calcium homeostasis *in utero* [keiver04]. It is unknown whether prenatal alcohol affects bone function later in life [snow07]. Depressed ossal growth rates definitely lead to permanent short stature in life. The mechanism behind these effects is still controversial. Recent experiments on rats suggest that EtOH inhibit ossal growth by interfering with the response to growth hormone. EtOH decreases skeletal expression of insulin-like growth factor-1 (IGF-1), an important skeletal growth factor under control from growth hormone [turner10]. Concerning pregnancy, it was found that ethanol acutely depresses maternal as well as fetal IGF-1 levels in sheep [gatford07].

## ETHANOL AND THE NEONATAL IMMUNE SYSTEM

Prenatal alcohol exposure may significantly affect the immune system of the offspring by various mechanisms. Human defense against xenobiotics is usually classified in either innate immunity or acquired immunity. The innate immunity involves all unspecific inflammatory reactions and is based on the action of the complement system, Mast cells, granulocytes, natural killer (NK) cells or macrophages. It is operational at partum. The acquired immunity is mobilized by exposure to specific antigens, and is based either on the release of antigenspecific immunoglobulins by B-lymphocytes (humoral immunity), or on the proliferation of T-lymphocytes carrying antigenspecific receptors (cellular immunity). This neonatal system of acquired immunity is only partially operational at partum, since it did not yet have the opportunity to develop. At birth, IgG is the only immunoglobulin present in the neonatal plasma in significant quantities. It dominates the secondary immune response and is the only maternal immunoglobulin that is sufficiently small to cross the placental barrier during gestation.

So far, studies in many different animals including primates have revealed only few, rather subtle effects of prenatal EtOH on the innate immune system: Prenatal EtOH leads to reduced white cell counts ([gauthier05] and other chapters in this volume), and predisposes adult rats to decreased hypothalamic IL-1β production and blunted febrile response to LPS-induced toxicity ([zhang05] and references therein). However, an interesting effect of EtOH on the protein content of lipid rafts has been noted in recent years [szabo07, goral08]. Such lipid rafts are detergent-resistant domains in the plasma membrane enriched in sphingomyelin and cholesterol. About half of all membrane lipid is incorporated in such rafts with sized from about ten to a few hundred nanometers in size (reviewed in [pike03]). Such rafts form preferred scaffolds for a variety of membrane proteins, including several receptors involved in innate immune signaling. A well documented case is formed by the Toll like receptors (TLR). This class of pattern recognition receptors trigger the cascade of innate immunity by initiating cytokine release and cellular activation. They are activated by binding of TLR-ligands of microbial origin, like lipopolysaccharide (LPS). Interestingly, physiological levels of EtOH affect this response via an interesting mechanism: EtOH acts antagonistically to the condensation of TLR-4 and CD14 into the lipid rafts ([szabo07, goral08] and references therein). At the moment, it appears unclear whether acute EtOH affects the expression of TLR (reduced as well as enhanced mRNA levels have been reported in the literature, cf [goral08]). As an independent mechanism, it was reported that prenatal EtOH predisposes to decreased cytotoxicity of the natural killer (NK) cells of the innate immune system in adult rats [arjona06]. Other sectors of the innate immune system are also damaged by high EtOH: It was recently shown that high levels of EtOH > 43 mM induce significant apoptosis in human HMC-1 Mast cells [nurmi09].

In spite of these effects on the innate immune signaling, the innate immune system itself appears functional and adequately competent at birth. In contrast, many studies document that prenatal EtOH induces marked chronic deficits in the acquired immunity system, and in its reponse to antigens (the older literature is reviewed in [gottesfeld91]). Children with FAS have enhanced susceptibility to fungal, viral and bacterial infections, suggesting that definitely T-cell and possibly B-cell mediated immunity are depressed ([zhang05] and references therein). *In vivo* studies of prenatally EtOH exposed peripubertal rats [gottesfeld95] showed marked suppression of the cellular (T-cell) response, whereas plasma immunoglobulin levels were normal at peripubertal age. Even a single maternal EtOH binge on the third day of pregnancy has irreversibly altered the immune response of the offspring after maturation: The immune cells in the peritoneal fluid had significantly depressed serotonin content (- 25 %) compared to controls [csaba06]. Although best known for its role as neurotransmitter, serotonin is important for immunity as well. It promotes activation of natural killer cells, release of chemotactic factors, and macrophages. It also functions in the coupling between the immune system and CNS ([csaba06] and references therein).

It was already mentioned above that EtOH consumption promotes depletion of maternal zinc stores by the combination of two effects: First, the inhibition of absorption of dietary Zn. Second, enhanced urinary excretion of Zn. Therefore, EtOH consumption during pregnancy carries significant risk of maternal Zn deficiency during a period of enhanced Zn demand. Zinc signaling is involved in cellular differentiation, and immunity. These signaling effects occur on acute timescales ('Zn waves') as well as on long timescales ('late Zn signaling') when based on changes in the expression of cellular Zn transporters. The many roles of Zn in the human immune system are reviewed in [hirota08].

Since the immune system develops rapidly after birth, it is necessary to distinguish immunity at later stages from that of the neonate. The neonate already received significant quantities of maternal IgG during gestation. After birth, lactation provides significant additional quantities of IgG. The IgG is absorbed from maternal milk and transferred to the neonatal circulation by the digestive system of the suckling. The capacity to absorb IgG from maternal milk has been found impaired in suckling rats that had been exposed to EtOH *in utero* [bhalla04]. There was a concomitant downregulation of IgG Fc receptors found on the cells of the innate immune system. It shows that the main pathway for neonatal immunity is impaired by prenatal EtOH exposure.

It had already been remarked above that the lipid composition of cell membranes has a large impact on the immunity response of T-cells. In particular, the membrane content of polyunsatured fatty acids and their metabolites has a big effect and motivated a large research effort in recent years. It has been noted that the presence of long-chain PUFA (LCPUFA) affects neonatal immunity via at least four separate mechanisms [calder06]: (1) decreasing synthesis of eicosanoids, thereby promoting the inflammatory response. (2) inhibiting expression of adhesion molecules like E-selectin, VCAM-1 or ICAM-1 [grimm02]; (3) inhibiting expression of inflammatory genes for IL-1α, TNFα and COX-2 ([sampath05] and references therein); (4) suppressing normal T-cell signaling [stulnig04, yacoob09]. Although many details of the mechanisms behind these actions are not yet understood, a mechanistic model plausibly argues that the intramembrane organization into lipid rafts modulates the T-cell response: It has been noted that incorporation of ω-6 LCPUFA alters lipid rafts and the protein composition of the cytosolic membrane leaflet, with significant suppression of the T-cell response [zeyda06, kabouridis06]. It is yet another example that the structural organization of lipid rafts play an important role in immune response (reviewed in [yacoob09]). For example, activation of Toll like receptor-4 (TLR-4) induces preferential concentration of TLR-4 and CD14 in lipid rafts of the outer membrane leaflet [szabo07]. The concentration or assembly of certain proteins inside such lipid rafts forms one of the steps in the signaling cascade initiated by Toll like receptors, and the antigen activation of B-cell receptors and T-cell receptors in the acquired immunity system [cheng01, kabouridis06, zeyda06]. Clearly, the adequate dietary supply of these essential fatty acids has large impact on the innate immunity system, and the proper balance between ω-3 and ω-6 PUFA in maternal diet during pregnancy and lactation seems important for neonatal immunity [harbige03, calder06, gottrand08, hanebutt08, chapkin09]. In addition to this effect on PUFA, we recall that EtOH also has an acute effect *per se* on the organization and protein content of lipid rafts in the cellular membranes (see above, and [szabo07]).

To conclude this section, we recall that the humoral immune system of human adults may be activated by aldehyde-derived adducts of proteins (see above). In the plasma of regular alcohol consumers, IgA and IgG isotype immunoglobulins with anti-AA adduct, anti-MDA adduct, and anti-MAA adduct specificity have been found [vidali08]. It seems plausible that similar activation will also take place in EtOH exposed near-term fetuses and neonates. However, the fetopathogenic significance of the immunoglobulin response against ethanol metabolites has not yet been investigated carefully.

## Conclusions and Implications for Fetal Health

Ethanol consumption during pregnancy exposes the fetus to a wide variety of phenotypic alterations including prenatal growth retardation, microcephaly and a distinctive pattern of craniofacial features. Recent research has provided a wealth of new insights on the primary mechanisms and biochemical pathways underlying such toxic effects. Not all children who are exposed prenatally to the same amount of alcohol will be affected and individual susceptibility, variations in dose exposures at different gestational timings and genetic factors involving the genes coding for alcohol metabolizing enzymes appear to be associated with abnormal outcome in child development. Many of the fetotoxic manifestations of ethanol intake can be attributed to acetaldehyde, the first metabolite of ethanol. This metabolite is highly reactive and may bind to proteins, DNA and other cellular constituents. This reactivity interferes with a broad spectrum of cellular functions and elicits immunological responses towards the aldehyde-modified epitopes in proteins. Ethanol metabolism also creates a variety of other metabolites with different pharmacological characteristics, tissue distributions and time dependence of clearance. The overall picture is that EtOH has many toxic side effects in human adults. During pregnancy, the fetus appears to be at triple risk of maternal alcohol consumption. First, the placenta allows free transfer of EtOH and toxic metabolites like AA into the fetus. The so called placental barrier is no barrier at all in this respect. Second, fetal tissues have an immature state with markedly lower capacities for clearance of ethanol and acetaldehyde. This results in longer and more intense exposure of the fetus than of the mother (cf fig 1). Third, the developing fetal nervous system seems particularly sensitive to ethanol toxicity. Proliferation, differentiation, systemic neuronal integration, network ripening, all major processes seem affected and very sensitive to detrimental effects of maternal alcohol. Effects of ethanol and its metabolites on purine metabolism and possible deficiencies in folate and zinc status also seem to fuel ethanol toxicity. The co-occurrence of low antioxidant levels and enhanced oxidative stress creates an unfavourable balance between production and scavenging of reactive oxygen species and accumulation of toxic lipid peroxidation products, such as MDA or 4-hydroxynonenal. These two products also react with proteins and accumulate in ethanol-exposed tissues. Altered cerebral neurotransmitter balance and signal transduction of many types of neurons and the devastating consequences on the developing nervous system have all been well documented. There may also be effects on the lipids of the central nervous system and on membrane structure and function. We note that most of these effects may be induced by rather modest doses of maternal ethanol.

Two aspects of fetal alcohol effects appear particularly striking: First, that exposure to alcohol during critical periods in the fetal stage may program the fetus for a disadvantaged destiny and irreversible damage that manifests itself only later in life. Second, that fetal alcohol effects occur at all, since they are completely preventable by parental self-discipline. In a way, the whole research effort described in this volume is perfectly superfluous. Fetal alcohol effects are currently believed not to be preventable by any other approach than abstinence of ethanol consumption. A major difficulty with alcohol-using pregnant women, is, however, underreporting of alcohol consumption in this context. Improved understanding of the primary mechanisms of fetal alcohol effects *in utero* may open new avenues for a more successful counselling of pregnant women and assist in preventing alcohol-induced fetotoxicity. Development of sensitive and accurate biological markers of fetal alcohol exposure and prediction of embryotoxicity is overdue.

## REFERENCES

[abman02] S Abman, J Kinsella. Inhaled ethyl nitrite gas for persistent pulmonary hypertension in infants. *Lancet* 360 (2002) 2076 – 2077.

[agarwal90] D Agarwal, H Goedde. Pharmacogenetics of alcohol dehydrogenase (ADH). *Pharmacol. Ther.* 45 (1990) 69 – 83.

[akbar06] M Akbar, J Baick, F Calderon, Z Wen, H-Y Kim. Ethanol promotes neuronal apoptosis by inhibiting phosphatidylserine accumulation. *J. Neurosci. Res.* 83 (2006) 432 – 440.

[alary03] J Alary, F Gueraud, J-P Cravedi. Fate of 4-hydroxynonenal in vivo: disposition and metabolic pathways. *Mol. Asp. Med.* 24 (2003) 177 – 187.

[alatalo09] P Alatalo, H Koivisto, J Hietala, R Bloigu, O Niemelä. Gender-dependent impacts of body mass index and moderate alcohol consumption on serum uric acid – an index of oxidant stress status? *Free Radic. Biol. Med.* 46 (2009) 1233 – 1238.

[alhomsi06] K Alhomsi, J Cluette-Brown, M Laposata. Fatty acid ethyl esters in human mononuclear cells: Production by endogenous synthesis greatly exceeds the uptake of preformed ethyl esters. *Alcohol Clin. Exp. Res.* 30 (2006) 560 – 566.

[alhomsi08] K Alhomsi, M Selig, T Sustic, E Katrangi, V Weissig, M Laposata. Induction of apoptosis and necrosis in human peripheral blood mononuclear cells by fatty acid ethyl esters. *Alcohol. Clin. Exp. Res.* 32 (2008) 534 – 543.

[antonio08] A Antonio, M Druse. Antioxidants prevent ethanol-associated apoptosis in fetal rhombencephalic neurons. *Brain Res.* 1204 (2008) 16 – 23.

[aradottir06] S Aradottir, G Asanovska, S Gjerss, P Hansson, C Alling. Phosphatidylethanol concentrations in blood are correlated to reported alcohol intake in alcohol-dependent patients. *Alcohol. Alcohol.* 41 (2006) 431 – 437.

[arevalo08] E Arevalo, S Shanmugasundararaj, M Wilkemeyer, X Dou, S Chen, M Charness, K Miller. An alcohol binding site on the neural cell adhesion molecule L1. *Proc. Natl. Acad. Sci. USA* 105 (2008) 371 – 375.

[arjona06] A Arjona, N Boyadjieva, P Kuhn, D Sarkar. Fetal ethanol exposure disrupts the daily rhythms of splenic granzyme B, IFN-γ, and NK cell cytotoxicity in adulthood. *Alchol. Clin. Exp. Res.* 38 (2006) 1039 – 1044.

[auten07] R Auten, S Mason, M Whorton, W Lampe, W Foster, r Goldberg, B Li, J Stamler, K Auten. Inhaled ethyl nitrite prevents hypoxia-impaired postnatal alveolar development in newborn rat. *Am. J. Respir. Crit. Care Med.* 176 (2007) 291 – 299.

[azara08] C Azara, I Maia, C Rangel, M Silva-Neto, R Serpa, E de Jesus, M Tavares do Carmo, E Fialho. Ethanol during lactation alters milk nutrient composition and growth and mineral status of rat pups. *Biol. Res.* 41 (2008) 317 – 330.

[azorin04] I Azorin, M Portoles, P Marin, f Lazaro-Dieguez, L Megias, G Egea, J Renau-Piqueras. Prenatal alcohol exposure alters the cytoskeleton and induces glycoprotein microheterogeneity in rat newborn hepatocytes. *Alchol. Alcohol.* 39 (2004) 203 – 212.

[badger05] T Badger, M Hidestrand, K Shankar, W D McGuinn, m Ronis. The effects of pregnancy on ethanol clearance. *Life Sci.* 77 (2005) 2111 – 2126.

[bailey04] C Bailey, J Brien, J Reynolds. Chronic prenatal alcohol exposure alters the proportion of GABAergic neurons in layers II/III of the adult guinea pig somatosensory cortex. *Neurotoxicol. Teratol.* 26 (2004) 59 – 63.

[bearer99] C Bearer, A Swick, M O'Riordan, G Cheng. Ethanol inhibits L1-mediated neurite outgrowth in postnatal rat cerebellar granule cells. *J. Biol. Chem.* 274 (1999) 13264 – 13270.

[bearer05] C Bearer, L Santiago, M O'Riordan, K Buck, S Lee, L Singer. Fatty acid ethyl esters: Quantitative biomarkers for maternal alcohol consumption. *J. Pediatr.* 146 (2005) 824 – 830.

[beblo05] S Beblo, K Stark, M Murthy, J Janisse, H Rockett, J Whitty, M Buda-Abela, S martier, R Sokol, J Hannigan, N Salem. Effect of alcohol intake during pregnancy on docosahexaenoic acid and arachidonic acid in umbilical cord vessels of black women. *Pediatr* 115 (2005) e194 – e203.

[beck03] O Beck, A Helander. 5-Hydroxytryptophol as a marker for recent alcohol intake. *Addiction* 98 (suppl 2) (2003) 63 – 72.

[bedard07] K Bedard, K-H Krause. The NOX family of ROS-generating NADPH oxidases: Physiology and pathophysiology. *Physiol. Rev.* 87 (2007) 245 – 313.

[benari07] Y Ben-Ari, J Gaiarsa, R Tyzio, R Khazipov. GABA: A pioneer transmitter that excites immature neurons and generates primitive oscillations. *Physiol. Rev.* 87 (2007) 1215 – 1284.

[berghaus98] T Berghaus, H demmelmair, B Koletzko. Fatty acid composition of lipid classes in maternal and cord plasma at birth. *Eur. J. Pediatr.* 157 (1998) 763 – 768.

[bhalla04] S Bhalla, K Kaur, A Mahmood, S Mahmood. Prenatal ethanol administration: Effects on IgG absorption during postnatal development in the rat intestine. *Biol. Neonate* 86 (2004) 10 – 14.

[bird06] D Bird, A Sato, D Knee, C Uyehara, D Person, J Claybaugh. Effects of prenatal alcohol exposure and sex on the arginine vasopressin response to hemorrhage in the rat. *A J. Physiol. Regul. Integr. Comp. Physiol.* 291 (2006) R77 – R82.

[blanco07] R Blanco, T Ziegler, B Carlson, P-Y Cheng, Y Park, G Cotsonis, C Jonas Accardi, D Jones. Diurnal variations in glutathione and cysteine redox states in human plasma. *Am. J. Clin. Nutr.* 86 (2007) 1016 – 1023.

[blom06] H Blom, G Shaw, M den Heijer, R Finnell. Neural tube defects and folate: A case case far from closed. *Nature Rev. Neurosci.* 7 (2006) 724 – 731.

[bookstein06] F Bookstein, A Streissguth, P Connor, P Sampsom. Damage to the human cerebellum from prenatal alcohol exposure: The anatomy of a simple biometrical explanation. *Anat. Rec. – New Anat.* 289B (2006) 195 – 209.

[bookstein07] F Bookstein, P Connor, j Huggins, H Barr, K Pimentel, A Streissguth. Many infants prenatally exposed to high levels of alcohol show one particular anomaly of the corpus callosum. *Alcohol. Clin. Exp. Res.* 31 (2007) 868 – 879.

[breese06] G Breese, H Criswell, M Carta, P Dodson, H Hanchar, R Khisti, M Mameli, Z Ming, A Morrow, R Olsen, T Otis, L Parsons, S Penland, M Roberto, G Siggins, C Valenzuela, M Wallner. Basis of the GABAmimetic profile of ethanol. *Alcohol. Clin. Exp. Res.* 30 (2006) 731 – 744.

[brien83] J Brien, C Loomis, J Tranmer, M McGrath. Disposition of ethanol in human maternal venous blood and amniotic fluid. *Am. J. Obstet. Gynecol.* 146 (1983) 181 – 186.

[brooks05] P J Brooks, JA Theruvathu. DNA adducts from acetaldehyde: implications for alcohol-related carcinogenesis. *Alcohol.* 35 (2005) 187 – 193.

[brzezinski99] M Brzezinski, H Boutelet-Bochan, R Person, A Fantel, M Juchau. *J. Pharmacol. Exp. Ther.* 289 (1999) 1648 – 1653.

[cancedda07] L Cancedda, H Fiumelli, K Chen, M Poo. Excitatory GABA action is essential for morphological maturation of cortical neurons *in vivo*. *J. Neurosci.* 27 (2007) 5224 – 5235.

[burd07] L Burd, D Roberts, M Olson, H Odendaal. Ethanol and the placenta: A review. *J. Mater-Fetal Neonat. Med.* 20 (2007) 361 – 375.

[caldeira04] J Caldeira, Y Wu, M Mameli, R Purdy, P Li, Y Akwa, D Savage, J Engen, C Valenzuela. Fetal alcohol exposure alters neurosteroid levels in the developing rat brain. *J. Neurochem.* 90 (2004) 1530 – 1539.

[calder06] P Calder. N-3 polyunsaturated fatty acids, inflammation, and inflammatory diseases. *Am. J. Clin. Nutr.* 83 (2006) 1505S – 1519S.

[cannizzaro10] C Cannizzaro, M La Barbera, F Plescia, S Cacace, G Tringali. Ethanol modulates corticotrophin releasing hormone release from rat hypothalamus: Does acetaldehyde play a role? *Alcohol. Clin. Exp. Res.* 34 (2010) 1-6.

[cao89] Q Cao, G Tu, H Weiner. Presence of cytosolic aldehyde dehydrogenase isozymes in adult and fetal rat liver. *Biochem. Pharmacol.* 38 (1989) 77 – 83.

[carey00] L Carey, P Coyle, J Philcox, A Rofe. Ethanol decreases zinc transfer to the fetus in normal but not metallothionein-null mice. *Alcohol. Clin. Exp. Res.* 24 (2000) 1236 – 1240.

[carlson99] S Carlson, M Neuringer. Polyunsaturated fatty acid status and neurodevelopment: A summary and critical analysis of the literature. *Lipids* 34 (1999) 171 – 178.

[carta04] M Carta, M Mameli, C Valenzuela. Alcohol enhances the GABA-ergic transmission to cerebellar granule cells via an increase in Golgi cell excitability. *J. Neurosci.* 24 (2004) 3746 – 3751.

[cazzaniga09] E Cazzaniga, A Bulbarelli, M Masserini. Alcohol and neural lipids. Ch 19 in Handbook of Neurochemistry and Molecular Neurobiology. Springer, 2009.

[cederqvist94] B Cederqvist, M Persson, L Gustafsson. Direct demonstration of NO formation *in vivo* from organic nitrites and nitrates, and correlation to effects on blood pressure and to i*n vitro* effects. *Biochem. Pharmacol.* 47 (1994) 1047 – 1053.

[chambon96] P Chambon, A decade of molecular biology of retinoic acid receptors. *FASEB J.* 10 (1996) 940 – 954.

[chan04] D Chan, B Knie, R Boskovic, G Koren. Placental handling of fatty acid ethyl esters: Perfusion and subcellular studies. *J. Pharmacol. Exp. Ther.* 310 (2004) 75 – 82.

[chapkin09] R Chapkin, W Kim, J Lupton, D McMurray. Dietary docosahexaenoic and eicosapentaenoic acid: emerging mediators of inflammation. *Prostagland Leukotr. Ess. Fatty Acids* 1 (2009) 187 – 191.

[chen00] S Chen, K Kulik. Iron-mediated free radical injury in ethanol-exposed mouse neural crest cells. *J. Pharmacol. Exp. Ther.* 294 (2000) 134 – 140.

[chen03] W-J Chen, S Maier, S Parnell, J West. Alcohol and the developing brain: Neuroanatomical studies. *Alcohol. Res. Health* 27 (2003) 174 – 180.

[chen06] C-P Chen, P Kuhn, K Chaturvedi, N Boyadjieva, D Sarkar. Ethanol induces apoptotic death of developing β-endorphin neurons via suppression of cyclic adenosine monophosphate production and activation of transforming growth factor-β1 linked apoptotic signalling. *Mol. Pharmacol.* 69 (2006) 706 – 717.

[chen08] S Chen, M Charness. Ethanol inhibits neuronal differentiation by disrupting activity-dependent neuroprotective protein signalling. *Proc. Natl. Acad. Sci.* 105 (2008) 1962 – 19967.

[cheng01] P Cheng, A Cherkuri, S Dykstra, T Malapati, M Sproul, R Chen, S Pierce. Floating the raft hypothesis: the roles of lipid rafts in B cell antigen receptor function. *Semin. Immuno.* 13 (2001) 107 – 114.

[choi08]I Choi, S Lee, C Rivier. Novel role of adrenergic neurons in the brain stem in mediating the hypothalamic-pituitary axis hyperactivity caused by prenatal alcohol exposure. *Neurosci* 155 (2008) 888 – 901.

[christiansen93] P Christiansen, P Toft, H Larsson, M Stubgaard, O Henriksen. The concentration of N-acetyl aspartate, creatine, phosphocreatine, and choline in different parts of the barin in adulthood and senium. *Magn. Reson. Im.* 11 (1993) 799 – 806.

[clagett02] M Clagett-Dame, H DeLuca. The role of vitamin A in mammalian reproduction and embryonic development. *Annu. Rev. Nutr.* 22 (2002) 347 – 381.

[cohen03] R Cohen-Kerem, G Koren. Antioxidants and fetal protection against ethanol teratogenicity I. Review of the experimental data and implications to humans. *Neurotoxicol. Teratol.* 25 (2003) 1 - 9.

[cortese06] B Cortese, G Moore, B Bailey, S Jacobson, V Delaney-Black, J Hannigan. Magnetic resonance and spectroscopic imaging in prenatal alcohol-exposed children: Preliminary findings in the caudate nucleus. *Neurotoxicol. Teratol.* 28 (2006) 597 – 606.

[costa00] E Costa, D Savage, C Valenzuela. A review of the effects of prenatal or early postnatal ethanol exposure on brain ligand-gated ion channels. *Alcohol. Clin. Exp. Res.* 24 (2000) 706 – 715.

[costa00b] E Costa, D Olivera, D Meyer, V Ferreira, E Soto, S Frausto, D Savage, M Browning, C Valenzuela. Fetal alcohol exposure alters neurosteroid modulation of hippocampal N-methyl-D-aspartate receptors. *J. Biol. Chem.* 275 (2000) 38268 – 38274.

[crabb04] D Crabb, M Matsumoto, D Chang, M You. Overview of the role of alcohol dehydrogenases and aldehyde dehydrogenase and their variants in the genesis of alcohol – related pathology. *Proc. Nutr. Soc.* 63 (2004) 49 – 63.

[crews09] F Crews, K Nixon. Mechanisms of neurodegeneration and regeneration in alcoholism. *Alcohol Alcohol* 44 (2009) 115 – 127.

[criswell08] H Criswell, Z Ming, K Kelm, G Breese. Brain regional differences in the effect of ethanol on GABA release from presynaptic terminals. *J. Pharmacol. Exp. Ther.* 326 (2008) 596 – 603.

[csaba06] G Csaba, P Kovacs, E Pallinger. Changes in the endorphin and serotonin content of rat immune cells during adulthood following maternal exposure to ethanol during pregnancy and lactation. *Alcohol* 38 (2006) 111 – 116.

[cuzon08] V Cuzon, P Yeh, Y Yanagawa, K Obata, H Yeh. Ethanol consumption during early pregnancy alters the dispositions of tangentially migrating GABAergic interneurons in the fetal cortex. *J. Neurosci.* 28 (2008) 1854 – 1864.

[dasgupta07] S Dasgupta, J Adams, E Hogan. Maternal alcohol consumption increases sphingosine levels in the brains of progeny mice. Neurochem Res 32 (2007) 2217 – 2224.

[de86] K De, D Sengupta. Ontogeny of human fetal catalase, superoxide dismutase and lipid peroxidation: A comparative study. *J. Biosci.* 10 (1986) 319 – 322.

[deelchand09] DK Deelchand, A Shestov, D Koski, K Ugurbil, P-G Henry. Acetate transport and utilization in the rat brain. *J. Neurochem.* 109 S1 (2009) 46 – 54.

[deng04] X-S Deng, P Bludeau, R Deitrich. Formation of ethyl nitrite in vivo after ethanol administration. *Alcohol* 34 (2004) 217 – 223.

[deng07] X-S Deng, R Deitrich. Ethanol metabolism and effects: nitric oxide and its interaction. *Curr. Clin. Pharmacol.* 2 (2007) 145 – 153.

[denkins00] Y Denkins, J Wood, J Whitty, J Hannigan, S Martier, R Sokol, N Salem. Effects of gestational alcohol exposure on fatty acid composition of umbilical cord serum in humans. *Am. J. Clin. Nutr.* 71 (2000) 300S – 306S.

[dianzani03] M Dianzani. 4-Hydroxynonenal from pathology to physiology. *Mol. Aspect Med.* 24 (2003) 263 – 272.

[dickerson10] D Dickerson, B Pittmann, E Ralevski, A Perrino, D Limoncelli, J Edgecombe, G Acampora, J Krystal, I Petrakis. Ethanol-like effects of thiopental and ketamine in healthy humans. *Psychopharm* 24 (2010) 203 – 211.

[dong10] J Dong, K Sulik, S-Y Chen. The role of NOX enzymes in ethanol-induced oxidative stress and apoptosis in mouse embryos. *Toxicol. Lett.* 193 (2010) 94 – 100.

[dotzler04] S Dotzler, R Digeronimo, B Yoder, T Siler-Khodr. Distribution of corticotrpoin releasing hormone in the fetus, newborn, juvenile and adult baboon. *Pediatr Res.* 55 (2004) 120 – 125.

[dubois06] C Dubois, M Naassila, M Daoust, O Pierrefiche. Early chronic ethanol exposure in rats disturbs respiratory network activity and increases sensitivity to ethanol. *J. Physiol.* 576 (2006) 297 – 307.

[dubois08] C Dubois, H Houchi, M Naassila, M Daoust, O Pierrefiche. Blunted response to low oxygen of rat respiratory network after perinatal ethanol exposure: Involvement of inhibitory control. *J. Physiol.* 586 (2008) 1413 – 1427.

[duester98] G Duester. Alcohol dehydrogenase as a critical mediator of retinoic acid synthesis from vitamin A in the mouse embryo. *J. Nutr.* 128 (1998) 459S – 462S.

[eggers04] E Eggers, A Berger. Mechanisms for the modulation of native glycine receptor channels by ethanol. *J. Neurophysiol.* 91 (2004) 2685 – 2695.

[elmore07] S Elmore. Apoptosis: A review of programmed cell death. *Toxicol. Pathol.* 35 (2007) 495.

[estonius96] M Estonius, S Svensson, J-O Höög. Alcohol dehydrogenase in human tissues: Localization of transcripts codimg for five classes of the enzyme. *FEBS Lett.* 397 (1996) 338 – 342.

[faassen07] *Radicals for life: The various forms of nitric oxide*. E. van Faassen and A. F. Vanin, eds. Elsevier, Amsterdam 2007.

[faassen09] E van Faassen, S Bahrami, M Feelisch, N Hogg, M Kelm, D Kim-Shapiro, A Kozlov, H Li, JO Lundberg, R Mason, H Nohl, T Rassaf, A Samouilov, A Slama-Schwok, S Shiva, A Vanin, E Weitzberg, J Zweier, M Gladwin. Nitrite as regulator of hypoxic signaling in mammalian physiology. *Med. Res. Rev.* 29 (2009) 683 – 741.

[fadok98] V Fadok, D Bratton, S C Frasch, M Warner, P Henson. The role of phophatidylserine in recognition of apoptotic cells by phagocytes. *Cell Death Differ.* 5 (1998) 551 – 562.

[farwell05] A Farwell, J Leonard. Nongenomic actions of thyroid hormone during fetal brain development. *Curr. Opin. Endocrin. Diabetes* 12 (2005) 17 – 22.

[fernandez04] J Fernandez-Solari, C Scorticati, C Mohn, A de Laurentiis, S Billi, A Franchi, S McCann, V Rettori. Alcohol inhibits luteinizing hormone-releasing hormone release by activating the endocannabinoid system. *Proc. Natl. Acad. Sci.* 101 (2004) 3264 – 3268.

[ferrani03] K Ferrani-Kile, P Randall, S Leslie. Acute ethanol affects phosphorylation state of the NMDA receptor complex.: implication of tyrosine phsphatases and protein kinase A. *Brain Res. Mol. Brain Res.* 115 (2003) 78 – 86.

[feyder10] M Feyder, M Camp, A Holmes, Y-C Chen. Ethanol and NMDA receptor interactions: Implications for pharmacotherapeutic treatments. *J. Med. Sci.* 30 (2010) 3 – 10.

[florent06] S Florent, C Malaplate-Armand, I Youssef, B Kriem, V Koziel et al. Docosahexaenoic acid prevents neuronal apoptosis induced by soluble amyloid-β oligomers. *J. Neurochem.* 96 (2006) 385 – 395.

[flynn81] A Flynn, S Miller, S Martier, N Golden, R Sokol, B del Villano. Zinc status of pregnant alcoholic women: A determinant of fetal outcome. *Lancet* 1 (1981) 572 – 651.

[foddai04] M Foddai, G Dosia, S Spiga, M Diana. Acetaldehyde increases dopaminergic neuronal activity in the VTA. *Neuropsychopharmacol.* 29 (2004) 530 – 536.

[freeman05] T Freeman, D Tuma, G Thiele, L Klassen, S Worrall, O Niemelä, S Parkkila, P Emery, V Preedy. Recent advances in alcohol-induced adduct formation. *Alcohol. Clin. Exp. Res.* 29 (2005) 1310 – 1316.

[fung97] E Fung, L Ritchie, L Woodhouse, R Roehl,J King. Zinc absorption in women during pregnancy and lactation: A longitudinal study. *Am. J. Clin. Nutr.* 66 (1997) 80 – 88.

[gabriel98] K Gabriel, C Hofmann, M Glavas, J Weinberg. The hormonal effects of alcohol use on the mother and fetus. *Alcohol Health Res. World* 22 (1998) 170 – 177.

[gago04] N Gago, M El-Etr, N Sananes, F Cadepont, D Samuel, V Avellana-Adalid, A Baron – van Evercooren, M Schumacher. Allopregnanolone and gamma-aminobutyric acid: autocrine/paracrine interactions in the control of neonatal PSA $^-$ NCAM$^+$ progenitor proliferation. *J. Neurosci. Res.* 78 (2004) 770 – 783.

[gago08] B Gago, T Nystrom, C Cavaleiro, B Rocha, R Barbosa, J Laranjinha, JO Lundberg. The potent vasodilator ethyl nitrite is formed upon the reaction of nitrite and ethanol under gastric conditions. *Free Radic. Biol. Med.* 45 (2008) 404 – 412.

[gao07] X Gao, L Qi, N Qiao, H Choi, G Curhan, K Tucker, A Ascherio. Intake of added sugar and ugar-sweetened drink and serum uric acid concentration in US men and women. *Hypertension* 50 (2007) 306 – 312.

[gardner03] J Gardner, A doi, R Pham, C Huisden, E Gallagher. Ontogenic differences in human liver 4-hydroxynonenal detoxification are associated with in vitro injury to fetal hematopoietic stem cells. *Toxicol. Appl. Pharmacol.* 191 (2003) 95 – 106.

[gatford07] K Gatford, P Dalizt, M Cock, R Harding, J Owens. Acute ethanol exposure in pregnancy alters the insulin-like growth factor axis of fetal and maternal sheep. *Am. J. Physiol. Endocrin. Metab.* 292 (2007) E494 – E500.

[gauthier05] T Gauthier, C Drews-Botsch, A Falek, C Coles, L-A Brown. Maternal alcohol use and neonatal infection. *Alcohol. Clin. Exp. Res.* 29 (2005) 1035 – 1043.

[gauthier10] T Gauthier, J Kable, L Burwell, C Coles, L-A Brown. Maternal alcohol use during pregnancy causes systemic oxidation of the glutathione redox system. *Alcohol. Clin. Exp. Res.* 34 (2010) 123 – 130.

[gavin94] C Gavin, B Kates, G Hoffman, P Rodier. Changes in the reproductive system following acute prenatal exposure to ethanol or methylazoxymethanol in the rat: I.Effects on immunoreactive LHRH cell number. *Teratol.* 49 (1994) 13 – 19.

[gemma07] S Gemma, S Vichi, E Testai. Metabolic and genetic factors contributing to alcohol induced effects and fetal alcohol syndrome. *Neurosci. Biobehav. Rev.* 31 (2007) 221 – 229.

[germain06] P Germain, P Chambon, G Eichele, R Evans, M Lazar, M Leid, A de Lera, R Lotan, D Mangelsdorf, H Gronemeyer. Retinoic acid receptors. *Pharmacol. Rev.* 58 (2006) 712 – 725.

[ghishan82] F Ghishan, R Padwarthan, H Greene. Fetal alcohol syndrome: inhibition of placental zinc transport as a potential mechanism for fetal growth retardation in the rat. *J. Lab. Clin. Med.* 100 (1982) 45 – 52.

[giglia06] R Giglia, C Binns. Alcohol and lactation: A systematic review. *Nutr. Diet* 63 (2006) 103 – 116.

[gill00] J Gill. The effects of moderate alcohol consumption on female hormone levels and reproductive function. *Alcohol. Alcohol.* 35 (2000) 417 – 423.

[goral08] J Goral, J Karavitis, E Kovacs. Exposure-dependent effects of ethanol on the innate immune system. *Alcohol* 42 (2008) 237 – 247.

[gottesfeld90] Z Gottesfeld, P Silverman. Developmental delays associated with prenatal alcohol exposure are recovered by thyroid hormone treatment. *Neurosci. Lett.* 109 (1990) 42 – 47.

[gottesfeld91] Z Gottesfeld, E Abel. Maternal and paternal alcohol use: effects on the immune system of the offspring. *Life Sci.* 48 (1991) 1 – 8.

[gottesfeld95] Z Gottesfeld, S Ullrich. Prenatal alcohol exposure selectively suppresses cell-mediated but not humoral immune responsiveness. *Int. J. Immunopharmac.* 17 (1995) 247 – 254.

[gottrand08] F Gottrand. Long-chain polyunsaturated fatty acids influence the immune system of infants. *J. Nutr.* 138 (2008) 1807S – 1812S.

[gowder09] S Gowder, K McMartin. Methods to evaluate the effect of ethanol on the folate analogue: fluorescein methotrexate uptake in human proximal tubular cells. *Adv. Pharmacol. Sci.* (2009) article ID 291349.

[gozes07] I Gozes. Activity-dependent neuroprotective protein: From gene to drug candidate. *Pharmacol. Ther.* 114 (2007) 146 – 154.

[green07] R.F. Green, J M Stoler. Alcohol dehydrogenase 1B genotype and fetal alcohol syndrome: a HuGE minireview. *Am. J. Obstet Gynecol.* (2007) 12 – 25.

[grimm02] H Grimm, K Mayer, P Mayser, E Eigenbrodt. Regulatory potential of (n-3) fatty acids in immunological and inflammatory processes. *Br. J. Nutr.* 87 (2002) S59 – S67.

[grobin03] A C Grobin, E Heenan, J Lieberman, L Morrow. Perinatal neurosteroid levels influence GABAergic interneuron localization in adult rat prefrontal cortex. *J. Neurosci.* 23 (2003) 1832 – 1839.

[guan03] K-L Guan, Y Rao. Signalling mechanisms mediating neuronal responses to guidance cues. *Nature Rev. Neurosci.* 4 (2003) 941 – 956.

[gubitosi07] R Gubitosi-Klug, C Larimer, C Bearer. L1 cell adhesion molecule is neuroprotective of alcohol induced cell death. *Neurotoxicol.* 28 (2007) 457 – 462.

[gupta09] S Gupta, N Aziz, L Sekhon, R Agarwal, G Mansour, J Li, A Agarwal. Lipid peroxidation and antioxidant status in preeclampsia: a systematic review. *Obstet Gynecol. Surv.* 64 (2009) 750 – 759.

[haggarty02] P Haggarty, D Abramovich, K Page. The effect of maternal smoking and ethanol on fatty acid transport by the human placenta. *Br. J. Nutr.* 87 (2002) 247 – 252.

[haley06] D Haley, N Handmaker, J Lowe. Infant stress reactivity nd prenatal alcohol exposure. *Alchol. Clin. Exp. Res.* 30 (2006) 2055 – 2064.

[halsted02] C Halsted, J Villanueva, A Devlin, O Niemelä, S Parkkila, T Garrow, L Wallock, M Shigenaga, S Melnyk, S James. Folate deficiency distrurbs hepatic methionine metabolism and promotes liver injury in the ethanol-fed micropig. *Proc. Natl. Acad. Sci. USA* 99 (2002) 10072 – 10077.

[hamby97] R Hamby-Mason, J Chen, S Schenker, A Perez, G Henderson. Catalase mediates acetaldehyde formation from ethanol in fetal and neonatal rat brain. *Alcohol. Clin. Exp. Res.* 21 (1997) 1063 – 1072.

[hamid09] A Hamid, J Kaur. Role of signalling pathways in the regulation of folate transport in ethanol-fed rats. *J. Nutr. Biochem.* 40 (2009) 291 – 297.

[han98] C Han, CS Liao, CW Wu, CL Hwong, AR Lee. Contribution to first pass metabolism of ethanol and inhibition by ethanol for retinol oxidation in human alcohol dehydrogenase family . Implications for etiology of fetal alcohol syndrome and alcohol related diseases. *Eur. J. Biochem.* 254 (1998) 25 – 31.

[handmaker06] N Handmaker, W Rayburn, C Meng, J Bell, B Rayburn, V Rappaport. Impact of alcohol exposure after pregnancy recognition on ultrasonographic fetal growth measures. *Alcohol. Clin. Exp. Res.* 30 (2006) 892 – 898.

[hanebutt08] F Hanebutt, H Demmelmair, B Schiessl, E Larque, B Koletzko. Long-chain polyunsaturated fatty acid (LC-PUFA) transfer across the placenta. *Clin. Nutr.* 27 (2008) 685 – 693.

[harbige03] L Harbige. Fatty acids, the immune response, and autoimmunity: a question of n-6 essentiality and the balance between n-6 and n-3 lipids. *Lipids* 38 (2003) 323 – 341.

[hard01] M Hard, T Einarson, G Koren. The role of acetaldehyde in pregnancy outcome after prenatal alcohol exposure. *Ther. Drug Monit.* 23 (2001) 427 – 434.

[hayward04] M Hayward, A Martin, J Brien, H Dringenberg, M Olmstead, J Reynolds. Chronic prenatal ethanol exposure impairs conditioned responding and enhances GABA release in the hippocampus of the adult guinea pig. *J. Pharmacol. Exp. Therap.* 308 (2004) 644 – 650.

[heaton06] M Heaton, M Paiva, I Madorski, K Siler-Marsilio, G Shaw. Effect of bax deletion on ethanol sensitivity in the neonatal rat cerebellum. *J. Neurobiol.* 66 (2006) 95 – 101. Note: the title states erroneously rats. In fact, mice were used.

[heck06] N Heck, W Kilb, P Reiprich, H Kubota, T Furukawa, A Fukuda, H Luhmann. $Gaba_A$ receptors regulate neocortical neuronal migration *in vitro* and *in vivo*. *Cereb. Cortex* 17 (2006) 138 – 148.

[hellemans10] K Hellemans, J Sliwowska, P Verma, J Weinberg. Prenatal alcohol exposure: fetal programming and later life vulnerability to stress, depression and anxiety disorders. *Neurosci. Biobehav. Rev.* 34 (2010) 791 – 807.

[henderson99] G Henderson, JJ Chen, S Schenker. Ethanol, oxidative stress, reactive aldehydes, and the fetus. *Frontiers Biosci.* 4 (1999) 541 – 550.

[hewitt10] A Hewitt, K Walker, S Mobus, M Poklewska – Koziell, J Reynolds, J Brien. Differential effects of chronic ethanol exposure on cytochrome P450 2E1 and the hypothalamic – pituitary – adrenal axis in the maternal-fetal unit of the guinea pig. *Neurotox. Terat* 32 (2010) 164 – 170.

[higuchi01] H Higuchi, M Adachi, S Miura, G Gores, H Ishii. The mitochondrial permeability transition contributes to acute ethanol-induced apoptosis in rat hepatocytes. *Hepatol.* 34 (2001) 320 – 328.

[hiney99] J Hiney, R Dearth, F Lara III, S Wood, V Srivastava, W L Dees. Effects of ethanol on leptin secretion and the leptin-induced luteinizing hormone (LH) release from late juvenile female rats. *Alcohol Clin. Exp. Res.* 23 (1999) 1785 – 1792.

[hirano08] T Hirano, M Murakami, T Fukada, K Nishida, S Yamasaki, T Suzuki. Roles of zinc and ainc signalling in immunity: zinc as an intracellular signalling molecule. *Adv. Immunol.* 97 (2008) 149 – 176.

[hirota08] T Hirota, M Murakami, T Fukada, K Nishida, S Yamasaki, T Suzuki. Roles of zinc and zinc signalling in immunity: Zinc as an intracellular signalling molecule. *Adv. Immunol.* 97 (2008) 149 – 176.

[hofmann07] C Hofmann, L Ellis, W Yu, J Weinberg. Hypothalamic-pituitary-adrenal responses to $5\text{-}HT_{1A}$ and $5\text{-}HT_{2A/C}$ agonists are differentially altered in female and male rats prenatally exposed to ethanol. *Alcohol. Clin. Exp. Res.* 31 (2007) 345 – 355.

[huang07] Z Huang, G di Cristo, F Ango. Development of GABA innervation in the cerebral and cerebellar cortices. *Nature Rev. Neurosci.* 8 (2007) 673 – 686.

[huisman00] A Huisman, A Vanin, E van Faassen, H Rijn, P Martasek, T Rabelink, E Stroes. Tetrahydrobiopterin shifts iNOS from a superoxide producing to a peroxynitrite producing enzyme. *Circulation* 102 (2000) 63 - 63 .

[ikonomidou01] C Ikonomidou, P Brittigau, C Koch, K Genz, F Hoerster, U Felderhoff-Mueser, T Tenkova, K Dikranian, J Olney. Neurotransmitters and apoptosis in the developing brain. *Biochem. Pharmacol.* 62 (2001) 401 – 405.

[isayama09] R Isayama, P Correa Leite, J-P Mendes Lima, D Uziel, E Yamasaki. Impact of ethanol on the developing GABAergic system. *Anat. Rec.* 292 (2009) 1922 – 1939.

[jansson03] N Jansson, S Greenwood, B Johansson, T Powell, T Jansson. Leptin stimulates the activity of the system A amino acid transporter in human placental villous fragments. *J. Clin. Endocrin. Metab.* 88 (2003) 1205 – 1211.

[jelski08] W Jelski, M Szmitkowski. Alcohol dehydrogenase (ADH) and aldehyde dehydrogenase (ALDH) in the cancer diseases. *Clin. Chim. Acta* 395 (2008) 1-5.

[john06] C John, E Theogaraj, H Christian, J Morris, S Smith, J Buckingham. Thime-specific effects of perinatal glucocorticoid treatment on anterior pituitary morphology, annexin 1 expression and adrenocorticotrophic hormone secretion in the adult female rat. *J. Endocrin.* 18 (2006) 949 – 959.

[jones07] H Jones, T Powell, T Jansson. Regulation of placental nutrient transport. *Placenta* 28 (2007) 763 – 774.

[jornvall00] H Jörnvall, J-O Höög, B Persson, X Peres. Pharmacogenetics of the alcohol dehydrogenase system. *Pharmacol.* 61 (2000) 184 – 191.

[joseph00] R Joseph. Fetal brain behaviour and cognitive development. *Development Rev.* 28 (2000) 81 – 98.

[kabouridis06] P Kabouridis. Lipid rafts in T cell receptor signalling. *Mol. Membr. Iol.* 23 (2006) 49 – 57.

[kapoor06] A Kapoor, E Dunn, A Kostaki, M Andrews, S Matthews. Fetal programming of the hypothalamo-pituitary-adrenal (HPA) function: Prenatal stress and glucocorticoids. *J. Physiol.* 572 (2006) 31 – 44.

[kapoor08] A Kapoor, S Petropoulos, S Matthews. Fetal programming of hypothalamic-pituitary-adrenal (HPA) axis function and behavior by synthetic glucocorticoids. *Brain Res. Rev.* 57 (2008) 586 – 595.

[karl88] P Karl, B Gordon, C Lieber, S Fisher. Acetaldehyde production and transfer by the perfused human placental cotyledon. *Science* 242 (1988) 273 – 275.

[kaur08] G Kaur, S Mishra, A Sehgal, R Prasad. Alterations in lipid peroxidation and antioxidant status in pregnancy with eclampsia. *Mol. Cell Biochem.* 313 (2008) 37 – 44.

[keen93] C Keen, M Taubeneck, G Datson, J Rogers, M Gershwin. Primary and secondary zinc deficiency as factors underlying abnormal CNS development. *Ann. N. Y. Acad. Sci.* 678 (1993) 37 – 47.

[keiver04] K Keiver, J Weinberg. Effect of duration of maternal alcohol consumption on calcium metabolism and bone in the fetal rat. *Alcohol Clin. Exp. Res.* 28 (2004) 456 – 467.

[keppen85] L Keppen, T Pysher, O Rennert. Zinc deficiency acts as a co-teratogen with alcohol in the fetal alcohol syndrome. *Pediatr Res.* 19 (1985) 944 – 947.

[kim03] H-Y Kim, M Akbar, A Lau. Effects of docosapentaenoic acid on neuronal apoptosis. *Lipids* 38 (2003) 453 – 457.

[kim08] H-Y Kim. Biochemical and biological functions of docosahexaenoic acid in the nervous system: modulation by ethanol. *Chem. Phys. Lipids* 153 (2008) 34 – 46.

[king00] J King. Determinants of maternal zinc status during pregnancy. *Am. J. Clin. Nutr.* 71 (2000) 1334S – 1343S.

[kinney05] K C Kinney. Human myelination and perinatal white matter disorders. *J. Neurol. Sci.* 228 (2005) 190 – 192.

[kiss01] J Kiss, S Vizi. Nitric oxide: a novel link between synaptic and nonsynaptic transmission. *Trends Neurosci.* 24 (2001) 211 – 215.

[kitson10] A Kitson, C Stroud, K Stark. Elevated production of docosahexaenoic acid in females: potential molecular mechanisms. *Lipids* 45 (2010) 2009 – 224.

[kiyoshi09] A Kiyoshi, W Weihuan, J Mostofa, K Mitsuru, I Toyoshi, K Toshihiro, K Kyoko, N Keiichi, I Iwao, K Hiroshi. Ethanol metabolism in ALDH2 knockout mice – blood acetate levels. *Legal. Med.* 11 (2009) 5413 – 5415.

[koeners07] M Koeners, E van Faassen, S Wesseling, M de Sain, H Koomans, B Braam, J A Joles. Maternal supplementation with citrulline has long-term antihypertensive effects in spontaneously hypertensive rats. *Hypertension* 50 (2007) 1077 – 1084.

[koop06] D R Koop. Alcohol metabolism's damaging effect on the cell: a focus on reactive oxygen generation by the enzyme cytochrome P450 2E1. *Alcoh. Res. Health* 29 (2006) 274 – 280.

[kumar04] S Kumar, R Fleming, L Morrow. Ethanol regulation of γ-aminobutyric $acid_A$ receptors: genomic and nongenomic mechanisms. *Pharmacol. Ter.* 101 (2004) 211 – 226.

[kurra09] V Kurra, A Eraranta, P Jolma, T Vehmas, A Riutta, E Moilanen, A Tahvanainen, J Kalliovalkama, O Niemelä, J Myllymäki, J Mustonen, I Pörsti. Hyperuricemia, oxidative stress, and carotid artery tone in experimental renal insufficiency. *Am. J. Hypertens.* 22 (2009) 964 – 970.

[lan09a] N Lan, K Hellemans, L Ellis, V Viau, J Weinberg. Role of testosterone in mediating prenatal ethanol effects on the hypothalamic – pituitary – adrenal activity in male rats. *Psychoneuroendocrin.* 34 (2009) 1314 – 1328.

[lan09b] N Lan, F Yamashita, A Halpert, J Sliwowska,V Viau, J Weinberg. Effects of prenatal ethanol exposure on hypothalamic – pituitary – adrenal function across the estrous cycle. *Alcohol. Clin. Exp. Res.* 33 (2009) 1075 – 1088.

[laposata02] M Laposata, A Hasaba, C Best, D Yoerger, b McQuillan, R Salem, M Refaai, B Soderberg. Fatty acid ethyl esters: recent observations. Prostagl Leukotr Ess Fatty Acids 67 (2002) 193 – 196.

[latvala05] J Latvala, J Hietala, H Koivisto, K Järvi, P Anttila, O Niemelä. Immune responses to ethanol metabolites and cytokine profiles differentiate alcoholics with or without liver disease. A, *J. Gastroenterol.* 100 (2005) 1303 – 1310.

[ledig90] M Ledig, R Misslin, P Kopp, E Vogel, G Tholey, P Mandel. Alcohol exposure before pregnancy: biochemical and behavioural effects on the offspring of rats. *Pharmacol. Biochem. Behav.* 36 (1990) 279 – 285.

[lee08] S Lee, I Choi, S Kang, C Rivier. Role of various neurotransmitters in mediating the long-term endocrine consequences of prenatal alcohol exposure. *Ann. N. Y. Acad. Sci.* 1144 (2008) 176 – 188.

[leunen03] K Leunen, D Hall, H Odendaal, D Grove. The profile and complications of women with placental abruption and intrauterine death. *J. Trop. Pediatr* 49 (2003) 231 – 234.

[licona09] H de Licona, B Karacay, J Mahoney, E McDonald, T Luang, D Bonthius. A single exposure to alcohol during brain development induces microencephaly and neuronal losses in genetically susceptible mice, but not in wild type mice. *Neurotoxicology* 30 (2009) 459 - 470,

[lieber04] S Lieber. The discovery of the microsomal ethanol oxidizing system and its physiologic and pathologic role .*Drug Metab. Rev.* 36 (2004) 511 – 529.

[lin91] G W-J Lin. Maternal-fetal folate transfer: effect of ethanol and dietary folate deficiency. *Alcohol* 8 (1991) 169 – 172.

[lisander06] B Lisander, O Lundvall, J Tomner, A Jones. Enhanced rate of ethanol elimination from blood after intravenous administration of amino acids compared with equicaloric glucose. *Alcohol. Alcohol.* 41 (2006) 39 – 43.

[littner07] Y Littner, C Bearer. Detection of alcohol consumption during pregnancy – Current and future biomarkers. *Neurosci Biobehav. Rev.* 31 (2007) 261 – 269.

[liu06] Z Liu, R Neff, D Berg. Sequential interplay of nicotinic and GABAergic signaling guides neuronal development. *Science* 314 (2006) 1610 – 1613.

[livy08] D Livy, A Elberger. Alcohol exposure during the first two trimesters-equivalent alters the development of corpus callosum projection neurons in the rat. *Alcohol* 42 (2008) 285 – 293.

[lu08] Y Lu, A Cederbaum. CYP2E1 and oxidative liver injury by alcohol. *Free Radic. Biol. Med.* 44 (2008) 723 – 738.

[lucock03] M Lucock, Z Yates, T Glanville, R Leeming, N Simpson, I Daskalakis. A critical role for B-vitamin nutrition in human developmental and evolutionary biology. *Nutr. Res.* 23 (2003) 1463 – 1475.

[luisi00] S Luisi, F Petraglia, C Benedetto, R Nappi, F Bernardi, M Fadalti, F Reis, M Luisi, A Gennazzani. Serum allopregnanolone levels in pregnant women: changes during pregnancy, at delivery, and in hypertensive patients. *J. Clin. Endicrin. Metab.* 85 (2000) 2429 – 2433.

[lundberg09] JO Lundberg, M Gladwin, A Ahluwalia et al. Nitrate and nitrite in biology, nutrition and therapeutics. *Nature Chem. Biol.* 5 (2009) 865 – 869.

[lye01] S Lye, J Challis. Ch 12 in *Fetal growth and development.* Eds A Bocking, R Harding. Cambridge University Press, Cambridge 2001.

[lyer09] S Lyer, C Accardi, T Ziegler, R Blanco, J Ritzenthaler, M Rojas, J Roman, D Jones. Cysteine redox potential determines pro-inflammatory IL-1β levels. *PLOS ONE* 4 (2009) e5017.

[lymar95] SV Lymar, JK Hurst. Rapid reaction between peroxynitrite ion and carbon dioxide: Implications for biological activity. *J. Am. Chem. Soc.* 117 (1995) 8867 – 8868.

[maden00] M Maden. The role of retinoic acid in embryonic and post-embrionic development. *Proc. Nutr. Soc.* 59 (2000) 65 – 73.

[maegher99] E Maegher, O Barry, A Burke, M Lucey, J Lawson, J Rokach, G FitzGerald. Alcohol-induced geberation of lipid peroxidation products in humans. *J. Clin. Invest.* 104 (1999) 805 – 813.

[maffi08] S Maffi, M Rathinam, P Cherian, W Pate, R Hamby-Mason, S Schenker, G Henderson. Glutathione content as a potential mediator of the vulnerability of cultured fetal cortical neurons to ethanol-induced apoptosis. *J. Neurosci. Res.* 86 (2008) 1064 – 1076.

[makrigiannakis04] A Makrigiannakis, E Zoumakis, S kalantaridou, G Chrousos. Endometrial and placental CRH as regulators of human embryo implantation. *Rev. Reprod. Immunol.* 62 (2004) 53 – 59.

[maldve02] R Maldve, T Zhang, K Ferrani-Kile, S Schreiber, M Lippmann, G Snyder et al. DARPP-32 and regulation of the ethanol sensitivity of NMDA receptors in the nucleus accumbens. *Nature Neurosci.* 5 (2002) 641 – 648.

[mandel08] S Mandel, I Spivak-Pohis, I Gozes. ADNP differential nucleus/cytoplasm localization in neurons suggests multiple roles in neuronal differentiation and maintenance. *J. Mol. Neurosci.* 35 (2008) 127 – 141.

[matthews02] S Matthews. Early programming of the hypothalamo-pituitary-adrenal axis. *Trends Endocrinol. Metab.* 13 (2002) 373 – 380.

[mennella01] J Mennella, P Garcia-Gomez. Sleep disturbances after acute exposure to alcohol in mother's milk. *Alcohol* 25 (2001) 153 – 158.

[mennella05] J Mennella, M Pepino, K Teff. Acute alcohol consumption disrupts the hormonal milieu of lactating women. *J.Clin. Endocrin. Metab.* 90 (2005) 1979 – 1985.

[miller02] M Miller, J Luo. Effects of ethanol and transforming growth factor β (TGFβ) on neuronal proliferation and nCAM expression. *Alcohol Clin. Exp. Res.* 26 (2002) 1281 – 1285.

[miller06] M Miller. Effect of prenatal exposure to ethanol on glutamate and GABA immunoreactivity in macaque somatosensory and motor cortices: critical timing of exposure. *Neurosci.* 138 (2006) 97 – 107.

[minko09] I Minko, I Kozekov, T Harris, C Rizzo, R S Lloyd, m Stone. Chemistry and biology of DNA containing 1,$N^2$-deoxyguanosine adducts of the α,β-unsaturated aldehydes acrolein, crotonaldehyde, and 4-hydroxynonenal. *Chem. Res. Toxicol.* 22 (2009) 759 – 778.

[moffett06] *N-acetylaspartate: A unique neuronal molecule in the central nervous system.* J Moffett, S Tieman, D Weinberger, J Cole, M Namboodiri, eds. Springer, New York, 2006.

[moneypenny05] C Moneypenny, E Callagher. 4-Hydroxynonenal inhibits cell proliferation and alters differentiation pathways in human fetal liver hematopoietic stem cells. *Biochem. Pharmacol.* 69 (2005) 105 – 112.

[monte09] S de la Monte, L Longato, M Tong, S DeNucci, J Wands. The liver-brain axis of alcohol-mediated neurodegeneration: Role of toxic lipids. *Int. J. Environ. Res. Public Health* 6 (2009) 2055 – 2075.

[montfort08] C von Montfort, J Beier, L Guo, J P Kaiser, G Arteel. Contribution of the sympathetic hormone epinephrine to the sensitizing effect of ethanol on LPS-induced liver damage in mice. *Am. J. Gastrointest Liver Physiol.* 294 (2008) G1227 – 1234.

[moriarty04] S Moriarty-Craige, D Jones. Extracellular thiols and thiol/disulfide redox in metabolism. *Annu. Rev. Nutr.* 24 (2004) 481 – 509.

[morreale04] G Morreale de Escobar, M Obregon, F Escobar del Rey. Maternal thyroid hormones early in pregnancy an dfetal brain development. *Best Pract. Res. Clin. Endocrin. Met.* 18 (2004) 225 – 248.

[morrow01] A Morrow, M van Doren, S Penland, D Matthews. The role of GABAergic neuroactive steroids in ethanol action, tolerance and dependence. *Brain Res. Rev.* 39 (2001) 98 – 109.

[morrow09] A morrow, G Biggio, M Serra, H Becker, M Lopez, P Porcu, S Alward, T O'Buckley. The role of neuroactive steroids in ethanol/stress interactions: Proceedings of symposium VII at the Volterra conference on alcohol and stress, May 2008. *Alcohol* 43 (2009) 521 – 530.

[moya02] M Moya, A Gow, R Califf, R Goldberg, J Stamler. Inhaled ethyl nitrite gas for persistent pulmonary hypertension of the newborn. *Lancet* 360 (2002) 141 – 143.

[murillo03] M Murillo-Fuentes, M Murillo, O Carreras. Effects of maternal ethanol consumption during pregnancy or lactation on intestinal absorption of folic acid in suckling rats. *Life Sci.* 73 (2003) 2199 – 2209.

[murillo10] M-L Murillo-Fuentes, R Artillo, M-L Murillo, O Carreras. Different effects on zinc redistribution if ethanol is consumed before or immediately after birth. *J. Trace El. Med.Biol.* 24 (2010) 200 – 206.

[murrey10] S Murrey, A Brecher. Interaction of biogenic amine hormones with acetaldehyde. *Dig. Dis. Sci.* 55 (2010) 21 - 27.

[myatt06] L Myatt. Placental adaptive responses and fetal programming. *J. Physiol.* 572 (2006) 25 – 30.

[nam09]C Nam, A Case, B Hostager, M S O'Dorisio. The role of vasoactive intestinal protein (VIP) in megakaryocyte proliferation. *J. Mol. Neurosci.* 37 (2009) 160 – 167.

[naseer10] M Naseer, H Lee, M Kim. Neuroprotective effect of vitamin C against the ethanol and nicotine modulation of $GABA_B$ receptor and PKA-α expression in prenatal rat brain. *Synapse* 64 (2010) 467 – 477.

[nava04] A Nava-Ocampo, Y Velazquez-Armenta, J Brien, G Koren. Elimination kinetics of ethanol in pregnant women. *Reproduct Toxicol.* 18 (2004) 613 – 617.

[neville01] M Neville. The anatomy and physiology of lactation. *Pediatr Clin. North Am.* 48 (2001) 13 – 34.

[naseer10] M Naseer, H Lee, M Kim. Neuroprotective effect of vitamin C against ethanol and nicotine modulation of $GABA_B$ receptor and PKA-α expression in prenatal rat brain. *Synapse* 64 (2010) 467 – 477.

[niemela91] O Niemelä, E Halmesmäki, O Ylikorkala. Hemoglobin-acetaldehyde adducts are elevated in women carrying alcohol-damaged fetuses. *Alcohol. Clin. Exp. Res.* 15 (1991) 1007 – 1010.

[niemela01] O. Niemelä. Distribution of ethanol-induced protein adducts in vivo: relationship to tissue injury. *Free Radic. Biol. Med.* 31 (2001) 1533 – 1538.

[niemela04] O Niemelä, S Parkkila. Alcoholic macrocytosis – is there a role for acetaldehyde and adducts? *Addict* Biol (2004) 3-10.

[niemela07] O. Niemelä. Biomarkers in alcoholism. Clin Chim Acta 377 (2007) 39 – 49.

[nowoslawski05] L Nowoslawski, B Klocke, K Roth. Molecular regulation of acute ethanol-induced neuron apoptosis. *J. Neuropath Exp. Neurol.* 64 (2005) 490 – 497.

[nurmi09] K Nurmi, T Methuen, T Mäki, K Lindstedt, P Kovanen, C Sandler, K Eklund. Ethanol induces apoptosis in human mast cells. *Life Sci.* 85 (2009) 678 – 684.

[okouchi07] M Okouchi, O Ekshyyan, M Maracine, T Y Aw. Neuronal apoptosis in neurodegenration. *Antiox. Redox. Sig.* 9 (2007) 1059 – 1096.

[orhan03] H Orhan, L Onderoglu, A Yucel, G Sahin. Circulating biomarkers of oxidative stress in complicated pregnancies. *Arch. Gynecol. Obstet.* 267 (2003) 239 – 241.

[patterson05] P Patterson-Buckendahl, L Kubovcakova, O Krizanova, L Pohorecky, R Kvetnansky. Ethanol consumption increases rat stress hormones and adrenomedullary gene expression. *Alcohol* 37 (2005) 157 – 166.

[polikandriotis05] J Polikandriotis, H Rupnow, C M Hart. Chronic ethanol exposure stimulates endothelial cell nitric oxide production through PI-3 kinase and hsp90 dependent mechanisms. *Alcohol. Clin. Exp. Res.* 29 (2005) 1932 – 1938.

[pollard08] T.D. Pollard, W.C. Earnshaw. Cell biology, 2nd edition. Saunders Elsevier, Philadelphia 2008.

[perez06] M Perez, A Velasco, M Monte, J Gozalez-Buitrago, J Marin. Maternal ethanol consumption during pregnancy enhances bile acid-induced oxidative stress and apoptosis in fetal rat liver. *Toxicol.* 225 (2006) 183 – 194.

[perrotta03] S Perrotta, B Nobili, F Rossi, D Di Pinto, V Cucciolla, A Borriello, A Oliva, F Della Ragione. Vitamin A and infancy: Biochemical, functional, and clinical aspects. *Vit. Horm.* 66 (2003) 457 – 591.

[pike03] L Pike. Lipid rafts: bringing order to chaos. *J. Lipid Res.* 44 (2003) 655 – 667.

[pikkarainen71] P Pikkarainen. Metabolism of ethanol and acetaldehyde in perfused human fetal liver. *Life Sci.* 10 (1971) 1359 – 1364.

[pitocco08] D Pitocco, S Di, F Romitelli, B Tavazzi, A Manto, S Caputo, T Musella, C Zuppi, S Santini, G Ghirlanda. Hypouricemia linked to an overproduction of nitric oxide is an early marker of oxidative stress in female subjects with type 1 diabetes. *Diabetes Metab. Res. Rev.* 24 (2008) 318 – 323.

[porcu08] P Porcu, T O'Buckley, AL Morrow, B Adinoff. Differential hypothalamic-pituitary-adrenal activation of the neuroactive steroids pregnenolone sulphate and deoxycorticosterone in healthy controls and alcohol-dependent subjects. *Psychoneuroendocrin.* 33 (2008) 214 – 226.

[powroszek09] T Powroszek, M Miller. Ethanol affects transforming growth factor β1 – initiated signals: cross-talking pathways in the developing rat cerebral wall. *J. Neurosci.* 29 (2009) 9521 – 9533.

[puddey01] I Puddey, R Zilkens, K Croft, L Beilin. Alcohol and endothelial function: A brief review. *Clin. Exp. Pharmacol. Physiol.* 28 (2001) 1020 – 1024.

[pueta08] M Pueta, P Abate, O Haymal, N Spear, J Molina. Ethanol exposure during late gestation and nursing in the rat: Effects upon maternal care, ethanol metabolism and infantile milk intake. *Pharmacol. Biochem. Behav.* 91 (2008) 21 – 31.

[purdy05] R Purdy, F Valenzuela, P Janak, D Finn, G Biggio, T Bäckström. Neuroactive steroids and ethanol. *Alchol. Clin. Exp. Res.* 29 (2005) 1292 – 1298.

[quertemont05] E Quertemont, S Tambour, E Tirelli. The role of acetaldehyde in the neurobehavioral effects of ethanol: A comprehensive review of animal studies. *Prog. Neurbiol.* 75 (2005) 247 – 274.

[quertemont06] E Quertemint, V Didone. Role fo acetaldehyde in mediating the pharmacological and behavioral effects of alcohol. *Alcohol. Res. Health* 29 (2006) 258 – 265.

[rakic90] P Rakic. Principles of neural cell migration. *Experientia* 46 (1990) 882 – 891.

[ramachandran01] V Ramachandran, A Perez, J Chen, D Senthil, S Schenker, G Henderson. In utero ethanol exposure causes mitochondrial dysfunction, which can result in apoptotic cell death in fetal brain: A potential role for 4-hydroxynonenal. *Alcohol. Clin. Exp. Res.* 25 (2001) 862 – 871.

[ramachandran03] V Ramachandran, L Watts, S Maffi, J Chen, S Schenker, G Henderson. Ethanol-induced oxidative stress precedes mitochondrially mediated apoptotic death of cultured fetal cortical neurons. *J. Neurosci. Res.* 74 (2003) 577 – 588.

[randall96] C Randall, U Ekblad, N White, J Cook. Increase in vasoactive prostaglandin E production after perfusion in human placental cotyledons. *Alcohol. Clin. Exp. Res.* 20 (1996) 1321 – 1328.

[rathinam06] M Rathinam, L Talley Watts, A Stark, L Mahimainathan, J Stewart, S Schenker, G Henderson. Astrocyte control of fetal cortical neuron glutathione homeostasis: up-regulation by ethanol. *J. Neurochem.* 96 (2006) 1289 – 1300.

[raza06] H Raza, A John. 4-Hydroxynoneal induces mitochondrial oxidative stress, apoptosis and expression of glutathione transferase A4-4 and cytochrome P450 2E1 in PC12 cells. *Toxicol. Appl. Pharmacol.* 216 (2006) 309 – 318.

[regan99] R Regan, Y Guo. Potentiation of excitotoxic injury by high concentrations of extracellular reduced glutathione. *Neurosci.* 91 (1999) 463 – 470.

[ron04] D Ron. Signaling cascades regulating NMDA receptor sensitivity to ethanol. *Neuroscientist* 10 (2004) 325 – 336.

[rosenberg09] M Rosenberg, C Wolff, A El-Emawy, M Staples, N Perrone-Bizzozero, D Savage. Effects of moderate drinking during pregnancy on placental gene expression. *Alcohol* (2009) 1- 18.

[saito05] M Saito, M Saito, T Cooper, C Vadasz. Ethanol-induced changes in the content of triglycerides, ceramides, and glucosylceramides in cultured neurons. *Alcohol. Clin. Exp. Res.* 29 (2005) 1374 – 1383.

[salinas08] P Salinas, Y Zou. Wnt signalling in neural circuit assembly. *Annu. Rev. Neurosci.* 31 (2008) 339 – 358.

[sampath05] H Sampath, J Ntambi. Polyunsaturated fatty acid regulation of genes of lipid metabolism. *Anny. Rev. Nutr.* 25 (2005) 317 – 340.

[sanghani03] P Sanghani, H Robinson, R Bennett-Lovsey, T Hurley, W Bosron. Structure-function relationships in human Class III alcohol dehydrogenase (formaldehyde dehydrogenase). *Chem. Biol. Interact.* 143 (2003) 195 – 200.

[sari06] Y Sari, I Gozes. Brain deficits associated with fetal alcohol exposure may be protected, in part, by peptides derived from activity-dependent neurotrophic factor and activity-dependent neuroprotective protein. *Brain Res. Rev.* 52 (2006) 107 – 118.

[sarkola02] T. Sarkola, M Iles, K Kohlenberg-Muller, C Peter Eriksson. Ethanol, acetaldehyde, acetate, and lactate levels after alcohol intake in white men and women: effect of 4-methylpyrazole. *Alcohol. Clin. Exp. Res.* 26 (2002) 239 – 245.

[schuchardt10] J Schuchardt, M Huss, M Strauss-Grabo, A Hahn. Significance of long-chain polyunsaturated fatty acids (PUFAs) for the development and behaviour of children. *Eur. J. Pediatr.* 169 (2010) 149 – 164.

[seitz06] H Seitz, P Meier. The role of acetaldehyde in upper digestive tract cancer in alcoholics. *Transl. Res.* 149 (2007) 293 – 297.

[sequerra07] E Sequerra, P Gardino, C Hedin-Pereira, F de Mello. Putresceine as an important source of GABA in the postnatal rat subventricular zone. *Neurosci.* 146 (2007) 489 – 493.

[seyfarth08] E Seyfarth, E Schleussner, U Markert. Impact of PUFA on early immune and fetal development. *Br. J. Nutr.* 100 (2008) 1158 – 1168.

[siegenthaler04] J Siegenthaler, M Miller. Transforming growth factor β1 modulates cell migration in rat cortex: Effects of ethanol. *Cereb. Cortex.* 14 (2004) 791 – 802.

[signore08] C Signore, S Aros, J Morrow, J Trundle, M Conley, E Flanigan, F Cassorla, J Mills. Markers of oxidative stress and systemic vasoconstriction in pregnant women drinking > 48 grams of alcohol per day. *Alcohol. Clin. Exp. Res.* 32 (2008) 1893 – 1898.

[sikkema01] J Sikkema, B van Rijn, A Franx, H Bruinse, R de Roos, E Stroes, E van Faassen. Placental superoxide is increased in preeclampsia. *Placenta* 22 (2001) 304 – 308.

[siler00] T Siler-Khodr, Y Yang, M Grayson, G Henderson, M Lee, S Schenker. Effect of ethanol on thromboxane and prostacyclin production in the human placenta. *Alcohol* 21 (2000) 169 – 180.

[simpson05] M Simpson, S Duggal, K Keiver. Prenatal alcohol exposure has differential effects on fetal growth and skeletal ossification. *Bone* 26 (2005) 521 – 532.

[sliwowska08] J Sliwowska, N Lan, F Yamashita, A Halpert, V Viau, J Weinbarg. Effects of ethanol exposure on regulation of the basal hypothalamic – pituitary - adrenal activity and hippocampal 5-$HT_{1A}$ receptor mRNA levels in female rats across the estrous cycle. *Psychoneuroendocrinol.* 33 (2008) 1111 – 1123.

[snow07] M Snow, K Keiver. Prenatal alcohol exposure disrupts the histological stages of fetal bone development. *Bone* 41 (2007) 181 – 187.

[sokol03] R Sokol, V Delaney-Black, B Nordstrom. Fetal alcohol spectrum disorder. *JAMA* 290 (2003) 2996 – 2999.

[spanagel09] R Spanagel. Alcoholism: A systems approach from molecular physiology to addictive behavior. *Physiol. Rev.* 89 (2009) 649 – 705.

[stevens05] R Stevens, R Cohen, M-B Terry, B Lasley, Pentti Siiteri, B Cohn. Alcohol consumption and serum hormone levels during pregnancy. *Alcohol.* 36 (2005) 47 – 53.

[stoler98] J Stoler, K Huntington, C Peterson, K Peterson, P Daniel, K Aboagye, E Lieberman, L Ryan, L Holmes. The prenatal detection of significant alcohol exposure with maternal blood markers. *J. Pediatr.* 133 (1998) 346 – 352.

[stroes00] E Stroes, E van Faassen, P Martasek, R Wever, P Boer, R Govers, T Rabelink. Folic acid reverts dysfunction of endothelial nitric oxide synthase. *Circ. Res.* 86 (2000) 1129 – 1134.

[stulnig04] T Stulnig, M Zeyda. Immunomodulation by polyunsaturated fatty acids: Impact on T-cell signaling. *Lipids* 39 (2004) 1171 – 1175.

[sulik05] K Sulik. (2005) Genesis of alcohol-induced craniofacial dysmorphism. *Exp. Biol. Med.* 230 (2005) 366-375.

[summers08] B Summers, C Henry, A Rofe, P Coyle. Dietary zinc supplementation during pregnancy prevents spatial and object recognition memory impairments caused by early prenatal ethanol exposure. *Behav. Brain Res.* 186 (2008) 230 – 238.

[szabo07] G Szabo, A Dolganiuc, Q Dai, S Pruett. TLR4, ethanol, and lipid rafts: A new mechanism of ethanol action with implications for other receptor-mediated effects. *J. Immunol.* 178 (2007) 1243 – 1249.

[takahama08] U Takahama, M Tanaka, S Hirota. Transformation of ethyl alcohol to ethyl nitrite in acidified saliva: Possibility of its occurrence in the stomach. *Arch. Biochem. Biophys.* 475 (2008) 135 – 139.

[tapiero03] H Tapiero, K Tew. Trace elements in human physiology and pathology: Zinc and metallothioneins. *Biomed. Pharmacother.* 57 (2003) 399 – 411.

[terragni08] J Terragni, J Graham, K Adams, M Schaffer, J Tullai, G Cooper. Phosphatidylinositol 3-kinase signalling in proliferating cells maintains an anti-apoptotic transcriptional program mediated by inhibition of FOXO and non-canonical activation of NFκB transcription factors. *BMC Cell Biol.* 9 (2008) 471-2121/9/6

[thomasson95] H Thomasson. Gender differences in alcohol metabolism. Physiological responses to ethanol. Ch 7 in *Recent developments in alcoholism Vol 12: Women and alcoholism.* Ed M Galanter, Plenum Press, New York 1995.

[thompson09] C Thompson, B Sonawane, R Grafström. The ontogeny, distribution and regulation of alcohol dehydrogenase 3: Implications for pulmonary physiology. *Drug Metab. Disp.* 37 (2009) 1565 – 1571.

[tollinger79] C Tollinger, H Vreman, M Weiner. Measurement of acetate in human blood by gas chromatography: effects of sample preparation, feeding and various diseases. *Clin. Chem.* 25 (1979) 1787 – 1790.

[traves95] C Traves, L Camps, D Lopez-Tejero. Liver alcohol dehydrogenase activity and ethanol levels during chronic ethanol intake in pregnant rats and their offspring. *Pharmacol. Biochem. Behav.* 52 (1995) 93 – 99.

[tsukamoto95] H Tsukamoto, W Horne, S Kamimura, O Niemelä, S Parkkila, S Ylä-Herttuala, G Brittenham. Experimental liver cirrhosis induced by alcohol and iron. *J. Clin. Invest.* 96 (1995) 620 – 630.

[tuma02] D J Tuma. Role of malondialdehyde – acetaldehyde adducts in liver injury. *Free Radic. Biol. Med.* 32 (2002) 303 – 308.

[turner10] R Turner, C Rosen, U Iwaniec. Effects of alcohol on skeletal response to growth hormone in hypophysectomized rats. *Bone* 46 (2010) 806 – 812.

[tyzio06] R Tyzio, R Cossart, I Khalilov, M Minlebaev, C Hübner, A Represa, Y Ben-Ari, R Khazipov. Maternal oxytocin triggers a transient inhibitory switch in GABA signaling in the fetal brain during delivery. *Science* 314 (2006) 1788 – 1792.

[uziel06] D Uziel, P Garcez, R Lent, C Peuckert, R Niehage, F Weth, J Bolz,. Connecting thalamus and cortex.: The role of ephrins. *Anat. Rec. A Discov. Mol. Cell Evol. Biol.* 288 (2006) 135 – 142.

[vidali08] M Vidali, J Hietala, G Occhino, A Ivaldi, S Sutti, O Niemelä, E Albano. Immune responses against oxidative stress-derived antigens are associated with increased circulating tumor necrosis factor-alpha in heavy drinkers. *Free Radic. Biol. Med.* 45 (2008) 306 – 311.

[wang05] J Wang, P Johnston, B Ball, R Diaz Brinton. The neurosteroid allopregnanolone promotes proliferation of rodent and human neural progenitor cells and regulates cell-cycle gene and protein expression. *J. Neurosci.* 25 (2005) 4706 – 4718.

[ward03] I Ward, O B Ward, J Affuso, W Long III, J French, S Hendricks. Fetal testosterone surge: specific modulations induced in male rats by maternal stress and/or alcohol consumption. *Hormones Behav.* 43 (2003) 531 – 539.

[warren05] K Warren, T Li. Genetic polymorphism: impact on the risk of fetal alcohol spectrum disorders. *Birth Defects Res. A Clin. Mol. Teratol.* 73 (2005) 195 – 203.

[watson98] A Watson, J Skepper, A Jauniaux, G Burton. Changes in concentration, localization and activity of catalase within the human placenta during early gestation. *Placenta* 19 (1998) 27 – 34.

[weinberg08] J Weinberg, J Sliwowska, N Lan, K Hellemans. Prenatal alcohol exposure.: foetal programming , the hypothalamic – pituitary – adrenal axis and sex differences in outcome. *J. Neuroendocrin.* 20 (2008) 470 – 488.

[wen04] Z Wen, H Kim. Alterations in hippocampal phospholipids profile by prenatal exposure to ethanol. *J. Neurochem.* 89 (2004) 1368 – 1377.

[wilcoxon04] J Slone Wilcoxon, E Redei. Prenatal programming of adult thyroid function by alcohol and thyroid hormones. *Am. J. Physiol. Endocrin. Metab.* 287 (2004) 318 – 326.

[wu03] D Wu, A Cederbaum. Alcohol, oxidative stress, and free radical damage. *Alcohol. Res. Health* 27 (2003) 277 – 284.

[wu05] D Wu, A Cederbaum. Oxidative stress mediated toxicity exerted by ethanol-inducible CYP2E1. *Toxicol. Appl. Pharmacol.* 207 (2005) 70 – 76.

[wu06] D Wu, A Cederbaum. Nitric oxide donors prevent while the nitric oxide synthase inhibitor L-NAME increases arachidonic acid plus CYP2E1 – dependent activity. *Toxicol. Appl. Pharmacol.* 216 (2006) 282 – 292.

[yacoob09] P Yacoob. The nutritional significance of lipid rafts. *Annu. Rev. Nutr.* 29 (2009) 257 – 282.

[yaka03] R Yaka, K Phamluong, D Ron. Scaffolding of Fyn kinase to the NMDA receptor determines brain region sensitivity to ethanol. *J. Neurosci.* 23 (2003) 3623 – 3632.

[yamamoto05] T Yamamoto, Y Moriwaki, S Takahashi. Effect of ethanol on metabolism of purine bases (hypoxanthine, xanthine and uric acid). *Clin. Chim. Acta* 356 (2005) 35 – 57.

[yan06] J Yan, B Hales. Depletion of glutathione induces 4-hydroxynonenal protein adducts and hydroxyurea teratogenicity in the organogenesis stage mouse embryo. *J. Pharmacol. Exp. Ther.* 319 (2006) 613 – 621.

[yeaney09] N Yeaney, M He, N Tang, A malouf, M O'Riordan, V Lemmon, C Bearer. Ethanol inhibits L1 cell adhesion molecule tyrosine phosphorylation and dephosphorylation and activation of pp60(src). *J. Neurochem.* 110 (2009) 779-790.

[yeh07] M Yeh, E Burnham, M Moss, L Brown. Chronic alcoholism alters systemic and pulmonary glutathione redox status. *Am. J. Respir. Crit. Care Med.* 176 (2007) 270 – 276.

[yin02] S-J Yin, C-F Chou, C-L Lai, S-L Lee, C-L Han. Human class IV alcohol dehydrogenase: kinetic mechanism, functional roles and medical relevance. *Chemico-Biol. Interact.* 143 (2002) 219 – 227.

[young03] C Young, B Klocke, T Tenkova, J Choi, J Labruyere, Y-Q Qin, D Holtzman, K Roth, J Olney. Ethanol-induced neuronal apoptosis in vivo requires BAX in the developing mouse brain. *Cell Death Differ.* 10 (2003) 1148 – 1155.

[zeyda06] M Zeyda, T Stulnig. Lipid rafts and Co: an integrated model of membrane organization in T-cell activation. *Prog. Lipid Res.* 45 (2006) 187 – 202.

[zhang05] X Zhang, J Sliwowska, J Weinberg. Prenatal alcohol exposure on hypothalamic-pituitary-adrenal responses and fetal programming: effects on neuroendicrine and immune function. *Exp. Biol. Med.* 230 (2005) 376 – 388.

[zhou04] F Zhou, Y Sari, T Powrozek, C Spong. A Neuroprotective peptide antagonizes fetal alcohol exposure-compromised brain growth. *J. Mol. Neurosci.* 24 (2004) 189 – 199.

[zhou05] F Zhou, Y Sari, T Powrozek. Fetal alcohol exposure reduces serotonin innervation and compromises development of the forebrain along the serotonergic pathway. *Alcohol. Clin. Exp. Res.* 29 (2005) 141 – 149.

[zhou08] F Zhou, Y Fang, C Goodlett. Peptidergic agonists of activity-dependent neurotrophic factor protect against prenatal alcohol-induced neural tube defects and serotonin neuron loss. *Alcohol. Clin. Exp. Res.* 32 (2008) 1361 – 1371.

[zink09]M Zink, G Arac, S Frank, P Gass, P Gebicke-Härter, R Spanagel. Perinatal exposure to alcohol reduces the expression of complexins I and II. *Neurotoxicol. Teratol.* 31 (2009) 400 – 405.

[zoeller00] R Zoeller, K Crofton. Thyroid hormone action in fetal brain development and potential for disruption by environmental chemicals. *Neurotoxicology* 21 (2000) 935 – 945.

In: Pregnancy and Alcohol Consumption
Editor: Joshua D. Hoffman, pp. 67-103
ISBN 978-1-61761-122-3


*Chapter 2*

# MECHANISMS OF FETAL TOXICITY TO ALCOHOL WITH SPECIAL CONSIDERATION TO FETAL ZINC DEFICIENCY

***P. Coyle, B. L. Summers-Pearce, C. J. Cowley, and A. M. Rofe***
SA Pathology, Institute of Medical and Veterinary Science, South Australia

## ABSTRACT

Alcohol use in pregnancy is associated with a wide range of adverse pregnancy outcomes and whilst the likelihood of these increases with heavy drinking patterns, morbidity to the fetus may nevertheless result from an acute episode of alcohol consumption (i.e. "binge-drinking"). Increased maternal age, genetic susceptibility to alcohol, low socio-economic status, tobacco smoking and illicit drug use have all been reported to contribute to increased risk from alcohol exposure in pregnancy. Fundamental to understanding the risks associated with alcohol consumption in pregnancy and to providing an insight into factors that may contribute to comorbidity, is a basic understanding of how alcohol causes fetotoxicity. In this chapter we will review the potential mechanisms causing alcohol-mediated damage to the fetus, including altered retinoic acid metabolism, excess prostaglandins, oxidative stress and alterations in placental structure and function, with a particular focus on the accumulating evidence that fetal zinc deficiency may underpin many of events that interrupt developmental processes. This chapter also includes new findings in regard to zinc homeostasis, including the roles of the metal binding protein metallothionein and zinc transporters, and the regulation of these by inflammatory mediators.

# INTRODUCTION

Alcohol exposure during pregnancy can impair fetal development, and is associated with an increased risk of spontaneous abortion, growth retardation, congenital malformations and central nervous system dysfunction [Jones *et al.* 1973; Streissguth *et al.* 1980]. These fetal abnormalities may not only result from the chronic consumption of alcohol at high intakes and frequency, but also from a single episode of alcohol intake, which is commonly referred to as "binge drinking or exposure" (> 4 drinks /occasion). The range of disorders caused by prenatal alcohol exposure, most accurately termed fetal alcohol spectrum disorders (FASD), extends from full fetal alcohol syndrome (FAS) through to a milder although often clinically significant form which can affect physical, learning and behavioural outcomes (e.g. partial FAS, alcohol related neurodevelopmental disorders (ARND) or alcohol related birth defects (ARBD)). Although all FASD would be prevented if women abstained from drinking alcohol during pregnancy, acceptance of this advice is not uniformly taken as not all women are motivated sufficiently to change their drinking patterns [Goransson *et al.* 2003; Kesmodel *et al.* 2003; Colvin *et al.* 2007; Urban *et al.* 2008]. In addition, various studies have reported that up to two-thirds of pregnancies are unplanned and this suggests that many women may unwittingly expose their fetus to alcohol before they recognise they are pregnant [Kesmodel *et al.* 2003; Colvin *et al.* 2007; Urban *et al.* 2008]. Taken together, these studies indicate that adverse fetal outcomes resulting from alcohol consumption during pregnancy will continue to be a major health concern in the foreseeable future.

Despite extensive research demonstrating the harm to the fetus associated with alcohol in pregnancy, there remains a paucity of studies which provide insight into how alcohol causes the range of birth anomalies associated with FASD. Such knowledge is essential in understanding factors that may contribute to co-morbidity and may be important in identifying potential intervention strategies that may help reduce or prevent fetal morbidity. The general dogma is that alcohol teratogenicity is likely to occur through multiple mechanisms working independently, or in combination, and are likely activated at different dose thresholds of exposure and different stages of development to produce the full spectrum of outcomes caused by alcohol. However, establishing the major pathways involved is complicated by the fact that alcohol interferes with numerous molecular, neurochemical and cellular events which occur during normal fetal development and causes a relatively wide variability in the type and severity of pathophysiological outcomes in the fetus. Over the last decade, investigations using animal models of FAS have provided new insight into primary events that may initiate the pathways leading to alcohol-related teratogenicity. The focus of this chapter is to review and discuss the evidence supporting several potential mechanisms which have been demonstrated to mediate the effects of alcohol. However, it is important to first review the maternal and environmental factors that are known to increase the vulnerability of the fetus to alcohol exposure, and potentially influence the mechanisms mediating alcohol teratogenicity and the type and severity of alcohol-related outcomes.

# RISK FACTORS INFLUENCING THE EFFECT OF ALCOHOL

## Patterns of Alcohol Exposure during Pregnancy

It has long been recognised that the incidence of mortality, malformations and behavioural impairments from prenatal alcohol increase in a dose-dependant manner [Randall and Taylor 1979; Streissguth *et al.* 1994; Sood *et al.* 2001]. This supports the view that the number of drinks per occasion or peak blood alcohol concentrations (pBAC), rather than solely the exposure to alcohol in utero, is the critical factor in producing defective embryos. In other words, the higher the quantity of alcohol and the quicker it is consumed, the higher the pBAC and the more likely that a teratogenic "threshold" is reached [Abel and Hannigan 1995]. However, this level has not yet been determined. The involvement of pBAC in the aetiology of FASD is reflected in a recent study where estimated pBAC in mothers of FAS children were higher in comparison to mothers where only partial FAS expression was observed [May *et al.* 2008]. As binge drinking results in high pBAC exposure to the fetus, this pattern of alcohol consumption has been demonstrated to be particularly harmful, even if the overall alcohol amount consumed is less than those of chronic intake patterns [West *et al.* 1990; Maier and West 2001]. In animal studies, a single acute dose of alcohol during pregnancy has been found to result in fetal malformations, neurodevelopmental anomalies and increased risk of post natal death [Sulik 1984; West *et al.* 1990; Summers *et al.* 2006; Summers *et al.* 2008; Summers *et al.* 2009]. In humans, children from binge-drinking mothers have been found to exhibit especially severe cognitive and behavioural deficits [Maier and West 2001]. A further study conducted on children exposed to binge drinking were found to be 1.7 times more likely to have IQ scores in the mentally retarded range and 2.5 times more likely to have delinquent behaviour [Bailey *et al.* 2004].

## Timing of Exposure during Pregnancy

The timing of exposure to alcohol during pregnancy is critical in determining the fetal phenotype and severity of outcome. This is because embryonic and fetal development occurs in a very structured and regulated pattern, with particular growth and developmental processes occurring at specific periods during pregnancy. However, these stages of development are not equally susceptible to the damaging effects of alcohol. A critical period of vulnerability to alcohol occurs during the organogenesis stage of gestation (i.e. 3-8 weeks of gestation in humans) where animal studies have demonstrated an increased incidence of craniofacial and brain pathologies; the most common malformations of FAS [Sulik 1984; Day *et al.* 1989; Becker *et al.* 1996; Goodlett *et al.* 2005]. In addition, windows of vulnerability to alcohol-induced cell death have been found to occur during the brain growth spurt [Guerri *et al.* 1990; Hamre and West 1993; Ikonomidou *et al.* 2000], where depletion of cells can explain the reduced brain mass and neurobehavioural disturbances that are associated with FAS [Ikonomidou *et al.* 2000].

## Maternal Factors

FAS is estimated to occur in only 4.3% of all live births in women who drink "heavily" during pregnancy (i.e. clinical diagnosis, reported consuming 5 or more drinks per occasion or an average of 2 or more drinks per day) [Abel 1995]. This low incidence in a population of women seeming at the highest risk of FAS and alcohol-related impairments would suggest that FAS is not equally manifested [Abel 1995], nor can the severity of fetal outcomes be fully determined by the level of alcohol exposure. These findings indicate that there are other maternal factors in addition to the pattern of alcohol consumption and the timing of exposure, which act to intercede or alter the actions of alcohol on the developing fetus.

### *Genetic and Ethnic Susceptibility*

Twin studies report similar FAS outcomes in identical twins but different outcomes in non-identical twins [Streissguth and Dehaene 1993], indicating that genetic factors can influence individual susceptibility to the effects of alcohol. Moreover, in studies with mice there is evidence that different genotypes have different sensitivity to alcohol [Crabbe and Harris 1991]. Variations in the metabolic capacity of the mother, which may be the result of genetic polymorphisms of genes encoding enzymes involved in alcohol metabolism, have been proposed to explain differences in the peak alcohol exposure of the fetus between individuals and have been implicated in the pathogenesis of FASD [Warren and Li 2005; Gemma *et al.* 2007]. In addition, genetic modulation of nitric oxide synthase expression has also been linked with neuronal injury caused by alcohol-induced oxidative stress (see section below on Oxidative Stress) [Haorah *et al.* 2008].

There is similarity in function of shared versions (alleles) of the gene that encodes alcohol dehydrogenase in some persons with shared ancestry (e.g. Native Americans) which may increase risk for alcohol dependence [Mulligan *et al.* 2003]. The incidence of FAS in populations characterised by African American or Native American background has been reported to be higher than those with a Caucasian background [Abel 1995]. Studies have shown that African Americans or Native Americans have higher rates of alcohol elimination compared with Caucasians, indicating that different susceptibility to alcohol toxicity may occur in different ethnic groups [Bosron *et al.* 1993]. However, inter-individual and ethnic variability in FASD may result from a combination of genetic and environmental factors which influence alcohol metabolism [Gemma *et al.* 2006]. Cultural factors such as drinking patterns and socioeconomic status (which is highly associated with race/ethnicity) may also contribute to differences in FAS between groups. Black, Hispanic, American Indian/Alaskan native and Asian/Pacific Islander women have all been reported as less likely to quit binge drinking while pregnant compared to Caucasian women [Tenkku *et al.* 2009].

### *Maternal Age*

Advancing age of the mother (>25 years of age at the time the child is born) has been identified as a maternal risk factor for FAS [May and Gossage 2001; May *et al.* 2009]. Jacobson and colleagues found that infants born to mothers drinking five or more drinks per occasion at least weekly, were 2 to 5 times more likely to be functionally impaired when the mother is 30 years of age or older. This outcome was not due to younger mothers having a lower level of alcohol consumption. Physiological changes, including an age-related increase in maternal body fat-to-water ratio and a faster rate of alcohol metabolism in chronic drinking mothers has been suggested to account for the increased vulnerability of children born to older mothers [Jacobson *et al.* 1996; Jacobson *et al.* 1998].

### *Low Socio-Economic Status*

Mothers with FAS children are more likely to live in impoverished or low socio-economic status (SES) areas [Bingol *et al.* 1987; Abel 1995; Abel and Hannigan 1995; May *et al.* 2009]. This is typically seen in South Africa women where the highest incidence of FAS is reported [May *et al.* 2000; Viljoen *et al.* 2005; May *et al.* 2007]. In a study comparing FAS in offspring of lower and upper middle class chronic alcoholic mothers, the incidence of FAS was significantly higher in offspring of lower SES mothers (70.9%) than offspring of upper-middle class mothers (4.5%). It is proposed that differences in FAS between socioeconomic groups are due to an interaction of genetic factors, social factors, poor nutrition and the cumulative effect of intergenerational maternal alcoholism in the low SES group [Bingol *et al.* 1987; May *et al.* 2009]. Undernutrition is commonly associated with chronic alcohol abuse and FAS [Abel and Hannigan 1995; Guerrini *et al.* 2007]. As alcohol replaces other energy sources in the diet, maternal undernutrition could contribute to the severity of alcohol-related outcomes by reducing the availability of nutrients to the fetus which are required for optimal development [Leis-Marquez and Guzman-Huerta 1999; Black 2001; Lozoff and Georgieff 2006; Antony 2007].

### *Smoking and Illicit Drug Use*

Smoking (tobacco) and drug use are commonly observed in women who consume alcohol during pregnancy [Flynn *et al.* 2003; Urban *et al.* 2008; Morojele *et al.* 2010]. A higher risk of prenatal alcohol abuse has been shown to be predicted by smoking status [Flynn *et al.* 2003; Morojele *et al.* 2010] and 80% of mothers of children with FAS were reported to currently smoke [Urban *et al.* 2008]. Similarly, drug users (use more than one illicit drug) from a cohort of low-income women, were more likely to report frequent drinking, binge-drinking and drinking during pregnancy compared with non-users [Sharpe and Velasquez 2008]. Smoking, cocaine and heroin can contribute to adverse pregnancy outcomes, particularly low birth-weight [Nakamura *et al.* 2004]. The risk of delivering a small for gestation age infant was found to be higher among women who reported both drinking and smoking compared to drinking without smoking [Aliyu *et al.* 2009]. It has been proposed that smoking and drugs may enhance the teratogenic effects of alcohol by reducing the levels of nutrients, or reducing fetal oxygenation (via effects on uterine blood flow) resulting in hypoxia and increased free radical formation [Young 1997].

## Mechanisms of Alcohol Teratogenicity

While identifying molecular pathways involved in alcohol teratogenicity has been complicated by an interaction of the maternal, environmental and genetic risk factors described, multiple mechanisms have been reported in the literature to mediate the effect of alcohol on the fetus. Alcohol may influence embryonic or fetal development directly by passing across the placenta and interacting with fetal cells, or indirectly, by causing biochemical or physiological changes in the mother which can be detrimental to the fetus. For example, nutritional and hormonal factors can be affected by maternal alcohol exposure and as these factors have a direct influence on embryonic development, any alterations can therefore influence organ formation and growth [Michaelis and Michaelis 1994]. The remainder of this chapter will review the potential mechanisms of alcohol teratogenicity which include direct effects of alcohol on the fetus, as well as indirect mechanisms, such as the effect of acetylaldehyde, oxidative stress, altered retinoic acid metabolism, excess prostaglandins, and impaired placental nutrient delivery on fetal development. Fetal Zn deficiency, as another potential mechanism mediating alcohol-related teratogenicity, will then be discussed in greater detail with evidence that this mechanism may be one of the underlying mediators interrupting fetal development in utero.

## Direct Effect of Alcohol on the Fetus

Many researchers have claimed that alcohol has a direct effect on fetal development. Impaired DNA myelination [Overholser 1990], decreased synthesis of DNA [Dreosti *et al.* 1981] altered protein synthesis, RNA transport [Henderson and Schenker 1977], cell membrane fluidity and composition, and impaired growth signalling [Schenker *et al.* 1990a] have all been purported to result from the direct effect of alcohol on these cellular processes. That alcohol alone is responsible for fetal damage is supported by the following evidence; (1) alcohol is able to cross the placenta into the fetal blood circulation and reach concentrations equal to that of maternal blood; (2) *in vitro* embryos cultured in alcohol causes dose dependent damage to the fetus which parallels that observed *in vivo*, (3) when products that block alcohol metabolism to acetaldehyde, via the inhibition of alcohol dehydrogenase, are added to culture with alcohol, teratogenic effects on the fetus are still observed, and (4) that tertiary-butanol, a form of alcohol but is not metabolised to acetaldehyde, causes some of the teratogenicity observed following exposure to alcohol.

### *Placental Alcohol Transfer*

The dynamics of placental alcohol transfer has been examined in many *in vivo* studies using both pregnant women [Nava-Ocampo *et al.* 2004] and experimental animals including sheep [Ng *et al.* 1982; Wilkening *et al.* 1982], mice [Blakley and Scott 1984b], rats [Hayashi *et al.* 1991] and guinea pigs [Clarke *et al.* 1986]. Alcohol, a small hydrophilic and lipophilic molecule, is known to freely and readily diffuse across the placenta and accumulate in the fetus [Overholser 1990]. In mouse dams treated with alcohol on day 10 of gestation, the appearance of alcohol in the embryo occurred 5 minutes after treatment, with maximal concentrations of alcohol occurring 1 hour following treatment, but still remained significantly lower than maternal blood concentrations [Blakley and Scott 1984b]. However, in a study in which an oral dose of alcohol was given to women at 16-18 weeks of pregnancy, amniotic fluid alcohol levels were observed to be nearly identical to maternal blood levels after 1.5 hours [Nava-Ocampo *et al.* 2004]. Similarly, in rats orally administered with alcohol, alcohol readily crossed the placenta and 2 hours following exposure maternal and fetal blood alcohol concentrations had equilibrated [Hayashi *et al.* 1991].

### *In Vitro Toxicity to Alcohol*

In order to remove the maternal influences that may confound the teratogenic effects of alcohol, many studies have focused on exposing embryos to alcohol in an *in vitro* culture system [Michaelis and Michaelis 1994]. In culture studies, the majority of damage was found in rat embryos undergoing organogenesis (gestation day (GD) 7-14) with the most prevalent abnormalities being growth retardation and the failure of the neural tube to close [Brown *et al.* 1979; Giavini *et al.* 1992]. There was also a strong relationship between alcohol dose and the incidence of malformations including open neural tube, failure of normal embryo rotation and defects of the heart. In studies on mouse embryos that were cultured *in vitro* with alcohol from GD9, severe growth retardation and fetal dysmorphology, including exencephaly and microcephaly, was observed [Higuchi and Matsumoto 1984]. In a more recent study, alcohol was found to inhibit brain development in GD8 cultured mouse embryos, with the most prevalent abnormality being the failure of cephalic neural tube closure [Jing and Li 2004]. Alcohol also affected cranial morphology, where embryos showed reduced forebrain and abnormal head shape. This study also found that in mid brain cell cultures at GD 12, alcohol inhibited neuronal differentiation and proliferation. However, whilst the findings from in vitro studies are indicative of a direct effect of alcohol there still remains doubt as to the physiological relevance of these experiments to whole body system where alcohol concentrations reaching the fetus are likely to be lower and more transient.

### *Inhibitors of Alcohol Metabolism*

In studies where alcohol dehydrogenase activity has been inhibited, preventing alcohol metabolism to acetaldehyde, embryo teratogenicity still occurs [Varma and Persaud 1979; Blakley and Scott 1984a]. The findings suggest that alcohol itself is the active agent responsible for the teratogenicity. Pyrazole and 4-methylpyrazole are both potent inhibitors of alcohol dehydrogenase which in turn significantly reduces the rate of alcohol metabolism [Goldberg and Rydberg 1969; Rydberg and Neri 1972]. When pyrazole was co-administered orally with an intraperitoneal injection of alcohol in rats on GD6, 9 and 12, fetal weight was significantly reduced for all three days of gestation examined [Varma and Persaud 1979]. There were also a high proportion of fetuses developing abnormalities following pyrazole and alcohol administration on GD9, compared with none or fewer observed on GD6 and 12, respectively. In mice co-treated orally with alcohol and 4-methylpyrazole on day 10 of gestation, a significant number of embryos developed fetal malformations, however, the authors did not mention the type of these abnormalities [Blakley and Scott 1984a]. Similarly, whilst the evidence for a direct effect of alcohol on the fetus is compelling, it does not take into account that inhibiting alcohol dehydrogenase activity may increase peroxisomal and microsomal metabolism of alcohol and result in acetaldehyde and reactive oxygen species that at least in part could account for the teratogenicity.

### *Teratogenicity Caused by Tertiary-Butanol*

Tertiary-butanol (*t*-butanol) is a form of alcohol which is not a substrate for alcohol dehydrogenase, and therefore unable to be metabolised to acetaldehyde [Daniel and Evans 1982; Faulkner *et al.* 1989]. It has been used in studies to differentiate between the direct effects of alcohol on the developing fetus, and those resulting from its metabolism or metabolites [Daniel and Evans 1982; Grant and Samson 1982; Faulkner *et al.* 1989]. In one study, it was observed that the administration of *t*-butanol to neonatal rats in the milk formula at the time of significant brain growth resulted in microcephaly, but did not cause alteration of myelin formation and protein synthesis as did alcohol administered at the same time [Grant and Samson 1982]. Tertiary-butanol was also found to be 4 to 5 times more potent than alcohol in producing behavioural deficits in postnatal mice whose mother's were treated with alcohol and *t*-butanol during pregnancy [Daniel and Evans 1982]. Conversely, when *t*-butanol was given to pregnant mice during the critical stages of pregnancy from day 6 to 18 no teratogenicity was observed [Faulkner *et al.* 1989]. Due to the differences in findings, and since the pharmacokinetics of *t*-butanol in the whole animal is sufficiently different to alcohol, there is reason for caution on any inference made concerning the direct effects of alcohol on the fetus.

## Formation of Acetaldehyde via Alcohol Metabolism

### *Metabolism of Alcohol*

In contrast to alcohol having a direct effect on the fetus, it has been argued that alcohol metabolism is necessary for the development alcohol-related birth defects. It is generally considered that the main site of alcohol metabolism is the liver with the rate-limiting step being the conversion of alcohol to acetaldehyde which is catalysed by the zinc (Zn) containing enzyme, alcohol dehydrogenase [Pawan 1972]. This process occurs in the cytoplasm with nicotinamide adenine dinucleotide (NAD) acting as a hydrogen acceptor. Acetaldehyde is a high unstable compound and is rapidly metabolised to acetic acid by aldehyde dehydrogenase. Excess alcohol can also be metabolised by the microsomal alcohol oxidising system (MEOS) system or within peroxisomes. Alcohol metabolism by the MEOS involves the P450 cytochromes CYP2E1, CYP1A2 and CYP3A4, with the former being of particular interest because it is inducible in hepatocytes and Kupffer cells at high alcohol concentrations [Tsutsumi *et al.* 1989; Koivisto *et al.* 1996]. CYP2E1 is markedly increased in alcoholics [Salaspuro and Lieber 1978] and after a single acute dose of alcohol [Ariyoshi *et al.* 1970]. Harmful effects of the MEOS result from the generation of superoxide radicals [Dai *et al.* 1993] which can be directly toxic, or by depleting GSH, making the body vulnerable to oxidative stress from other agents [Lieber 2004]. The MEOS also produces acetaldehyde from alcohol which is more concentrated in Kupffer cells than in hepatocytes, and has its own level of toxicity. Peroxisomal metabolism also plays a role in the overall degradation of alcohol and may be important in teratogenicity as metabolism by catalase generates hydrogen peroxide which is a source of other oxygen radicals [Lieber 1990]. Acute administration of alcohol leads to increase in hepatic respiration, which in turn increases alcohol metabolism. The mechanism is thought to involve both facilitation of NAD dependent alcohol dehydrogenase as well as enhanced catalase dependent peroxisomal oxidation of alcohol [Bradford *et al.* 1999]. Additionally, liberation of peripheral fatty acids via activation of an adrenergic response to alcohol provides added substrate for peroxisomes further accelerating alcohol metabolism. Alcohol ingestion, particularly in excess, also causes the release of endotoxin, with activation of Kupffer cells [Bradford 2007]. The importance of alcohol-induced reactive oxygen species, and interactions with toll like receptor 4 (TLR 4) pathways in macrophages leading to inflammation is becoming increasingly evident [Mandrekar and Szabo 2009]. While alcohol elicits a range of effects subsequent to its metabolism, the link with the bacterial endotoxin lipopolysaccharide (LPS), macrophages and inflammatory mediators provides a new direction for understanding alcohol effects on the fetus via maternal Zn redistribution (see section on Zn deficiency).

***Teratogenicity from Acetaldehyde***

The premise that acetaldehyde is responsible for the teratogenicity observed following alcohol administration remains in question. Studies examining the dynamics of acetaldehyde transfer from mother to fetus have been inconsistent, though the general dogma is that acetaldehyde does not cross the placenta as readily as alcohol [Blakley and Scott 1984a]. When alcohol was administered to mice at a concentration of 7 g/kg on day 10 of gestation, acetaldehyde was detectable in the maternal blood at a high concentration at 5 minutes following treatment, and whilst acetaldehyde was also observed in the embryo and yolk sac, the concentrations were extremely low [Blakley and Scott 1984a]. However, Karl *et al.* [1988] observed that the perfused human term placenta can transfer acetaldehyde to the fetus and reach concentrations of about 50% of the maternal perfusate concentration, indicating that significant amounts of acetaldehyde can reach the fetal circulation.

Controversy also exists in regard to the concentration of acetaldehyde that is necessary to cause teratogenicity in both *in vivo* and *in vitro* studies. Some studies have demonstrated teratogenic effects at low concentrations [Sreenathan *et al.* 1982; Campbell and Fantel 1983; Higuchi and Matsumoto 1984], whilst others have reported no teratogenicity at all [Priscott 1985], or only when concentrations were so high that they are unlikely to be achieved physiologically [O'Shea and Kaufman 1979; Dreosti *et al.* 1981; Padmanabhan *et al.* 1983; Blakley and Scott 1984a]. In the studies that demonstrated teratogenicity following acetaldehyde treatment, anomalies including an increase in resorptions [O'Shea and Kaufman 1979; Dreosti *et al.* 1981; Sreenathan *et al.* 1982; Padmanabhan *et al.* 1983], fetal malformations such as microcephaly, micrognathia, exencephaly and micromelia [O'Shea and Kaufman 1979; Sreenathan *et al.* 1982; Padmanabhan *et al.* 1983], growth retardation [O'Shea and Kaufman 1979; Campbell and Fantel 1983; Padmanabhan *et al.* 1983; Higuchi and Matsumoto 1984] and neural tube defects [O'Shea and Kaufman 1979; Higuchi and Matsumoto 1984] were observed.

Whilst acetaldehyde has demonstrated teratogenicity as an independent agent it seems unlikely that the concentrations of acetaldehyde in a physiological setting would reach a level comparable to that administered in these studies. It has been reported the peak acetaldehyde concentrations are approximately 1000-fold less than corresponding alcohol concentrations after alcohol administration [Brien and Loomis 1983]. Even when blood acetaldehyde concentrations were artificially raised using disulfiram, an inhibitor of acetaldehyde dehydrogenase, no further increase in fetal malformations were observed following treatment with alcohol. [Webster *et al.* 1983].

## Oxidative Stress

Embryonic oxidative stress in relation to fetal teratogenicity has been recently reviewed [Cohen-Kerem and Koren 2003; Orny 2007]. In the general sense, oxidative stress refers to the damage caused to membranes, lipids, proteins, receptors and chromosomes (essentially cellular integrity) by short lived reactive oxygenated free radicals including superoxide anion, hydroxyl radical, singlet oxygen and hydrogen peroxide. These are normally produced in respiring cells when extra electrons from the mitochorial cytochromes associate with oxygen. Peroroxisomal oxidation may also be particularly relevant with regard to hydrogen peroxide generation through flavin catalysed reactions [Bradford 2007]. The rapid metabolism of alcohol also has a central effect on the cellular redox state due to the marked change in the NAD+/NADH ratio, impacting on many cellular events In the intact animal, alcohol can cause ischemia and hypoxia; however the damage cause by alcohol generated free radicals appears to be independent of this as alcohol causes damage to embryos in culture [Priscott 1982].

Fetal cells appear to be more sensitive to free radical damage as they posses lower levels of superoxide dismutase and antioxidants such as selenium vitamin E [Davis *et al.* 1990]. Rat hippocampal cells in culture are protected from the deleterious effects of alcohol by the addition of vitamin E and β-carotene [Mitchell *et al.* 1999]; a finding replicated with Vitamin E treatment in vivo [Wentzel *et al.* 2006]. Some of the other free radical scavenging systems require the trace elements Zn and Mg (superoxide dismutase) and selenium (glutathione peroxidase). Zn treatment protects against the fetal alcohol effects in mice, an effect attributed to the correction of a transient Zn deficiency; however Zn treatment also eliminated the background levels of abnormalities seen in control (saline treated) mice, a finding consistent with an antioxidant effect [Carey *et al.* 2000b].

The susceptibility of the fetus to alcohol has also been linked to genetic polymorphism [Warren and Li 2005; Gemma *et al.* 2007], with a much higher concordance rate for FAS amongst identical twins compared to fraternal twins [Streissguth and Dehaene 1993]. Recent attentions has focused on the gene responsible for neuronal nitric oxide synthase (nNOS), with brain cell cultures from nNOS knockout mice being more susceptible than wild type cells to alcohol induced cell death [Bonthius *et al.* 2008].

While it is clear from animal studies that treatment with antioxidants can limit the developmental abnormalities associated with agents like alcohol that increase the formation of reactive oxygen species, extension of these findings into the clinical setting of human pregnancy where alcohol consumption is a risk factor is the new challenge.

## Interference of Retinoid Metabolism by Alcohol

Retinoic acid (RA) is the oxidized form of retinol (also known as Vitamin A) that acts as a transcriptional regulator by binding to specific receptors, signalling the initiation of a cascade of events that affect gene expression and, ultimately, controls anterior and posterior patterning in early developmental stages [Maden *et al.* 1989; Mark *et al.* 1999]. RA is particularly high in the developing embryo where RA-signalling occurs through Hox genes that in turn regulate large networks of other genes that affect organogenesis and the development of the CNS [Marshall *et al.* 1996]. It has been argued that teratogenicity can result when embryos are subjected to RA concentrations either too low or in excess [McCaffery *et al.* 2003; Yelin *et al.* 2005]. RA-teratogenicity shares many of the phenotypic manifestations of FAS including heart defects, craniofacial malformations and CNS abnormalities [Duester 1991; Kessel 1992; Clagett-Dame and DeLuca 2002; Yelin *et al.* 2007; Kot-Leibovich and Fainsod 2009]. Thus, it has been proposed that alcohol teratogenicity may in part be caused by an effect of alcohol on RA metabolism. Various mechanisms have been proposed and these include alcohol (or its metabolites) competing with enzymes involved in RA synthesis, altering levels of cellular RA binding proteins, and/or disrupting RA receptors [Grummer and Zachman 1995; Liu *et al.* 2002]. Presumably, these mechanisms are not mutually exclusive and may act alone or in combination depending on the location and/or time of gestation.

### *Alcohol a Cause of Retinoic Acid Deficiency*

Evidence that alcohol affects RA-signalling by causing RA deficiency comes from studies conducted in zebrafish, frog and mouse, where RA supplements have been found to prevent developmental defects in alcohol-treated embryos [Yelin *et al.* 2005; Johnson *et al.* 2007; Marrs *et al.* 2009]. In animal cells, retinol is required to produce RA. The conversion of retinol to RA occurs in a two-step enzymatic process whereby retinol is first oxidised to retinal, then retinal to RA, with the conversion of retinol to retinal being the rate-limiting step. Once retinol is absorbed, it attaches to Retinol Binding Protein in the serum which transports it to receptors on the cell surface mediating its uptake. Within the cell, retinol is carried by Cellular Retinol Binding Protein (CRBP) where it is oxidised to RA. Alcohol dehydrogenase catalyses the conversion of retinol to retinal, whilst aldehyde dehydrogenase controls the oxidation of retinal to RA [Connor and Smit 1987]. The detoxification of alcohol also requires the same two oxidation steps as RA metabolism, but with acetaldehyde being the intermediate metabolite and acetic acid the end product. Therefore, a competition with retinoids could result since alcohol dehydrogenase could use either alcohol or retinol as a substrate. It has been argued that in the presence of alcohol, a competitive inhibition of RA synthesis may occur.

However, mutation studies on both dehydrogenases have indicated that the aldehyde dehydrogenase-2 (RALDH2) is the key enzyme controlling the synthesis of RA in early embryogenesis [Niederreither *et al.* 1999; Chen *et al.* 2001]. Furthermore, in recent studies on embryos of Xenopus laevis expressing a reporter for RA-signalling, reduced RALDH2 activity was found to be the main cause of alcohol-mediated decrease in RA-signalling and teratogenicity. In those studies, partial inhibition of RALDH2 activity resulted in developmental defects characteristic of high alcohol exposure when low concentrations of alcohol were used. Over-expression of the message for RALDH2 resulted in higher RA-signalling levels and rescued the developmental malformations induced by high alcohol presumably by providing sufficient enzyme levels for both alcohol detoxification and RA biosynthesis. In addition, when RALDH2 activity was decreased in knockdown studies, a similar reduction in RA-signalling was found when this was carried out alone or in combination with alcohol treatment, evidence that further supports RALDH2 being the main target for alcohol [Kot-Leibovich and Fainsod 2009].

Retinol binding proteins may also be altered by alcohol exposure and may contribute to defective RA-signalling. In studies in rats that were chronically exposed to alcohol during pregnancy, an increase in the abundance of mRNA for CRBP was found in 12 day embryos, while in the fetal brain at gestational day 20 there was elevated levels of CRBP as well as its nuclear receptors (RARs) [Grummer and Zachman 1995]. While RA levels were not measured in this study, it seems plausible that the increased CRBP following alcohol could result in the sequestration of retinol within the cell preventing its oxidation to RA.

***Alcohol a Cause of Excess Retinoic Acid***

The majority of studies, however, which provide evidence that deficiency of RA is the cause of alcohol-mediated teratogenicity, have used indirect measurements of RA rather than quantitative assessments. In studies where the effects of alcohol on all-*trans*-retinoid concentration was investigated in pregnant mice fed normal levels of vitamin-A, acute alcohol administration was found to increase RA levels in the fetal hippocampus (1.6-fold), liver (2.4-fold) and testes (1.5-fold) or had no effect on RA levels in other fetal tissues. However, 20-fold and 50-fold increases were found in fetal hippocampus and cortex, respectively after chronic alcohol feeding [Kane *et al.*]. This data suggests that super-physiological levels of RA and not low levels of RA may contribute to deleterious effects on neurodevelopment.

An area that has received little attention is the potential for alcohol to affect RA degradation. RA levels are a balance between the rate of synthesis and degradation with the latter being controlled by the level of P450 enzyme, CYP26, in cells. Knockout mice lacking CYP26 have been found to have elevated RA and lack the uneven distribution of RA that normally occurs along the anterior-posterior axis, which is required for patterning the hindbrain, vertebrae and tailbud [Sakai *et al.* 2001]. However, whether alcohol alters the rate of RA degradation through CYP26 requires further investigation.

Clearly, there is accumulating evidence that alcohol causes dysregulation of RA-signalling. However, whether this is due to deficient or excessive cellular RA levels, the mechanism by which this occurs, and, additionally, whether this is relevant to doses of alcohol encountered in animal models of FAS, requires further investigation in future studies.

## Altered Prostanoid Metabolism

Prostanoids are peroxidation products of membrane phospholipid that have hormone-like properties, but unlike hormones act locally with a short biological half-life to mediate a diverse range of physiological functions. Prostanoids are synthesised from polyunsaturated fatty acids via a pathway that involves the synthesis of arachidonic acid, which is then converted by two cyclooxygenases (COX-1 and COX-2) to form the endoperoxides prostaglandin (PG) $G_2$ and $PGH_2$. These are further converted by a specific family of microsomal synthetases to either the stabile active prostaglandins (PGEs including; $PGE_2$, $PGF_{2\alpha}$, $PGD_2$, $PGJ_2$) or to labile prostacyclin (PGI) or thromboxane (TX) [Grylewski 2008]. These prostanoids have divergent vasoactive roles and regulate the contraction or relaxation of smooth muscle. In most cell types, PGEs, PGI and TX are differentially regulated by controlling the expression COX-enzyme levels. COX-1 is constitutively produced in all cell types whereas COX-2 is induced by inflammatory stimuli including cytokines and bacterial endotoxin and in endothelial cells by shear stress [Okahara *et al.* 1998; Caughey *et al.* 2001]. TX is vasoconstrictive and a promoter of platelet aggregation while the opposite is the case for PGI which is a vasodilator and an inhibitor of platelet aggregation. An imbalance of TX and PGI levels during pregnancy has been linked to the pathogenesis of high blood pressure. In women with preeclampsia, an increase in TX production and decrease in PGI has been found and this has lead to the premise that placental vasoconstriction may occur unopposed resulting in maternal hypertension and decreased utero-placental blood flow [Walsh 2004]. It is argued that oxidative stress manifested by increased lipid peroxidation and decreased antioxidant protection may be the cause of the altered prostanoid metabolism. In normal pregnancy, however, prostenoids have critical roles in implantation, fetal growth, neurodevelopment, and in the initiation of labour [Goldberg and Ramwell 1975; Keirse 1978; Persaud 1978; Challis and Patrick 1980].

It has long been recognised that PGEs are teratogenic in various animals models if administered at high dose [Hilbelink and Persaud 1981; Liebgott and Wiley 1985]. However, the relevance of birth defects caused by pharmacological doses of PGEs has been questioned as they are unlikely to be achieved by challenge with physiological stressors [Abel and Hannigan 1995]. Nonetheless, interest in prostenoids as potential mediators of the detrimental effects of prenatal alcohol originated from studies in animal models of FAS. In an chicken egg model, which exclude maternal and placental influences, alcohol was found to decrease the weight of the chick brain by 19% and this was prevented by administering the non-steroidal anti-inflammatory drug (NSAID), indomethacin, a non-selective COX-1 and COX-2 inhibitor [Pennington and Kalmus 1987]. In studies in pregnant mice administered alcohol on GD10, high levels of TX and PGE were found in uterine/embryo tissue which was associated with an increased incidence of prenatal mortality and number of malformed pups. Interestingly, the deleterious effects on the fetus were attenuated by pre-treatment with indomethacin or aspirin (a selective COX-1 inhibitor) [Randall and Anton 1984; Randall *et al.* 1987; Anton *et al.* 1990]. In studies in near-term pregnant ewes, alcohol administration suppressed the rate of fetal breathing that was observed concurrent with increased $PGE_2$ and TX levels in maternal and fetal plasma and CSF. Administration of indomethacin shortly after the alcohol treatment increased the rate of fetal breathing which was then reversed by administration of $PGE_2$. These findings indicate that prostenoids may mediate the alcohol-induced suppression of fetal breathing and this might result in hypoxia sufficient to cause fetal damage [Smith *et al.* 1990; Smith *et al.* 1991]. That this may occur in humans is supported by the observation that raised levels of prostanoid metabolites have been found in the urine of pregnant women after consuming alcohol [Ylikorkala *et al.* 1988]. Others have associated maternal alcohol exposure with foetal hypoxaemia [Mukherjee and Hodgen 1982], as well as decreased transfer of amino acids [Lin 1981] and glucose [Singh *et al.* 1989] which might all be explained by an alcohol-prostanoid interaction on maternal/fetal blood flow.

However, the evidence supporting a prostanoid-mediated mechanism by which alcohol causes fetal damage is mostly circumstantial since it is primarily based upon either the association of raised prostanoid levels in maternal/fetal tissues after maternal alcohol administration and/or the protection offered by NSAIDs against alcohol-related birth defects. In regard to the former, while elevated levels of prostenoids are found in the mother and fetus, it is not yet possible to determine whether this is the cause of cytotoxicity or a response to damage from excessive alcohol consumption. For instance, PGEs may rise in response to changes in blood flow caused by a range of inflammatory mediators such as reactive oxygen species released in the microsomal oxidation of alcohol. Moreover, it is difficult to equate the biological activity of prostenoids measured in blood, urine or in uterine/embryo systems with activity that is relevant to specific tissues, where local rates of synthesis and degradation dictate their paracrine or autocrine action. The mechanism of protection against alcohol related birth defects offered by aspirin and indomethacin has also been questioned [Abel and Hannigan 1995]. It has been argued that protection may result from their ability to chelate free iron rather than through cyclooxgyenase inhibition. Both aspirin and indomethacin are strong iron chelators and could prevent damage to the fetus by reducing the number of Fenton reactions resulting in the production of reactive oxygen species that would be detrimental to the fetus [Abel and Hannigan 1995].

In summary, the role that prostenoids play in alcohol-mediated fetal damage remains unclear. Further studies are required to examine the effect of acute and chronic alcohol exposure on maternal/fetal blood flow and the extent that this might have on hypoxia and the transfer of specific nutrients to the fetus. Advances in anti-inflammatory drugs that inhibit specific cytokines and non-prostanoid components as well as knockdown studies on specific prostanoid-producing synthetases may further help clarify the potential involvement of individual prostenoids in alcohol-related birth defects.

## Impaired Placental Nutrient Delivery

Over the past 30 years, a significant number of human and animal studies have investigated the potential role of abnormalities of placental growth and function in the aetiology of alcohol-related birth defects [Fisher *et al.* 1982; Burd *et al.* 2007]. The fetus is dependent on efficient placental function for the delivery of oxygen and essential nutrients (e.g. amino acids, fatty acids, glucose, vitamins, and trace metals) from the mother. Thus, any interference in the delivery of these nutrients is likely to have a detrimental effect on fetal growth and development. Prenatal alcohol exposure has been demonstrated to impair placental transport of a number of these important nutrients to the fetus (reviewed by Burd *et al.* 2007).

### *Amino Acids*

Acute, and especially chronic, maternal alcohol exposure has been shown to depress the in vitro placental uptake of a variety of amino acids in animal studies, including alpha-aminoisobutyric acid (AIB), cycloleucine, L-alanine, L-leucine, L-lysine, valine [Henderson *et al.* 1982; Fisher *et al.* 1983]. In human studies, where placental perfusion systems were utilised, transport of AIB and histidine was shown to be relatively resistant to the inhibitory effects of acute alcohol exposure in the maternal perfusate [Schenker *et al.* 1989; Fisher and Karl 1990], suggesting that placental transport of amino acids may be altered primarily after chronic alcohol consumption.

### *Vitamins*

Water-soluble vitamins are required for the actions of many enzymes and metabolic reactions, and are therefore essential for fetal growth and development. Schenker and colleagues performed several studies using perfused single cotyledons from term human placentas to examine the effect of short-term term exposure to 400 mg/dL alcohol on vitamin transfer. Alcohol inhibited the transport of pyridoxal (B6) across the placenta by 42% [Schenker *et al.* 1992], but had no effect on maternal to fetal compartment transfer of thiamine [Schenker *et al.* 1990b]. The rate-limiting transfer of biotin by human placenta was also not inhibited by alcohol [Schenker *et al.* 1993]. However, biotin was found to be moderately inhibited in a later study where the basal membrane vesicles of the syncytiotrophoblast were exposed to alcohol, which could lead to decreased availability to the fetus of drinking mothers [Hu *et al.* 1994]. Uptake of [$^3$H] folic acid by a human trophoblast cell line and human cultured cytotrophoblasts was reduced by chronic exposure to alcohol [Keating *et al.* 2008], which may be due in part to a reduced folate receptor activity in the placenta following chronic exposure [Fisher *et al.* 1985].

### *Fatty Acids*

Fatty acids are important for maintaining the fluidity, permeability and conformation of membranes, and as precursors of prostacyclins, prostaglandins and thromboxanes [Burd *et al.* 2007]. The presence of alcohol in the perfusate of term human placentas at a concentration of 2mg/dL was demonstrated to reduce the absolute transfer rate of two n-3 polyunsaturated fatty acids, alpha-linolenic and docosahexaenoic acid, suggesting that alcohol could decrease polyunsaturated fatty acid availability to the developing fetus [Haggarty *et al.* 2002]. Lipid phosphorus and free fatty acid production rates were significantly increased by 780% and 897% respectively, following alcohol administration in term placentas [Rice *et al.* 1986].

### *Glucose*

Glucose is essential as an energy source in all cells and is required for the production of various important types of molecules, including DNA and RNA building blocks, fat molecules and hormones [Goodlett and Horn 2001]. Impaired glucose transport to the fetus has been suggested to play a significant role in the growth restriction observed in fetuses exposed to alcohol. The consumption of alcohol throughout pregnancy in rats (30% alcohol derived calories) reduced fetal body, liver, lung and brain weights, reduced placental uptake by the placenta and fetal brain, and placental transfer of [$^3$H] 2-deoxy-D-glucose. Most importantly, a significant correlation was demonstrated between fetal weights and 2-deoxy-D-glucose transfer and with fetal plasma $^3$H activity [Snyder *et al.* 1986; Singh *et al.* 1989].

The impairments in placental nutrient transfer observed following alcohol exposure could be accounted for by alcohol-induced placental dysmorphology and dysfunction (reviewed by Burd *et al.* 2007). In 13 alcoholic women, placental weights at term were significantly lower (526 +/- 116) compared to controls (653 +/- 77 g) [Andersson *et al.* 1989]. Similarly, in mice fed 0%, 10%, 15 % or 20% alcohol (v/v) in their drinking water from GD 11-18, placental weight decreased with increasing alcohol exposure [Kennedy 1984]. While several studies have found no gross or microscopic structural changes from alcohol exposure in placentas [Sokol *et al.* 1980; Rice *et al.* 1986], others have reported abnormal placental histopathology. Chronic alcohol exposure during pregnancy in rodents was shown to impair or prevent the physiological conversion of uterine vessels required for expansion of maternal circulation into the placenta (a critical process for adequate placentation) [Gundogan *et al.* 2008], and revealed advanced degenerative changes in the basal zone [Kennedy 1984]. Abnormal placental membranes were shown to be more prevalent in a group of alcohol-exposed women from an alcohol treatment program, compared to control women [Hollstedt *et al.* 1983]. Villus infarction and the presence of intervillous thrombi were also more common in alcohol-exposed pregnancy, with 22% of alcohol abuse cases displaying villitis, a condition associated with intrauterine growth restriction [Baldwin *et al.* 1982].

Functional changes in placental and umbilical cord blood flow following alcohol exposure may alternatively influence nutrient transfer to the fetus during development. Chronic alcohol exposure in pregnant rats has been shown to redistribute blood, decreasing the supply to the placenta [Jones *et al.* 1981]. Alcohol exposure in human placentas induced placental vasoconstriction in a dose-dependent manner and increased fetal-placental vascular resistances and perfusion pressure [Taylor *et al.* 1994; Acevedo *et al.* 1997]. A transient but marked collapse in umbilical vasculature in pregnant monkeys was observed within 15 minutes after intravenous injection of alcohol, producing severe hypoxia and acidosis in the fetus [Mukherjee and Hodgen 1982]. Furthermore, alcohol caused dose-dependent contractions in isolated human segments of umbilical cord veins and arteries, lasting as long as the alcohol was present [Altura *et al.* 1982; Savoy-Moore *et al.* 1989], suggesting that alcohol may increase umbilicoplacental resistance, decreasing maternal-fetal blood flow. Alcohol therefore has multiple adverse effects on placental growth, function, and nutrient transport to the fetus, which could contribute to the aetiology of FASD.

## Zinc Deficiency

### *A Link between Prenatal Alcohol Exposure and Fetal Zinc Deficiency*

Zinc is an essential trace element that is required for a wide range of biological processes in both animals and humans. It is currently estimated that more than 1000 enzymes and proteins require Zn for their function, where Zn is critical for their catalytic activity or structural stability (see reviews [Vallee and Falchuk 1993; Zalewski *et al.* 1994]). These Zn-binding proteins play a pivotal role, not only in general metabolic processes (e.g. reproduction, vision, taste, immune function and cognitive behaviour), but also in the regulation of growth and development. Thus, at the cellular level, Zn participates in protein, nucleic acid, carbohydrate and lipid metabolism, the control of gene transcription and the regulation of cell proliferation, differentiation and apoptosis [Vallee and Falchuk 1993; Zalewski *et al.* 1994]. Consequently, Zn is critical for fetal growth and development and this is reflected by an increase in Zn requirements throughout gestation paralleling the growth of the fetus. Therefore, it is not surprising that maternal Zn deficiency during pregnancy can be detrimental to fetal development. In rodents, a single day on a Zn deficient diet can be sufficient to reduce the maternal plasma Zn levels in a pregnant dam by 30% [Hurley and Swenerton 1966; Dreosti *et al.* 1968]. Since the maternal plasma is the major source of Zn for placental/fetal interchange, any reduction in its concentration can potentially limit that available to the fetus.

Animal studies have been valuable in demonstrating the link between fetal Zn deficiency and teratology [Hurley and Swenerton 1966; Beach *et al.* 1982; Dreosti *et al.* 1986; Halas *et al.* 1986; da Cunha Ferreira *et al.* 1989]. Long-term Zn deficiency in rats fed a diet containing less than 0.5 mg/kg of Zn throughout pregnancy (compared with 35 mg Zn /kg control) impairs reproduction and decreases fetal body weight, with 90% of the fetuses demonstrating gross malformations affecting every organ system [Hurley *et al.* 1971]. Short-term Zn deficiency is also teratogenic, but with altered incidences of abnormalities depending upon the timing of the deficiency relative to the stage of development. In early pregnancy, Zn deficiency is associated with defects of the head region, including the eyes, facial structures and brain. Later in pregnancy, Zn deficiency results in a more frequent incidence of skeletal malformations [Hurley and Swenerton 1966] and with defects in uro-genital system and tail. A number of studies have reported that Zn deprivation during pregnancy and lactation can result in poor fetal activity, newborn motor development, learning, long-term, short-term and working memory in adult offspring [Lokken *et al.* 1973; Halas and Sandstead 1975; Halas *et al.* 1977; Halas *et al.* 1979; Halas *et al.* 1983; Halas *et al.* 1986; Golub *et al.* 1995].

There is considerable experimental evidence linking alterations in Zn homeostasis with the teratogenic effects of alcohol. In rodents, there are striking similarities in fetal outcome between Zn-deficient and alcohol-exposed dams. These include increased fetal resorptions, low birth weight, anophthalmia, exencephaly, clefts of the lip and palate, major skeletal defects and impairments in neurodevelopment resulting cognitive anomalies in offspring [Hickory *et al.* 1979; Randall and Taylor 1979; Sulik *et al.* 1981; Keppen *et al.* 1985; Dreosti *et al.* 1986; Keen and Hurley 1987; Sauerbier 1987; Boehm *et al.* 1997; Summers *et al.* 2006; Summers *et al.* 2009]. Moreover, Zn deficiency and alcohol both cause programmed cell death in specific embryonic cell populations [Rogers *et al.* 1995; Jankowski-Hennig *et al.* 2000; Dunty *et al.* 2001]. It has also been noted that short or long term exposure of rodents to Zn deficiency and alcohol simultaneously during pregnancy is synergistic with an increased incidence of fetal abnormalities compared to either insult alone [Ruth and Goldsmith 1981; Keppen *et al.* 1985].

One question which has been the topic of much discussion is how Zn deficiency in the fetus is caused by the mother drinking alcohol. As previously discussed, reactive oxygen species formed by microsomal metabolism of alcohol might cause prostanoid release that could restrict placental transport of nutrients by inhibiting maternal/fetal blood flow. However, such a mechanism would be expected to cause a multi-nutrient deficiency in the fetus rather than one pertaining to a single element. In an early study, placental Zn transport was found to be inhibited by 40%, and fetal Zn uptake by 30% when rats were chronically administered alcohol throughout pregnancy or when given as an acute dose late in gestation [Ghishan *et al.* 1982]. It was argued that alcohol interferes with placental Zn transport, although the mechanism was not determined. In a later study with isolated term human placenta, placental Zn transport was found to be bidirectional, require ligand binding, did not occur against a concentration gradient of Zn, and proceeded at a slow rate that was only 6% of that of a freely diffusible marker [Beer *et al.* 1992]. In that study, placental Zn transport was not found to be inhibited directly by alcohol. It is possible that species differences may explain the different findings in the rat and human placenta, however, it can also be argued that human term placenta is free from systemic factors that may be released by alcohol and alter placental nutrient uptake or blood flow. The answer to how Zn deficiency may arise in fetus prenatally exposed to alcohol came from studies of Daston and colleagues. They demonstrated that metallothionein (MT), a zinc binding protein, was induced in the mother's liver by a variety of xenobiotics including alcohol. Once induced, MT sequestered Zn from the maternal blood into the maternal liver, thus reducing the amount in blood which limits the placental/fetal transport of Zn [Daston *et al.* 1991].

MT is a low molecular weight (6-7KDa), cysteine rich, intracellular protein that can bind 7 gram atoms of Zn per molecule of protein. In rodents, MT is expressed as one of four isoforms. MT-1 and -2 predominate by being expressed in all tissues, and are highly inducible, especially in the liver, pancreas, small intestine and kidneys. While MT-1 and -2 concentrations are low in the unstressed setting, they rapidly increase when homeostasis is disrupted. In the setting of maternal Zn deficiency, MT-1 and -2 have been shown to provide a reproductive advantage as surviving embryos of MT-1 and MT-2 KO mice show greater morphological abnormalities [Andrews and Geiser 1999]. Endogenous regulators (IL-6, glucocorticoids, Zn) and exogenous compounds (endotoxins, alcohols including alcohol) induce MT expression independently and synergistically (for reviews see [Cousins 1985; Hidalgo *et al.* 2001; Coyle *et al.* 2002]). In the seminal work of Daston and coworkers, the injection of urethane into pregnant rats on GD11 was found to significantly induce maternal liver MT, decrease maternal plasma Zn concentrations by 30%, and inhibit the transfer of $^{65}$Zn into the fetus by 50% [Daston *et al.* 1991]. The induction of MT and subsequent decrease in fetal Zn supply resulted in fetuses that exhibited decreased weight and delayed skeletal ossification when examined on GD18. A range of other teratogenic compounds with different pharmacological actions, such as α-hederin, TNF-α, 2-ethylhexanoic acid, arsenic, and alcohol, were later demonstrated to have similar effects on MT, Zn distribution and fetal outcome [Daston *et al.* 1994; Taubeneck *et al.* 1994; Taubeneck *et al.* 1995; Bui *et al.* 1998]. Our group extended these findings in a C57BL/6 mouse model. In one study, a single binge of alcohol, whereby blood alcohol levels reached 0.2-0.3% over 8h, administered at the beginning of organogenesis (GD8) was found to increase maternal liver MT by 20-fold and decrease maternal plasma Zn concentrations by up to 65% within 16h [Carey *et al.* 2000b]. When fetuses were large enough to be examined on GD12, this alcohol-mediated decrease in maternal plasma Zn was found to markedly impair $^{65}$Zn transfer to the fetus and cause a 20% reduction in total fetal Zn content, 3h after an acute alcohol intake [Carey *et al.* 2000a].

Perhaps the most compelling evidence linking MT with alcohol-mediated teratogenicity came from findings obtained using our colony of MT-knockout (MT-/-) mouse which has allowed us to closely examine the effects of maternal MT with regard to fetal Zn homeostasis. The MT-/- mouse was derived by Michalska and Choo [1993] and lacks the two inducible genes MT-1 and MT-2. It serves as the absolute control in all comparisons with the wild type (MT+/+) mouse, in which both MT-1 and -2 genes are expressed, where the primary variable is Zn balance. In studies where we injected alcohol in MT+/+ or MT-/- mice on GD8, an increased incidence of birth abnormalities (27%) were observed in the MT+/+ animals which was associated with a decreased plasma Zn concentration.

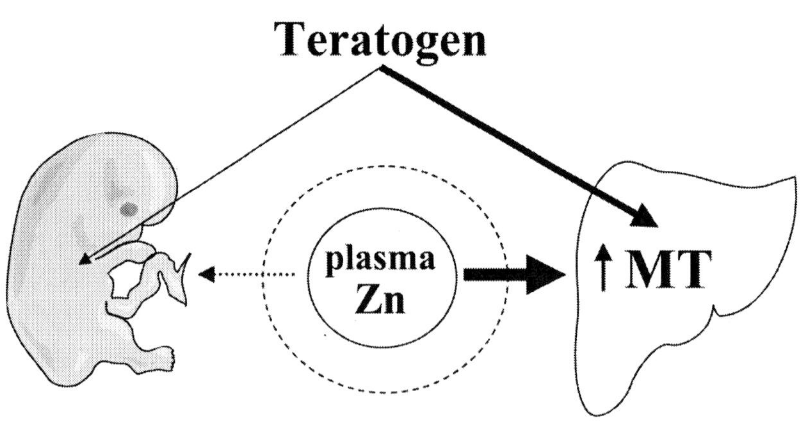


Figure 1. The effect of teratogens (alcohol, stress hormones, cytokines) on maternal-fetal zinc homeostasis. Alcohol induces maternal liver metallothionein (MT) causing a flux of zinc (Zn) out of the plasma compartment into the liver where it is bound by MT. There is a resultant decrease in plasma zinc concentration. As the plasma zinc falls the delivery of zinc to the fetus is impaired. The transient zinc deficiency is either detrimental in itself or exacerbates the direct effects of alcohol on the fetus. Zinc is essential for growth and development of the brain where it is required for a plethora of functions including functional roles in many enzymes and transcription factors.

Abnormalities pertaining to the eye contributed 50% of the total abnormalities in the MT+/+ alcohol fetuses. However, MT-/- fetuses exhibited fewer abnormalities than saline-treated controls (2.2%) [Carey *et al.* 2000b]. In addition, in MT-/- mice, plasma Zn levels increased rather than fell following alcohol exposure, and this resulted from a direct effect of alcohol on muscle and skin which causes the release of Zn. In other studies, $^{65}$Zn transfer to MT-/- fetuses was found to be unaffected by alcohol administration in comparison to the impairment observed in MT+/+ controls [Carey *et al.* 2000a]. While Zn limitation of less than one day is sufficient to cause fetal malformations in mice this period can only be surmised in humans. In this regard, the half-life of MT is approximately 20 hours, so the critical period in the human could be up to 48 hours.

Our studies, where the mother's Zn status was elevated on challenge with alcohol, provide further evidence that fetal Zn insufficiency is the underlying cause of the alcohol-mediated teratogenicity. Here, subcutaneous injection of Zn at the time of alcohol exposure, or supplementation of the mother's diet with Zn from conception to the time of alcohol administration, was found to prevent the depression of plasma Zn concentration associated with alcohol-induction of liver MT. Most importantly, both forms of Zn treatment were found to be effective and prevent birth defects [Carey *et al.* 2003; Summers *et al.* 2006; Summers *et al.* 2008; Summers *et al.* 2009]. These studies indicate that maternal plasma Zn levels are important in the aetiology of alcohol-related impairments and can be manipulated by Zn treatment.

### *Zinc Transporters*

Our understanding of how cells and organelles transport Zn has seen major advances in the last decade, through the application of molecular techniques and the production of transgenically modified cells and animals. Lichten and Cousins [2009] have recently published an extensive review of this area. The two groups of proteins which act to transport zinc are the ZnT family of transporters, which function to decrease intracellular Zn levels, and the ZIP family, which do the reverse by increasing intracellular Zn levels. Within cells, ZnTs increase Zn movement into organelles such as lysosomes, vesicles and secretory granules, while ZIP proteins transport Zn from the lumen of organelles into the cytoplasm. These proteins are essential for zinc homeostasis, including the primary functions intestinal zinc transport (ZnT1, Zip4, Zip5), renal zinc re-absorption (ZnT1, Zip10) and pancreatic release of Zn (ZnT1, ZnT2, Zip5).

The example of Zip4 protein is particularly instructive in relation to Zn and the fetus due to its central role in the disease acrodermatititis enteropathica. This rare autosomal recessively inherited disorder is primarily the result of intestinal Zn malabsorption, now shown to be the result of different types of mutations in the hZip4 gene (SLC39A4). Andrews and coworkers [Andrews 2008] have studied this protein extensively, including the investigation of a Zip4 knockout (KO) mouse. In one study, they determined that the homozygous fetuses do not proceed past gestational day 8-10 [Dufner-Beattie *et al.* 2007], which importantly, is the critical period of organogenesis. The deformities seen in these fetuses are consistent with those seen with Zn deficiency and indeed FAS. Interestingly, oral Zn or i.p. Zn was ineffective in rescuing the Zip4 KO fetuses, whereas we have shown that such treatments protect against FAS in the mouse. Heterozygous Zip4 KO mice were particularly sensitive to Zn deficiency and showed growth retardation and physical abnormalities.

In the context of altered Zn homeostasis during pregnancy, the studies of Dufner-Beattie *et al.* [2006] using Zip1 and Zip3 KO mice highlight the importance of Zn supply to the fetus. When dietary Zn was adequate in pregnant Zip1 and Zip3 KO mice, fetal development was normal. However, when a Zn deficient diet was fed from day 8 of pregnancy, fetuses showed a range of developmental malformations including missing digits and cranial and facial malformations. It was concluded that these transporters, which are predominantly expressed in the kidney, liver, intestine and pancreas, may function by altering the redistribution and retention of Zn, rather than facilitating absorption from the diet. It is of interest that the nature of the fetal malformations seen in Zip1 and Zip3 KO fetuses are similar to those seen when alcohol is administered to pregnant mice at gestational day 8 [Carey *et al.* 2003].

Another transporter that may be of particular interest to understanding the effects of alcohol on the fetus is Zip14 as this transporter is involved in the hypozincaemia of inflammation. In a study using IL-6 KO mice, it was clearly demonstrated that IL-6 was the primary inducer of Zip14 in the liver [Liuzzi *et al.* 2005]. The inflammatory mediators used in this study were LPS and turpentine, acting through IL-6 and other cytokines. The mediators of alcohols actions in the inflammatory process may well include IL-6. It is also known that hepatic MT is a major player in eliciting the hypozincaemia of inflammation; an event driven by either IL-6 or Zn influx. Liuzzi *et al.* [2005] demonstrated that while MT induction by LPS was markedly decreased in IL-6 KO mice, it was not completely abolished. Further studies are required to understand the interrelationships between transporters and metal binding proteins as they relate to the major redistribution of Zn that occurs during inflammation; with alcohol consumption having all the hallmarks of an inflammatory event.

### *Prenatal Alcohol and Brain Development*

Damage to brain development is the least visible but most socially and economically disruptive problem related to FAS and ARND. Furthermore, there is evidence that cognition may be more affected by alcohol in early rather than late pregnancy. Offspring of macaque monkeys who were fed alcohol weekly during their pregnancies were most affected (developmentally delayed) in infants of mothers whose drinking began in week 1 of pregnancy compared to those who began drinking in week 5. Even infants whose mothers had been given higher doses of alcohol beginning week 5 had fewer developmental deficiencies than infants exposed to lower doses of alcohol throughout gestation [Clarren *et al.* 1988; Astley *et al.* 1999]. Studies in rodents [Becker *et al.* 1996; Berman and Hannigan 2000] and monkeys [Clarren *et al.* 1988; Astley *et al.* 1999] have shown that prenatal alcohol exposure has a marked effect on brain growth and cognitive function. The deficits in cognition appear mainly due to degenerative changes occurring in the basal forebrain, neocortex and hippocampus (for review see [Arendt 1994]). Reduced numbers of neurones, lower dendritic spine density on pyramidal neurons and changes in synaptic activity have been reported [Arendt 1994]. Our C57BL/6 mouse model shows the full range of birth defects and is particularly sensitive to neurological change [Boehm *et al.* 1997; Carey *et al.* 2003; Summers *et al.* 2006; Summers *et al.* 2008; Summers *et al.* 2009]. In addition to determining a specific link between alcohol ingestion and physical birth abnormalities, we have shown that memory deficits are also apparent in the offspring that appear to have no visible abnormalities. These memory deficits were found in adult offspring that were randomly selected from litters produced by dams treated on acute alcohol on GD8, and tested using both a water cross maze task to assess for spatial learning and memory and an object recognition task that measures a non-spatial form of short-term memory [Summers *et al.* 2006; Summers *et al.* 2008]. A most interesting finding, however, was that offspring from dam's given alcohol and a diet supplemented with Zn throughout pregnancy had normal scores, demonstrating that dietary Zn supplementation can prevent alcohol-related cognitive deficits [Summers *et al.* 2008]. Zinc treatment may also prevent some of the post-natal morbidity associated with prenatal alcohol exposure [Summers *et al.* 2006]. In a study where we assessed perinatal survival, we found that acute alcohol exposure on GD8 did not affect the number of fetal resorptions or pre- or post-natal weight, however, there were more stillbirths with alcohol alone. In addition, cumulative postnatal mortality was significantly higher in offspring exposed to alcohol alone (35 % deaths) compared to control (10% deaths) or alcohol + dietary zinc supplementation (12 % deaths) [Summers *et al.* 2009]. Taken together, our findings indicate that dietary Zn supplementation throughout pregnancy ameliorates much of the teratogenicity, postnatal mortality and cognitive impairments associated with acute alcohol exposure in early pregnancy.

While our data suggests that cognitive anomalies caused by prenatal alcohol are mediated through a mechanism involving MT-induction and fetal Zn deficiency this needs to be confirmed in our MT-knockout mouse. Zn may influence many processes independent of MT including protection and repair mechanisms through well described antioxidant and anti-apoptotic properties (reviewed by [Vallee and Falchuk 1993; Coyle *et al.* 2002]). If MT is important in alcohol-mediated cognitive deficits then the MT-knockout mouse should be resistant to the levels of alcohol that cause these defects in the wild type mouse.

Studies are also warranted to determine how alcohol induces MT. Early studies with cultured rat hepatocytes demonstrated that alcohol is not a direct inducer of MT but that its induction might be caused by alcohol-mediated glucocorticoid or catecholamine release. However, adrenergic blockers did not prevent MT induction from alcohol [Bracken and Klaassen 1987]. Other potential mediators include cytokines, presumably released when alcohol levels are sufficiently high to cause inflammatory damage, or reactive oxygen species as a result of the microsomal metabolism of the alcohol when the dehydrogenase pathway is overloaded. A response element in the promoter region of the MT-gene has been identified which is sensitive to ROS and their involvement in MT induction might in part explain why antioxidants are effective in protecting the embryo against alcohol-mediated birth defects [Lee *et al.* 2004; Orny 2007; Memon and Pratten 2009].

### *Predisposing Factors for Co-Teratogenicity*

Although the evidence supporting a MT-mediated mechanism for teratogenicity to prenatal alcohol is currently drawn from animal models there are indicators that this mechanism may apply, at least in part, to humans. Firstly, it has long been reported that alcoholic mothers have significantly lower plasma Zn levels than non-alcoholic women and that an inverse relationship occurs between maternal plasma Zn levels and expression of FAS [Flynn *et al.* 1981]. Secondly, induction of liver MT in humans is a well recognised cause of hypozincaemia related to infection, inflammation and chronic disease. Consequently, the promoter region on the MT-gene is activated by a range of factors including reactive oxygen species, inflammatory cytokines (IL-1$\beta$, TNF-$\alpha$ and IL-6), corticosteroids and xenobiotics (including alcohol) [Cousins 1985; Hidalgo *et al.* 2001; Coyle *et al.* 2002]. Thus MT is an acute phase reactant responding to systemic inflammatory or infectious events. While the primary function of MT is still a matter for debate, the net effect of its induction is a change in whole body Zn homeostasis whereby the exchangeable pool of Zn in the plasma is redistributed to the liver where it is incorporated into the nascent MT protein.

While MT induction is a cause of hypozincaemia, it has yet to be directly associated with binge alcohol intake in humans. Nonetheless, if it is relevant to alcohol-related teratogenicity in humans, then based upon the evidence found in animal models, one might speculate on predisposing factors that could increase the overall risk from alcohol intake in pregnancy. Over the last decade, evidence has accumulated that bacterial or viral infections during pregnancy may be the cause of the birth defects which include neuropathological and behavioural abnormalities in offspring [McDermott *et al.* 2000; Borrell *et al.* 2002; Shi *et al.* 2003; Fortier *et al.* 2004; Golan *et al.* 2005; Offenbacher *et al.* 2005; Opler and Susser 2005; Ashdown *et al.* 2006; Meyer *et al.* 2006]. Although it remains unclear how a broad range of infectious agents might trigger this teratogenicity, accumulating evidence suggests that the damage may be due to the maternal immune response rather than the infectious agent itself [Ashdown *et al.* 2006; Meyer *et al.* 2006]. Early in infection, inflammatory cytokines mediate a complex change in acute-phase reactants in the host's liver. Induction of MT is a component of this acute phase response and we have now evidence linking this with altered Zn homeostasis in the mother. Nutritional status will have many aspects, but the lack of certain trace elements, Zn in particular, will have a compounding effect on alcohol teratogenicity [Keen *et al.* 2010]. In studies where we gave LPS, on GD8 to pregnant mice, we found that MT induction and hypozincaemia over the subsequent 24h was associated with an marked increase in the frequency of fetal malformations on GD18 in MT+/+ fetuses but not in their MT-/- counterparts [Carey *et al.* 2000b]. In addition, we found that the frequency of LPS-related abnormalities was inversely proportional to the amount of Zn in the diet of pregnant dams [Chua *et al.* 2006]. In our most recent study, we confirmed that Zn supplementation throughout pregnancy prevented the aberrant behaviour of adult offspring of dams exposed to LPS in early pregnancy [Coyle *et al.* 2009]. Although the findings support a mechanism involving fetal Zn deficiency in the teratogenic process the observation that neurodevelopmental outcomes while not identical with LPS and prenatal alcohol would suggest that teratogenic phenotype may depend upon the nature and/or concentration of teratogen that directly or indirectly induces MT.

In summary, if the mechanism of teratogenicity involving MT is relevant to humans, it will provide further evidence that it is essential to abstain from alcohol consumption during pregnancy, as hormones released during severe stress, and/or cytokines released in infection could work in synergy with alcohol to induce MT and therefore be co-teratogenic. It would also be predicted that poor Zn nutrition in the pregnant mother would exacerbate an MT-driven fetal Zn deficiency. In this regard, it is perhaps not a coincidence that where FAS and ARND are over represented in some indigenous communities, substance abuse, chronic infections and poor nutrition are also endemic.

## CONCLUSION

This chapter provides researchers with evidence supporting the latest mechanisms that are thought to be involved in alcohol-related teratogenicity. While none of these mechanisms can currently be excluded, some would appear to more important than others. Direct effects of alcohol, or its metabolite acetaldehyde, will largely depend on the dose that reaches the fetus, the length of exposure, the amount of maternal/fetal metabolism of alcohol and potentially any number of complex interactions that may alter the ability of alcohol to reach or affect critical cellular processes. Such an array of factors cannot be mirrored in *in vitro* systems. However, the findings that alcohol-mediated teratogenicity can be prevented using various intervention strategies points to several mechanisms that may dominate. Prime examples of these are the anti-teratogenic benefits of supplementing the mother with antioxidants, retinol or zinc before alcohol exposure. The finding that the MT-knockout mouse is protected from teratogenicity after acute alcohol exposure during the critical period of organogenesis is compelling evidence that MT underpins much of the fetal morbidity from alcohol exposure. One might, therefore, speculate that the primary event leading to alcohol-teratogenicity is induction of MT in the mother's liver which results in maternal hypozincaemia and a reduction in the amount of Zn that is available to the developing fetus. As the fetus does not store Zn, a transient interruption in Zn supply is likely have catastrophic consequences, as multiple processes could be affected resulting in dysfunctional programming of biological processes that would normally proceed in a defined order. Secondary mechanisms of fetal damage are then likely to interplay with processes weakened by the absence of zinc (e.g. antioxidant or anti-apoptotic defence mechanisms) and together with maternal and environmental risk factors interact to be expressed in the extent of the fetal morbidity. A recent review on the potential influence of zinc status contributing to FASD has been published [Keen *et al.* 2010].

However, caution is needed in attempting to attribute the importance of one mechanism above another. Different animal models and experimental conditions can confound the interpretation, as factors such as the timing of alcohol exposure relative to the stage of gestation, the pattern of alcohol exposure e.g. acute or chronic and the composition of the nutrition offered to animals may significantly influence the findings in various studies. It should also be mentioned that some of the mechanisms may not be mutually exclusive. For instance, zinc has antioxidant and anti-apoptotic properties and therefore may play a role in modulating the effect of reactive oxygen species or on repair mechanisms independent of Zn interaction with MT. Moreover, care must be taken when relating these mechanisms to FAS as there are functional differences between the mouse and human placenta which can affect the relative uptake of nutrients, alcohol and the protection offered by antioxidant systems [Burton *et al.* 2002]. This may be particularly apparent in the first trimester, where in certain species, histiotrophic nutrition through the yolk sac and other uterine glands may operate well into gestation before the placenta is fully functional. The placenta is thought to operate very early in human pregnancy but may coexist with that from uterine glands throughout the first trimester [Burton *et al.* 2002].

Nonetheless, if MT induction by alcohol is a primary mechanism underpinning the symptoms of FAS, it can be predicted that if other inflammatory and infectious events coincide with alcohol exposure and further induce MT, this will exacerbate the damage caused by alcohol in pregnancy. This has an important health implication because, although there is evidence linking chronic or intermittent high level alcohol intake with adverse pregnancy outcomes, there still remains uncertainty about potential harm to the fetus from low-level alcohol intake in pregnancy. While maternal and fetal genetics, cigarette smoking and polydrug have been identified as factors that might contribute to this fetal morbidity, the fact that intercurrent infections and/or poor Zn nutrition may also increase the overall risk from alcohol further strengthens the debate supporting strict abstinence from alcohol in pregnancy. Moreover, the finding in animals that dietary Zn supplementation may help prevent or reduce alcohol-related teratogenicity identifies a treatment regimen which in the long-term could contribute to the protection against episodic prenatal alcohol exposure in high-risk communities.

## References


Abel, EL. An update on incidence of FAS: FAS is not an equal opportunity birth defect. *Neurotoxicol. Teratol.* 1995 Jul-Aug;17(4):437-43.

Abel, EL, Hannigan, JH. Maternal risk factors in fetal alcohol syndrome: provocative and permissive influences. *Neurotoxicol. Teratol*. 1995 Jul-Aug;17(4):445-62.

Acevedo, CG, Huambachano, AM, Bravo, I, Contreras, E. Endogenous nitric oxide attenuates ethanol-induced vasoconstriction in the human placenta. *Gynecol. Obstet Invest.* 1997;44(3):153-6.

Aliyu, MH, Wilson, RE, Zoorob, R, Brown, K, Alio, AP, Clayton, H, et al. Prenatal alcohol consumption and fetal growth restriction: potentiation effect by concomitant smoking. *Nicotine Tob. Res.* 2009 Jan;11(1):36-43.

Altura, BM, Altura, BT, Carella, A, Chatterjee, M, Halevy, S, Tejani, N. Alcohol produces spasms of human umbilical blood vessels: relationship to fetal alcohol syndrome (FAS). *Eur. J. Pharmacol.* 1982 Dec 24;86(2):311-2.

Andersson, S, Halmesmaki, E, Koivusalo, M, Lapatto, R, Ylikorkala, O. Placental alcohol metabolism in chronic alcohol abuse. *Biol. Neonate*. 1989;56(2):90-3.

Andrews, GK. Regulation and function of Zip4, the acrodermatitis enteropathica gene. *Biochem. Soc. Trans*. 2008 Dec;36(Pt 6):1242-6.

Andrews, GK, Geiser, J. Expression of the mouse metallothionein-I and -II genes provides a reproductive advantage during maternal dietary zinc deficiency. *J. Nutr.* 1999 Sep;129(9):1643-8.

Anton, RF, Becker, HC, Randall, CL. Ethanol increases PGE and thromboxane production in mouse pregnant uterine tissue. *Life Sci.* 1990;46(16):1145-53.

Antony, AC. In utero physiology: role of folic acid in nutrient delivery and fetal development. *Am. J. Clin. Nutr*. 2007 Feb;85(2):598S-603S.

Arendt, T. Impairment in memory function and neurodegenerative changes in the cholinergic basal forebrain system induced by chronic intake of ethanol. *J. Neural Transm. Suppl.* 1994;44:173-87.

Ariyoshi, T, Takabatake, E, Remmer, H. Drug metabolism in ethanol-induced fatty liver. *Life Sci*. 1970 Apr 8;9(7):361-9.

Ashdown, H, Dumont, Y, Ng, M, Poole, S, Boksa, P, Luheshi, GN. The role of cytokines in mediating effects of prenatal infection on the fetus: implications for schizophrenia. *Mol. Psychiatry* 2006 Jan;11(1):47-55.

Astley, SJ, Magnuson, SI, Omnell, LM, Clarren, SK. Fetal alcohol syndrome: changes in craniofacial form with age, cognition, and timing of ethanol exposure in the macaque. *Teratology* 1999 Mar;59(3):163-72.

Bailey, BN, Delaney-Black, V, Covington, CY, Ager, J, Janisse, J, Hannigan, JH, et al. Prenatal exposure to binge drinking and cognitive and behavioral outcomes at age 7 years. *Am. J. Obstet. Gynecol.* 2004 Sep;191(3):1037-43.

Baldwin, VJ, MacLeod, PM, Benirschke, K. Placental findings in alcohol abuse in pregnancy. *Birth Defects Orig. Artic Ser.* 1982;18(3 Pt A):89-94.

Beach, RS, Gershwin, ME, Hurley, LS. Reversibility of development retardation following murine fetal zinc deprivation. *J. Nutr.* 1982 Jun;112(6):1169-81.

Becker, HC, Diaz-Granados, JL, Randall, CL. Teratogenic actions of ethanol in the mouse: a minireview. *Pharmacol. Biochem. Behav.* 1996 Dec;55(4):501-13.

Beer, WH, Johnson, RF, Guentzel, MN, Lozano, J, Henderson, GI, Schenker, S. Human placental transfer of zinc: normal characteristics and role of ethanol. *Alcohol. Clin. Exp. Res.* 1992 Feb;16(1):98-105.

Berman, RF, Hannigan, JH. Effects of prenatal alcohol exposure on the hippocampus: spatial behavior, electrophysiology, and neuroanatomy. *Hippocampus.* 2000;10(1):94-110.

Bingol, N, Schuster, C, Fuchs, M, Iosub, S, Turner, G, Stone, RK, et al. The influence of socioeconomic factors on the occurrence of fetal alcohol syndrome. *Adv. Alcohol. Subst. Abuse.* 1987 Summer;6(4):105-18.

Black, RE. Micronutrients in pregnancy. *Br. J. Nutr.* 2001 May;85 Suppl 2:S193-7.

Blakley, PM, Scott, WJ, Jr. Determination of the proximate teratogen of the mouse fetal alcohol syndrome. 1. Teratogenicity of ethanol and acetaldehyde. *Toxicol. Appl. Pharmacol.* 1984a Feb;72(2):355-63.

Blakley, PM, Scott, WJ, Jr. Determination of the proximate teratogen of the mouse fetal alcohol syndrome. 2. Pharmacokinetics of the placental transfer of ethanol and acetaldehyde. *Toxicol. Appl. Pharmacol.* 1984b Feb;72(2):364-71.

Boehm, SL, 2nd, Lundahl, KR, Caldwell, J, Gilliam, DM. Ethanol teratogenesis in the C57BL/6J, DBA/2J, and A/J inbred mouse strains. *Alcohol* 1997 Jul-Aug;14(4):389-95.

Bonthius, DJ, Bonthius, NE, Li, S, Karacay, B. The protective effect of neuronal nitric oxide synthase (nNOS) against alcohol toxicity depends upon the NO-cGMP-PKG pathway and NF-kappaB. *Neurotoxicology* 2008 Nov;29(6):1080-91.

Borrell, J, Vela, JM, Arevalo-Martin, A, Molina-Holgado, E, Guaza, C. Prenatal immune challenge disrupts sensorimotor gating in adult rats. Implications for the etiopathogenesis of schizophrenia. *Neuropsychopharmacology* 2002 Feb;26(2):204-15.

Bosron, WF, Ehrig, T, Li, TK. Genetic factors in alcohol metabolism and alcoholism. *Semin. Liver Dis.* 1993 May;13(2):126-35.

Bracken, WM, Klaassen, CD. Induction of hepatic metallothionein by alcohols: evidence for an indirect mechanism. *Toxicol. Appl. Pharmacol.* 1987 Feb;87(2):257-63.

Bradford, BU. Role of peroxisomes in the swift increase in alcohol metabolism. *J. Gastroenterol. Hepatol.* 2007 Jun;22 Suppl 1:S28-30.

Bradford, BU, Enomoto, N, Ikejima, K, Rose, ML, Bojes, HK, Forman, DT, et al. Peroxisomes are involved in the swift increase in alcohol metabolism. *J. Pharmacol. Exp. Ther.* 1999 Jan;288(1):254-9.

Brien, JF, Loomis, CW. Pharmacology of acetaldehyde. *Canadian Journal of Physiology and Pharmacology* 1983;61:1-22.

Brown, NA, Goulding, EH, Fabro, S. Ethanol embryotoxicity: direct effects on mammalian embryos in vitro. *Science* 1979 Nov 2;206(4418):573-5.

Bui, LM, Taubeneck, MW, Commisso, JF, Uriu-Hare, JY, Faber, WD, Keen, CL. Altered zinc metabolism contributes to the developmental toxicity of 2-ethylhexanoic acid, 2-ethylhexanol and valproic acid. *Toxicology* 1998 Feb 20;126(1):9-21.

Burd, L, Roberts, D, Olson, M, Odendaal, H. Ethanol and the placenta: A review. *J. Matern. Fetal. Neonatal. Med.* 2007 May;20(5):361-75.

Burton, GJ, Watson, AL, Hempstock, J, Skepper, JN, Jauniaux, E. Uterine glands provide histiotrophic nutrition for the human fetus during the first trimester of pregnancy. *J. Clin. Endocrinol. Metab.* 2002 Jun;87(6):2954-9.

Campbell, MA, Fantel, AG. Teratogenicity of acetaldehyde in vitro: relevance to the fetal alcohol syndrome. *Life Sci.* 1983 Jun 6;32(23):2641-7.

Carey, LC, Coyle, P, Philcox, JC, Rofe, AM. Ethanol decreases zinc transfer to the fetus in normal but not metallothionein-null mice. *Alcohol. Clin. Exp. Res.* 2000a Aug;24(8):1236-40.

Carey, LC, Coyle, P, Philcox, JC, Rofe, AM. Maternal ethanol exposure is associated with decreased plasma zinc and increased fetal abnormalities in normal but not metallothionein-null mice. *Alcohol. Clin. Exp. Res.* 2000b Feb;24(2):213-9.

Carey, LC, Coyle, P, Philcox, JC, Rofe, AM. Zinc supplementation at the time of ethanol exposure ameliorates teratogenicity in mice. *Alcohol. Clin. Exp. Res.* 2003 Jan;27(1):107-10.

Caughey, GE, Cleland, LG, Penglis, PS, Gamble, JR, James, MJ. Roles of cyclooxygenase (COX)-1 and COX-2 in prostanoid production by human endothelial cells: selective up-regulation of prostacyclin synthesis by COX-2. *J. Immunol.* 2001 Sep 1;167(5): 2831-8.

Challis, JR, Patrick, JE. The production of prostaglandins and thromboxanes in the feto-placental unit and their effects on the developing fetus. *Semin. Perinatol.* 1980 Jan;4(1):23-33.

Chen, Y, Pollet, N, Niehrs, C, Pieler, T. Increased XRALDH2 activity has a posteriorizing effect on the central nervous system of Xenopus embryos. *Mech. Dev.* 2001 Mar;101(1-2):91-103.

Chua, JS, Rofe, AM, Coyle, P. Dietary zinc supplementation ameliorates LPS-induced teratogenicity in mice. *Pediatr Res.* 2006 Mar;59(3):355-8.

Clagett-Dame, M, DeLuca, HF. The role of vitamin A in mammalian reproduction and embryonic development. *Annu. Rev. Nutr.* 2002;22:347-81.

Clarke, DW, Steenaart, NA, Slack, CJ, Brien, JF. Pharmacokinetics of ethanol and its metabolite, acetaldehyde, and fetolethality in the third-trimester pregnant guinea pig for oral administration of acute, multiple-dose ethanol. *Can. J. Physiol. Pharmacol.* 1986 Aug;64(8): 1060-7.

Clarren, SK, Astley, SJ, Bowden, DM. Physical anomalies and developmental delays in nonhuman primate infants exposed to weekly doses of ethanol during gestation. *Teratology* 1988 Jun;37(6):561-9.

Cohen-Kerem, R, Koren, G. Antioxidants and fetal protection against ethanol teratogenicity. I. Review of the experimental data and implications to humans. *Neurotoxicol. Teratol.* 2003 Jan-Feb;25(1):1-9.

Colvin, L, Payne, J, Parsons, D, Kurinczuk, JJ, Bower, C. Alcohol consumption during pregnancy in nonindigenous west Australian women. *Alcohol. Clin. Exp. Res.* 2007 Feb;31(2):276-84.

Connor, MJ, Smit, MH. Terminal-group oxidation of retinol by mouse epidermis. Inhibition in vitro and in vivo. *Biochem. J.* 1987 Jun 1;244(2):489-92.

Cousins, RJ. Absorption, transport, and hepatic metabolism of copper and zinc: special reference to metallothionein and ceruloplasmin. *Physiol. Rev.* 1985 Apr;65(2):238-309.

Coyle, P, Philcox, JC, Carey, LC, Rofe, AM. Metallothionein: the multipurpose protein. *Cell Mol. Life Sci.* 2002 Apr;59(4):627-47.

Coyle, P, Tran, N, Fung, JN, Summers, BL, Rofe, AM. Maternal dietary zinc supplementation prevents aberrant behaviour in an object recognition task in mice offspring exposed to LPS in early pregnancy. *Behav. Brain Res.* 2009 Jan 30;197(1):210-18.

Crabbe, JC, Harris, RA. The genetic basis of alcohol and drug actions. New York: Plenum Press; 1991.

da Cunha Ferreira, RM, Marquiegui, IM, Elizaga, IV. Teratogenicity of zinc deficiency in the rat: study of the fetal skeleton. *Teratology* 1989 Feb;39(2):181-94.

Dai, Y, Rashba-Step, J, Cederbaum, AI. Stable expression of human cytochrome P4502E1 in HepG2 cells: characterization of catalytic activities and production of reactive oxygen intermediates. *Biochemistry* 1993 Jul 13;32(27):6928-37.

Daniel, MA, Evans, MA. Quantitative comparison of maternal ethanol and maternal tertiary butanol diet on postnatal development. *J. Pharmacol. Exp. Ther.* 1982 Aug; 222(2): 294-300.

Daston, GP, Overmann, GJ, Baines, D, Taubeneck, MW, Lehman-McKeeman, LD, Rogers, JM, et al. Altered Zn status by alpha-hederin in the pregnant rat and its relationship to adverse developmental outcome. *Reprod. Toxicol.* 1994 Jan-Feb;8(1):15-24.

Daston, GP, Overmann, GJ, Taubeneck, MW, Lehman-McKeeman, LD, Rogers, JM, Keen, CL. The role of metallothionein induction and altered zinc status in maternally mediated developmental toxicity: comparison of the effects of urethane and styrene in rats. *Toxicol. Appl. Pharmacol.* 1991 Sep 15;110(3):450-63.

Davis, WL, Crawford, LA, Cooper, OJ, Farmer, GR, Thomas, DL, Freeman, BL. Ethanol induces the generation of reactive free radicals by neural crest cells in vitro. *J. Craniofac. Genet Dev. Biol.* 1990;10(3):277-93.

Day, NL, Jasperse, D, Richardson, G, Robles, N, Sambamoorthi, U, Taylor, P, et al. Prenatal exposure to alcohol: effect on infant growth and morphologic characteristics. *Pediatrics* 1989 Sep;84(3):536-41.

Dreosti, IE, Ballard, FJ, Belling, GB, Record, IR, Manuel, SJ, Hetzel, BS. The effect of ethanol and acetaldehyde on DNA synthesis in growing cells and on fetal development in the rat. *Alcohol. Clin. Exp. Res.* 1981 Summer;5(3):357-62.

Dreosti, IE, Buckley, RA, Record, IR. The teratogenic effect of zinc deficiency and accompanying feeding patterns in mice. *Nutr. Res.* 1986;6:159-66.

Dreosti, IE, Tao, SH, Hurley, LS. Plasma zinc and leukocyte changes in weaning and pregnant rats during zinc deficiency. *Proc. Soc. Exp. Biol. Med.* 1968 May;128(1):169-74.

Duester, G. A hypothetical mechanism for fetal alcohol syndrome involving ethanol inhibition of retinoic acid synthesis at the alcohol dehydrogenase step. *Alcohol. Clin. Exp. Res.* 1991 Jun;15(3):568-72.

Dufner-Beattie, J, Huang, ZL, Geiser, J, Xu, W, Andrews, GK. Mouse ZIP1 and ZIP3 genes together are essential for adaptation to dietary zinc deficiency during pregnancy. *Genesis* 2006 May;44(5):239-51.

Dufner-Beattie, J, Weaver, BP, Geiser, J, Bilgen, M, Larson, M, Xu, W, et al. The mouse acrodermatitis enteropathica gene Slc39a4 (Zip4) is essential for early development and heterozygosity causes hypersensitivity to zinc deficiency. *Hum. Mol. Genet.* 2007 Jun 15;16(12):1391-9.

Dunty, WC, Jr., Chen, SY, Zucker, RM, Dehart, DB, Sulik, KK. Selective vulnerability of embryonic cell populations to ethanol-induced apoptosis: implications for alcohol-related birth defects and neurodevelopmental disorder. *Alcohol. Clin. Exp. Res.* 2001 Oct; 25(10): 1523-35.

Faulkner, TP, Wiechart, JD, Hartman, DM, Hussain, AS. The effects of prenatal tertiary butanol administration in CBA/J and C57BL/6J mice. *Life Sci.* 1989;45(21):1989-95.

Fisher, SE, Atkinson, M, Burnap, JK, Jacobson, S, Sehgal, PK, Scott, W, et al. Ethanol-associated selective fetal malnutrition: a contributing factor in the fetal alcohol syndrome. *Alcohol. Clin. Exp. Res.* 1982 Spring;6(2):197-201.

Fisher, SE, Atkinson, M, Jacobson, S, Sehgal, P, Burnap, J, Holmes, E, et al. Selective fetal malnutrition: the effect of in vivo ethanol exposure upon in vitro placental uptake of amino acids in the non-human primate. *Pediatr. Res.* 1983 Sep;17(9):704-7.

Fisher, SE, Inselman, LS, Duffy, L, Atkinson, M, Spencer, H, Chang, B. Ethanol and fetal nutrition: effect of chronic ethanol exposure on rat placental growth and membrane-associated folic acid receptor binding activity. *J. Pediatr Gastroenterol. Nutr.* 1985 Aug; 4(4): 645-9.

Fisher, SE, Karl, PI. Histidine transfer across the human placenta: characteristics in the isolated perfused human placenta and the effect of ethanol. *Placenta* 1990 Mar-Apr;11(2):157-65.

Flynn, A, Miller, SI, Martier, SS, Golden, NL, Sokol, RJ, Del Villano, BC. Zinc status of pregnant alcoholic women: a determinant of fetal outcome. *Lancet* 1981 Mar 14;1(8220 Pt 1):572-51.

Flynn, HA, Marcus, SM, Barry, KL, Blow, FC. Rates and correlates of alcohol use among pregnant women in obstetrics clinics. *Alcohol. Clin. Exp. Res.* 2003 Jan;27(1):81-7.

Fortier, ME, Joober, R, Luheshi, GN, Boksa, P. Maternal exposure to bacterial endotoxin during pregnancy enhances amphetamine-induced locomotion and startle responses in adult rat offspring. *J. Psychiatr. Res.* 2004 May-Jun;38(3):335-45.

Gemma, S, Vichi, S, Testai, E. Individual susceptibility and alcohol effects:biochemical and genetic aspects. *Ann. Ist. Super Sanita.* 2006;42(1):8-16.

Gemma, S, Vichi, S, Testai, E. Metabolic and genetic factors contributing to alcohol induced effects and fetal alcohol syndrome. *Neurosci. Biobehav. Rev.* 2007;31(2):221-9.

Ghishan, FK, Patwardhan, R, Greene, HL. Fetal alcohol syndrome: inhibition of placental zinc transport as a potential mechanism for fetal growth retardation in the rat. *J. Lab. Clin. Med.* 1982 Jul;100(1):45-52.

Giavini, E, Broccia, ML, Prati, M, Bellomo, D, Menegola, E. Effects of ethanol and acetaldehyde on rat embryos developing in vitro. *In Vitro Cell Dev. Biol.* 1992 Mar;28A(3 Pt 1):205-10.

Golan, HM, Lev, V, Hallak, M, Sorokin, Y, Huleihel, M. Specific neurodevelopmental damage in mice offspring following maternal inflammation during pregnancy. *Neuropharmacology* 2005 May;48(6):903-17.

Goldberg, L, Rydberg, U. Inhibition of ethanol metabolism in vivo by administration of pyrazole. *Biochem. Pharmacol.* 1969 Jul;18(7):1749-62.

Goldberg, VJ, Ramwell, PW. Role of rostaglandins in reproduction. *Physiol. Rev.* 1975 Jul;55(3):325-51.

Golub, MS, Keen, CL, Gershwin, ME, Hendrickx, AG. Developmental zinc deficiency and behavior. *J. Nutr.* 1995 Aug;125(8 Suppl):2263S-71S.

Goodlett, CR, Horn, KH. Mechanisms of alcohol-induced damage to the developing nervous system. *Alcohol. Res. Health* 2001;25(3):175-84.

Goodlett, CR, Horn, KH, Zhou, FC. Alcohol teratogenesis: mechanisms of damage and strategies for intervention. *Exp. Biol. Med.* (Maywood). 2005 Jun;230(6):394-406.

Goransson, M, Magnusson, A, Bergman, H, Rydberg, U, Heilig, M. Fetus at risk: prevalence of alcohol consumption during pregnancy estimated with a simple screening method in Swedish antenatal clinics. *Addiction* 2003 Nov;98(11):1513-20.

Grant, KA, Samson, HH. Ethanol and tertiary butanol induced microcephaly in the neonatal rat: comparison of brain growth parameters. *Neurobehav. Toxicol. Teratol.* 1982 May-Jun;4(3):315-21.

Grummer, MA, Zachman, RD. Prenatal ethanol consumption alters the expression of cellular retinol binding protein and retinoic acid receptor mRNA in fetal rat embryo and brain. *Alcohol. Clin. Exp. Res.* 1995 Dec;19(6):1376-81.

Grylewski, RJ. Prostacyclin among prostenoids. *Pharmacological Reports* 2008;60:3-11.

Guerri, C, Saez, R, Sancho-Tello, M, Martin de Aquilera, E, Renau-Piqueras, J. Ethanol alters astrocyte development: a study of critical periods using primary cultures. *Neurochem. Res.* 1990 May;15(5):559-65.

Guerrini, I, Thomson, AD, Gurling, HD. The importance of alcohol misuse, malnutrition and genetic susceptibility on brain growth and plasticity. *Neurosci. Biobehav. Rev.* 2007; 31(2): 212-20.

Gundogan, F, Elwood, G, Longato, L, Tong, M, Feijoo, A, Carlson, RI, et al. Impaired placentation in fetal alcohol syndrome. *Placenta* 2008 Feb;29(2):148-57.

Haggarty, P, Abramovich, DR, Page, K. The effect of maternal smoking and ethanol on fatty acid transport by the human placenta. *Br. J. Nutr.* 2002 Mar;87(3):247-52.

Halas, ES, Eberhardt, MJ, Diers, MA, Sandstead, HH. Learning and memory impairment in adult rats due to severe zinc deficiency during lactation. *Physiol. Behav.* 1983 Mar; 30(3): 371-81.

Halas, ES, Heinrich, MD, Sandstead, HH. Long term memory deficits in adult rats due to postnatal malnutrition. *Physiol. Behav.* 1979 May;22(5):991-7.

Halas, ES, Hunt, CD, Eberhardt, MJ. Learning and memory disabilities in young adult rats from mildly zinc deficient dams. *Physiol. Behav.* 1986;37(3):451-8.

Halas, ES, Reynolds, GM, Sandstead, HH. Intra-uterine nutrition and its effects on aggression. *Physiol. Behav.* 1977 Nov;19(5):653-61.

Halas, ES, Sandstead, HH. Some effects of prenatal zinc deficiency on behavior of the adult rat. *Pediatr Res.* 1975 Feb;9(2):94-7.

Hamre, KM, West, JR. The effects of the timing of ethanol exposure during the brain growth spurt on the number of cerebellar Purkinje and granule cell nuclear profiles. *Alcohol. Clin. Exp. Res.* 1993 Jun;17(3):610-22.

Haorah, J, Ramirez, SH, Floreani, N, Gorantla, S, Morsey, B, Persidsky, Y. Mechanism of alcohol-induced oxidative stress and neuronal injury. *Free Radic. Biol. Med.* 2008 Dec 1;45(11):1542-50.

Hayashi, M, Shimazaki, Y, Kamata, S, Kakiichi, N, Ikeda, M. Disposition of ethanol and acetaldehyde in maternal blood, fetal blood, and amniotic fluid of near-term pregnant rats. *Bull. Environ. Contam. Toxicol.* 1991 Aug;47(2):184-9.

Henderson, GI, Patwardhan, RV, McLeroy, S, Schenker, S. Inhibition of placental amino acid uptake in rats following acute and chronic ethanol exposure. *Alcohol. Clin. Exp. Res.* 1982 Fall;6(4):495-505.

Henderson, GI, Schenker, S. The effect of maternal alcohol consumption on the viability and visceral development of the newborn rat. *Res. Commun. Chem. Pathol. Pharmacol.* 1977 Jan;16(1):15-32.

Hickory, W, Nanda, R, Catalanotto, FA. Fetal skeletal malformations associated with moderate zinc deficiency during pregnancy. *J. Nutr.* 1979 May;109(5):883-91.

Hidalgo, J, Aschner, M, Zatta, P, Vasak, M. Roles of the metallothionein family of proteins in the central nervous system. *Brain Res. Bull.* 2001 May 15;55(2):133-45.

Higuchi, Y, Matsumoto, N. Embryotoxicity of ethanol and acetaldehyde: Direct effects of mouse embryo in vitro. *Congenital Anomalies* 1984;24:9-28.

Hilbelink, DR, Persaud, TV. Teratogenic effects of prostaglandin E2 in hamsters. *Prog. Lipid Res.* 1981;20:241-2.

Hollstedt, C, Dahlgren, L, Rydberg, U. Outcome of pregnancy in women treated at an alcohol clinic. *Acta Psychiatr Scand.* 1983 Apr;67(4):236-48.

Hu, ZQ, Henderson, GI, Mock, DM, Schenker, S. Biotin uptake by basolateral membrane vesicles of human placenta: normal characteristics and role of ethanol. *Proc. Soc. Exp. Biol. Med.* 1994 Sep;206(4):404-8.

Hurley, LS, Gowan, J, Swenerton, H. Teratogenic effects on short term and transitory zinc deficiency in rats. *Teratology* 1971;4:199-204.

Hurley, LS, Swenerton, H. Congenital malformations resulting from zinc deficiency in rats. *Proc. Soc. Exp. Biol. Med.* 1966 Dec;123(3):692-6.

Ikonomidou, C, Bittigau, P, Ishimaru, MJ, Wozniak, DF, Koch, C, Genz, K, et al. Ethanol-induced apoptotic neurodegeneration and fetal alcohol syndrome. *Science* 2000 Feb 11;287(5455):1056-60.

Jacobson, JL, Jacobson, SW, Sokol, RJ. Increased vulnerability to alcohol-related birth defects in the offspring of mothers over 30. *Alcohol. Clin. Exp. Res.* 1996 Apr;20(2):359-63.

Jacobson, JL, Jacobson, SW, Sokol, RJ, Ager, JW, Jr. Relation of maternal age and pattern of pregnancy drinking to functionally significant cognitive deficit in infancy. *Alcohol. Clin. Exp. Res.* 1998 Apr;22(2):345-51.

Jankowski-Hennig, MA, Clegg, MS, Daston, GP, Rogers, JM, Keen, CL. Zinc-deficient rat embryos have increased caspase 3-like activity and apoptosis. *Biochem. Biophys. Res. Commun.* 2000 Apr 29;271(1):250-6.

Jing, H, Li, Y. Effects of ethanol on mouse embryonic brain development and heat shock protein 73 expression. *Toxicology in vitro* 2004;18:601-7.

Johnson, CS, Zucker, RM, Hunter, ES, 3rd, Sulik, KK. Perturbation of retinoic acid (RA)-mediated limb development suggests a role for diminished RA signaling in the teratogenesis of ethanol. *Birth Defects Res. A Clin. Mol. Teratol.* 2007 Sep;79(9):631-41.

Jones, KL, Smith, DW, Ulleland, CN, Streissguth, P. Pattern of malformation in offspring of chronic alcoholic mothers. *Lancet* 1973 Jun 9;1(7815):1267-71.

Jones, PJ, Leichter, J, Lee, M. Placental blood flow in rats fed alcohol before and during gestation. *Life Sci.* 1981 Sep 14;29(11):1153-9.

Kane, MA, Folias, AE, Wang, C, Napoli, JL. Ethanol elevates physiological all-trans-retinoic acid levels in select loci through altering retinoid metabolism in multiple loci: a potential mechanism of ethanol toxicity. *Faseb J.* Mar;24(3):823-32.

Karl, PI, Gordon, BH, Lieber, CS, Fisher, SE. Acetaldehyde production and transfer by the perfused human placental cotyledon. *Science* 1988 Oct 14;242(4876):273-5.

Keating, E, Lemos, C, Goncalves, P, Martel, F. Acute and chronic effects of some dietary bioactive compounds on folic acid uptake and on the expression of folic acid transporters by the human trophoblast cell line BeWo. *J. Nutr. Biochem.* 2008 Feb;19(2):91-100.

Keen, CL, Hurley, LS. Effects of zinc deficiency on prenatal and postnatal development. *Neurotoxicology* 1987 Fall;8(3):379-87.

Keen, CL, Uriu-Adams, JY, Skalny, A, Grabeklis, A, Grabeklis, S, Green, K, et al. The plausibility of maternal nutritional status being a contributing factor to the risk for fetal alcohol spectrum disorders: The potential influence of zinc status as an example. *Biofactors* 2010 Mar 23.

Keirse, MJ. Biosynthesis and metabolism of prostaglandins in the pregnant human uterus. *Adv. Prostaglandin Thromboxane Res.* 1978;4:87-102.

Kennedy, LA. Changes in the term mouse placenta associated with maternal alcohol consumption and fetal growth deficits. *Am. J. Obstet Gynecol.* 1984 Jul 1;149(5):518-22.

Keppen, LD, Pysher, T, Rennert, OM. Zinc deficiency acts as a co-teratogen with alcohol in fetal alcohol syndrome. *Pediatric Research* 1985 Sep;19(9):944-7.

Kesmodel, U, Kesmodel, PS, Larsen, A, Secher, NJ. Use of alcohol and illicit drugs among pregnant Danish women, 1998. *Scand. J. Public Health* 2003;31(1):5-11.

Kessel, M. Respecification of vertebral identities by retinoic acid. *Development* 1992 Jun;115(2):487-501.

Koivisto, T, Mishin, VM, Mak, KM, Cohen, PA, Lieber, CS. Induction of cytochrome P-4502E1 by ethanol in rat Kupffer cells. *Alcohol. Clin. Exp. Res.* 1996 Apr;20(2):207-12.

Kot-Leibovich, H, Fainsod, A. Ethanol induces embryonic malformations by competing for retinaldehyde dehydrogenase activity during vertebrate gastrulation. *Dis. Model Mech.* 2009 May-Jun;2(5-6):295-305.

Lee, BE, Hong, YC, Lee, KH, Kim, YJ, Kim, WK, Chang, NS, et al. Influence of maternal serum levels of vitamins C and E during the second trimester on birth weight and length. *Eur. J. Clin. Nutr.* 2004 Oct;58(10):1365-71.

Leis-Marquez, MT, Guzman-Huerta, E. [Maternal nutrition effect on fetus development and pregnant women's health]. *Ginecol. Obstet Mex.* 1999 Mar;67:113-28.

Lichten, LA, Cousins, RJ. Mammalian zinc transporters: nutritional and physiologic regulation. *Annu. Rev. Nutr.* 2009;29:153-76.

Lieber, CS. Interaction of ethanol with drugs, hepatotoxic agents, carcinogens and vitamins. *Alcohol. Alcohol.* 1990;25(2-3):157-76.

Lieber, CS. The discovery of the microsomal ethanol oxidizing system and its physiologic and pathologic role. *Drug Metab. Rev.* 2004 Oct;36(3-4):511-29.

Liebgott, B, Wiley, MJ. Prenatal hamster development following maternal administration of PGE2 at midterm. *Prostaglandins Leukot. Med.* 1985 Mar;17(3):309-18.

Lin, GW. The effect of ethanol consumption during gestation on maternal-fetal amino acid metabolism in the rat. *Curr. Alcohol.* 1981;8:479-83.

Liu, C, Chung, J, Seitz, HK, Russell, RM, Wang, XD. Chlormethiazole treatment prevents reduced hepatic vitamin A levels in ethanol-fed rats. *Alcohol. Clin. Exp. Res.* 2002 Nov;26(11):1703-9.

Liuzzi, JP, Lichten, LA, Rivera, S, Blanchard, RK, Aydemir, TB, Knutson, MD, et al. Interleukin-6 regulates the zinc transporter Zip14 in liver and contributes to the hypozincemia of the acute-phase response. *Proc. Natl. Acad. Sci. USA* 2005 May 10;102(19):6843-8.

Lokken, PM, Halas, ES, Sandstead, HH. Influence of zinc deficiency on behavior. *Proc. Soc. Exp. Biol. Med.* 1973 Nov;144(2):680-2.

Lozoff, B, Georgieff, MK. Iron deficiency and brain development. *Semin. Pediatr. Neurol.* 2006 Sep;13(3):158-65.

Maden, M, Ong, DE, Summerbell, D, Chytil, F. The role of retinoid-binding proteins in the generation of pattern in the developing limb, the regenerating limb and the nervous system. *Development* 1989;107 Suppl:109-19.

Maier, SE, West, JR. Drinking patterns and alcohol-related birth defects. *Alcohol. Res. Health* 2001;25(3):168-74.

Mandrekar, P, Szabo, G. Signalling pathways in alcohol-induced liver inflammation. *J. Hepatol.* 2009 Jun;50(6):1258-66.

Mark, M, Ghyselinck, NB, Wendling, O, Dupe, V, Mascrez, B, Kastner, P, et al. A genetic dissection of the retinoid signalling pathway in the mouse. *Proc. Nutr. Soc.* 1999 Aug;58(3):609-13.

Marrs, JA, Clendenon, SG, Ratcliffe, DR, Fielding, SM, Liu, Q, Bosron, WF. Zebrafish fetal alcohol syndrome model: effects of ethanol are rescued by retinoic acid supplement. *Alcohol* 2009 Dec 24.

Marshall, H, Morrison, A, Studer, M, Popperl, H, Krumlauf, R. Retinoids and Hox genes. *Faseb J.* 1996 Jul;10(9):969-78.

May, PA, Brooke, L, Gossage, JP, Croxford, J, Adnams, C, Jones, KL, et al. Epidemiology of fetal alcohol syndrome in a South African community in the Western Cape Province. *Am. J. Public Health* 2000 Dec;90(12):1905-12.

May, PA, Gossage, JP. Estimating the prevalence of fetal alcohol syndrome. A summary. *Alcohol. Res. Health* 2001;25(3):159-67.

May, PA, Gossage, JP, Kalberg, WO, Robinson, LK, Buckley, D, Manning, M, et al. Prevalence and epidemiologic characteristics of FASD from various research methods with an emphasis on recent in-school studies. *Dev. Disabil. Res. Rev.* 2009;15(3):176-92.

May, PA, Gossage, JP, Marais, AS, Adnams, CM, Hoyme, HE, Jones, KL, et al. The epidemiology of fetal alcohol syndrome and partial FAS in a South African community. *Drug Alcohol. Depend.* 2007 May 11;88(2-3):259-71.

May, PA, Gossage, JP, Marais, AS, Hendricks, LS, Snell, CL, Tabachnick, BG, et al. Maternal risk factors for fetal alcohol syndrome and partial fetal alcohol syndrome in South Africa: a third study. *Alcohol. Clin. Exp. Res.* 2008 May;32(5):738-53.

McCaffery, PJ, Adams, J, Maden, M, Rosa-Molinar, E. Too much of a good thing: retinoic acid as an endogenous regulator of neural differentiation and exogenous teratogen. *Eur. J. Neurosci.* 2003 Aug;18(3):457-72.

McDermott, S, Callaghan, W, Szwejbka, L, Mann, H, Daguise, V. Urinary tract infections during pregnancy and mental retardation and developmental delay. *Obstet Gynecol.* 2000 Jul;96(1):113-9.

Memon, S, Pratten, MK. Developmental toxicity of ethanol in chick heart in ovo and in micromass culture can be prevented by addition of vitamin C and folic acid. *Reprod. Toxicol.* 2009 Sep;28(2):262-9.

Meyer, U, Schwendener, S, Feldon, J, Yee, BK. Prenatal and postnatal maternal contributions in the infection model of schizophrenia. *Exp. Brain Res.* 2006 Aug;173(2):243-57.

Michaelis, EK, Michaelis, ML. Cellular and molecular bases of alcohol's teratogenic effects. *Alcohol Health and Research World* 1994;18:601-7.

Michalska, AE, Choo, KH. Targeting and germ-line transmission of a null mutation at the metallothionein I and II loci in mouse. *Proc. Natl. Acad. Sci. USA* 1993 Sep 1;90(17):8088-92.

Mitchell, JJ, Paiva, M, Heaton, MB. The antioxidants vitamin E and beta-carotene protect against ethanol-induced neurotoxicity in embryonic rat hippocampal cultures. *Alcohol.* 1999 Feb;17(2):163-8.

Morojele, NK, London, L, Olorunju, SA, Matjila, MJ, Davids, AS, Rendall-Mkosi, KM. Predictors of risk of alcohol-exposed pregnancies among women in an urban and a rural area of South Africa. *Soc. Sci. Med.* 2010 Feb;70(4):534-42.

Mukherjee, AB, Hodgen, GD. Maternal ethanol exposure induces transient impairment of umbilical circulation and fetal hypoxia in monkeys. *Science* 1982 Nov 12;218(4573):700-2.

Mulligan, CJ, Robin, RW, Osier, MV, Sambuughin, N, Goldfarb, LG, Kittles, RA, et al. Allelic variation at alcohol metabolism genes ( ADH1B, ADH1C, ALDH2) and alcohol dependence in an American Indian population. *Hum. Genet.* 2003 Sep;113(4):325-36.

Nakamura, MU, Alexandre, SM, Kuhn dos Santos, JF, de Souza, E, Sass, N, Auritscher Beck, AP, et al. Obstetric and perinatal effects of active and/or passive smoking during pregnancy. *Sao Paulo Med. J.* 2004 May 6;122(3):94-8.

Nava-Ocampo, AA, Velazquez-Armenta, Y, Brien, JF, Koren, G. Elimination kinetics of ethanol in pregnant women. *Reprod. Toxicol.* 2004 Jun;18(4):613-7.

Ng, PK, Cottle, MK, Baker, JM, Johnson, B, van Muyden, P, van Petten, GR. Ethanol kinetics during pregnancy. Study in ewes and their fetuses. *Prog. Neuropsychopharmacol. Biol. Psychiatry* 1982;6(1):37-42.

Niederreither, K, Subbarayan, V, Dolle, P, Chambon, P. Embryonic retinoic acid synthesis is essential for early mouse post-implantation development. *Nat. Genet.* 1999 Apr;21(4):444-8.

O'Shea, KS, Kaufman, MH. The teratogenic effect of acetaldehyde: implications for the study of the fetal alcohol syndrome. *J. Anat.* 1979 Jan;128(Pt 1):65-76.

Offenbacher, S, Riche, EL, Barros, SP, Bobetsis, YA, Lin, D, Beck, JD. Effects of maternal Campylobacter rectus infection on murine placenta, fetal and neonatal survival, and brain development. *J. Periodontol.* 2005 Nov;76(11 Suppl):2133-43.

Okahara, K, Sun, B, Kambayashi, J. Upregulation of prostacyclin synthesis-related gene expression by shear stress in vascular endothelial cells. *Arterioscler. Thromb Vasc. Biol.* 1998 Dec;18(12):1922-6.

Opler, MG, Susser, ES. Fetal environment and schizophrenia. *Environ. Health Perspect.* 2005 Sep;113(9):1239-42.

Orny, A. Embryonic oxidative stress as a mechanism of teratogenesis with special emphasis on diabetic embryopathy. *Reprod. Toxicol.* 2007;24:31-41.

Overholser, JC. Fetal alcohol syndrome: A review of the disorder. *Journal of Contemporary Psycgotherapy* 1990;20:163-76.

Padmanabhan, R, Sreenathan, RN, Singh, S. Studies on the lethal and teratogenic effects of acetaldehyde in the rat. *Congenital Anomalies* 1983;23:13-23.

Pawan, GL. Metabolism of alcohol (ethanol) in man. *Proc. Nutr. Soc.* 1972 Sep;31(2):83-9.

Pennington, S, Kalmus, G. Brain growth during ethanol-induced hypoplasia. D*rug Alcohol. Depend.* 1987 Nov 30;20(3):279-86.

Persaud, TV. Prostaglandins and organogenesis. A*dv. Prostaglandin. Thromboxane Res.* 1978;4:139-56.

Priscott, PK. The effects of ethanol on rat embryos developing in vitro. *Biochem. Pharmacol.* 1982 Nov 15;31(22):3641-3.

Priscott, PK. The effects of acetaldehyde and 2,3-butanediol on rat embryos developing in vitro. *Biochem. Pharmacol.* 1985 Feb 15;34(4):529-32.

Randall, CL, Anton, RF. Aspirin reduces alcohol-induced prenatal mortality and malformations in mice. *Alcohol. Clin. Exp. Res.* 1984 Nov-Dec;8(6):513-5.

Randall, CL, Anton, RF, Becker, HC. Effect of indomethacin on alcohol-induced morphological anomalies in mice. *Life Sci.* 1987 Jul 20;41(3):361-9.

Randall, CL, Taylor, WJ. Prenatal ethanol exposure in mice: teratogenic effects. *Teratology* 1979 Jun;19(3):305-11.

Rice, PA, Nesbitt, RE, Jr., Cuenca, VG, Zhang, W, Gordon, GB, Kim, TJ. The effect of ethanol on the production of lactate, triglycerides, phospholipids, and free fatty acids in the perfused human placenta. *Am. J. Obstet Gynecol.* 1986 Jul;155(1):207-11.

Rogers, JM, Taubeneck, MW, Daston, GP, Sulik, KK, Zucker, RM, Elstein, KH, et al. Zinc deficiency causes apoptosis but not cell cycle alterations in organogenesis-stage rat embryos: effect of varying duration of deficiency. *Teratology* 1995 Sep;52(3):149-59.

Ruth, RE, Goldsmith, SK. Interaction between zinc deprivation and acute ethanol intoxication during pregnancy in rats. *J. Nutr.* 1981 Nov;111(11):2034-8.

Rydberg, U, Neri, A. 4-Methylpyrazole as an inhibitor of ethanol metabolism: differential metabolic and central nervous effects. *Acta Pharmacol. Toxicol.* (Copenh). 1972;31(5):421-32.

Sakai, Y, Meno, C, Fujii, H, Nishino, J, Shiratori, H, Saijoh, Y, et al. The retinoic acid-inactivating enzyme CYP26 is essential for establishing an uneven distribution of retinoic acid along the anterio-posterior axis within the mouse embryo. *Genes. Dev.* 2001 Jan 15;15(2):213-25.

Salaspuro, MP, Lieber, CS. Non-uniformity of blood ethanol elimination: its exaggeration after chronic consumption. *Ann. Clin. Res.* 1978 Oct;10(5):294-7.

Sauerbier, I. Circadian modification of ethanol damage in utero to mice. *Am. J. Anat.* 1987 Feb;178(2):170-4.

Savoy-Moore, RT, Dombrowski, MP, Cheng, A, Abel, EA, Sokol, RJ. Low dose alcohol contracts the human umbilical artery in vitro. *Alcohol. Clin. Exp. Res.* 1989 Feb;13(1):40-2.

Schenker, S, Becker, HC, Randall, CL, Phillips, DK, Baskin, GS, Henderson, GI. Fetal alcohol syndrome: current status of pathogenesis. *Alcohol. Clin. Exp. Res.* 1990a Oct;14(5): 635-47.

Schenker, S, Dicke, JM, Johnson, RF, Hays, SE, Henderson, GI. Effect of ethanol on human placental transport of model amino acids and glucose. *Alcohol. Clin. Exp. Res.* 1989 Feb;13(1):112-9.

Schenker, S, Hu, ZQ, Johnson, RF, Yang, Y, Frosto, T, Elliott, BD, et al. Human placental biotin transport: normal characteristics and effect of ethanol. *Alcohol. Clin. Exp. Res.* 1993 Jun;17(3):566-75.

Schenker, S, Johnson, RF, Hoyumpa, AM, Henderson, GI. Thiamine-transfer by human placenta: normal transport and effects of ethanol. *J. Lab. Clin. Med.* 1990b Jul;116(1):106-15.

Schenker, S, Johnson, RF, Mahuren, JD, Henderson, GI, Coburn, SP. Human placental vitamin B6 (pyridoxal) transport: normal characteristics and effects of ethanol. *Am. J. Physiol.* 1992 Jun;262(6 Pt 2):R966-74.

Sharpe, TT, Velasquez, MM. Risk of alcohol-exposed pregnancies among low-income, illicit drug-using women. *J. Womens Health* (Larchmt). 2008 Oct;17(8):1339-44.

Shi, L, Fatemi, SH, Sidwell, RW, Patterson, PH. Maternal influenza infection causes marked behavioral and pharmacological changes in the offspring. *J. Neurosci.* 2003 Jan 1;23(1):297-302.

Singh, SP, Snyder, AK, Pullen, GL. Maternal alcohol ingestion inhibits fetal glucose uptake and growth. *Neurotoxicol. Teratol.* 1989 May-Jun;11(3):215-9.

Smith, GN, Brien, JF, Homan, J, Carmichael, L, Treissman, D, Patrick, J. Effect of ethanol on ovine fetal and maternal plasma prostaglandin E2 concentrations and fetal breathing movements. *J. Dev. Physiol.* 1990 Jul;14(1):23-8.

Smith, GN, Sinervo, KR, Carmichael, L, Patrick, J, Bocking, AD, Brien, JF. The effects of indomethacin and prostaglandin E2 on the ethanol-induced suppression of ovine fetal breathing movements. *J. Dev. Physiol.* 1991 Oct;16(4):239-42.

Snyder, AK, Singh, SP, Pullen, GL. Ethanol-induced intrauterine growth retardation: correlation with placental glucose transfer. *Alcohol. Clin. Exp. Res.* 1986 Mar-Apr;10(2):167-70.

Sokol, RJ, Miller, SI, Reed, G. Alcohol abuse during pregnancy: an epidemiologic study. *Alcohol. Clin. Exp. Res.* 1980 Apr;4(2):135-45.

Sood, B, Delaney-Black, V, Covington, C, Nordstrom-Klee, B, Ager, J, Templin, T, et al. Prenatal alcohol exposure and childhood behavior at age 6 to 7 years: I. dose-response effect. *Pediatrics* 2001 Aug;108(2):E34.

Sreenathan, RN, Padmanabhan, R, Singh, S. Teratogenic effects of acetaldehyde in the rat. *Drug Alcohol. Depend.* 1982 Aug;9(4):339-50.

Streissguth, AP, Dehaene, P. Fetal alcohol syndrome in twins of alcoholic mothers: concordance of diagnosis and IQ. *Am. J. Med. Genet.* 1993 Nov 1;47(6):857-61.

Streissguth, AP, Landesman-Dwyer, S, Martin, JC, Smith, DW. Teratogenic effects of alcohol in humans and laboratory animals. *Science* 1980 Jul 18;209(4454):353-61.

Streissguth, AP, Sampson, PD, Olson, HC, Bookstein, FL, Barr, HM, Scott, M, et al. Maternal drinking during pregnancy: attention and short-term memory in 14-year-old offspring--a longitudinal prospective study. *Alcohol. Clin. Exp. Res*. 1994 Feb;18(1):202-18.

Sulik, KK. Critical periods for alcohol teratogenesis in mice, with special reference to the gastrulation stage of embryogenesis. *Ciba Found Symp*. 1984;105:124-41.

Sulik, KK, Johnston, MC, Webb, MA. Fetal alcohol syndrome: embryogenesis in a mouse model. *Science* 1981 Nov 20;214(4523):936-8.

Summers, BL, Henry, CM, Rofe, AM, Coyle, P. Dietary zinc supplementation during pregnancy prevents spatial and object recognition memory impairments caused by early prenatal ethanol exposure. *Behav. Brain Res*. 2008 Jan 25;186(2):230-8.

Summers, BL, Rofe, AM, Coyle, P. Prenatal zinc treatment at the time of acute ethanol exposure limits spatial memory impairments in mouse offspring. *Pediatr Res*. 2006 Jan;59(1): 66-71.

Summers, BL, Rofe, AM, Coyle, P. Dietary zinc supplementation throughout pregnancy protects against fetal dysmorphology and improves postnatal survival after prenatal ethanol exposure in mice. *Alcohol. Clin. Exp. Res*. 2009 Apr;33(4):591-600.

Taubeneck, MW, Daston, GP, Rogers, JM, Gershwin, ME, Ansari, A, Keen, CL. Tumor necrosis factor-alpha alters maternal and embryonic zinc metabolism and is developmentally toxic in mice. *J. Nutr*. 1995 Apr;125(4):908-19.

Taubeneck, MW, Daston, GP, Rogers, JM, Keen, CL. Altered maternal zinc metabolism following exposure to diverse developmental toxicants. *Reprod. Toxicol*. 1994 Jan-Feb; 8(1): 25-40.

Taylor, SM, Heron, AE, Cannell, GR, Florin, TH. Pressor effect of ethanol in the isolated perfused human placental lobule. *Eur. J. Pharmacol*. 1994 Aug 3;270(4):371-4.

Tenkku, LE, Morris, DS, Salas, J, Xaverius, PK. Racial disparities in pregnancy-related drinking reduction. *Matern Child Health J*. 2009 Sep;13(5):604-13.

Tsutsumi, M, Lasker, JM, Shimizu, M, Rosman, AS, Lieber, CS. The intralobular distribution of ethanol-inducible P450IIE1 in rat and human liver. *Hepatology* 1989 Oct;10(4):437-46.

Urban, M, Chersich, MF, Fourie, LA, Chetty, C, Olivier, L, Viljoen, D. Fetal alcohol syndrome among grade 1 schoolchildren in Northern Cape Province: prevalence and risk factors. *S. Afr. Med. J*. 2008 Nov;98(11):877-82.

Vallee, BL, Falchuk, KH. The biochemical basis of zinc physiology. *Physiol. Rev*. 1993 Jan;73(1):79-118.

Varma, PK, Persaud, TV. Influence of pyrazole, an inhibitor of alcohol dehydrogenase on the prenatal toxicity of ethanol in the rat. *Res. Commun. Chem. Pathol. Pharmacol*. 1979 Oct;26(1):65-73.

Viljoen, DL, Gossage, JP, Brooke, L, Adnams, CM, Jones, KL, Robinson, LK, et al. Fetal alcohol syndrome epidemiology in a South African community: a second study of a very high prevalence area. *J. Stud. Alcohol*. 2005 Sep;66(5):593-604.

Walsh, SW. Eicosanoids in preeclampsia. Prostaglandins Leukot Essent Fatty Acids. 2004 Feb;70(2):223-32.

Warren, KR, Li, TK. Genetic polymorphisms: impact on the risk of fetal alcohol spectrum disorders. *Birth Defects Res. A Clin. Mol. Teratol*. 2005 Apr;73(4):195-203.

Webster, WS, Walsh, DA, McEwen, SE, Lipson, AH. Some teratogenic properties of ethanol and acetaldehyde in C57BL/6J mice: implications for the study of the fetal alcohol syndrome. *Teratology* 1983 Apr;27(2):231-43.

Wentzel, P, Rydberg, U, Eriksson, UJ. Antioxidative treatment diminishes ethanol-induced congenital malformations in the rat. *Alcohol. Clin. Exp. Res.* 2006 Oct;30(10):1752-60.

West, JR, Goodlett, CR, Bonthius, DJ, Hamre, KM, Marcussen, BL. Cell population depletion associated with fetal alcohol brain damage: mechanisms of BAC-dependent cell loss. *Alcohol. Clin. Exp. Res.* 1990 Dec;14(6):813-8.

Wilkening, RB, Anderson, S, Martensson, L, Meschia, G. Placental transfer as a function of uterine blood flow. American Journal of Physiology: *Heart and Circulatory Physiology* 1982;242:H429-H36.

Yelin, R, Kot, H, Yelin, D, Fainsod, A. Early molecular effects of ethanol during vertebrate embryogenesis. *Differentiation* 2007 Jun;75(5):393-403.

Yelin, R, Schyr, RB, Kot, H, Zins, S, Frumkin, A, Pillemer, G, et al. Ethanol exposure affects gene expression in the embryonic organizer and reduces retinoic acid levels. *Dev. Biol.* 2005 Mar 1;279(1):193-204.

Ylikorkala, O, Halmesmaki, E, Viinikka, L. Urinary prostacyclin and thromboxane metabolites in drinking pregnant women and in their infants: relations to the fetal alcohol effects. *Obstet. Gynecol.* 1988 Jan;71(1):61-6.

Young, NK. Effects of alcohol and other drugs on children. *J. Psychoactive Drugs* 1997 Jan-Mar;29(1):23-42.

Zalewski, PD, Forbes, IJ, Seamark, RF, Borlinghaus, R, Betts, WH, Lincoln, SF, et al. Flux of intracellular labile zinc during apoptosis (gene-directed cell death) revealed by a specific chemical probe, Zinquin. *Chem. Biol.* 1994 Nov;1(3):153-61.

In: Pregnancy and Alcohol Consumption
Editor: Joshua D. Hoffman, pp. 105-127 ISBN 978-1-61761-122-3


*Chapter 3*

# ALCOHOL USE PRE- AND LATE-PREGNANCY: EPIDEMIOLOGY AND COMMENTS FROM POSTPARTUM SURVEYS

***Diana Cheng[1], Laurie Kettinger[1], Douglas D'Agati[2], Paula J. Lockhart[3] and Lee Hurt[1]***

1. Center for Maternal and Child Health,
Maryland Department of Health and Mental Hygiene
2. University of Maryland School of Medicine
3. Kennedy Krieger Institute,
Johns Hopkins University School of Medicine, USA

## ABSTRACT

*Background:* Avoidance of maternal alcohol consumption during pregnancy is the only way to prevent the harmful effects of alcohol on the fetus known as fetal alcohol spectrum disorder (FASD).

*Objective:* To assess the prevalence of pre- and late-pregnancy alcohol consumption among women and to determine maternal opinions about prenatal alcohol use.

*Methods:* Data were obtained from a stratified random sample of 12,611 Maryland mothers who delivered live born infants during the years 2001-2008 and completed the Maryland Pregnancy Risk Assessment Monitoring System (PRAMS) survey. Univariable and bivariable analyses were conducted using Proc Surveyfreq in SAS v9.2. Multivariable logistic regression analysis, using Proc Surveylogistic in SAS, was used to control for potential confounding factors. Maternal quotes about alcohol use were taken verbatim from mothers who wrote comments either next to the survey questions or on the last blank page of the survey.

*Results:* Nearly 8% of Maryland mothers reported any alcohol consumption during the last three months of pregnancy. Alcohol consumption occurred most frequently among mothers who were white non-Hispanic, 35+ years of age, college graduates, and married. Less than 1% of mothers reported binge drinking during the last three months of pregnancy. Binge drinking occurred most frequently among mothers who were under 20 years of age and unmarried. During the three months before pregnancy, 51% of women reported consuming alcohol and 16% reported binge drinking. Alcohol use and binge drinking increased significantly between 2001 and 2008.

Many mothers voiced their opinions about the adverse consequences of alcohol use during pregnancy. Some urged mothers not to drink, others wanted to help mothers stop drinking, a few thought women were selfish to continue drinking during pregnancy and several thought this was a form of child abuse. It was clear that many mothers were not assessed for alcohol use during their prenatal visits and some went so far as to say that their physicians sent mixed messages about alcohol use. Among mothers who reported alcohol use during pregnancy, most wanted to minimize its use by conveying that the amount consumed was small or for a special occasion. Some confirmed that they drank during early pregnancy before the pregnancy was confirmed.

*Conclusion:* Pre and late-pregnancy alcohol use was common among women—especially those who are usually at low risk for adverse pregnancy outcomes such as college graduates. Screening all women for alcohol use before and during pregnancy will improve identification of women who need help or treatment for alcohol use reduction. This will facilitate the achievement of an alcohol-free pregnancy—theoretically the only sure way to prevent FASD.

## 1. Introduction

Alcohol consumption during pregnancy is a serious public health concern worldwide. Scientific evidence clearly demonstrates that many permanent cognitive and behavioral disabilities are due to prenatal alcohol exposure. In the USA alone, it has been estimated that 9.1 in 1000 newborns or approximately 1% of offspring have a prenatal alcohol related disability or a Fetal Alcohol Spectrum Disorder (FASD) [1]. FASD, is the non-diagnostic umbrella term for the following diagnosable disorders due to prenatal alcohol exposure; these disorders are: Fetal Alcohol Syndrome (FAS), Partial Fetal Alcohol Syndrome (pFAS), Alcohol-Related Neurodevelopmental Disorder (ARND) and Alcohol-Related Birth Defects (ARBD). These disorders are totally preventable.

The importance of educating reproductive aged women on the dangers of even mild to moderate alcohol consumption during any phase of pregnancy cannot be overestimated. Prenatal alcohol exposure affects individuals selectively across numerous areas of cognitive function that most individuals take for granted for living independently and responsibly in our modern society [2]. Since the majority of the individuals affected have borderline intelligence or above and have no physical signs of the disorder they go unnoticed as having a life altering brain disorder. Binge drinking however, once or twice per week during pregnancy, even without other alcohol use during the week, can lead to severe cognitive and physical disabilities in the offspring and the worse cases of FAS [3].

Affected individuals can suffer from mild to profoundly serious behavioral and emotional disorders, academic disability, speech and language problems, fine and gross motor skills deficits, sensory integration problems, uneven development of adaptive living skills, problems in judgment, memory, insight, "cause and effect" reasoning, and social skills [2]. For some individuals, their disability is mild enough for environmental and academic accommodations to help the person to be successful. But a large number of individuals are destined, by virtue of the extremeness of their disability, to live out their lives being cared for by unaffected family members, group homes, residential treatment centers, state hospitals, detention centers, homeless shelters, jails and prisons. Often their FASD cognitive disability is never uncovered. It is estimated that the lifetime costs of caring for one baby with FASD is 1.4 - 1.5 million dollars and more in the most complicated cases [4].

Despite the evidence of fetal effects from prenatal alcohol exposure since Jones, et al first published their report in the U.S. in 1973 [5] the rate of alcohol use during pregnancy remains high. Recent national multi-state survey data of alcohol use during pregnancy have reported a range of 10.6% to 30.3% for any alcohol use and 1.8% to 5.7% for binge drinking (defined as 5 or more drinks on one occasion) [6-10]. Wide state to state variations existed within each survey method utilized.

Our objective in this Maryland study was to estimate the prevalence of preconceptional and late-pregnancy alcohol consumption and to determine characteristics of women at high risk of alcohol use. Comments from postpartum mothers about alcohol use were also analyzed to further our understanding of women's views about alcohol use during pregnancy.

## 2. Methods

We examined data collected from a random sample of postpartum mothers in Maryland who delivered live births between 2001 and 2008 and completed the Pregnancy Risk Assessment Monitoring System (PRAMS) survey two to nine months after delivery. The Maryland Department of Health and Mental Hygiene conducts the survey under a cooperative agreement with the Centers for Disease Control and Prevention (CDC). Stratified random sampling is used to oversample mothers 35 years of age or older and women who delivered low birth weight (<2500 grams) infants. The annual sample, determined by the CDC for each PRAMS state, is large enough for estimating statewide risk factor proportions within 3.5% at a 95% confidence level. PRAMS is a mixed-mode surveillance system supported by the CDC that asks women about their experiences before, during, and after pregnancy in an attempt to improve the future health outcomes of mothers and babies. Mothers are sent up to three surveys followed by telephone interviews if no response is received by mail. Survey data are linked with birth certificate data to provide additional demographic, medical and pregnancy information. The 12,611 responses to the survey received during the study years were weighted to make the results representative of all Maryland women delivering live born infants during the study period and to account for non-response. The overall response rate for the survey during this study period was 72%, with annual response rates over 70%.

Alcohol consumption during pregnancy was assessed by response to the following two survey questions:

> "During the last 3 months of your pregnancy, how many alcoholic drinks did you have in an average week? (A drink is 1 glass of wine, wine cooler, can or bottle of beer, shot of liquor or mixed drink)."
>
> a) 14 drinks or more a week
> b) 7 to 13 drinks a week
> c) 4 to 6 drinks a week
> d) 1 to 3 drinks a week
> e) Less than 1 drink a week
> f) I didn't drink then

"During the last 3 months of your pregnancy, how many times did you drink 5 alcoholic drinks or more in one sitting?"

a) 6 or more times
b) 4 to 5 times
c) 2 to 3 times
d) 1 time
e) I didn't have 5 drinks or more in 1 sitting
f) I didn't drink then

These same questions were used to ask mothers about their preconception alcohol use and binge drinking episodes "during the three months before you got pregnant". Birth certificate data were used for maternal race, ethnicity, age, education level, and marital status. Use of Medicaid coverage at delivery was part of the PRAMS survey.

The PRAMS survey collects mainly quantitative data on the mothers' behaviors and experiences before, during and after pregnancy. However, it also collects qualitative data in the form of maternal comments written throughout the survey. PRAMS mothers are given the opportunity to share information on the back page of the survey booklet with the prompt, "Please use this space for any additional comments you would like to make about the health of mothers and babies in Maryland". Many of the mothers also write comments in the margins of the survey booklet relating to particular questions. All back page and margin comments are entered into a database for future review. Women who complete the survey by phone instead of mail are also given the opportunity to share "back page" comments. All comments are recorded verbatim and the phone interviewer can break off from the survey at any time to enter a comment if the mother has more to say about a particular question before getting to the back page comment section (i.e., analogous to margin comments in the mail survey).

Univariable and bivariable analyses were conducted using Proc Surveyfreq in SAS v9.2. Multivariable logistic regression analysis, using Proc Surveylogistic in SAS was used to control for potential confounding factors. The Maryland Department of Health and Mental Hygiene Institutional Review Board qualified this project as exempt research.

## 3. Results

Self-reported alcohol consumption and binge drinking decreased from 50.6% and 15.2% pre-pregnancy to 7.7% and 0.5% during late-pregnancy [Table 1 and 2]. During pregnancy, teens had the lowest reported alcohol use of any age group (3.6%) but had the highest reported rate of binge drinking episode (1.2%) [Table 2]. The highest prevalence for any alcohol consumption before and during pregnancy was reported by mothers who were White non-Hispanic, college graduates, 35 years of age or more, married and not using Medicaid for their delivery [Table 1 and 2]. The 50.6% of mothers who consumed alcohol pre-pregnancy included 43.1% of mothers who reported drinking <4 drinks/week, 5.0% 4-6 drinks/week and 2.5% $\geq$7 drinks/week. Pre-pregnancy, adolescents less than 20 years of age reported the lowest alcohol use rates of any age group that we studied - 30.2% reported any alcohol use before pregnancy and 11.1% reported binge drinking before pregnancy [Table 1].

The 7.7% of mothers who reported drinking during the last three months of pregnancy included 6.3% who reported consuming <1 drink/week and 1.4% who reported ≥1 drink/week. Preconceptional binge drinking was reported most commonly by women who were White non-Hispanic, under 25 years old, and unmarried [Table 1]. The 15.2% of mothers who reported preconceptional binge included 6.0% who reported one episode, 6.5% two to three episodes and 2.6% four or more episodes. Binge drinking during late-pregnancy was reported most commonly by women who were Black, under 20 years of age, unmarried and not college-educated [Table 2]. The 0.5% of women who reported binge drinking during late pregnancy included 0.2% who reported one episode, 0.2% two to three episodes and 0.1% four or more episodes. The number of Asian and Hispanic women who reported any alcohol use or binge drinking during pregnancy was small (n<15 for 1 or more drinks/week or 1 or more episodes of binge drinking over the eight year period) therefore the prevalence rates for these women are not shown.

**Table 1. Pre-Pregnancy Alcohol Consumption**

| *Factor* | *Any alcohol use* | *Binge drinking* |
|---|---|---|
| | % | % |
| *Total* | 50.6 | 15.2 |
| *Race/Ethnicity* | | |
| White, Non-Hispanic | 66.8 | 21.0 |
| Black, Non-Hispanic | 39.5 | 9.8 |
| *Age, years* | | |
| <20 | 30.2 | 11.1 |
| 20-24 | 52.8 | 21.3 |
| 25-29 | 49.1 | 16.5 |
| 30-34 | 54.7 | 13.4 |
| 35+ | 55.0 | 11.3 |
| *Education* | | |
| High school or less | 39.5 | 15.6 |
| Some college | 54.0 | 16.1 |
| College graduate | 61.6 | 14.3 |
| *Marital status* | | |
| Married | 54.5 | 13.4 |
| Unmarried | 44.4 | 18.1 |
| *Medicaid, delivery* | | |
| Yes | 37.2 | 14.8 |
| No | 56.7 | 15.4 |

*P values are <0.05 for all categories except binge drinking by education and Medicaid status.

The prevalence of pre-pregnancy binge drinking has generally increased each year from 13.2% in 2001 to 19.7% in 2007 and decreased to 18.2% in 2008 [Figure 3]. There was an increase in pre- and late-pregnancy alcohol use and binge drinking between 2001 and 2008. However this increase was statistically significant only for pre-pregnancy rates for reported consumption of four or more drinks per week, any binge drinking, and two or more episodes of binge drinking. The increase in alcohol use and binge drinking rates during late pregnancy was not statistically significant [Table 3].

**Table 2. Alcohol Consumption, Last Three Months of Pregnancy**

| *Factor* | *Any alcohol use* | *Binge drinking* |
|---|---|---|
| | % | % |
| *Total* | 7.7 | 0.5 |
| *Race/Ethnicity* | | |
| White, Non-Hispanic | 10.9 | 0.2 |
| Black, Non-Hispanic | 4.3 | 0.9 |
| *Age, years* | | |
| <20 | 3.6 | 1.2 |
| 20-24 | 4.6 | 0.4 |
| 25-29 | 5.6 | 0.4 |
| 30-34 | 10.0 | 0.3 |
| 35+ | 13.4 | 0.8 |
| *Education* | | |
| High school or less | 4.4 | 0.9 |
| Some college | 7.7 | 0.5 |
| College graduate | 11.3 | 0.1 |
| *Marital Status* | | |
| Married | 9.4 | 0.2 |
| Unmarried | 5.1 | 1.1 |
| *Medicaid, delivery* | | |
| Yes | 4.0 | 1.0 |
| No | 9.4 | 0.3 |

*P values are <0.05 for all categories except binge drinking by age.

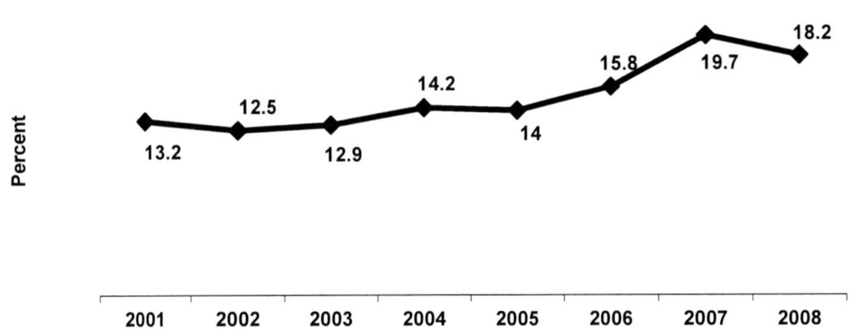


Figure 1. Pre-Pregnancy Binge Drinking Rates

## Comments from PRAMS Mothers

From 2001-2008, we reviewed 205 comments pertaining to alcohol use that were made by mothers. Several recurrent themes emerged and the comments were classified by two coders into the following categories: (1) Affirmation of non-drinking status, (2) Feelings about alcohol use, (3) Admit drinking alcohol with only minimal use or minimization of use, (4) Admit drinking alcohol, (5) No preconception thought given, (6) Preconception thought given, (7) Doctor asked about or discussed alcohol use, (8) Doctor did not discuss alcohol use and/or gave misleading advice, and (9) Want legal action taken.

**Table 3. Alcohol Use and Binge Drinking, Pre- and Late-Pregnancy.**

| Alcohol consumption | 2001 % | 2008 % | Change % |
|---|---|---|---|
| Pre-pregnancy | | | |
| Any alcohol use | 51.5 | 52.8 | +2.5 |
| 4 or more drinks/week | 4.9 | 10.6 | +116.3* |
| Binge drinking, any | 13.2 | 18.2 | +37.8* |
| 2 or more episodes | 7.4 | 11.1 | +50.0* |
| Late pregnancy | | | |
| Any alcohol use | 8.1 | 8.8 | +8.6 |
| Binge drinking, any | 0.6 | 1.0 | +66.7 |

*difference is significant [$p < 0.05$].

We'll now take a closer look at each theme, giving examples using comments in the respondents' own words.

### *Affirmation of Non-Drinking Status*

Many women (n=58) made comments that they do not drink. Some reported that they have never had a drink in their life.

- "I do not drink at all."
- "Nunca e tomado bebida alcoholicas." (I never drink alcoholic drinks)
- "don't drink ever"

### *Opinions about Alcohol Use*

Some mothers (n=52) did not like the notion that mothers would jeopardize their babies' health by drinking during pregnancy. Most commented that women simply should not drink during pregnancy while others went on to discuss how alcohol can affect the baby. A few commented on how the system could help mothers who drink.

- "Mothers should not drink or smoke during pregnancy. It can affect the baby."
- "Women should not drink or use alcohol during pregnancy. Some women may still have a healthy baby, but it is taking a chance."
- "I think the most important thing…no drinking and of course no drugs. Be responsible and realize that you are growing a human in your belly and that baby is counting on you for everything. Just think of how you would want to be treated."
- "Alas madres que no fumen ni tomar vevidas alcoholicas son malas para su bebe." (mothers should not smoke or take alcoholic drinks as they are bad for the baby)
- "I think all women-rich or poor, black, white or purple know what they need to do to have a healthy baby. Some of them choose not to do those things. It is not rocket science to figure out that drugs and booze are bad for the baby..."

- "Not all babies born premature are a result of drugs or alcohol or to low income families."
- "I notice that this questionnaire had questions about alcohol use and not drug use… that makes a difference too."
- "…I have a friend that got pregnant and was scared. Hence, she took Sudafed and dry gin in an attempt to get rid of the pregnancy…Things like this will not be disclosed by mothers. What…will help is more education and encouragement."
- "Not all women want officials to know the circumstances in which they find themselves when they are pregnant (i.e. addicted to alcohol or drugs, homeless, battered). Maybe as a state we could do a better job of seeking out these people without imposing a penalty."

### *Minimal Use or Minimization of Use*

A number of women (n=46) expressed that they only used alcohol sparingly during or before pregnancy. These women often used words in their comments such as "only", "once or twice", "occasionally" or they named a special occasion when they had a drink.

- "I would have an alcoholic beverage occasionally."
- "Didn't drink a lot."
- "I am not an alcoholic. I would drink a glass of wine at dinner."
- "I did drink only on Christmas or holidays. I don't drink."
- "maybe 1-2 drinks only."
- "I barely drink any alcohol [only] >1 week."
- "only on special occasions"
- "During my pregnancy I drank just a little bit because I was craving beer."

### *Admit Drinking Alcohol*

Several mothers (n=14) reported that they used alcohol without trying to show minimal use.

- "1 pt. of liquor, 5 to 7 days a week"
- "…as for the alcoholic drinks when I'm with family (well, they are drinkers), I didn't want them to know that I was with child."
- "I had 3 drinks the night my daughter was conceived."
- "…mostly have drinks all in one sitting when I drink."

### *Preconception thought Given*

A few mothers (n=3) commented that they gave up drinking when they decided to try to get pregnant.

- "I avoided alcohol while trying to get pregnant, while pregnant and while breastfeeding"

- "When I decided to get pregnant, I made a point of eliminating certain toxins from my body. I stopped drinking, increased my water intake and fruit/veggies."

### *No Preconception thought Given*

A few mothers (n=9) reported that they stopped or decreased drinking once they found out that they were pregnant. This category is distinct from the 'Preconception thought given' where the mothers mention ceasing alcohol use before they became pregnant.

- "...I learned I was pregnant a month later. From that point forward, I had a few sips of wine or champagne during my pregnancy, but only on rare occasion."
- "I went on vacation and was drinking...then I came home and found I was pregnant."
- "...before my first child I was a very bad drinker, but when I found out I was 'pregnant' I stopped."
- "Never drank once I found out I was pregnant."

### *Doctor Asked about or Discussed Alcohol Use*

Several mothers (n=7) commented that their doctor asked them about alcohol use during pregnancy however some mothers reported that their doctors only screened them once—and sometimes with a previous pregnancy.

- "They asked initially if I smoked or drank, but I was never asked again."
- "My doctor gave me information regarding the effects of alcohol, cigarettes and drugs. It was discussed with my first child, but I don't recall with my second."
- "I don't drink or smoke so I think that when they asked, it was dropped."
- "I have been going to her [doctor] years prior to my pregnancy and she knew my lifestyle."

### *Doctor did not Ask about Alcohol Use and/or Gave Misleading Advice*

A few mothers (n=7) mentioned that their doctor did not ask them about alcohol use while they were pregnant and a couple actually reported that their doctor told them they could drink while pregnant.

- "... I was instructed by my doc to [have one] drink at night...to stop me from going into labor."
- "they said I could have a drink after the 3rd trimester... "
- "My ob/gyn did not speak to me about alcohol and drug usage because she knows my religious beliefs."

### *Want Alcohol Use during Pregnancy Punished by Legal System*

Four mothers (N=4) felt strongly that women who drink while they are pregnant should have legal action taken against them for endangering the unborn child.

- "I feel that mothers who are expecting should be prosecuted for smoking, drinking or using/abusing drugs or illegal substances for child abuse/neglect."
- "I wish we needed a license to get pregnant because smokers, drinkers, and drug users should not be having kids. It is...child abuse. I'd like to see that legislation!!"
- "I think all mothers should be drug tested when admitted to the hospital and immediate action should be taken against these women who expose their unborn child to drugs...Our children are brought into this world without a chance."
- "I think...information on the risks of smoking, drinking, and drugs on the baby... should be a mandatory [high school] class. Let them see babies who are suffering the effects of these issues. They should...be drug tested when they are pregnant in order for them to receive welfare. That might knock some sense into these teenagers so their babies are born healthy."

Half of the PRAMS respondents (50.7%) who wrote a comment pertaining to alcohol either denied using alcohol and/or tried to minimize the amount they drank. Seven percent (7%) of the mothers' comments stated that they drank before and/or during pregnancy.

When prompted to relay "additional comments about the health of mothers and babies in Maryland", one fourth of the women (25.4%) gave advice about not drinking while pregnant. They discussed avoiding alcohol use in order to have a healthy pregnancy and baby and the potential side effects that alcohol can have on the unborn child.

Four percent (4%) of the women who wrote comments pertaining to alcohol use admitted no preconception thought about alcohol use while one percent (1%) of the women mentioned that they consciously decreased or stopped alcohol consumption when deciding to get pregnant. An equal number of comments (3%) were made by mothers stating that their doctor asked them about alcohol use during pregnancy as by those who made comments that it was not discussed by a doctor or other healthcare provider. Two percent (2%) of the women wrote comments suggesting legal action be taken against women who use alcohol during pregnancy.

# 4. DISCUSSION

## Prevalence

*"I had a drink every now and then."*

Our data from Maryland PRAMS reported lower levels of alcohol use (7.7%) and binge drinking (0.5%) during pregnancy than most national studies. The most widely used data for alcohol use comes from the National Survey on Drug Use and Health (NSDUH) [8]. This dataset uses audio computer assisted self-interview techniques conducted at interviewee residences. Their 2007-2008 survey results reported that 10.6% of pregnant women aged 15 to 44 had consumed at least one drink and 4.5% had 5 or more drinks on the same occasion in the past 30 days. Another widely used dataset is the Behavioral Risk Factor Surveillance System (BRFSS). The BRFSS uses random-digit-dialed telephone surveys of the civilian population aged $\geq$18 years. Data from 2001-2005 reported that 11.2% of pregnant women had at least one drink in the past 30 days and 1.8% reported binge drinking [6]. Differences between Maryland PRAMS and NSDUH or BRFSS most likely reflect the methodology used.

Whereas Maryland PRAMS only asks about alcohol consumption during the last three months of pregnancy, NSDUH and BRFSS data is representative of all gestational ages, including the 1st month when few women realize they are pregnant and have not changed their alcohol use patterns.

## Early Pregnancy Alcohol Use

*"...I was a very bad drinker, but when I found out I was 'pregnant' I stopped."*

Many women will decrease their drinking consumption after they learn they are pregnant. In a computer-assisted telephone survey of postpartum women, the National Birth Defects Prevention Study reported alcohol consumption rates from eight stages of preconception and pregnancy including the 1$^{st}$, 2$^{nd}$, and 3$^{rd}$ month before conception, the 1$^{st}$, 2$^{nd}$, and 3$^{rd}$ month of pregnancy, and the 2$^{nd}$ and 3$^{rd}$ trimester [7]. The NBDPS data from the 3$^{rd}$ trimester of pregnancy reported similar results of any alcohol use (7.9%) and binge drinking (0.5%) to PRAMS data (7.7% and 0.5%). NBDPS reported that 30.3% of women consumed alcohol during pregnancy and 5.7% reported binge drinking. These women represented the control group of the NBDPS from eight states who delivered live born infants without birth defects during 1997-2002. Similar to the decrease in alcohol consumption rates from early to late pregnancy, NSDUH data reported alcohol consumption rates that decreased from 25.2% during the 1$^{st}$ trimester to 7.9% during the 3$^{rd}$ trimester [8]. It is possible that the rates of early pregnancy alcohol consumption in Maryland were 2-3 times greater than that reported for the 3$^{rd}$ trimester. Drinking rates just before pregnancy may be a more accurate indication of drinking rates during early pregnancy before pregnancy confirmation [11].

## Is Maryland Data Comparable to U.S. Data?

Maryland is a diverse state, with a larger Black and smaller Hispanic population, and a larger proportion of mothers 35 and older than the U.S. average. In 2005, there were 74,880 births in Maryland. Of the mothers who delivered, 49% were White non-Hispanic, 33% Black, 6% Asian, and 12% Hispanic, 9% under age 20 years, and 19% age 35 years or over [12]. In the U.S., mothers of 2005 births were 55% White non-Hispanic, 15% Black, 6% Asian, 24% Hispanic, 10% under age 20 years, and 14% age 35 years or over [13]. Maryland women at highest risk for any alcohol use before or during pregnancy were White non-Hispanic and college graduates. This profile was the same in national studies [6-8]. Rates for alcohol use during pregnancy were not analyzed using Maryland PRAMS data for the Asian and Hispanic population because of the small numbers who reported drinking.

Most national data have reported wide variations in alcohol consumption among different states. For 2006-2007, the NSDUH reported any alcohol use within the past 30 days was 51.04% in the U.S., with a range of 30.85% in Utah to 67.05% in RI and 54.03% in Maryland. Binge drinking rates for U.S. were 23.15%, with a range of 15.64% Utah to 32.01% ND and 21.06% in Maryland [14]. The NBDPS study [7], using data from eight states, reported alcohol use during pregnancy that ranged from 23.3% (AR) to 37.6% (NY), and binge drinking during pregnancy ranged from 5.6% (CA) - 12.7% (IA).

A report of PRAMS surveillance results of 2004 births from 27 states showed that Maryland's rate of alcohol use during late pregnancy was in the middle third of the states that were surveyed [9]. The average for alcohol use during the last three months of pregnancy for all 27 states was 5.6%, with a range of 2.0% (WVA) -11.6% (VT). Maryland's rate was 6.6% and was 18th highest of the 27 states. Maryland was also in the middle third of 2004 preconceptional alcohol use with the 14th highest rate (50.9%) of 26 reporting areas (average 50.1%), ranging from 25.3% (UT) to 66.8% (VT).

## Healthy People 2010 Objectives about Alcohol Use during Pregnancy

The Healthy People Objectives are a set of evidence-based disease prevention and health promotion objectives to identify and track the most significant preventable health threats in the U.S. These objectives are created by the Department of Health and Human Services with input from multiple local and federal partners from various health fields. These objectives were initiated as Healthy People 2000 and are meant to be updated every ten years. The main goals of HP 2010 are to decrease health disparities and to increase the quality and length of life.

There are two HP 2010 objectives for alcohol use during pregnancy [15]:

1. Objective 16-17a: increase abstinence from alcohol among pregnant women to 94%.
2. Objective 16-17b: increase abstinence from binge drinking among pregnant women to 100%.

So far, Maryland has not met either HP 2010 objective. Although the Maryland PRAMS data reported rates of abstinence from alcohol (92.3%) and binge drinking (0.5%) during pregnancy were close to HP 2010 objectives, it should be remembered that Maryland data only reflects alcohol use during the 3rd trimester and that drinking rates were probably considerably higher during early pregnancy. Both the American College of Obstetricians and Gynecologists and the American Academy of Pediatrics recommend that all pregnant women and women planning a pregnancy should abstain completely from alcohol to prevent the birth defects and behavioral problems associated with FASD, essentially raising both objectives to 100%. However, the two HP 2010 objectives on alcohol use during pregnancy will likely be retained for HP 2020.

## Maryland Trend 2001-2008 - Increasing Rates of Alcohol Consumption

Pre-pregnancy binge drinking rates showed a fairly steady increase from 13.2% in 2001 to 19.7% in 2007 before declining to 18.2% in 2008, with the largest increases from previous years in 2006 and 2007 (Figure 3); rates for two or more pre-pregnancy binge episodes increased even more significantly, from 7.4% to 11.1% (Table 3).

The Maryland BRFSS reported a similar increase in binge drinking rates among non-pregnant women aged 18-44 years, going from 8.8% (2001) and 11.1% (2002) to 14.9% (2008). Rates for drinking one or more drinks per week did not show any increase (5.7% in 2001 to 4.9% in 2008) [16].

National data from NSDUH showed a similar increase in any alcohol use before pregnancy among women aged 15-44 years from 49.8% (2000-2001) to 54.0% (2007-2008), and a smaller increase in binge drinking rates 20.4 (2000-2001) to 24.2% (2007-2008) than

Maryland [17]. Maryland pre-pregnancy rates are for the three months just before pregnancy and the NSDUH rates are any time outside of pregnancy.

## Binge Drinking

*"(I drank) 1 pt. of liquor, 5 to 7 days a week."*

Even though the threshold amount of prenatal alcohol necessary to cause fetal effects is not known, there is little doubt that the risk to the fetus increases as the amount of alcohol consumed per sitting increases [3]. Consuming seven drinks in one episode per week is much more risky than consuming that same amount over the course of a week even though the net amount consumed during the week is identical. Long term studies have shown behavioral and cognitive abnormalities among children whose mothers had binged during pregnancy [18,19]. In 2004, the National Institute on Alcohol Abuse and Alcoholism (NIAAA) revised the definition of binge drinking for women to 4 or more drinks per occasion [20]. Previously, the definition for binge drinking was set at 5 drinks per occasion for both sexes. At risk drinking also differs by gender. For males, it is defined as more than two drinks per day and for females it is more than one drink per day. Of course during pregnancy, any drinking is considered at risk.

## Screening Women for Alcohol Use

*"My ob/gyn did not speak to me about alcohol and drug usage because she knows my religious beliefs."*

Various stereotypes about who develops a cognitive disability continue to lull many pregnant women and their physicians into a state of complacency. Physicians are an essential component in helping uninformed pre-pregnant and pregnant women view alcohol as an equal opportunity "neurotoxin" capable of rendering a perfectly healthy fetal brain into one that has had its normal developmental trajectory diverted into abnormal directions, regardless of social standing, educational attainment, race, ethnicity or religion.

One-third of mothers commented that they had consumed alcohol during pregnancy. Most of these mothers (66.7%) reported minimal use of alcohol, using words such as "only" and "just" as if to reiterate the slight amount used. The majority of comments were from women who denied alcohol use or made a point of affirming their non-drinking status. Four percent reported alcohol use during early pregnancy prior to pregnancy confirmation. Some mothers commented that their doctors did not screen them for alcohol use because they already "knew" that they didn't drink.

One of the recommendations towards "Reducing Alcohol-Exposed Pregnancies" from a 2009 report of the National Task Force on Fetal Alcohol Syndrome and Fetal Alcohol Effect is to use validated instruments to establish formal screening for all women of childbearing age [21]. However, the identification of individuals [22], especially women [23], who have problems with alcohol use is difficult for physicians. The social stigma associated with prenatal alcohol consumption encourages denial or minimization of use by women [24]. In addition, health care providers are more apt to suspect men of an alcohol problem since it is more commonly seen in men. This makes screening very difficult. Buchsbaum and colleagues reported that 67% of men vs. 24% of women with alcohol problems were diagnosed correctly by residents at an outpatient urban university teaching hospital [25].

One widely used screening tool T-ACE, a validated 4-question assessment tool, was the first tool specifically developed for use with pregnant women, but it can also be used for non-pregnant women:

1. **Tolerance (T)**: How many drinks does it take to make you feel high?
2. **Annoyed (A):** Have people annoyed you by criticizing your drinking?
3. **Cut Down (C):** Have you ever felt you ought to cut down on your drinking?
4. **Eye Opener (E):** Have you ever had a drink first thing in the morning to steady your nerves or get rid of a hangover?

Reprinted with permission from American Journal of Obstetrics and Gynecology [26]

Each affirmative reply is scored as one point for the A, C, E questions. The T question is scored 2 points if the respondent answers more than 2 drinks. The T-ACE is considered positive for at-risk alcohol use, defined as one ounce or more per day, with a total score of 2 or more. Consistent use of T-ACE resulted in dramatically increased identification of pre-pregnancy alcohol use, with a sensitivity of 74.3 and specificity of 71.4 and prenatal use sensitivity of 60.0 and specificity of 66.9 [27,28]. The developer of the T-ACE screening tool found that the Tolerance question was answered more truthfully than direct inquiry because it did not trigger a guilt or denial response. Another screening tool, the 5P's [29] was adapted from the 4Ps [30], and was targeted for pregnant women. The 5P's was developed through funding from the Maternal and Child Health Bureau and is in the public domain:

1. **Parents:** Do either of your parents have a problem with using alcohol or drugs?
   (Yes/No/No answer)
2. **Peers:** Do any of your friends have a problem with using alcohol or drugs?
   (Yes/No/No answer)
3. **Partner:** Does your partner have a problem with drug or alcohol use?
   (Yes/No/No answer)
4. **Past:** Before you knew you were pregnant, how often did you drink beer, wine, wine coolers or liquor?
   (Not at all, rarely, sometimes, frequently)
5. **Present:** In the past month how often did you drink beer, wine, wine coolers or liquor?
   (Not at all, rarely, sometimes, frequently)

This five-question screen can be used to detect cigarette, alcohol and illicit drug use. For alcohol and other drug use, it can identify not only high levels of use but also small amounts of use. These screening tools may be self-administered or asked by a provider.

Improvement in disclosure rates can be increased if screening is done universally, regardless of race or economic status, and if the questions are part of the routine medical history.

Other screens such as TWEAK [31] or AUDIT-C [32] may also be used. Screening tools are not diagnostic and only indicate that a woman may be at-risk for alcohol use or misuse. The NIAAA recommends asking women about the exact quantity and frequency of alcohol and drug use so that at-risk drinkers could be identified and receive help before their drinking progressed towards misuse or dependence [33].

1. Do you drink?
2. Do you use drugs?
3. On average, how many days per week do you drink alcohol (beer, wine, liquor)?
4. On a typical day when you drink, how many drinks do you have?

[positive score = >7 drinks/week for non-pregnant women]

5. What is the maximum number of drinks you had on any given occasion during the past month? [positive score = >3 for non-pregnant women]

Drug testing has not been performed routinely by most providers to detect alcohol during pregnancy or at delivery. The American College of Obstetricians and Gynecologists states in a Committee Opinion that "state laws that require physicians to report the nonmedical use of controlled substances by a pregnant woman or that require toxicology tests after delivery when there is evidence of possible use of a controlled substance...may unwittingly result in pregnant women not seeking prenatal care or concealing drug use from their obstetricians" [34].

## Screening for other Substances

*"I notice this questionnaire had questions about alcohol use and not drug use."*
*"I did stop smoking weed [during pregnancy].*

The CDC PRAMS survey includes questions about tobacco and alcohol use and does not include questions about other drug use. Therefore there are no data about illicit drug use. Alcohol and tobacco are the most common substances that are abused during pregnancy. However, use of other illegal drugs such as marijuana, cocaine and heroin are more common in women who report tobacco and alcohol use than women who don't smoke or drink [34]. The same screens that are used for alcohol can also be used for other drugs.

## Interventions for Prenatal Alcohol Use

*"It is not rocket science to figure out that drugs and booze are bad for the baby"*
*"Women should not drink or use alcohol during pregnancy... it is taking a chance."*

Comments from Maryland PRAMS mothers about not drinking currently or ever (28%) and opinions—mostly negative—about prenatal drinking (25%) made up the majority of comments about alcohol use. It seemed that mothers either wanted to affirm that they didn't drink alcohol during pregnancy or wanted to deny that they did. Women may be more apt to deny a problem with alcohol because of the social stigma of female alcohol use. During pregnancy, when drinking may adversely affect the fetus, women may feel especially guilty about alcohol use and have great difficulty disclosing use.

Alcohol is the most common teratogen that women consume during pregnancy. High levels of alcohol use and binge drinking among women of reproductive age and high rates of unintended pregnancy in the U.S. may cause unintentional exposure to alcohol before pregnancy is confirmed. The most critical period for morphologic birth defects is during the first 3-8 weeks of pregnancy when organ formation occurs. Drinking in the last trimester should not be perceived as any safer for the fetus. Late pregnancy alcohol exposure has been associated with massive apoptosis of neurons or "cell death" during this period of rapid synaptogenesis. This can be associated with multiple adverse behavioral and cognitive outcomes.

Brief interventions and advice from health care providers for women who screen positive have been shown to result in decreased alcohol use and less physical adverse outcomes [35-37]. Screening also allows for timely referrals to treatment facilities. Since neonates with a FASD are usually not routinely identified, having the rates of those affected provide a clue as to the need for better surveillance in the newborn nursery and later in well baby check-ups. Having the rates of alcohol use both before and during pregnancy give an estimate of how many offspring will be affected by FASD. Potentially affected individuals can be provided with appropriate monitoring and early intervention. The most severe outcomes occur in those individuals who are not identified early, are subjected to adverse environmental conditions such as abuse and neglect, and lack environmental and academic accommodations. Unidentified individuals live with the primary disability and the secondary impact of attempting to function without the cognitive and social tools to negotiate the complex demands society places on the young.

## Prosecution of Prenatal Alcohol Use

> *"...mothers who are expecting (and drinking) should be prosecuted...for child abuse/neglect."*

The majority (57%) of PRAMS survey comments came from mothers who either reported that they did not consume any alcohol during pregnancy or made a point of advising women not to drink alcohol during pregnancy. Most of the admonitions about drinking during pregnancy warned that abstinence was needed to have a healthy baby. However some respondents were indignant that women would use alcohol and a few were hostile —calling for legal action to protect the fetus from harm or to prosecute the mother for "child abuse."

Currently no state legislatures have passed laws that specifically criminalize prenatal drug or alcohol use [38]. Many states have tried to prosecute women on the basis of drug possession, underage drinking, providing drugs to minor children [i.e. fetuses] through the umbilical cord, assault with a deadly weapon [alcohol/drugs], or contributing to the delinquency of a minor [39]. Three states, Minnesota, South Dakota, and Wisconsin, have used punitive policies such as civil commitment of pregnant women. Other states have requirements to report women who use alcohol during pregnancy to law enforcement or child welfare agencies, and initiation of child welfare proceedings to temporarily remove children from mothers or terminate parental rights. In cases where infants with positive drug tests have died soon after birth, women have even been charged with homicide. The judicial system has upheld that pregnant women may not be subject to non-consensual drug testing and no state expects physicians to use medical evidence of addiction for criminal prosecution or to act as agents of the criminal justice system [39].

The first time a pregnant woman was charged with child abuse for drinking during pregnancy involved a 29 year old woman who was physically abused by her husband and went to a Wyoming hospital for care. After her blood tests at the hospital were positive for alcohol, she was arrested and charged with child abuse. A Wyoming trial judge dismissed the charges because the prosecution could not demonstrate that the fetus had suffered injury [40].

Prosecutions of women for a variety of crimes based on their alleged drug use during pregnancy have been rejected by most courts in the U.S. and in the Supreme Court (Commonwealth vs. Welch, 864 S.W.2d 280, Ky. 1993) each finding that such acts were not in the purview of criminal law.

## Non-Criminalization of Prenatal Alcohol Use

*"What I think will help is more education and encouragement."*

The medical approach to prenatal drug use primarily utilizes drug treatment and education. Non-prosecution of drug use is endorsed by most health organizations because the potential threat of criminal prosecution or having their children taken away from them will deter women from obtaining prenatal care and substance abuse treatment. The American College of Obstetricians and Gynecologists, American Academy of Pediatrics, American Medical Association, American Nurses Association, American Public Health Association, and American Society of Addiction Medicine, Institute of Medicine, the March of Dimes, and National Council on Alcoholism and Drug Dependence have all voiced their concern about the criminalization of drug use during pregnancy. Many states have established treatment programs, coordinated services, given pregnant women priority for treatment, encouraged health providers to screen for substance abuse, and have passed laws requiring places that sell alcoholic beverages to post warnings about fetal alcohol spectrum disorder effects directed to pregnant women who drink. Incarceration has not been effective in reducing alcohol use and may even worsen the health of women and their families [41]. ACOG states that legally mandated testing or reporting of substance use "may endanger the relationship of trust between physician and patient, place the obstetrician in an adversarial relationship with the patient and possibly conflict with the therapeutic obligation. If pregnant women become reluctant to seek medical care because they fear being reported for alcohol or illegal drug use, these strategies will actually increase the risks for the woman and the fetus rather than reduce the consequences of substance abuse" [34].

## Maryland Approach to FASD Prevention

*"Maybe as a state we could do a better job of seeking out these people (e.g. drinkers) without imposing a penalty".*

Maryland does not specifically consider alcohol consumption during pregnancy to be child abuse under civil child-welfare statutes or grounds for civil commitment. No testing for alcohol is required during pregnancy or postpartum and health providers are not mandated to report alcohol use to government officials. Maryland does not have legislation that mandates the placement of warning signs about drinking during pregnancy in public facilities that serve alcohol.

Since 1990, Maryland has mandated that pregnant and postpartum (within one year of delivery) women must receive priority admission for public-funded substance abuse treatment programs. These programs must also have referral systems in place for linked medical and social services. In 2004, House Bill 1274, titled, "Fetal Alcohol Syndrome Prevention – Public Awareness Campaign" was signed by the Governor to establish and promote a statewide public information campaign on FASD and the effects of prenatal alcohol exposure. The 2005 Title V Maternal and Child Health Needs Assessment identified the prevention of alcohol use during pregnancy as a priority need in Maryland. A new state performance measure was established to track the prevalence of pregnant women who consumed alcohol during pregnancy. A Maryland State Fetal Alcohol Spectrum Disorder Coalition was established the following year to increase public awareness of FASD and to create a state plan to prevent and treat FASD.

## Pregnancy Planning

*"I wish we needed a license to get pregnant because smokers, drinkers, and drug users should not be having kids"*

An important group to target for the prevention of FASD is the preconception population. These women may be using alcohol in the early weeks of pregnancy before they realize they are pregnant. Similarly, these women may opt to use contraception to delay pregnancy until their alcohol use is manageable. In a randomized controlled trial, the Project CHOICES Intervention Group reported that 68.5% of women decreased their risk for an alcohol-exposed pregnancy [42]. The improvement in risk was due to either a decrease in alcohol use or an increase in effective contraception use or both that occurred after brief four-session interventions that included motivational interviewing and contraception counseling. Similar success with this dual-focused intervention was shown for decreasing alcohol use on a college campus [43].

## Alcohol Use among Adolescents

*"Most of the time it [drinking] will be young girls who don't know any better."*

The drinking age in every state in the U.S is 21. However, alcohol use among adolescents is common. Maryland PRAMS reported late-pregnancy binge drinking rates among teens were three to four times higher than rates among women aged 20-34. And although pre-pregnancy drinking rates were lowest of any age group for teens (11.1%), the rates nearly doubled (21.3%) for women aged 20-24, the age group with the highest rate of binge drinking. National data showed similar high rates of drinking among adolescents.

The 2008 NSDUH [8] reported that 3.4% of 12-13 year olds, 13.1% of 14-15 year olds, 26.2% of 16-17 year olds, 48.7% of 18-20 year olds and 69.5% of 21-25 year olds had at least one drink in the past 30 days or were current users. Rates of binge alcohol use were 1.5% among 12-13 year olds, 6.9% among 14-15 year olds, 17.2% among 16-17 year olds, 33.7% among 18-20 year olds and 46% among 21-25 year olds. Rates of current alcohol use were also similar by gender, 27.1% for males and 25.8% for females aged 12 to 20. Binge drinking rates were higher for males (19.2%) than females (15.5%). Binge drinking during the first trimester was reported by 4.5% of pregnant women aged 15-44 over 2007-2008.

Similar rates for underage alcohol use were reported by the Maryland Youth Risk Behavior Survey (YRBS), a survey of high school students in grades 9-12, which is part of the Youth Risk Behavior Surveillance System (YRBSS) developed in 1990 by the Centers for Disease Control and Prevention (CDC). According to the 2007 Maryland YRBS [44], 75% of females have tried alcohol at least one time in their lives and 20% of females surveyed had their first drink before age 13. Forty-five percent of females reported they were current drinkers (defined as having at least one drink of alcohol in past 30 days) and 22% had at least one episode of binge drinking (defined as 5 or more drinks in a row) within the past 30 days. More females than males were current drinkers (45% vs. 40%) and more males than females were binge drinkers (25% vs. 22%). From the 9$^{th}$ to 12$^{th}$ grade, the rate of current binge drinking increased from 18% to 36%.

Data from the 1991 to 2005 Behavioral Risk Factor Surveillance System (BRFSS) telephone survey indicated that 11.1% of pregnant U.S. women ages 18-44 reported alcohol use and 1.8% reported binge drinking in the previous month of their pregnancy [6]. The BRFSS rate for any alcohol use is higher than the Maryland PRAMS rate (11.1% vs. 7.7%) and probably reflects responses from women during different trimesters of pregnancy, whereas the PRAMS rate only asks about the last three months of pregnancy. Alcohol use is much lower than during the 1$^{st}$ trimester, when many women consume alcohol before they realize they are pregnant. Preconceptional alcohol use was also similar. BRFSS data reported 54.6% any alcohol use and 12.6% binge drinking in the previous month among non-pregnant women aged 18-44 years.

## Limitations

Maryland PRAMS uses survey response data that is completed by mothers two to nine months after delivery. Mothers may not accurately remember their drinking behavior that occurred months ago. Self-report data is also subject to social desirability bias. Most women feel guilt, shame, and social stigmatization about drinking during pregnancy and may not admit to any negative behaviors. There may also be unfounded fears of repercussions such as child welfare involvement or even incarceration due to their drinking. Because the outcome of pregnancy was known at the time of survey, mothers whose infant had a less than optimal outcome may have been less inclined to disclose accurate levels of prenatal alcohol. Underestimation of amount of alcohol used is likely. The heaviest drinkers may not have been accessible to the survey, participation in which required that the respondent have an address or phone. Heavy drinkers may also choose not to respond to surveys. It should be noted that the definition for female binge drinking was changed in 2005 to four or more drinks on one occasion. Until 2009 births, the PRAMS survey used 5 or more drinks on one occasion in their survey about binge drinking. The estimation of binge drinking is therefore lower than it should be.

Lastly, PRAMS samples only women who have delivered a live infant. Women who have had a non-viable pregnancy such as stillbirth, ectopic pregnancy, and spontaneous or therapeutic abortion were not surveyed. The prevalence of binge drinking and alcohol use during pregnancy therefore only reflects those pregnancies that have survived through the delivery.

## 5. Conclusion

Unlike most other congenital birth defects, FASD is entirely preventable. In Maryland, and in most other national studies, preconceptional alcohol use (and therefore most probably early pregnancy use) is prevalent in the majority (51%) of women and is common among all racial, ethnic, age, and sociodemographic groups. Even by the last three months of pregnancy, nearly 8% of women reported alcohol consumption. Binge drinking was reported by 15% of women preconceptionally.

It is clear from many comments of mothers in Maryland that alcohol use during pregnancy is a controversial issue with comments ranging from mothers ambivalent about their alcohol use to those who think that women who drink should be prosecuted for child abuse. The U.S. Services Task Force (USPSTF) "recommends screening and behavioral counseling interventions to reduce misuse by adults, including pregnant women, in primary care settings" [45]. Because the actual amount of prenatal alcohol consumption needed to produce adverse fetal effects is unknown, most experts caution women to abstain completely from alcohol during pregnancy. According to the U.S. Surgeon General (2005), "health professionals should inquire routinely about alcohol consumption by women of childbearing age and inform them of the risks of alcohol consumption during pregnancy, and advise them not to drink alcoholic beverages during pregnancy" [46]. The lack of any effective treatment for FASD, places the onus of dealing with the disorder on prevention of alcohol consumption. A number of screening tests such as T-ACE are validated tools for the identification of alcohol consumption during pregnancy, however, it remains difficult to obtain an accurate drinking history from many women during pregnancy due to guilt and denial. For this reason, education about the effects of prenatal alcohol exposure on the fetus should be discussed with all patients with or without a positive screen. For women with a positive screen, brief interventions reduced alcohol use and improved infant outcomes [47,48]. Criminalization of alcohol use during pregnancy by prosecution of women who exposed their pregnancies to drugs or alcohol is not supported by any medical organization. Instead, education, interventions and treatment are endorsed and found to be helpful.

In addition to screening women during pregnancy, identification of women at risk for alcohol abuse before pregnancy may be the most effective method in preventing FASD. As one Maryland mother commented, "if [drinking alcohol] can be controlled before you get pregnant, that is a good thing". Most respondents confirmed their non-drinking status on the comments section of the survey however one mother reported that her doctor told her to have a "drink every night". Women were divided about how to handle mothers who drink during pregnancy, ranging from "education and encouragement" to "legal action…for endangering the unborn child". As these comments reveal, qualitative data can provide insight into the behaviors and experiences of survey respondents. While it cannot be generalized, such data are a valuable resource to identify and describe mothers' perceptions, attitudes, and experiences regarding alcohol use before, during and after pregnancy that might not be captured with quantitative data collection methods.

Considering the cost in terms of lives lost to mental and cognitive disorders, the savings to society by the primary prevention of FASD would be massive. With the steadily rising rates of alcohol use and binge drinking in recent years, especially among adolescent young women, there is much work to be done.

## REFERENCES


[1] Sampson PD, Streissguth AP, Bookstein FL, Little RE, Clarren SK, Dehaene P, Hanson JW, Graham JM Jr. Incidence of fetal alcohol syndrome and prevalence of alcohol-related neurodevelopmental disorder. *Teratology* 1997; *56*(5):317-326.

[2] Nash K, Sheard E, Rovet J, Koren G. Understanding fetal alcohol spectrum disorders (FASDs): toward identification of a behavioral phenotype. *ScientificWorldJournal* 2008;21:873-882.

[3] Maier SE, West JR. Drinking patterns and alcohol-related birth defects. *Alcohol Research and Health* 2001;25(3):168-174.

[4] Lupton C, Burd L, Harwood R. Cost of fetal alcohol spectrum disorders. *Amer. J. Med. Genetics* 2004;127C:42-50.

[5] Jones K, Smith D, Ulleland C, Streissguth P. Pattern of malformation in offspring of chronic alcoholic mothers. *Lancet* 1973;1(7815):1267-71.

[6] Centers for Disease Control and Prevention. Alcohol use among pregnant and nonpregnant women of childbearing age—United States, 1991-2005. *MMWR Morb. Mortal. Wkly Rep.* 2009;58(19):529-532.

[7] Ethen MK, Canfield MA, Romitt PA. Alcohol consumption by women before and during pregnancy. *Matern. Child Health J.* 2009;13:274-285.

[8] Substance Abuse and Mental Health Services Administration. Results from the 2008 national Survey on Drug Use and Health: National Findings. Rockville MD: Office of Applied Studies; 2008.NSDUH Series H-36, HHS Publications No. SMA 09-4434.

[9] D'Angelo D, Williams L, Morrow B, Cox S, Harris N, Harrision L, Posner SF, Hood JR, Zapata L. Preconception and interconception health status of women who recently gave birth to a live-born infant—Pregnancy Risk Assessment Monitoring System (PRAMS), United States, 26 reporting areas, 2004. *MMWR Surveill Summ.* 2007; 56(10):1-35.

[10] Naimi TS, Lipscomb LE, Brewer RD, Gilbert BC. Binge drinking in the preconception period and the risk of unintended pregnancy: implications for women and their children. *Pediatrics* 2003;111:1136-1141.

[11] Day NL, Cottreau CM, Richardson GA. Epidemiology of alcohol, marijuana and cocaine use among women of childbearing age and pregnant women. *Clin. Obstet. Gynecol.* 1993;26:237-245.

[12] Vital Statistics Administration (2006). Maryland Vital Statistics Annual Report 2005. Baltimore, MD:Maryland Department of Health and Mental Hygiene.

[13] Martin JA, Hamilton BE, Sutton PD, Ventura SJ, Menacker F, Kirmeyer S, Munson ML. (2007). Births: Final data for 2005. National vital statistics reports; vol 56 no 6. Hyattsville, MD: National Center for Health Statistics.

[14] Office of Applied Studies, SAMHSA. State estimates of the 2006-2007 NSDUH. Accessed April 4, 2010 at http://www.oas.samhsa.gov/2k7state/Ch1.htm.

[15] U.S. Department of Health and Human Services. *Healthy People 2010*. 2nd ed. With Understanding and Improving Health and Objectives for Improving Health. 2 vols. Washington, DC: U.S. Government Printing Office, November 2000.

[16] Office of Health Policy and Planning. Maryland Department of Health and Mental Hygiene. Maryland BRFSS. Accessed April 4, 2010 at www.marylandbrfss.org/

[17] Office of Applied Studies, SAMHSA. NSDUH Reports. Accessed 4/1/10 at http://www.oas.samhsa.gov/NSDUH.HTM

[18] Streissguth AP, Barr HM, Olson HC, et al. Drinking during pregnancy decreases word attack and arithmetic scores on standardized tests: Adolescent data from a population-based prospective study. *Alcohol. Clin. Exp. Res.* 1994;18:248-255.

[19] Jacobson JL, Jacobson SW, Sokol RJ, Ager JW,Jr. Relation of maternal age and pattern of pregnancy drinking to functionally significant cognitive deficit in infancy. *Alcohol. Clin. Exp. Res.* 1998;22:345-351.

[20] Department of Health and Human Services. National Institute on Alcohol Abuse and Alcoholism. NIAAA council approves definition of binge drinking. NIAAA Newsletter No 3. HIN Publication No. 04-5346. Winter 2004. Available at: http://pubs.niaaa.nih.gov/publications/Newsletter/winter2004/Newsletter_Number3.htm

[21] Barry KL, Caetano R, Chang G, DeJoseph MC, Miller LA, O'Connor MJ, Olson HC, Floyd RL, Weber MK, DeStefano F, Dolina S, Leeks K. National Task Force on Fetal Alcohol Syndrome and Fetal Alcohol Effect. Reducing alcohol-exposed pregnancies: a report of the National Task Force on Fetal Alcohol Syndrome and Fetal Alcohol Effect. Atlanta,, GA: Centers for Disease Control and Prevention; March 2009.

[22] Fiellin DA, Reid MC, O'Connor PG. Screening for alcohol problems in primary care: A systematic review. *Arch. Intern. Med.* 2000;160(13):1977-89.

[23] Wilson L, Kahan M, Liu E, Brewster Jm, Sobell MB, Sobell LC. Physician behavior towards male and female problem drinkers: a controlled study using simulated patients. *J. Addict. Dis.* 2002;21(3)87-99.

[24] Ernhart CB, Morrow-Tlucak M, Sokol RJ, Martier S, Ager J. Underreporting of alcohol use in pregnancy: relationship to alcohol problem history. *Alcohol. Clin. Exp. Res.* 1989;13:399-401.

[25] Buchsbaum DG, Buchanan RG, Poses RM, Schnoll SH, Lawton MJ. Physician detection of drinking problems in patients attending a general medicine practice. *J. Gen. Intern. Med.* 1992;7(5):517-21.

[26] Sokol RJ, Martier SS, Ager JW. 1989. The T-ACE questions: Practical prenatal detection of risk drinking. *Am. J. Obstet. Gynecol.* 160(4):863-70.

[27] Chang G, Wilkins-Haug L, Berman S, Goetz MA, Behr H, Hiley A. Alcohol use and pregnancy: improving identification. *Obstet. Gynecol.* 1998;91(6):773-83.

[28] Chang G. Alcohol-screening instruments for pregnant women. *Alcohol Res. Health* 2001;25 (3):204-209.

[29] Kennedy C, Finkelstein N, Hutchins E, Mahoney J. Improving screening for alcohol use during pregnancy: the Massachusetts ASAP program. *Matern. Child Health J.* 2004; 8(3):137-147.

[30] Ewing, H. A Practical Guide to Intervention in Health and Social Services with Pregnant and Postpartum Addicts and Alcoholics: Theoretical Framework, Brief Screening Tool, Key Interview Questions, and Strategies for Referral to Recovery Resources. State of California Grant for Training and Cross-Training in Health, Social Services, and Alcohol/Drug Services, 1990.

[31] Russell M, Martier SS, Sokol RJ, Mudar P, Bottoms S, Jacobson S, Jacobson J. Screening for pregnancy risk-drinking. *Alcohol. Clin. Exp. Res.* 1994;18(5):1156-61.

[32] Dawson DA, Grant BF, Stinson FS, Zhou Y. Effectiveness of the derived Alcohol Use Disorders Identification Test (AUDIT-C) in screening for alcohol use disorders and risk drinking in the US general population. *Alcohol. Clin. Exp. Res.* 2005;29(5):844-54.
[33] National Institute on Alcohol Abuse and Alcoholism (2005). Helping People Who Drink Too Much – A Clinician's Guide.
[34] American College of Obstetricians and Gynecologists. ACOG Committee Opinion No. 422. At-risk drinking and illicit drug use: ethical issues in obstetric and gynecologic practice. *Obstet. Gynecol.* 2008;112:1449-60.
[35] Chang G, Goetz MA, Wilkins-Haug L, Berman S. A brief intervention for renatal alcohol use: an in-depth look. *J. Subst. Abuse Treat* 2000;18:365-9.
[36] Manwell LB, Fleming MF, Mundt MP, Stauffacher EA, Barry KL. Treatment of problem alcohol use in women of childbearing age: results of a brief intervention trial. *Alcohol. Clin. Exp. Res.* 2000;24:1517-24.
[37] Project Choices Intervention Research Group. Reducing the risk of alcohol-exposed pregnancies: a study of a motivational intervention in community settings. *Pediatrics* 2003;111:1131-1135.
[38] American College of Obstetricians and Gynecologists. ACOG Committee Opinion No. 321. Maternal Decision Making, Ethics, and the Law. *Obstet. Gynecol.* 2005;106:1127-44.
[39] Harris LH, Paltrow L. The status of pregnant women and fetuses in US criminal law. *JAMA* 2003;289(13):1697-1699.
[40] Schrodel JR, Peretz P. A gender analysis of policy formation: the case of fetal abuse. *J. Health Polit. Policy Law*. 1994; 19: 335-360.
[41] Drug exposed infants: recommendations. Center for the Future of Children. *Future Child* 1991;1:8-9.
[42] Floyd RL, Sobell M, Velasquez MM, Ingersoll K, Nettleman M, Sobell LS, Mullen PD, Ceperich S, von Sternberg K, Bolton B, Skarpness B, Nagaraja J. Preventing alcohol-exposed pregnancies. *Am. J. Prev. Med.* 2007;32(1):1-10.
[43] Ingersoll KS, Ceperich SD, Nettleman MD, Karanda K, Brocksen S, Johnson BA. Reducing alcohol-exposed pregnancy risk in college women: initial outcomes of a clinical trial of motivational intervention. *J. Subst. Abuse Treat.* 2005;29(3):173-80.
[44] Maryland State Department of Education (2008). 2007 Maryland Youth Risk Behavior Survey. September 2008. Accessed 4/4/10 at http://www.marylandpublicschools.org/NR/rdonlyres/707B5FB5-9A0C-4A06-A741-92D16DC7B2E7/18502/2007_MD_YRBS_Report_Oct_1.pdf
[45] U.S. Preventive Services Task Force. Screening and behavioral counseling interventions in primary care to reduce alcohol misuse: recommendation statement. *Ann. Intern. Med.* 2004;140:554-556.
[46] U.S. Department of Health and Human Services (2005). Office of Surgeon General Advisory on Alcohol Use and Pregnancy. Accessed 4/4/10 at http://www.hhs.gov/surgeongeneral/pressreleases/sg02222005.html
[47] Chang G. Alcohol screening instruments for pregnant women. *Alcohol. Res. Health* 2001;25:204-209.
[48] O'Connor, MJ, Whaley SE. Brief intervention for alcohol use with pregnant women in the WIC setting. *Am. J. Public Health* 2007;97(2):252-8.

In: Pregnancy and Alcohol Consumption
Editor: Joshua D. Hoffman, pp. 129-153
ISBN 978-1-61761-122-3


*Chapter 4*

# MEDAKA (*ORYZIAS LATIPES*) AS A MODEL TO STUDY FETAL ALCOHOL SPECTRUM DISORDER

***Yuhui Hu, Minghui Wu, Ikhlas A. Khan, and Asok K. Dasmahapatra****

National Center for Natural Product Research,
Environmental Toxicology Research Program,
Department of Pharmacology, University of Mississippi,
University, MS, USA

## ABSTRACT

Alcohol abuse during pregnancy produces permanent brain damage in the fetus and is associated with the development of a life-long behavioral, social, and cognitive disorder known as fetal alcohol spectrum disorder (FASD). Fetal alcohol syndrome (FAS) is the most clinically recognizable form of FASD and is characterized by a set of facial dysmorphogenesis, mental dysfunction, growth retardation, cardiovascular and limb defects. Human studies of FAS are very limited because of ethical constraints. However, several non-human vertebrate and invertebrate animal models are currently used, and our major understanding about FASD is mainly based on the studies on these animals. We have used Japanese medaka (*Oryzias latipes*) as a non-mammalian vertebrate model to elucidate the mechanism(s) of FASD. We have demonstrated that fertilized medaka embryos exposed to ethanol developed several phenotypic features in cardiovascular, craniofacial, and skeletal systems which are comparable to the FASD features observed in human. Moreover, the effects at the cellular level have shown that ethanol is able to reduce total protein, RNA, and DNA contents of the embryos in a dose- and time-dependent manner. The alcohol metabolizing enzyme mRNA expression such as alcohol dehydrogenase (ADH5 and ADH8) and aldehyde dehydrogenase ( Aldh1A2 and Aldh9A) mRNAs also showed a developmental stage-specific reduction after alcohol treatment. Our studies indicate that medaka embryogenesis might be used as an

* Address for Correspondence: Asok Dasmahapatra, National Center for Natural Product Research, School of Pharmacy, University of Mississippi, University, MS 38677, e-mail: asok @olemiss.edu.

alternative non-mammalian model for investigating the molecular mechanisms involved in FASD.

## INTRODUCTION

Alcohol is a systemic toxin. Alcohol abuse and dependency, together known as alcohol use disorder (AUD), are one of the major health problems in the United States and many other countries. Almost one third of Americans consume enough alcohol to be considered at risk for alcohol dependence. Approximately, 100,000 US citizens die each year due to alcohol-related causes, including traffic collisions and cirrhosis (http://www.cdc.gov/ncipc/fact). The direct and indirect cost of AUD was estimated to be more than $276 billion per year (Miller and Spear, 2006). Thus, AUD costs the American economy more than the combined costs of cancer, heart disease, and diabetes (Miller and Spear, 2006). Epidemiological, experimental and clinical investigations have shown a strong relationship between alcohol abuse, cardiomyopathy, hypertension, brain anomalies and other disorders. Alcohol abuse during pregnancy produces permanent brain damage in the fetus and is associated with the development of a life-long behavioral, social, and cognitive disorder known as fetal alcohol spectrum disorder (FASD) (Goodlett et al., 2005). Fetal alcohol syndrome (FAS) is the most clinically recognizable form of FASD and is characterized by a set of facial dysmorphogenesis, mental dysfunction, growth retardation, cardiovascular and limb defects (Abel, 1998). According to the Centers for Disease Control Study on the prevalence of alcohol consumption among women of childbearing age, 50% appear to consume alcohol. Forty five percent are defined as light drinkers (≤ 30 drinks/month), 3% as moderate (30-60 drinks per month) and 2% as heavy drinkers (≥60 drinks/month). The rate of drinking in North America, Europe and Australia are similar (Abel, 1998). Although significant efforts have been made to educate women about the toxic effects of alcohol during pregnancy, the incidence of FAS remains unchanged (Cook et al., 1990; Goodlett et al., 2005). It is estimated that in the USA about 1 to 3% of the children are born with FASD, but the incidence of FAS is 1-2 per 1000 live births (Duimstra et al., 1993; Sampson et al., 1997). In some selected populations such as in native American communities, FAS is 10.3 per 1000 live births (Abel and Sokol, 1992; Burd and Moffatt, 1994; May et al., 2004; Russo et al., 2004). In fact, FAS is the principal known cause of mental retardation in the USA (Sulik, 2005).

Although the fetotoxic effects of maternal ethanol consumption have been documented for more than forty years (Lemoine et al., 1968; Jones and Smith, 1973), the ways by which ethanol affects biochemical processes and cellular structures have been the focus of extensive research and they are still far from being completely understood (Sant'Anna and Tosello, 2006; Mao et al., 2009). Moreover, studies have shown that FASD depend on several other variables including the timing, frequency, the quantity of alcohol consumed by the mother during pregnancy, the health status of the mother, and the genetic make-up of the mother and fetus (Sulik et al., 1981, 1986; Sant'Anna and Tosello, 2006; Kaminen-Ahola et al., 2010). Due to ethical constraints, human studies of FAS are very limited. Several animal models from round worms to nonhuman primates, including mouse, rat, *Caenorhabditis elegans*, *Drosophila*, zebrafish (*Danio rerio*), and *Xenopus* have been used and our major understanding about FASD is mainly based on studies on these animals. In fact, it is very difficult to find a single animal model that accurately mimics the human conditions. Every model is unique and has individual strengths and weaknesses (Cudd, 2005). Also, the choice of animal model is very important, because prenatal alcohol exposure causes damage to the embryo by multiple mechanisms, depending on dose, pattern, and time of ethanol exposure (Goodlett, 2005). Therefore, to understand the molecular mechanism of FASD, studies in multiple models is necessary.

*Medaka as a model of FASD study :* The use of fish models, particularly zebrafish (*Danio rerio*) and Japanese medaka (*Oryzias latipes*), as alternatives to mammalian models is currently emerging because of their easy availability, low maintenance cost, short life cycle, and also their accessibility to the study of gene function (Wittbrodt et al., 2002; Furutani-Seiki and Wittbrodt, 2004). Fertilization and embryonic development in these fish are external (develop directly in the outside environment). The embryos are covered by a transparent egg chorion which allows direct observation of the development without interfering with normal embryogenesis. Large-scale mutagenic screens in both zebrafish and medaka have identified several ortholog genes which are closely related to those involved in human genetic diseases (Wittbrodt et al., 2002; Nurse et al., 2004). The response of zebrafish embryos to ethanol has been studied by a number of investigators (Bilotta et al., 2002, 2004; Carvan et al., 2004; Lookwood et al., 2004; Reimers et al., 2004, 2006; Prang et al., 2007). Ethanol causes cyclopia, affects visual functions, inhibits photoreceptor development and causes hypoplasia of the optic nerves, induces pericardial edema and otolith defects, lowers heart rate, disrupts the formation of hypochord and dorsal aorta, reduces eye diameter, induces axial malformations, delays development and produces axial blistering in zebrafish (Bilotta et al., 2002, 2004; Reimers et al., 2004; Qian et al., 2005; Arenzana et al., 2006; Matsui et al., 2006; Dlugos and Rabin, 2007; Kashyap et al., 2007; Loucks et al., 2007; Parng et al., 2007). In addition, ethanol exposure alters gene expression in the ventral aspects of the fore- and mid- brain, inhibits acetylcholinesterase activity and reduces nucleoside triphosphate diphosphohydrolases (NDTPases) 1 and 2 mRNA levels in brain (Blader and Strahle, 1998; Rico et al., 2007, 2008). Furthermore, ethanol induces heat shock proteins (Krone et al., 1997; Lele et al., 1997), produces developmental abnormalities of the notochord and spinal cord, and malformations of the body trunk (Baumann and Sander, 1984). The effects of ethanol were found to be strain-dependent in zebrafish and showed in modulated aggression and other social behavior (Dlugos and Rabin, 2003; Carvan et al., 2004; Lookwood et al., 2004; Gerlai, 2003; Gerlai et al., 2006, 2008; Macphail et al., 2009). Microarray analysis using whole brain RNA samples of ethanol-treated zebrafish identified a number of genes that are implicated in drug dependency (Kily et al., 2008). A proteomic analysis identified several novel proteins which are either up or down regulated in the brain of adult zebrafish chronically exposed to ethanol (Damodaran et al., 2006; Kily et al., 2008).

Although zebrafish is a more well-known and established model system, development of another fish model for comparative studies provides increased confidence and opportunities for advancement. Medaka have generated increasing interest with regard to developmental biology and toxicology (Wittbrodt et al., 2002; Carvan et al., 2007). We are evaluating medaka as a non-mammalian vertebrate model to study FASD (Dasmahapatra, 2005; Wang et al., 2006, 2007a,b; Wu et al., 2008; Hu et al., 2008, 2009). These two fish species (zebrafish and Japanese medaka) were separated from a common ancestor about 140 million years ago (Wittbrodt et al., 2002) and have developed several distinct features that are species specific. Although the normal embryonic development in medaka (7-10 days) is significantly slower than zebrafish (3-4 days), the reproductive maturity in both fish is within three months of age. Some medaka mutations are unique, ensuring that the medaka and zebrafish are complementary model systems (Shimada et al., 2008). The whole genome sequence of medaka is known (http://dolphin.nig. ac.jp/medaka), and the spectrum and phenotypes of induced mutations in medaka is often different from those found in zebrafish (Ishikawa, 2000; Loosli et al., 2000; Naruse et al., 2004). During neurogenesis, the overall pattern of the longitudinal fiber systems in medaka brain is more like that of mouse than that of zebrafish (Ishikawa et al., 2004). Moreover, the cardiovascular morphology of zebrafish embryo differs from mammals during development, but medaka embryos follow the common vertebrate embryonic circulatory patterns (Fujita et al., 2006). The structural anatomy of the head skeleton of these two fish species is also different. The trabecular cartilages (TC) in the neurocranium of zebrafish hatchlings are fused caudally with polar cartilages (PC), however, in medaka the caudal end of TC remain separated from PC (Langille and Hall, 1987). Both zebrafish and medaka embryos absorbed alcohol though their chorion when exposed in an alcohol containing medium(Reimers et al., 2004; Bradfield et al., 2006; Oxendine et al., 2006; Wang et al., 2006). Our laboratory is able to demonstrate that medaka embryos exposed to ethanol for first 48 hour post fertilization (hpf) produced craniofacial, skeletal, and cardiovascular abnormalities which are analogous to the FAS phenotypic features observed in human (Wang et al., 2006; Hu et al., 2008, 2009). Another group has shown several other phenotypic features including body length, head width, and caspase 3/7 activity are affected by ethanol during medaka embryogenesis (Oxendine et al., 2006). Therefore, medaka can be used as a unique non-mammalian vertebrate model for identifying the mechanisms related to FASD development.

*Medaka embryos require more waterborne ethanol to induce FASD :* To get a measurable effects of alcohol on medaka development we have determine the lethal concentration of ethanol that is required to induce 50% mortality ($LC_{50}$). Fertilized medaka eggs (Iwamatsu stage ~ 10) were exposed to ethanol for 48 h and then maintained in clean hatching solution until hatching (Wang et al., 2006). The calculated $LC_{50}$ as on 10 day post fertilization (dpf) is 568 mM which is equivalent to 3.2% of ethanol. In a later study, Oxendine et al (2006) observed that medaka embryos maintained in 2% (344 mM) or more ethanol containing medium for 8 dpf were unable to complete normal morphogenesis.We have also observed that medaka embryos in late developmental stages (specifically after the onset of circulation; Iwamatsu stage 25 and above ) were more resistant to ethanol than the embryos of early developmental stages (Iwamatsu stage ~ 10). Compared to rat and mouse (Priscott, 1982; Higuchi and Matsumoto, 2008; Liu et al., 2009), the $LC_{50}$ of ethanol in medaka embryos seems to be very high. It is likely that fish embryos due to the presence of chorion require more waterborne ethanol than mammalian models to induce an observable effect. We therefore determine the embryonic ethanol concentration in medaka embryos at different times points of ethanol exposure during first 48 h of development (Wang et al., 2006).

Fertilized medaka eggs (Iwamatsu stage ~10) were exposed to 100 and 400 mM of ethanol and harvested at 3, 8, 24, 30, and 48 h after treatment. After removal from the culture the embryos were washed in 1 ml cold 3.5% perchloric acid twice to remove any residual alcohol from the outside of the chorion (Wang et al., 2006). Using an enzyme based assay (Reimers et al., 2004), it was observed that embryos exposed to 400 mM of ethanol have significantly higher amount of embryonic ethanol than the embryos exposed to 100 mM. Moreover, throughout the exposure period embryos maintained a steady-state level of ethanol and the embryonic ethanol concentration in both groups (100 and 400 mM) was only 15-20% of the waterborne ethanol (Wang et al., 2006). Studies by Oxendine et al (2006) showed that medaka embryos exposed to ethanol for 3 days at different stages of development (0-3 dpf, 3-6 dpf, 6-9 dpf) absorbed 60-70% of the waterborne ethanol. Compared to medaka, zebrafish following a 45 h ethanol exposure require 340 mM of waterborne ethanol (1.98%) to cause 50% mortality (Reimers et al., 2004). However, after 4 h exposure, embryonic ethanol concentration is only 30% of waterborne ethanol (Reimers et al., 2004). In another experiment, dechorinated zebrafish embryos (4 hpf) exposed to 50 and 500 mM of ethanol achived 70% that of the exposure medium within 3 h as determined by gas chromatography and radiometry (Bradfield et al. 2006). In a later study zebrafish embryos (24 hpf) exposed to 0.25-1% ethanol for 2 h achieved only 1/25- 1/30 of the external concentration (Fernandes and Gerlai, 2009). Taken together, it may be concluded that fish embryos due to the presence of chorion and yolk require more ethanol than mammals to induce FASD.

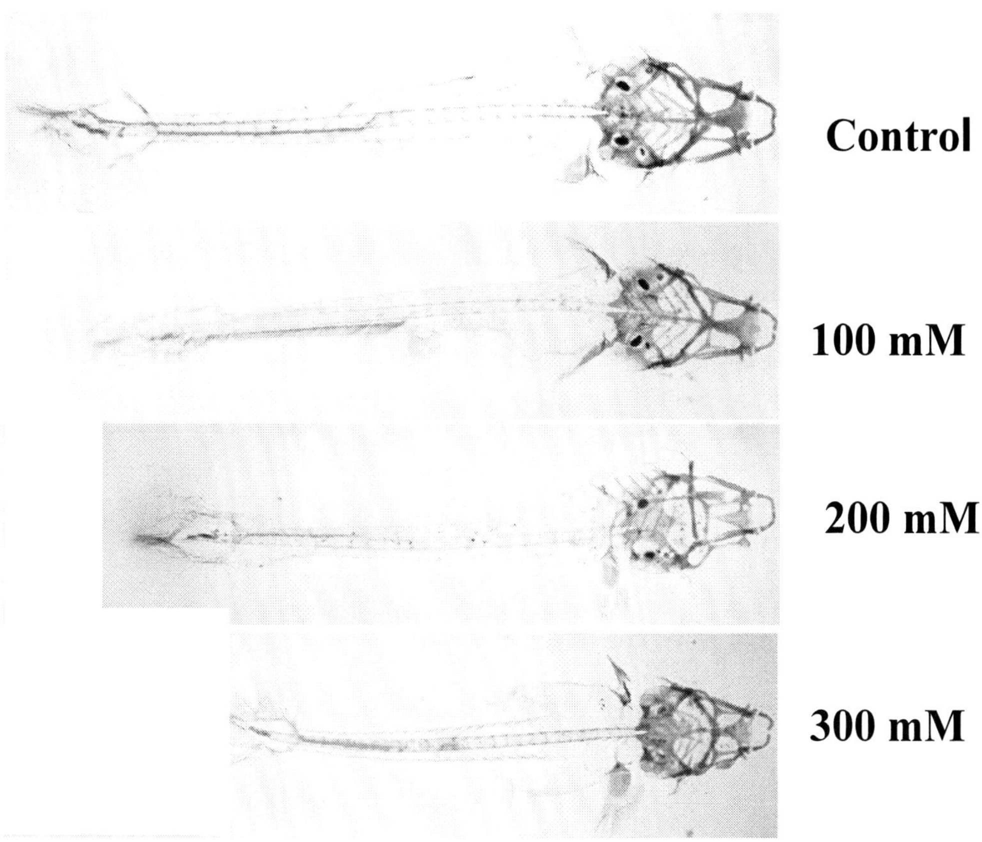


Figure 1. Representative photomicrograph of the skeleton of medaka hatchlings 10 dpf. Medaka embryos were exposed to ethanol (100-300 mM) for first 48 h of development (group A) and then transferred to clean hatching solution. Controls were maintained in clean hatching solution throughout the experiment. Hatchlings (10 dpf) were stained in Alcian Blue after Carvan et al (2004). Ethanol dose-dependently reduced the total length of the skeleton.

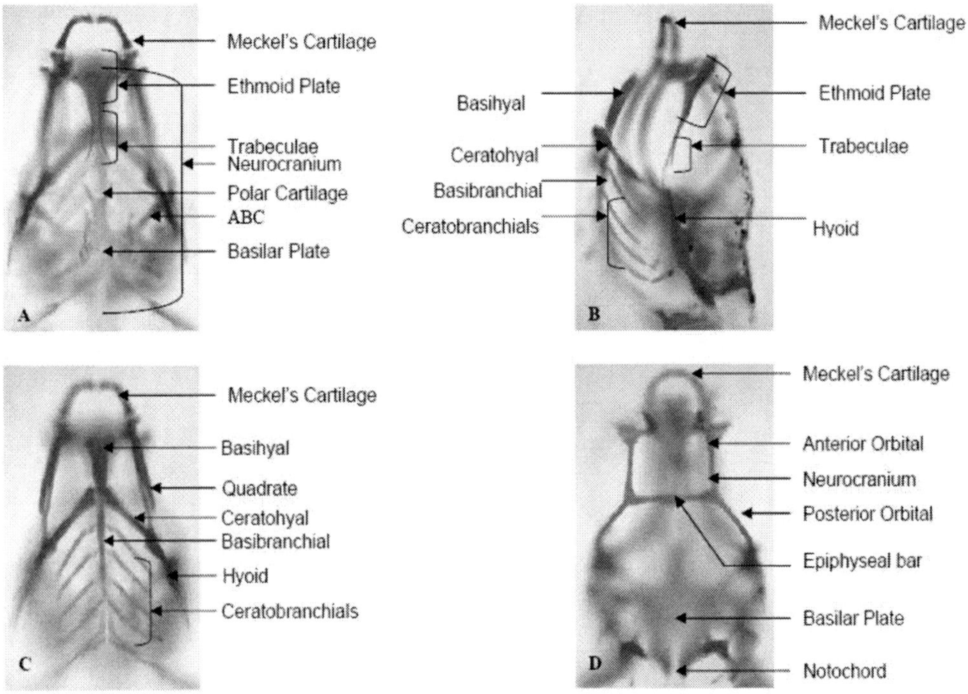


Figure 2. Representative photomicrographs of neurocranial cartilages of medaka hatchlings (10 dpf). The hatchlings (10 dpf) were stained with Alcian Blue and pictures (40X) were taken with an Olympus B-Max 40 microscope. A= neurocranium (dorsal view); B= neurocranium (lateral view); C= splanchnocranium (dorsal view); D= neurocranium (dorsal view focusing orbital cartilages). The ethmoid plate and trabeculae are seen in dorsal (A) and lateral (B) views of neurocranium. The orbital cartilages (D) are further up in position with regard to ethmoid plate.

## CHANGES IN SKELETAL STRUCTURE

The craniofacial morphology appears to be the most significant phenotypic defects observed in FASD. We, therefore, examined the neurocranial cartilage morphology of medaka hatchlings treated with ethanol during embryogenesis. Fertilized medaka eggs at five different time points of development [ group A= 0-48 hour post fertilization (hpf), group B= 24-72 hpf, Group C= 48-96 hpf, group D= 72-120 hpf, group E= 96-144 hpf ] were exposed to 0 (control), and 100-400 mM of ethanol in hatching solution (17 mM NaCl, 0.4 mM KCl, 0.36 mM $CaCl_2$ and 0.6 mM $MgSO_4$) for 48 h, then transferred to fresh hatching solution with no ethanol. The development of neurocranial cartilages and skeleton were examined in hatchlings (10 dpf) after staining with Alcian Blue . In the neurocranium, the ethmoid plate (EP) with lamina orbitonasalis, paired trabeculae (TB), anterior orbital cartilage (AOC), posterior orbital cartilage (POC), epiphyseal bar (EB), basilar plate (BP) with anterior (ABC) and posterior (PBC) basicranial commissures, hypophyseal plate (HP) with paired polar cartilages (PC), and auditory capsules in the neurocranium are clearly visible in hatchlings. In the splanchnocranium, Meckel's cartilage (MC) and lower jaw, pterygoid processes (PT), quadrate (QU), hyosymplectic (HYS), hyoid (HYO), basihyal (BH), ceratohyal (CH), 4 basibranchials (BB), 3 pair hypobranchials (HBR), 5 pair ceratobranchial (CBR), $4^{th}$

epibranchial (EBR) and 4th hypobranchial (HBR) are also identifiable (Figures 1A-D). The nomenclature of the cartilages used in this review is after Langille and Hall (1987).

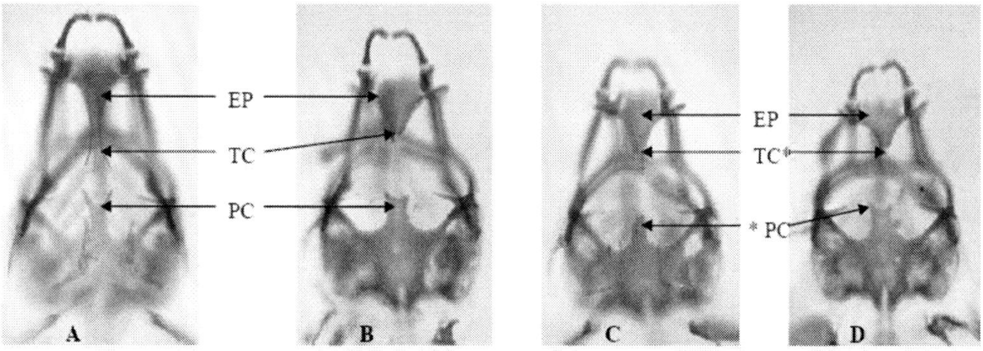


Figure 3. Representative photomicrographs of the neurocranium (dorsal view) of medaka hatchlings showing the disruption in chondrification of neurocranial cartilages by ethanol during development. The embryos were exposed to ethanol (300 mM) 48 hpf and transferred to fresh hatching solution. The hatchlings (10 dpf) were stained with Alcian Blue. It was observed that chondrification of ethmoid plate (EP), trabecular cartilages (TC) and polar cartilages (PC) are disrupted by ethanol (B-D). A= control (no ethanol); B, C, and D= 300 mM ethanol (0-48 hpf).In A, a normal EP, TC and PC are seen; in B, C, and D various levels of disrupted chondrification in EP, TC and PC are seen (B= reduced EP with tiny TC and unequal PC; C=reduced EP with short and unequal TC and absence of *PC; D=reduced EP with no TC* and unequal PC).

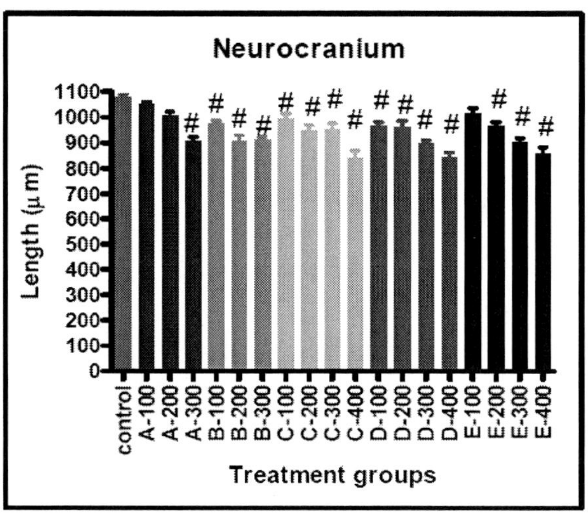


E.

Figure 3E. Effect of ethanol on linear length of neurocranium in medaka hatchlings. The embryos were exposed to ethanol (100-400 mM) during development (A=0-48 hpf; B=24-72 hpf; C=48-96 hpf; D=72-120 hpd; E=96-144 hpf) and transferred to fresh hatching solution. The hatchlings (10 dpf) were stained with Alcian Blue and the pictures were taken with an Olympus B-Max 40 microscope. Photomicrographs (40X) of the neurocranium were measured using Optimas 6 image analysis software (Media Cybernetics, Silver Springs, MD). The data were statistically analyzed by ANOVA followed by post-hoc Tukey's multiple comparison test. Each bar is the mean ±S.E.M. of 10 observations and $p<0.05$ considered as significant. Bar head with pound symbol (#) indicates that the mean data is significantly different from controls.

It was observed that total length of the skeleton (Figure 1) and several skeletal elements in the neurocranium and splanchnocranium (Figures 2 and 3) were affected by ethanol in a dose- and developmental stage-specific manner. Moreover, the chondrification of the neurocranial cartilages, specifically the EP, TC and polar cartilages (PC), were disrupted by ethanol (Figure 3). In some of the hatchlings TC and PC are very tiny, or absent (Figures 3B-3D). The average length of the neurocranium compared to control was reduced in ethanol-treated embryos (100-400 mM) in a dose and developmental stage-specific manner (Figure 3E). From these observations, we predict that ethanol induces inhibition in normal growth of the embryos and ethanol-induced abnormalities in neurocranial cartilages are the result of discrepancies in normal patterning and migration of neural crest (NC) cells from the developing central nervous system. NC cells, as in other vertebrates, form most of the cartilages and bones in the skull of medaka.

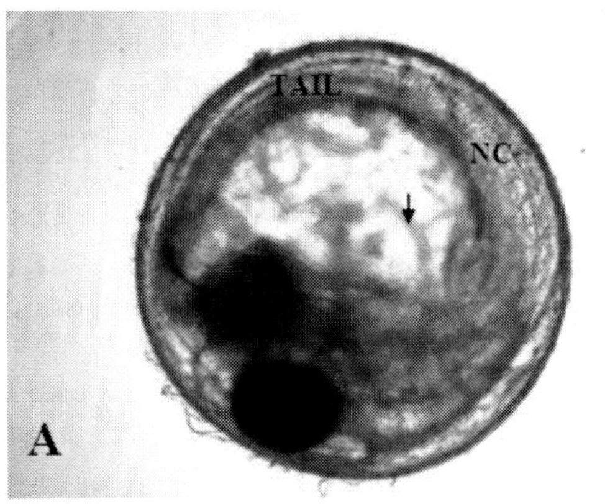


CONTROL

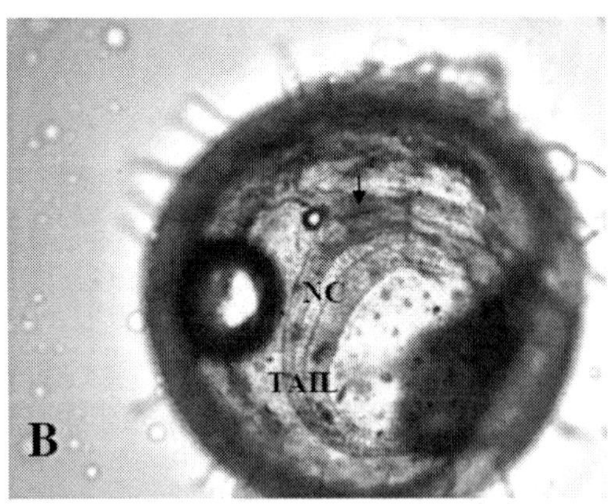


ETHANOL (400 mM)

Figure 4. Representative photomicrographs of medaka embryos showing blood clots in the circulating vessels. Group F embryos (0-24 hpf treatment) were photographed at 96 hpf. A= control (no ethanol); B= 400 mM ethanol (0-24 hpf). Arrow (→ ) represent the area near to the blood island where the first sign of blood clots seen (B) absent in control (A). NC indicates the notochord and TAIL indicates the tail of the embryo.

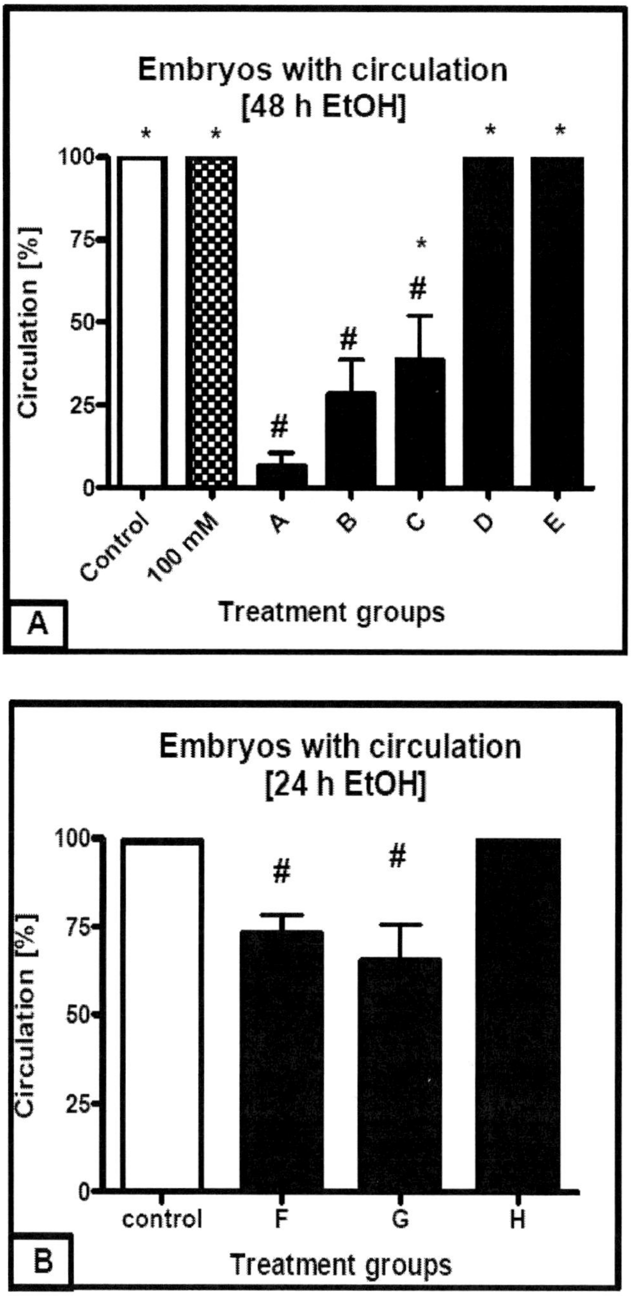


Figure 5. Effect of ethanol on circulation status of medaka embryos during development. Embryos were exposed to 100 or 400 mM ethanol for 48 h in groups A, B, C, D and E, and 400 mM ethanol for 24 h in groups F, G and H. Parallel groups with no ethanol served as controls. For group details see text. Circulation status of the embryos was examined and analyzed on 6 dpf. Each group contained 6-8 embryos per treatment. Each bar is the mean± SEM of 15 to 20 separate treatment repetitions. Bar head with pound symbol (#) indicates that the data are significantly different ($p < 0.05$) from corresponding controls (no ethanol) and asterisks (*) indicates the difference ($p < 0.05$) with group A. Panel marked A= Embryos were exposed to ethanol (100 or 400 mM) for 48 h, and marked B= embryos exposed to ethanol (400 mM) for 24 h. The values of A, B and C in panel A are significantly different from the corresponding values of F, G, and H of panel B.

## Changes in Cardiovascular Structure

In FASD phenotypes the cardiovasculature is also affected by embryonic ethanol exposure. We, therefore, focused on cardiovascular development of medaka embryos exposed to ethanol developmentally. In normal development, the heart formation in medaka was initiated at ~38 hpf (Iwamatsu stage 23) and the embryos initiate circulation by 50 hpf (Iwamatsu Stage 25). We exposed the embryos to ethanol (100 and 400 mM) for two consecutive days (with one-time change of ethanol after 24 h) before (groups A, B and C; Iwamatsu stage 4-24) and after (groups D and E, Iwamatsu stage 25-30) the onset of circulation. It was observed that control embryos were able to maintain the normal circulation in 6 dpf without any cardiovascular developmental deformities. Moreover, the embryos exposed to 100 mM ethanol (groups A-E) also exhibited normal circulation status. In contrast, a significant number of embryos of groups A, B and C treated with 400 mM of ethanol were unable to initiate normal circulation on 6 dpf (compared to control and 100 mM) and majority of them developed blood clots (one to many) in different parts of the circulating vessels (Figure 4). The heart either remained straight (tube heart) or unable to loop completely. Further analysis of the data showed that the number of embryos with disrupted circulation was significantly higher in group A than group C (Figure 5). The embryos of groups D and E treated with equal ethanol concentration (400 mM) were able to maintain their normal circulation status as in controls and 100 mM ethanol-treated embryos (Figure 5A).

In order to determine the critical period of ethanol effect in cardiovascular development of medaka, fertilized embryos at three different stages of development were exposed to ethanol for 24 h [ group F= 0 -24 hpf embryos, Iwamatsu stages ~ 10; group G= 24-48 hpf embryos, Iwamatsu stages 15-20; group H= 48-72 hpf, Iwamatsu stages 23-24]. All of these embryos were in a non-circulating stage at the beginning of the ethanol treatment (Iwamatsu stages 4-24). These embryos were exposed to 400 mM of ethanol only for 24 h and examined on 6 dpf. It was observed that the number of embryos with circulation in groups F and G (Figure 5B) were significantly increased in comparison with the embryos treated with two consecutive days ethanol (Group A, B or C), however, those with disrupted circulation had blood clots and cardiac deformities. All embryos of group H (Iwamatsu stage 23-24; no circulation) treated with 400 mM ethanol (2 dpf- 3 dpf) were able to initiate circulation in 6 dpf as in controls (Figure 5B).

## Biochemical Parameters

To find a suitable biochemical marker that reflects the normal developmental pattern of medaka during embryogenesis and altered by ethanol, we have measured the nucleic acid (DNA and RNA) and protein contents in medaka embryos (group A embryos) exposed to ethanol (100 and 400 mM for first 48 h of development, then transferred to clean hatching solution) at zero, 2, 4 and 6 dpf. The data were expressed as the concentration of macromolecules (ng for DNA and RNA and μg for protein)/ embryo. The nucleic acid concentrations of the embryos were determined from the embryos with intact chorion and yolk materials (Wu et al., 2008), however, for protein embryos after required period of treatment fixed in 4% paraformaldehyde containing 0.1% Tween 20 for 4 h at room temperature. After fixation, the chorion and yolk were removed from the embryos and both yolk and embryos used separately for protein estimation (Wu et al., 2008). The DNA and protein contents of the embryos considered as zero day were prepared from the embryos at early blastula stage (Iwamatsu stage 10), but for total RNA the embryos of earlier developmental stages (Iwamatsu stages 3-4) were used.

As the cleavage continued, the amount of DNA in embryos in 2dpf was found to be increased in all groups (0, 100 and 400 mM) compared to the embryos of zero dpf, however, the values were not significantly different. Also, the increase in 2 dpf was statistically equal in all three groups (Figure 6A). On day 4, when ethanol was no longer present in the medium, DNA contents of the embryos were increased further, and the enhancement in control (no ethanol) and 100 mM group were statistically significant from the corresponding control and 100 mM groups of 2 dpf embryos, but not in 400 mM group (where the values were not significantly different from 400 mM group of 2dpf).

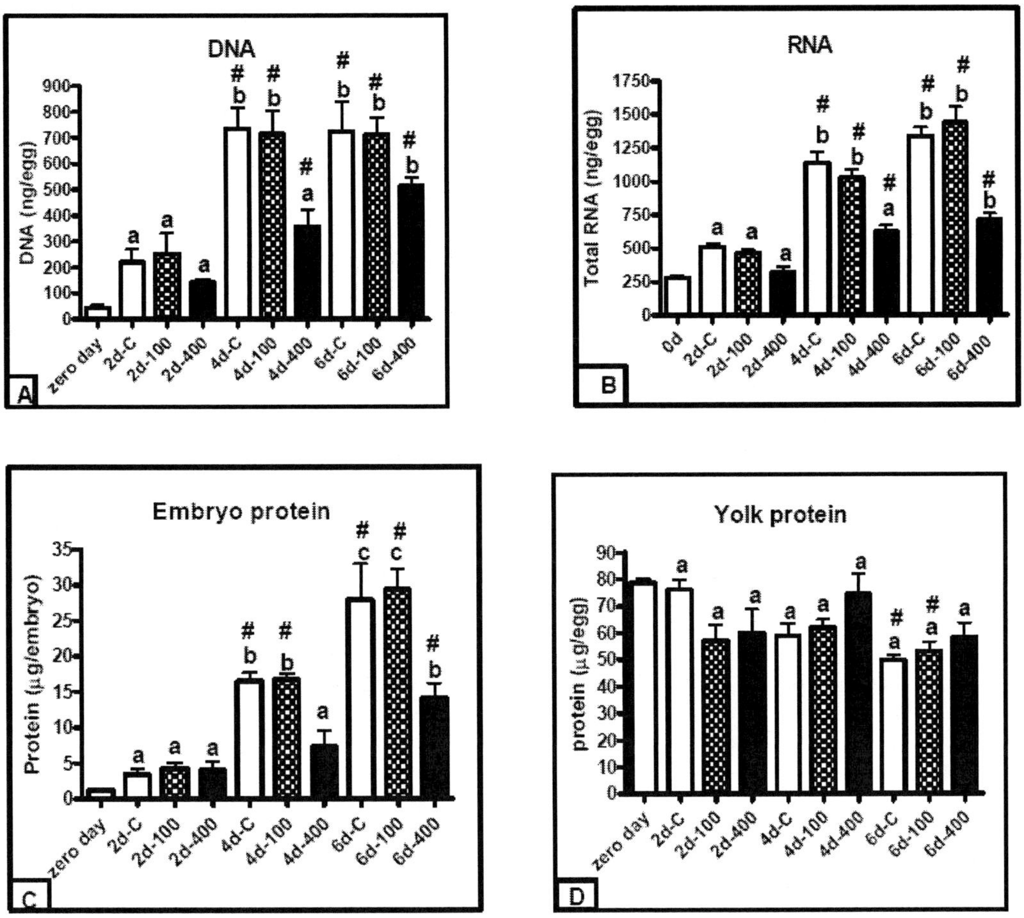


Figure 6. Effect of ethanol on DNA, RNA and protein contents of the medaka embryo during development. Each bar represents the mean± SEM of four to six separate experiments. Bar head with pound symbol (#) indicates that the results are significantly different ($p<0.05$) from zero dpf; different lower case letters (a, b and c) represent the data are significantly different from the corresponding control, 100 or 400 mM groups at 2dpf. A= DNA, B= RNA, C= embryo protein D= Yolk protein.

Moreover, the DNA contents of control embryos at 4 dpf also showed significantly higher amount of DNA than the embryos exposed to 400 mM ethanol. On day 6, no further increase of embryonic DNA was noticed in control, 100 and 400 mM groups with regard to the corresponding embryos of 4dpf, however, the value of 400 mM group was found to be significantly different from the 400 mM group of 2dpf (Figure 6A).

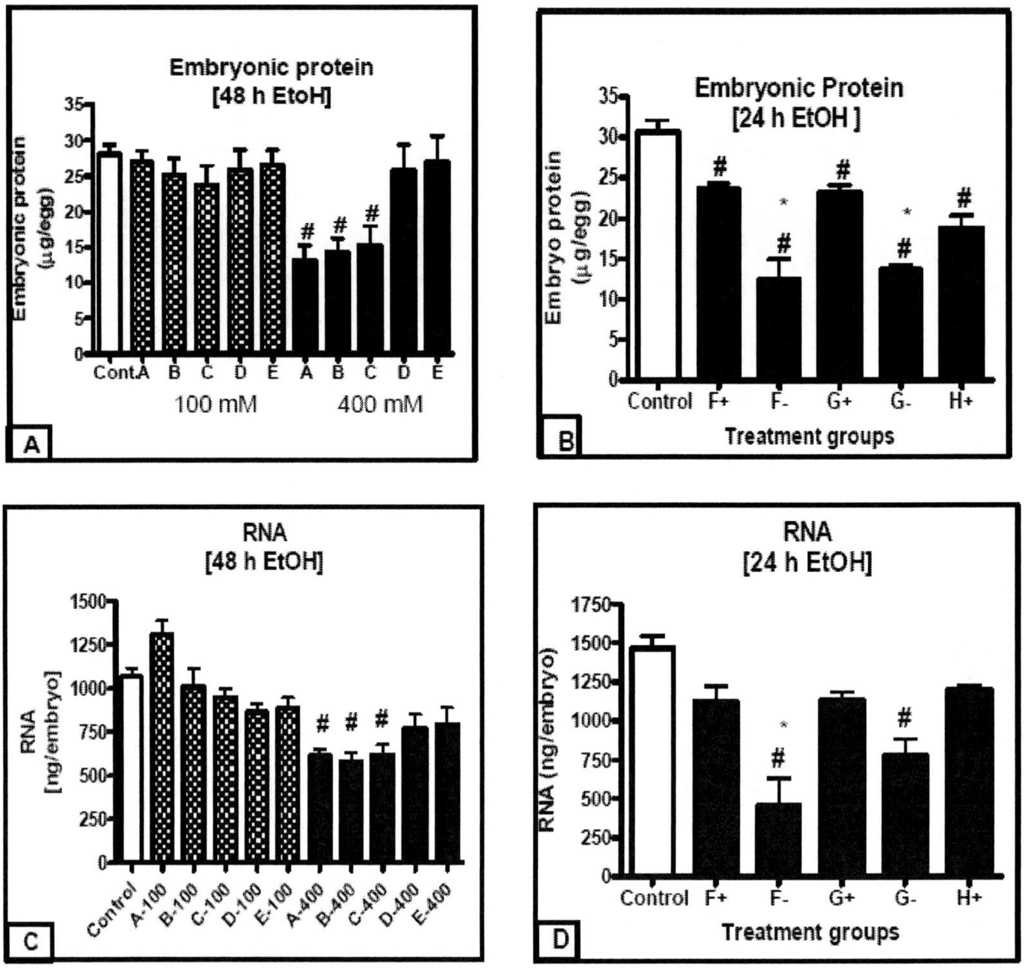


Figure 7. Embryos were exposed to 100 or 400 mM ethanol for 48 h in groups A, B, C, D, and E, and 400 mM ethanol for 24h in groups F, G and H. Parallel groups with no ethanol serve as control. For group details see text. Viable embryos were sacrificed on 6 dpf and were used for protein (panels A and B) and RNA (panels C and D) analysis. The circulating embryos from the same group were separated from the non-circulating ones before protein and RNA assay in groups F and G. Each group consists of 6-8 embryos per treatment. Each bar is the mean ±SEM of 4-6 separate treatment repetitions. Bar head with pound symbol (#) indicates the data are significantly different ($p<0.05$) from the corresponding control and with asterisk (*) indicate that the data are different from the circulating embryos. Panels A and B= Protein; Panels C and D= RNA. In panels B and D, the group (F, G and H) marked '+' indicate that the embryos were in circulation on 6 dpf and marked '-'indicate that the embryos were unable to initiate circulation.

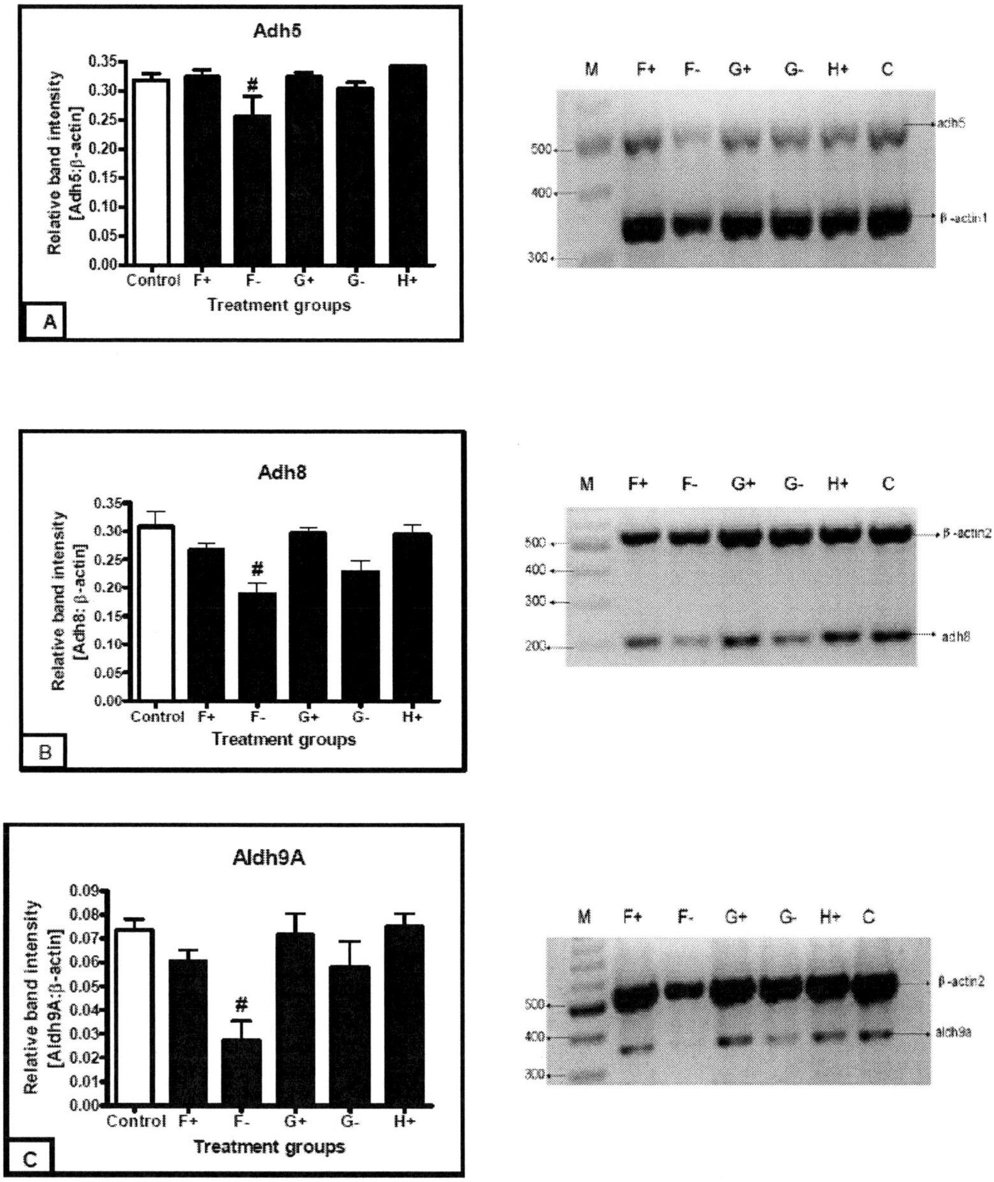


Figure 8. Effect of ethanol on Adh 5, Adh8 and Aldh9A mRNA expression in medaka embryos developmentally exposed to ethanol. Total RNA was prepared from 6-8 pooled medaka embryos on 6 dpf, reverse transcribed and analyzed by rRT-PCR using β-actin primers as internal control. The results were expressed as the ratio of relative band intensity of target gene: β-actin. The data obtained were log transformed and used for one way ANOVA followed by post-hoc Tukey's multiple comparison test. Each entry is the mean ±S.E.M. of 4-6 separate experiments and $p < 0.05$ considered as significant. F, G and H represents the groups of medaka embryos exposed to ethanol for a specific development period [F= 0-24 hpf, G= 24-48 hpf, H=48-72 hpf]; '+' indicates that the embryos were in circulation and '-' indicates the embryos were unable to initiate circulation on 6 dpf. A= Adh5, B=Adh8, C= Aldh9A. Bar head with pound symbol (#) indicates that the mean data is significantly different from the controls. Representative gel pictures of the rRT-PCR analysis are presented on the right side of the panel A (Adh5), B (Adh8) and C (Aldh9A) in which 'M' indicates 100 bp ladder and 'C' for controls (no ethanol).

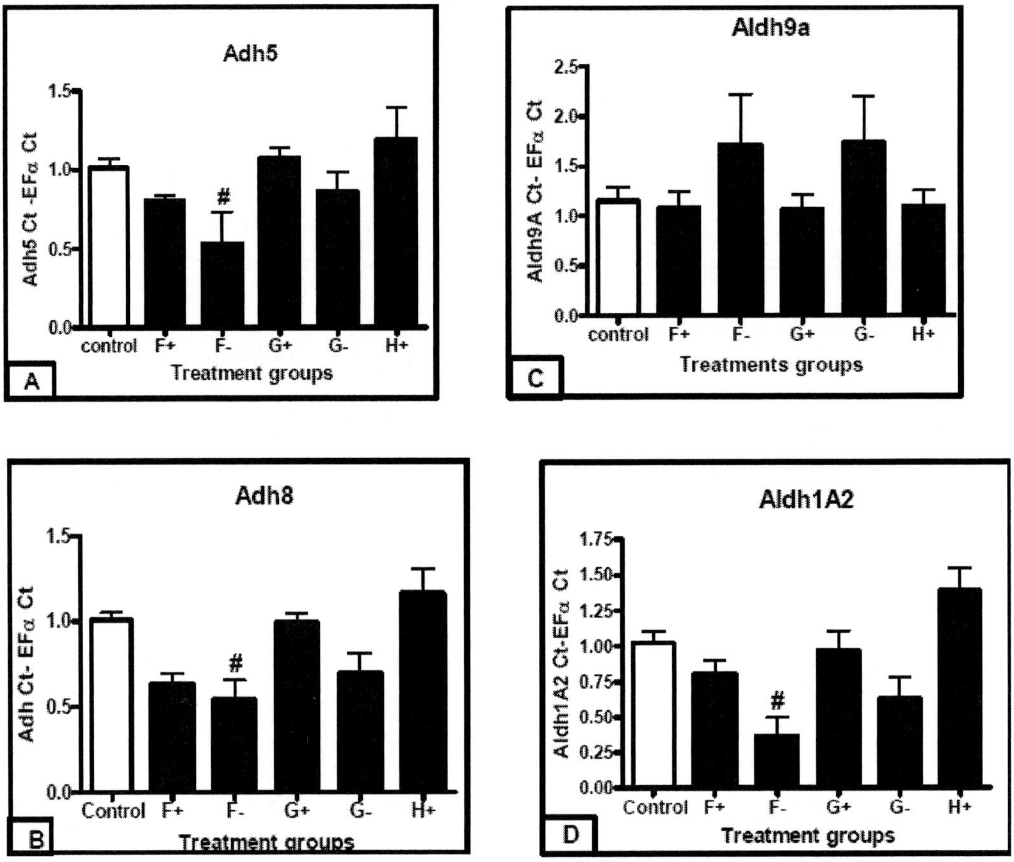


Figure 9. Effect of ethanol on Adh 5, Adh8 and Aldh9A mRNA expression in medaka embryos developmentally exposed to ethanol. Total RNA was prepared from 6-8 pooled medaka embryos on 6 dpf, reverse transcribed and analyzed by qRT-PCR. For each sample, the threshold cycle for internal standard (EF1α) amplification (Ct, EF1α) was subtracted from the threshold cycle of the corresponding enzyme mRNA amplification (Ct, enzyme) to yield ΔCt. For each treatment group, the data are the mean of ΔCt of control samples was subtracted from each individual samples to yield individual ΔΔCt. Fold induction relative to control samples was calculated with $2^{-\Delta\Delta Ct}$. The data obtained were log transformed and used for one way ANOVA followed by post-hoc Tukey's multiple comparison test; $p< 0.05$ was considered as significant. Each data are the mean ±S.E.M. of 3-4 separate experiments. F, G and H represents the groups of medaka embryos exposed to ethanol for a specific development period [F= 0-24 hpf, G= 24-48 hpf, H=48-72 hpf]. Group with '+' indicates that the embryos were in circulation and '-' indicates the embryos were unable to initiate circulation on 6 dpf. A= Adh5, B=Adh8, C= Aldh9A, D=Aldh1A2. Bar head with pound symbol (#) indicates that the mean data is significantly different from the controls.

The concentration of RNA, like DNA, was also increased in embryos with the advancement of embryogenesis. However, RNA contents of 2 dpf embryos (control, 100 and 400 mM) remained at the same level as in zero dpf group (Figure 6B). In 4 dpf, the RNA concentrations of the embryos of control and 100 mM group were significantly increased in comparison with the embryos of zero and 2 dpf, but in 400 mM group the enhancement was significantly different only from the embryos at zero dpf, but not from 2 dpf. Further analysis of the data indicates that in 4 dpf embryos the RNA content of control and 100 mM ethanol-treated groups have more amount of RNA than the embryos exposed to 400 mM ethanol. In

6dpf, no further enhancement of this macromolecule was noticed in control, 100 mM and 400 mM group with regard to the corresponding embryos of 4 dpf, however, in 400 mM group, the increase was significantly higher than the embryos of 2 dpf exposed to similar ethanol concentration (Figure 6B). Further comparison of RNA data in 6 dpf samples indicate that both control and 100 mM ethanol-treated groups have more RNA than the embryos exposed to 400 mM ethanol.

The embryonic protein showed the most significant change during the advancement of development (Figure 6C). Both in control and treated embryos, this cellular constituent showed a sharp rise over time and by day 6 the increase was more than 20-fold in control and 100 mM groups compared to the embryos of zero dpf. Like DNA and RNA, the enhancement of embryonic protein in 2 dpf embryos was not significantly different from zero dpf (stage 10) samples. The embryos of 4 dpf showed a significant rise of this macromolecule over zero dpf and corresponding 2 dpf groups in both control and 100 mM ethanol-treated embryos, but in 400 mM group the enhancement remained at the same level as in zero or 2 dpf groups. The embryonic protein was increased further in all groups in 6 dpf embryos. In control and 100 mM groups the values were significantly higher than the corresponding embryos of 4 dpf. The embryos treated with 400 mM ethanol also have higher amount of protein, and the increase was significantly different from the corresponding 2 dpf embryos, but not from 4 dpf. Also the values were significantly lower than the values observed in control and 100 mM groups on 6 dpf. The total embryonic yolk proteins remained almost unaltered during development, but was significantly reduced in control and 100 mM group in 6 dpf compared to the embryos of zero dpf (Figure 6D).

Total protein and RNA content of the medaka embryos developmentally exposed to ethanol were further analyzed with regard to circulation status of the embryos (Figure 7). The cellular constituents (protein and RNA) taken from fish embryos exposed to ethanol for two consecutive days (groups A-E) were pooled irrespective of their circulation status. Those exposed for one day (groups F, G and H) were separated into non-circulating embryos (F- and G-) and circulating embryos (F+, G+, H+) prior to be being pooled. It was observed that ethanol at 400 mM concentration significantly reduced the total protein and RNA contents of the embryos from groups A, B and C at 6 dpf in comparison with the controls and 100 mM groups. However, no significant differences in these macromolecular components (total protein and RNA) were observed in groups D and E embryos (Figures 7A and 7C) exposed to 0 (control), 100 or 400 mM ethanol. In groups F, G and H, embryonic protein content was significantly lower in the ethanol-treated embryos. Further, embryos without circulation (F- and G-) had significantly less protein than the embryos with circulation (F+ and G+) (Figure 7B). In case of RNA, the results were slightly different. Those embryos which had failed to initiate circulation on 6 dpf (F- and G-) due to ethanol treatment (400 mM for 24 h) had significantly less RNA than the embryos with circulation (controls or F+, G+ or H+ groups). No significant difference on 6 dpf embryos was observed in the RNA contents of the control and the ethanol-treated embryos with circulation (F+, G+ and H+) (Figure 7D).

## Alcohol Metabolizing Enzymes

Previously we have observed that medaka embryos (0 dpf) exposed to ethanol (100 and 400 mM) 48 hpf and measured *adh5*, *adh8* and *aldh9A* mRNA on 2, 4 and 6 dpf were unable to alter these mRNA content with regard to control embryos (no ethanol) (Wang et al., 2006). To investigate the influence of circulation status, both *adh* and *aldh* mRNAs (*adh5, adh8, aldh9A* and *aldh1A2*) were measured separately in circulating (groups F+, G+ and H) and non-circulating (F-, G-) embryos. We used rRT-PCR for *adh5*, *adh8* and *aldh9A* mRNAs (Figure 8) and qRT-PCR for *adh5*, *adh8*, *aldh9A* and *aldh1A2* mRNA (Figure 9) for analysis. The data obtained by rRT-PCR showed that the embryos treated with ethanol and have circulation (group F+, G+ and H+) were able to maintain equal amounts of *adh* and *aldh* mRNAs on 6dpf as in controls. However, embryos without circulation (F- and G-) showed developmental stage specific response (reduction). Embryos of group F- (embryos at Iwamatsu stages 4-10 exposed to 400 mM of ethanol for 24h and without circulation on 6 dpf) showed significant reduction in these mRNA (*adh5*, *adh8* and *aldh9*) levels with respect to controls, however, embryos of G- group (Iwamatsu stages 17-20, exposed to 400 mM ethanol 24h and without circulation on 6 dpf) had the same level of the mRNAs mentioned above as in controls (Figures 8A, B, and C). In qRT-PCR analysis, *adh5*, *adh8* and *aldh1A2* mRNA expression (Figures 9A, 9B and 9D) showed similar nature of changes (decreased in F- and remained at the same level in F+, G+, G- and H+) as in rRT-PCR, however, *aldh9A* (Figure 9C) mRNA level in F, G and H groups were remained at the same level as in controls regardless of the circulation status of the embryo.

## Discussion

Fetal alcohol syndrome (FAS) is a pattern of developmental anomalies found in children born to alcohol abusing mothers who consumed alcohol during pregnancy. This was first noticed in France (Lemoine et al., 1968), and in the USA, Jones and Smith (1973) correlated FAS phenotypes with maternal alcohol ingestion. Since then many studies have been done to understand the mechanism, however, very limited success has been achieved. The problem is complicated because of the pleiotropic nature of ethanol action at the cellular level during embryogenesis (Dunty et al., 2001; Goodlett et al., 2005; Sant'Anna and Tosello, 2006). As FAS studies in human is not possible due to ethical reason, many animal models are used. Moreover, it is very difficult to find a single animal model that can reflect human conditions. Therefore, studies in more models are necessary.

FAS phenotypes in human are physically identified by examining the facial features, such as the smooth philtrum, thin vermilion border of the upper lip, and short palpebral fissures. In addition to these soft tissues, the facial dysmorphology by ethanol can be observed in facial bones with a small head circumference (microcephaly), apparent flattening of the nasal bridge and midface, micrognathia (small jaw), facial asymmetry, and cleft palate (Su et al., 2001; Naidoo et al., 2005). In animal models, such as rat, chicken and zebrafish, prenatal ethanol exposure also produced a pattern of abnormal craniofacial defects (Guerrero, 1990; Su et al., 2001; Ahlgren et al., 2002; Carvan et al., 2004). The molecular mechanism of these defects has been proposed to be due to the induction of apoptosis in the neural crest (NC) cells (the precursor of many craniofacial cartilages and bones) during development.

Our studies of the effects of ethanol during medaka embryogenesis indicate that ethanol at early stages of development (Iwamatsu stages 4-24; embryos without circulation) induces abnormalities in craniofacial, cardiovascular and skeletal development followed by reduction in protein and RNA content (Figures1-7). Further analysis of *adh* and *aldh* mRNAs also indicates that embryos at early stages of development are more sensitive to ethanol than the embryos at late stages (Figures 8-9). Our previous studies showed that exposure to ethanol disrupted the circulation status of the embryos in a dose-dependent manner (Wang et al., 2006). Other morphological parameters such as craniofacial, cardiovascular and skeletal deformities by ethanol were also found to be dose-specific in medaka (Wang et al., 2006). The critical period of teratogenic action of alcohol during embryonic development of medaka was not known to us. We therefore followed a strategy to determine the critical phase of ethanol toxicity in medaka embryogenesis and used circulation status as morphological and macromolecular contents (RNA and Protein) as biochemical markers of ethanol teratogenesis.

Ethanol exposure of the embryos during prenatal development disrupts craniofacial and neurocranial cartilage development in other species including human, mouse, rat, chick, Xenopus and zebrafish (Nakatsuji, 1983; Sulik et al., 1988; Webster and Ritchie, 1991; Smith 1997; Roda-Moreno et al., 2000; Ahlgren et al., 2002; Loucks and Carvan, 2004). The primary cause of this defect is the induction of apoptosis in NC cells which are destined to give rise to facial structure (Smith 1997). In our model we have also observed a phenomenon of microcephaly due to the reduction of linear length of many chondrocranial cartilages. Moreover, TC and PC are the major cartilages where the disruptions are very prominent, and in many ethanol-treated (200-400 mM) embryos of groups A-D, complete absence of TC and PC in the neurocranium have been observed (Figures 3A-D). During embryogenesis, TC in medaka arises as two C-shaped rods at the anterolateral border of the head, and curve backward and inward to lie adjacent to each other along the midline (Langille and Hall, 1987). Later they fuse anteriorly to form EP and remain separated posteriorly. The PC arises as paired rods, flanking the hypophyseal fenestrae, fusing with the BP posteriorly and separating from each other anteriorly. The anterior ends of medaka PC, unlike zebrafish, do not fuse with the caudal ends of TC (Figure 2A). There is another diamond shaped membrane bone, the parasphenoid (remained unstained by Alcian Blue), which remains within TC and PC underlies the hypophyseal fenestrae with its flattened portion and the top and bottom corners elongated into thin rods. The anterior rod lies between the TC but does not reach the rostrum, the posterior rod extends below the BP, ending before the notochord (Langille and Hall, 1987).

The majority of the chondrocranial cartilages of medaka examined are formed after the migration of NC cells from the developing CNS (Langille and Hall, 1988). Neural crestectomies in mesencephalon and preotic rhombencephalon are able to disrupt EP and TC formation; however, formation of PC is not affected by NC extirpations (Langille and Hall, 1988). Therefore, from the present data it is also evident that the neurocranial cartilages, which are not affected by neural crestectomy (PC), are also disrupted by ethanol. Ethanol metabolism generates oxidative stress which is cytotoxic as well as apoptotic. Complete or partial loss of TC or PC in ethanol–treated embryos further indicate that oxidative stress may induce abnormalities in the migration pattern of NC cells or target the expression of a gene which is specifically expressed only in TC and PC precursor cells. Alternatively, oxidative stress induces apoptosis which may disrupt gene expression in the precursor cells of TC and PC due to some unknown specificity. As a result, mediolateral polarity in the neurocranium of medaka embryo is also affected after ethanol exposure. Studies in other models indicate that the members of common signaling pathways such as sonic hedgehog (shh), fibroblast growth factor (fgf), wingless (wnt) and bone morphogenic protein (bmp) have significant impact in NC survival, proliferation, differentiation and thus craniofacial development (Tapadia et al., 2005). Therefore, in medaka, as in other vertebrates, ethanol may be able to alter the functions of these signaling molecules and induce dysmorphogenesis in neurocranial and splanchnocranial cartilage development.

The cardiovascular development in medaka embryo has been studied by several investigators (Iwamatsu, 2004: Fujita et al., 2006). The heart becomes visible under a microscope ~38 hpf (Iwamatsu stage 22). The blood vessels (Cuvierian ducts and vitello-caudal vein or marginal vein) and the intermediate cell mass (ICM) or blood island are pronounced in Iwamatsu stage 23 (~41 hpf). The heart starts beating at ~ 44 hpf (Iwamatsu stage 24) with a very low heart rate (32-64 beats/min); the embryonic erythrocytes and hemangioblasts are aggregated in ICM during this period. During ~50 hpf (Iwamatsu stage 25) the heart rate increase (70-80 beats/min) and the globular blood cells come out from the ICM (onset of circulation). At ~64 hpf (Iwamatsu stage 28) the blood cells appear to be flattening (Iwamatsu, 2004). The differentiation of embryonic heart into atrium, ventricle, sinus venosus and bulbous aorta begins ~74 hpf (Iwamatsu stage 29). Branching of arteries to supply blood to trunk muscles, gills and brain starts at ~ 82 hpf (Iwamatsu stage 30) and the circulation to the pectoral fins occurs at ~ 121 hpf (Iwamatsu stage 34). Looping of the heart is complete at ~144 hpf (Iwamatsu stage 36).

In our experimental design the embryos belonging to group A were exposed to ethanol from very early stages of development (early to late blastula) to the stage prior to the onset of blood circulation (0-48 hpf). In group B, ethanol treatment started at early neurula stage and continued to the stage of heart chamber formation (24-72 hpf); in group C, embryos were exposed to ethanol prior to the onset of circulation and the treatment was continued to the beginning of the blood supply to the organs (48-96 hpf). In group D (72-120 hpf) and E (96-144 hpf), embryos were exposed to ethanol when the circulation was already started. With these treatment conditions we observed that embryos exposed to 100 mM of ethanol were able to initiate circulation as in controls; however, significant numbers of embryos exposed to 400 mM of ethanol in groups A, B and C were unable to initiate circulation on 6 dpf. If the embryos were exposed to ethanol after the onset of circulation, no alteration in the circulation status of the embryos was observed on 6 dpf (groups D and E). We therefore conclude that onset of circulation can be used as a hallmark of ethanol toxicity in medaka embryogenesis. We have also observed that some of the ethanol-treated embryos were able to establish circulation in later stages of development and were able to survive with FAS features like craniofacial disorders (Wang et al., 2006) after hatching. However, the embryos that were unable to establish circulation due to ethanol treatment, majority of them (specifically group A) died prior to, or after hatching.

To find the critical phase of ethanol toxicity we reduced the alcohol exposure window to 24 h. Embryos of groups A, B and C treated with 400 mM ethanol were removed from ethanol after 24 h (group F, ethanol: 0-24hpf, no sign of cardiovascular development; group G, ethanol: 24-48 hpf, heart and blood vessel development phase; group H, ethanol: 48-72 hpf, onset of circulation phase). It was observed that more embryos were able to initiate circulation on 6 dpf in groups F, G and H compared to the corresponding A, B and C groups. Moreover, in group H, all embryos were able to recover from ethanol stress (all stresses were located within the circulatory system). It is therefore further concluded that the effects of ethanol on cardiovascular development of medaka are specific to the dose, duration, and developmental status of the embryos. Ethanol at 100 mM concentration (48 h duration) had no effect in altering circulation status of the embryos, however, those exposed to 400 mM ethanol either for 48 h (groups A, B and C) or for 24 h (groups F and G) have a significantly disrupted circulation status depending upon the stage of ethanol treatment (Figure 5A). Embryos of group D and E were non-responsive to ethanol with regard to their circulation status. Analysis of protein and RNA content of the embryo further support our hypothesis that alterations in circulation status during embryogenesis were reflected in the reduction of cellular protein and RNA content in the embryonic body (Figures 6B and 6C) which ultimately can cause growth retardation in embryo, a major phenotypical feature observed in FASD babies. The yolk is the only source of nutrients during embryo development in medaka, and supply of nutrients from the yolk to the embryo occurs through circulation. Therefore, disruption in circulation/ circulatory system by ethanol inhibited the normal growth of the embryo. Moreover, from the present data it may also be concluded that medaka embryos are more sensitive to ethanol in early stages of development before the onset of circulation (Iwamatsu stages 4-24) than the embryos in late stages with circulation (stages 25-30).

One of the potential mechanisms of ethanol toxicity is the production of oxidative stress due to ethanol metabolism by ADH and ALDH enzymes (Dennery, 2007). The oxidative stress can generate either free radicals or highly reactive aldehydes that damage macromolecules (Reimers et al., 2004). Moreover, oxidative stress and redox signaling are essential for normal developmental processes (Dennery, 2007). In chick embryo, ethanol altered the early vascular development in area vasculosa in a concentration-dependent manner (Tufan and Satiroglu-Tufan, 2003). The mechanisms proposed for the disruption were the generation of reactive oxygen species, perturbation of retinoic acid signaling, and alteration in the expression of growth regulatory vasculogenic factors and their receptors (Tufan and Satiroglu-Tufan, 2003). Previously, we were unable to demonstrate any significant difference in *adh5*, *adh8* and *aldh9A* mRNA contents in the embryos on 6 dpf exposed to ethanol 48 hpf with controls (Wang et al., 2006, 2007b). However, the expression of *adh5*, *adh8*, and *aldh9A* mRNA was developmentally regulated (Dasmahapatra et al., 2005; Wang et al., 2007a, 2007b). The *aldh9* mRNA data presented here were obtained by rRT-PCR and qRT-PCR which were not identical. However, we were still able to demonstrate a significant dose- and developmental stage-specific reduction in *adh* and *aldh* mRNA level by ethanol during medaka embryogenesis (Figures 8 and 9). The reduction may be related to the growth retardation rather than inhibition in the synthesis of these enzymes during development. Previously we have reported that the expression of *adh8*, *aldh9A*, and *aldh1A2* was developmentally regulated and the level of mRNAs was increased with the advancement of morphogenesis (Wang et al., 2007a). Therefore, the reduced level of *adh* and *aldh* mRNAs in medaka embryogenesis by ethanol is probably due to the inhibition in morphogenesis.

Taken together, it may be concluded that medaka embryo with regard to craniofacial and cardiovascular development can be used as a unique non-mammalian vertebrate model to study ethanol teratogenesis and thus FASD. The embryos were very sensitive to ethanol before the onset of circulation than in later phases. Medaka embryos from Iwamatsu stage 25 onwards can be likened to a fetus. These embryos (stage 25 and onwards) have well developed heart with circulation, several organs including brain (organogenesis), pectoral fin buds, which can be compared with the features found in a human fetus. Therefore, in medaka, embryos are more ethanol-sensitive than in the fetal-like stages and the critical ethanol-sensitive phase was the embryonic phase.

## ACKNOWLEDGMENTS

We are grateful to Doris Powe for her generous help during the preparation of the manuscript. We are thankful to Elsevier for giving us permission to include some of the data previously published in Comparative Biochemistry and Physiology part B (149B, 191-201, 2008) and C (148C, 273-280, 2008; 150C, 495-502, 2009). This study was supported partially by the National Center for Natural Product Research, and the National Institute on Alcohol Abuse and Alcoholism (Grant Number RO3AA016915). The content is solely the responsibility of the authors and does not necessarily represent the official views of the National Institute on Alcohol Abuse and Alcoholism or the National Institute of Health. This publication was made possible by NIH grant number RR016476 from the MFGN INBRE Program of the National Center for Research Resources.

## REFERENCES

Abel EL. Fetal alcohol syndrome : the American Paradox. *Alcohol Alcohol.* 33:195-201(1998).

Abel EL, Sokol RJ. A revised conservative estimate of the incidence of FAS and economic impact. *Alcohol. Clin. Exp. Res.* 15:514-524(1992).

Ahlgren SC, Thakur V, Bronner-Fraser M. Sonic hedgehog rescues cranial neural crest from cell death induced by ethanol exposure. *Proc. Nat. Acad. Sci. USA,* 99:10476-10481(2002).

Arenzana FJ, Carvan MJ, III, Sanchez-Gonzalez R, Arevalo R, Porteros A. Teratogenic effects of ethanol exposure on zebrafish visual system development. *Neurotoxicol. Teratol.* 28:342-348(2006).

Baumann M. Sander K. Bipartite axiation follows incomplete epiboly in zebrafish embryos treated with chemical teratogens. *J. Exp. Zool.* 230:363-376(1984).

Bilotta J, Barnett JA, Hancock L, Saszik S. Ethanol exposure alters zebrafish development: A novel model of fetal alcohol syndrome. *Neurotox. Terato.* 26: 737-743(2004).

Bilotta J, Saszik S, Givin CM, Hardesty HR, Sutherland SE. Effects of embryonic exposure to ethanol on zebrafish visual function. *Neurotoxicol. Teratol.* 24:759-766(2002).

Blader P, Strahle U. Ethanol impairs migration of the prechordal plate in the zebrafish embryo. *Dev. Biol.* 201:185-201(1998).

Bradfield JY, West JR, Maier SE. Uptake and elimination of ethanol by young zebrafish embryos. *Neurotoxicol. Teratol.* 28:629-633(2006).

Burd L, Moffatt ME. Epidemiology of fetal alcohol syndrome in American Indians, Alaskan Natives, and Canadian Aboriginal peoples: a review of the literature. *Public Health Rep.* 109:688-693(1994).

Carvan MJ,III Loucks E, Weber DN, Williams FE. Ethanol effects on the developing zebrafish: neurobehavior and skeletal morphogenesis. *Neurotox. Terato.* 26: 757-768 (2004).

Carvan MJ, III, Gallagher EP, Goksoyr A, Hahn ME, Larsson DG. Fish models in toxicology. *Zebrafish*, 4:9-20(2007).

Cook PS, Petersen RC, Moore DT: Alcohol, tobacco and other drugs may harm the unborn. Publicatin no ADM 90-1711, p 17, US Department of Health and Human services, Bethesda, MD (1990).

Cudd TA. Animal model systems for the study of alcohol teratology. *Exp. Biol. Med.* 230: 389-393 (2005).

Damodaran S, Dlugos CA, Wood TD, Rabin RA. Effects of chronic ethanol administration on brain protein levels: a proteomic investigation using 2-D DIGE system. *Eur. J. Pharmacol.* 547:75-82(2006).

Dasmahapatra AK, Wang X, Haasch ML. Expression of Adh8 mRNA is developmentally regulated in Japanese medaka (Oryzias latipes). *Comp. Biochem. Physiol.* 140B: 657-664 (2005).

Dennery PA. Effects of oxidative stress on embryonic development. *Birth Defects Res.* 81C:155-162(2007)

Dlugos CA, Rabin RA. Ethanol effects on three strains of zebrafish: model system for genetic investigations. *Pharm. Biochem. Behav.* 74:471-480(2003).

Dlugos CA , Rabin RA. Ocular deficits associated with alcohol exposure during zebrafish development. *J. Comp. Neurol.* 502:497-506(2007).

Duimstra C, Johnson D, Kutsch C, Wang B, Zentner M, Kellerman S, Welty T. A fetal alcohol syndrome surveillance pilot project in American Indian communities in the Northern Plains. Public Health Rep. 108:225-229(1993).

Dunty WC Jr., Chen SY, Zucker RM, Dehart DB, Sulik KK. Selective vulnerability of embryonic cell populations to ethanol-induced apoptosis: implications for alcohol-related birth defects and neurodevelopmental disorder. *Alcohol. Clin. Exp. Res.* 25:1523-1535(2001).

Fernandes Y, Gerlai R. Long-term behavioral changes in response to early developmental exposure to ethanol in zebrafish. *Alcohol. Clin. Exp. Res.* 33:601-609(2009).

Fujita M, Isogai S, Kudo A. Vascular anatomy of the developing medaka, Oryzias latipes: a complementary fish model for cardiovascular research on vertebrates. *Dev. Dyn.* 235: 734-746(2006).

Furutani-Seiki M, Wittbrodt J. Medaka and zebrafish: an evolutionary twin study. *Mech. Dev.* 121:629-637 (2004).

Gerlai R. Zebrafish: An uncharted behavior genetic model. *Behav. Gent.* 33:461-468(2003).

Gerlai R, Lee V, Blaser R. Effects of acute and chronic ethanol exposure on the behavior of adult zebrafish (Danio rerio). *Pharmacol. Biochem. Behav.* 85:752-761(2006).

Gerlai R, Ahmad F, Prajapati S. Differences in acute alcohol-induced behavioral responses among zebrafish populations. *Alcohol. Clin. Exp. Res.* 32:1763-1773(2008).

Goodlett CR, Horn KH, Zhou FC. Alcohol teratogenesis: mechanisms of damage and strategies for invention. *Exp. Biol. Med.* 230:394-406(2005).

Guerrero JCH. Morphologic effects of maternal alcohol intake on skull, mandible and tooth of the offspring in mice, *Jpn. J. Oral. Biol.* 32 : 460–46 (1990).

Higuchi Y, Matsumoto N. Embryotoxicity of ethanol and acetaldehyde: Direct effects of mouse embryo in vitro. *Congen. Anom.* 24:9-28(2008).

Hu Y, Khan IA, Dasmahapatra AK. Disruption of circulation by ethanol promotes fetal alcohol spectrum disorder (FASD) in medaka (Oryzias latipes) embryogenesis. *Comp. Biochem. Phyisol.* 148C:273-280(2008).

Hu Y, Willett KL, Khan IA, Scheffler BE, Dasmahapatra AK. Ethanol disrupts chondrification of the neurocranial cartilages in medaka embryos without affecting aldehyde dehydrogenase 1A2 (Aldh1A2) promoter methylation. *Comp. Biochem. Physiol.* 150C: 495-502(2009).

Ishikawa Y. Medaka fish as a model system for vertebrate developmental genetics. *Bioessays* 22: 487- 495 (2000).

Ishikawa Y, Kage T, Yamamoto N, Yoshimoto M, Yasuda T, Matsumoto A, Maruyama K, Ito H. Axonogenesis in the medaka embryonic brain. *J. Comp. Neurol.* 476:240-253(2004).

Iwamatsu T. Stages of normal development in the medaka Oryzias latipes, *Mech. Dev.* 121:605-618 (2004).

Jones KL, Smith DW. Recognition of the fetal alcohol syndrome in early infancy. *Lancet* 2, 999-1001 (1974).

Kaminen-Ahola N, Ahola A, Maga M, Mallitt K-A, Fahey P, Cox TC, Whitelaw E, Chong S. Maternal alcohol consumption alters the epigenotype and the phenotype of offspring in a mouse model. *PLoS Genetics*, 6:e1000811(2010).

Kashyap B, Frederickson LC, Stenkamp DL. Mechanisms for persistent microphthalmia following ethanol exposure during retinal neurogenesis in zebrafish embryos. *Vis. Neurosci.* 24:409-431(2007).

Kily LJ, Cowe YC, Hussain O, Patel S, McElwaine S, Cotter FE, Brennan CH. Gene expression changes in a zebrafish model of drug dependency suggest conservation of neuro-adaptation pathway. *J. Exp. Biol.* 211:1623-1634(2008).

Krone PH, Lele Z, Sass JB. Heat shock genes and the heat shock response in zebrafish embryos. *Biochem. Cell. Biol.* 75:487-497(1997).

Langille RM, Hall BK. Development of the head skeleton of the Japanese medaka, Oryzias latipes(Teleostei). *J. Morphol.* 193:135-158(1987).

R.M. Langille RM, Hall BK. Role of the neural crest in development of the cartilaginous cranial and visceral skeleton of the medaka, Oryzias latipes (Teleostei), *Anat. Embryol.* 177: 297-305 (1988).

Lele Z, Engel S, Krone PH. Hsp47 and hsp70 gene expression is differentially regulated in a stress- and tissue-specific manner in zebrafish embryos. *Dev. Genet.* 21:123-133 (1997).

Lemoine P., Harousseau H, Borteyru JP, Menuet JC, Les enfants des parents alcoholiques: anomolies observees a propos de 127 cas (the children of alcoholic parents : anomalies observed in 127 cases) *Quest Medical* 25, 476-482(1968).

Liu Y, Balaraman Y, Wang G, Nephew KP, Zhou FC. Alcohol exposure alters DNA methylation profiles in mouse embryos at early neurulation. *Epigenetics*, 4:500-511(2009).

Lockwood B, Bjerke S, Kobayashi K, Guo S. Acute effects of alcohol on larval zebrafish: a genetic system for large-scale screening. *Pharmacol. Biochem. Behav.* 77: 647-654(2004).

Loosli F, Koster RW, Carl M, Kuhnlein R, Henrich T, Mucke M, Krone A, Wittbrodt JA. Genetic screen for mutations affecting embryonic development in medaka fish (Oryzias latipes). *Mech. Dev.* 97: 133-139 (2000).

Loucks EJ, Schwend T, Ahlgren SC. Molecular changes associated with teratogen-induced cyclopia. *Birth Def. Res.* 79A:642-651(2007).

MacPhail RC, Brooks J, Hunter DL, Padnos B, Irons TD, Padilla S. Locomotion in larval zebrafish: influence of time of day, lighting and ethanol. *Neurotoxicol.* 30:52-58(2009).

Mao H, Diehl AM, Li YX. Sonic hedgehog ligand partners with caveolin-1 for intracellular transport. *Lab. Invest.* 89:290-300(2009).

Matsui JI, Egana AL, Sponholtz TR, Adolph AR, Dowling JE. Effects of ethanol on photoreceptors and visual function in developing zebrafish. *Invest Ophthalmol. Vis. Sci.* 47:4589-4597(2006).

May PA, Gossage JP, White-Country M, Goodhart K, Decoteau S, Trujillo PM, Kalberg WO, Viljeon DL, Hoyme HE. Alcohol consumption and other maternal risk factors for fetal alcohol syndrome among three distinct samples of women before, during, and after pregnancy: the risk is relative. *Am. J. Med. Genet.*, 127:10-20(2004).

Miller MW, Spear LP: The alcoholism generator. *Alcohol. Clin. Exp. Res.* 30: 1466-1469 (2006).

Naidoo,S, Chikte,U, Laubscher R, Lombard, C. Fetal alcohol syndrome: anthropometric and oral health status, *J. Contemp. Dent. Pract.* 6:101-115 (2005).

Nakatsuji, N. Craniofacial malformation in Xenopus laevis tadpoles caused by the exposure of early embryos to ethanol, *Teratology* 28: 299–305 (1983)

Naruse K, Tanaka M, Mita K, Shima A, Postlethwait J, Mitani H. A medaka gene map: the trace of ancestral vertebrate protochromosomes revealed by comparative gene mapping. *Gen. Res.* 14: 820-828 (2004).

Oxendine SL, Cowden J, Hinton DE, Padilla S. Vulnerable windows for developmental ethanol toxicity in the Japanese medaka fish (Oryzias latipes). *Aquat. Toxicol.* 80:396-404(2006).

Parng C, Roy NM, Ton C, Lin Y, McGrath P. Neurotoxicity asseeement using zebrafish. *J. Pharmacol. Toxicol. Met.* 55:103-112(2007).

Priscott PK. The effects of ethanol on rat embryos developing in vitro. *Biochem. Pharmacol.* 31:3641-3643(1982).

Qian L, Wang Y, Jiang Q, Zhong T, Song H. Ethanol disrupts the formation of hypochord and dorsal aorta during the development of embryonic zebrafish. *Sci. China C. Life Sci.* 48:608-615(2005).

Reimers MJ, Flocktom AR, Tanguay RL. Ethanol- and acetaldehyde-mediated developmental toxicity in zebrafish. *Neurotox. Terato.* 26: 769-781(2004a).

Reimers MJ, La Du JK, Periera CB, Giovanini J, Tanguay RL. Ethanol-dependent toxicity in zebrafish is partially attenuated by antioxidants. Neurotoxicol. Teratol. 28:497-508(2006).

Rico EP, Rosemberg DB, Dias RD, Bogo MR, Bonan CD. Ethanol alters acetylcholinesterase activity and gene expression in zebrafish brain. *Toxicol. Lett.* 174:25-30(2007).

Rico EP, Rosemberg DB, Senger MR, Arizi M. de B, Dias RD, Souto AA, Bogo MR, Bonan CD. Ethanol and acetaldehyde alter NTDPase and 5'-nucleotidase from zebrafish brain membranes. *Neurochem. Int.* 52, 290-296(2008).

Roda-Moreno JA, Pascual-Morenilla MT, Roda-Murillo O, Lopez-Soler M,Arrebola-Nacle F. Action of ethanol on different skull and brain parameters in the chick embryo, *J. Craniofac. Genet. Dev. Biol.* 20:44-48 (2000).

Russo D, Purohit V, Foudin L, Salin M. Workshop on alcohol use and health disparities 2002: a call to arms. *Alcohol,* 32:37-43(2004).

Sampson PD, Streissguth AP, Bookstein FL, Little RE, Clarren SK, Dehaene P, Hanson JW, Graham JM Jr. Incidence of fetal alcohol syndrome and prevalence of alcohol-related neurodevelopmental disorder. *Teratology* , 56:317-326(1997).

Sant'Anna LB, Tosello DO. Fetal alcohol syndrome and developing craniofacial and dental structures-a review. *Orthod. Craniofac. Res.* 9:172-185(2006).

Shimada A, Yabusaki M, Niwa H, Yokoi H, Hatta K, Kobayashi D, Takeda H. Maternal-zygotic medaka mutants for fgfr1 reveal its essential role in the migration of the axial mesoderm but not the lateral mesoderm. *Development*, 135:281-290(2008).

Smith SM, Alcohol-induced cell death in the embryo, *Alcohol. Res. Health* 21:287-297 (1997).

Sulik KK. Genesis of alcohol-induced craniofacial dysmorphism. *Exp. Biol. Med.* 230: 366-375 (2005).

Sulik KK, Johnston M, Webb M. Fetal alcohol syndrome: embryogenesis in a mouse model. *Science*, 214:936-938(1981).

Sulik KK, Cook CS, Webster WS, Teratogens and craniofacial malformations: relationships to cell death, *Development* 103:213-231(1988).

Sulik K, Johnston M, Daft P, Russell W, Dehart D. Fetal alcohol syndrome and DiGeorge anomaly: critical ethanol exposure periods for craniofacial malformations as illustrated in an animal model. *Am. J. Med. Genet suppl.* 2:97-112(1986).

Su B, Debelak KA, Tessmer LL, Cartwright MM, Smith SM. Genetic influences on craniofacial outcome in an avian model of prenatal alcohol exposure. *Alchol. Cli. Exp. Res.* 25:60-69(2006).

Tapadia MD, Cordero DR, Helms JA. It's all your head: new insights into craniofacial development and deformation, *J. Anat.* 207:461-477 (2005).

Tufan AC, satiroglu-Tufan NL. The effect of ethanol exposure on extraembryonic vascular development in chick area vasculosa. *Cells Tissues Organs*, 175:84-97(2003).

Wang X, Williams E, Haasch ML, Dasmahapatra AK. Japanese medaka (Oryzias latipes): developmental model for the study of alcohol teratology. *Birth Def. Res.* 77: 29-39(2006).

Wang X, Zhu S, Khan IA, Dasmahapatra AK. Etanol attenuates Aldh9 mRNA expression in Japanese medaka (Oryzias latipes) embryogenesis. *Comp. Biochem. Physiol.* Part B 146:357-363 (2007 a).

Wang X, Khan IA, Dasmahapatra AK. Developmental regulation of ethanol metabolizing enzyme mRNA expression in Japanese medaka (Oryzias latipes). In Leading- Edge messenger RNA research communication, Ostrovskiy MH, ed. NOVA publishers: P169-181 (2007b).

Webster WS, Ritchie HE. Teratogenic effects of alcohol and isotretinoin on craniofacial development: an analysis of animal models, *J. Craniofac. Genet. Dev. Biol.* 11:296-302(1991).

Wittbrodt J, Shima A, Schart M. Medaka- a model organism from the far east. *Nature Rev. Genetics,* 3:53-64 (2002).

Wu M, Chaudhary A, Khan IA, Dasmahapatra AK. Ethanol teratogenesis in Japanese medaka: effects at the cellular level. *Comp. Biochem. Physiol.* 149B:191-201(2008).

In: Pregnancy and Alcohol Consumption
Editor: Joshua D. Hoffman, pp. 155-173
ISBN 978-1-61761-122-3


*Chapter 5*

# RESEARCH ON INTERVENTIONS TO PREVENT ALCOHOL CONSUMPTION DURING PREGNANCY

***Katrina Kully-Martens, Katy Wyper and Carmen Rasmussen****
University of Alberta, Alberta, Canada

Prenatal alcohol exposure (PAE) has been directly implicated in a wide range of deficits that adversely influence the development of affected individuals. Fetal Alcohol Spectrum Disorder (FASD) is an umbrella term referring to a continuum of effects that occur in individuals who were prenatally exposed to alcohol (Chudley, Conry, Cook, Loock, Rosales, and LeBlanc, 2005). FASD is a permanent birth defect, and a leading cause of mental retardation and developmental delay in North America (Chudley et al., 2005; Canadian Paediatric Society, 2002). In the United States and Canada, approximately 1 of every 100 children is affected with FASD (AADAC, 2004; Health Canada, 2006;, May and Gossage, 2001; Sampson et al., 1997).

Individuals affected by FASD may require lifetime support and extensive services related to health, social services, education and training, addictions, justice, and family supports due to various neuropsychological, physical, and behavioral sequelae, which are often costly and difficult to treat (Government of Alberta, 2005; Health Canada, 2006). The annual cost of FASD in Canada for individuals aged 0 to 53 is estimated at $5.3 billion, with an annual cost per individual of nearly $22,000 (Stade et al., 2009). Further, U.S. estimates place the lifetime cost of a child with FASD at $2 million (Lupton, Burd, and Harwood, 2004). These costs reflect, among other factors, the increased use of the above-mentioned services, as well as externalizing behaviors and lost personal or caregiver productivity. The overwhelmingly negative effects that PAE has on affected individuals and their families, combined with

* Correspondence concerning this article should be addressed to Dr Carmen Rasmussen at 266, Glenrose Rehabilitation Hospital, 10230-111 Ave, Edmonton, Alberta, T5G 0B7, Phone: (780) 735-7999 ext 15631, Fax: (780) 735-7907, E-mail: carmen@ualberta.ca.

enormous societal costs and the fact that FASD is, in theory, entirely preventable, make research on the efficacy of FASD prevention programs vital. In this chapter we will review research on selective and indicated FASD prevention strategies. The strategies reviewed include screening methods, brief interventions with and without motivational features, and longer-term prevention programs including enhanced case management.

## ALCOHOL CONSUMPTION DURING PREGNANCY

Despite bottle labeling, public health awareness campaigns, and the fact that no safe limit for alcohol intake during pregnancy has been consistently established, a surprising number of women continue to consume alcohol while pregnant. Rates of alcohol consumption for both pregnant and non-pregnant women have remained fairly stable for over a decade (Denny,Tsai, Floyd, and Green, 2009). Every year, approximately 500,000 (or 1 in 8) pregnant women in the U.S. consume at least one drink per week during pregnancy (Floyd and Sidhu, 2004). According to a national U.S. survey, about 12.9% of parturient women reported drinking alcohol while pregnant, and 4.6% reported binge drinking during their pregnancy (SAMHSA, 2002). Among non-pregnant women of childbearing age, over half consume alcohol and 1 in 8 binge drink (Floyd and Sidhu, 2004). In addition, nearly half of all pregnancies in North America are unplanned and the majority of women do not know they are pregnant for the first four to six weeks after conception, a critical period of embryonic development (Floyd, Decoufle, and Hungerford, 1999). In fact, half of the women surveyed drank alcohol in the 3 months prior to pregnancy recognition. These findings underscore the need for effective prevention of alcohol-exposed pregnancies for both at-risk pregnant and non-pregnant women of childbearing age.

Women who are at risk of giving birth to a child with FASD are a heterogeneous and complex group of individuals whose risk of having alcohol-exposed pregnancies is increased by various factors. Numerous studies have implicated several major mediating factors including: cigarette smoking and multiple drug use (Astley, Bailey, Talbot and Clarren, 2000; Day, Cottreau, and Richardson, 1993; Godel, Pabst, Hodges, Johnson, Froese, and Joffres, 1992; Greenfield, Rehm, and Rogers, 2002; Serdula, Williamson, Kendrick, Anda, and Byers, 1991) diagnosis of psychiatric illness (e.g. major depressive disorder, post traumatic stress disorder) (Astley et al., 2000; Svikis and Reid-Quiñones, 2003) or inpatient mental health treatment (Project CHOICES Research Group, 2002), history of physical, sexual, or emotional abuse, (Astley et al., 2000; Haynes, Dunnagan, and Christopher, 2003; Leonardson and Loudenburg, 2003; Project CHOICES Research Group, 2002; Svikis and Reid-Quiñones, 2003), having a previous child with FAS (May, Hymbaugh, Aase, and Samet, 1983), and a history of drinking or binge drinking (Chang, Behr, Goetz, Hiley, and Bigby, 1997; Day et al., 1993; Godel et al., 1992) especially with early age of onset (Smith and Coles, 1991; Smith, Lancaster, Moss-Wells, Coles, and Falek, 1987) or during a previous pregnancy (Project CHOICES Research Group, 2002). The majority of at-risk women also tend to be unmarried, unemployed, have lower levels of education (i.e., high school or less), and lower IQs; although higher socioeconomic status women who are married, employed, and are college educated have also been shown to be at-risk (Astley et al., 2000; Chang, Goetz, Wilkins-Haug, and Berman, 2000; Chang et al., 2005; Chang, Wilkins-Haug, Berman, and

Goetz, 1999; Haynes et al., 2003). Most research samples of women at-risk have been disproportionately Caucasian or Native American, with other ethnicities less likely to be identified as at-risk populations (Astley et al., 2000; Chang et al., 2000, 2005, 1999; Haynes et al., 2003; Project CHOICES Research Group, 2002).

Many prevention efforts at varying levels of specificity are currently in place. The broadest efforts, or *universal prevention*, are aimed at preventing maternal alcohol abuse by educating the public about the consequences and risks of drinking during pregnancy. This is achieved through the distribution of various didactic materials, such as pamphlets or poster campaigns, or simpler means such as alcoholic beverage bottle labeling. *Selective prevention* efforts target a narrower population, such as all women of reproductive age who consume alcohol. Examples of this include screening of pregnant women in primary care settings. The most narrowly focused efforts, *indicated prevention*, are directed at women who have been defined as 'high-risk.' This includes women who have already given birth to a child with FASD, or who continue to drink in the absence of effective birth control. Indicated interventions tend to focus on treating alcohol abuse in pregnant women, or preventing pregnancy in high risk women by encouraging sexual abstinence or effective use of birth control.

## SCREENING FOR PRENATAL ALCOHOL USE

Timely identification of women who are at risk of having alcohol-exposed pregnancies is necessary in order to be able to apply intervention and prevent more serious consequences such as FASD. Some studies have suggested that applying screening tools alone, such as the T-ACE, can decrease prenatal alcohol consumption (Sokol, Martier, and Ager, 1989). This reduction in alcohol use following screening, which has been found both in risk-drinkers in the regular population as well as in pregnant women, may occur because screening may promote individual awareness and reflection on problem drinking (Nilsen, 2009). Several brief interventions (discussed later in this chapter), which often begin with a screening method or very basic preliminary assessment questions, have also shown this so-called 'screening effect' (e.g. Chang et al., 2000, 2005, 1999; Handmaker, Miller, and Manicke, 1999).

Many screening tools used for detecting alcohol abuse in pregnant or periconceptional women have their origins in tools used to detect alcohol abuse in the general population, such as the Alcohol Use Disorders Identification Test (AUDIT) and the CAGE (described below). These early techniques were mainly validated for use in males (Floyd, Weber, Denny, and O'Connor, 2009). In response, several screening methods were created or adapted for use in female populations, and, more specifically, in pregnant women. Although clinical interviews for alcohol abuse or dependence in primary care settings mainly focus on questions about current frequency or quantity of alcohol intake, these types of questions do not tend to provide helpful information in prenatal populations. This can be attributed to a variety of reasons including: (1) underreporting of alcohol consumption, with up to 40% of pregnant women underestimating their alcohol intake (Ernhart, Morrow-Tlucak, Sokol, Martier, and Ager, 1989), (2) changing patterns of alcohol consumption, since many women will reduce their alcohol consumption temporarily upon pregnancy confirmation, yet subsequent drinking behavior is predicted more reliably by drinking that occurred before knowledge of the pregnancy (Chang, 2001), and (3) inconsistent screening by primary care physicians, with only 1/3 of women in prenatal care being routinely screened for alcohol use (Chang et al., 2000). Therefore, approaches that focus on past alcohol use and de-emphasize social consequences tend to give more reliable estimates of risk in pregnant women.

Two common screening tools for alcoholism, the MAST (Michigan Alcoholism Screening Test) and the CAGE, have poor specificity in these populations. However, they can still be used as part of a clinical interview (Chang, 2001). More importantly, these questionnaires have provided a basis for current tools used for screening of risk-drinking during pregnancy. The CAGE is a 4-item questionnaire used for identifying at-risk drinkers (Ewing, 1984). Its questions address the individual's need to Cut down, their Annoyance at criticisms levied by other's about the individual's drinking behavior, Guilty feelings about drinking, and the need for an Eye opener (a drink first thing in the morning). The MAST is a yes-no questionnaire that addresses more severe consequences of drinking, such as legal problems, hospitalization and family strife.

Screening tools that have been developed specifically for use in pregnant women in obstetric-gynecological practice include the inaugural T-ACE (Tolerance, Annoyance, Cut-down, Eye-opener) (Sokol et al., 1989) and the TWEAK (Tolerance, Worry, Eye-opener, Amnesia, K/Cut down) (Russell, 1994). Both tools incorporate elements from the CAGE (Annoyance, K/Cut down, and Eye opener), and add a new dimension, a question about Tolerance, or how many drinks the individual can hold (maximum level of alcohol intake). The tolerance element defines the tool's utility, and is therefore given double the weight during administration. Since 'tolerance' addresses alcohol use indirectly, and because most women are not sure of socially-desirable tolerance levels, the tendency of patients to underreport alcohol use is minimized and periconceptional risk-drinkers can be identified more accurately (Russell, Martier, and Sokol, 1996). The TWEAK additionally incorporates questions about Worry from family or relatives (which is also given double weight) and Amnesia after drinking. Both the T-ACE (scored out of five) and the TWEAK (scored out of seven) indicate risk-drinkers who should be afforded further evaluation at scores of two or more. Risk-drinking is defined as seven standard drinks per week, which is considered to be the point at which most fetal neurobehavioral implications begin to occur (Jacobson andJacobson, 1994).

Interestingly, Russell et al. (1996) found that the sensitivity of the T-ACE decreased when it was administered individually to pregnant women than when it was included as part of a broader clinical interview that included the CAGE and the MAST. The authors hypothesized that this may be due to a 'conditioning effect,' whereby after completing the MAST, which addresses the more severe consequences of drinking such as legal problems, hospitalization and family strife, the more benevolent questions on the T-ACE are more likely to be answered honestly. This suggests that the ability to accurately detect periconceptional risk-drinking can be optimized by including the CAGE and MAST alongside the T-ACE or even the TWEAK.

There are a few clinical issues with using screening measures in prenatal populations. Most importantly, screening tools do not diagnose alcohol problems; they are only suggestive of their probability. Another obvious limitation, as is common with many self-report interview methods, is that the individual's response in a clinical interview can be influenced by the perceived social desirability or stigma of certain answers. Thornberry et al. (2002)

examined the feasibility of administering screening methods, including the TWEAK, via computer, rather than through traditional face-to-face interviews. The computerized method used in their study detected a higher prevalence of risky drinking behavior compared to studies with similar populations that used interview or paper and pencil administration. The authors also found that women overwhelmingly liked the computerized screening tests and did not find the questions difficult to answer (Thornberry et al., 2002). Alvik, Haldorsen, and Lindemann (2005) hypothesized that anonymity in questionnaire completion (the T-ACE in this study) is typically associated with more accurate reporting of socially-sensitive behaviors and, when compared with confidentiality in questionnaire completion, would yield higher reports of alcohol consumption during pregnancy (presumably closer to the actual amount consumed). However, they did not find significant group differences between the anonymous and confidential groups.

Despite being brief, easy to administer, and effective at accurately detecting heavy alcohol use in pregnant women, neither the TWEAK nor the T-ACE are routinely included as part of the clinical interview. It has been hypothesized that this could be due to clinician discomfort with asking screening questions face-to-face with their patients (Arborelius and Damström Thakker, 1995; Diekman, Floyd, Decoufle, Schulkin, Ebrahim, and Sokol, 2000). Mengel, Searight, and Cook (2006) review several other barriers that seem to prevent clinicians from administering screening (and brief interventions, which we will discuss later). These include physician attitudes (e.g., treatment is ineffective, other health problems are more pressing, not a clinical health concern, etc), inadequate knowledge or skills (e.g., insufficiency of reference material, lack of training), lack of time and poor compensation, and intervention barriers (e.g., lack of tools, protocols, referral resources).

Additionally, pregnant women who are heavy or binge drinkers, and are thereby more likely to have a child affected by alcohol (compared to those who drink more lightly), have been found to be at risk for delaying prenatal care until after the first trimester (Stratton, Howe, and Battaglia, 1996). Since screening is typically administered in primary care settings where prenatal care occurs, the potential effectiveness of these tools may be severely limited if they cannot be timely implemented.

Screening is an important and essential first step in prenatal settings to determine which patients warrant further assessment, and potentially, intervention. A common intervention delivered in primary care facilities, subsequent to screening, are brief interventions. The next section will review several studies examining the efficacy of brief interventions in at-risk pregnant and non-pregnant women.

## Brief Intervention

The use of brief intervention to assist in preventing alcohol consumption during pregnancy, and thus FASD, has its roots in findings that brief interventions can be just as effective as longer, more intensive interventions in a variety of health related domains including problem alcohol and tobacco use (see Nilsen, 2009, for a review). The evidence base supporting the efficacy of brief intervention for alcohol use in pregnant women is modest, but growing. A number of randomized controlled trials have been conducted both in pregnant and non-pregnant women of childbearing age identified as risk-drinkers (selective brief intervention), and women who have a history of drinking during pregnancy and/or have previously given birth to a child with FASD (indicated brief intervention). Brief interventions also vary in duration. Typically, the shortest types of interventions are single five or 15-minute sessions, and the longest are multi-contact sessions generally up to 15-minutes each (see Mengel et al., 2006, for a review). Mengel et al. (2006) suggest that interventions with multi-contact sessions are typically the most beneficial and can be easily integrated into typical prenatal care, since many pregnant women visit primary care facilities routinely.

*Selective brief intervention in at-risk pregnant women.* Since 1999, a number of randomized clinical studies have addressed the efficacy of brief intervention for reducing alcohol consumption in pregnant women identified as risk-drinkers. Chang et al. (1999) conducted a randomized clinical trial examining the effect of a brief intervention on prenatal alcohol consumption in 250 pregnant women seeking prenatal care. The women had received a positive test result for risk-drinking on the T-ACE, were less than 28 weeks pregnant, had consumed alcohol in the six months before pregnancy, and were not currently seeking substance abuse treatment. Forty percent met the requirements for DSM-III-R lifetime alcohol abuse or dependence diagnoses and 43% drank while pregnant. However,, pregnancy recognition occurred at a mean of 4.2 weeks, suggesting that many more of these women may have been consuming alcohol prior to confirming their pregnancies. The ASI (Addiction Severity Index) was also administered among several other measures of alcohol use. Participants were randomly divided into an assessment-only control group (n = 127) and a brief-intervention experimental group (n = 123) which also included an assessment phase. The brief intervention, which lasted about 45 minutes per patient, consisted of reviewing the participant's health and lifestyle changes during their pregnancy, identifying drinking goals while pregnant and the motivation behind these goals, the circumstances under which the subject might feel compelled to drink, and possible alternatives to alcohol. The subjects were also given take-home information advocating for abstinence during pregnancy. Participants were followed-up postpartum with an interview about their drinking. Women in both groups experienced a decrease in prenatal alcohol consumption. However, there was not a significant difference between the two groups for the decrease in the average number of drinks, which suggests screening assessment alone may be effective at reducing alcohol consumption during pregnancy. The authors also identified patient characteristics that were associated with success, which included pre-assessment abstinence. The results of this study are potentially limited by the relatively high socio-economic status and social stability of the participants. These demographic characteristics may forecast better outcomes for women no matter the intervention (Chang et al., 1999).

In a subsequent study, Chang et al. (2000) applied a similar intervention to 123 women of a comparable demographic who were in their 16$^{th}$ week of pregnancy and screened positive on the T-ACE for risk-drinking. The intention of the study was to determine the relationship between drinking goals set during the brief intervention, the motivation behind these goals, and participant's ensuing gestational alcohol use. At post-partum follow up, 70% of participants reported abstinence following the brief intervention. The most commonly set goal was abstinence during pregnancy (77%), which was shown to be significantly motivated (at the time of assessment) by considering the infant's health; however, this reason was not significantly tied to subsequent abstinence. Women who selected abstinence as their goal were more likely to reduce alcohol consumption after intervention, a finding that held true for women who were current drinkers as well as women who had been abstinent since confirming their pregnancy. Further, 29% of participants reported being motivated to alter their drinking behavior because of knowledge of FASD; these participants also reduced their prenatal alcohol consumption. This study also examined the relationship between self-reported situations that increased drinking and later alcohol use. The most common situation that participants felt would induce risk of alcohol consumption was social events (54%), although 26% of participants reported that there were no situations that would compel them to drink. The subjects who reported the latter opinion were more likely to be abstinent following the intervention.

A further study by Chang et al. (2005) investigated the effectiveness of a single session brief intervention delivered to 304 pregnant women who had tested positive on the T-ACE, and a support partner of the subject's choosing. Following enrollment in the study, prenatal alcohol use decreased in both the control and treatment groups. However, women who reported the heaviest alcohol consumption pre-intervention reduced their post-intervention drinking significantly compared to controls. Additionally, effects of the intervention were maximized when a participant's support partner was involved. As in Chang et al. (2000), participants were more likely to be unsuccessful at reducing alcohol consumption post-intervention if they reported being tempted to drink in social situations.

The majority of brief intervention studies in this domain have been conducted in primary care or hospital settings using middle-class, more highly educated Caucasian women. However, a recent randomized clinical study examined the efficacy of a community-based brief intervention for alcohol use by 250 lower-income minority (i.e. Hispanic, African-American) pregnant women who reported drinking alcohol (O'Connor and Whaley, 2007). The intervention, which was delivered by non-medical professionals in 10- to 15-minute sessions, sought to examine the efficacy of this intervention by examining outcome variables related to neonatal health. The authors found that women who completed the brief intervention were five times more likely to be abstinent following the intervention compared to the control subjects (who had received assessment only). Additionally, the newborns of the experimental group subjects had higher birth weights and mortality rates that were three times lower than control participants. The findings of this study are important as they highlight the potential for brief intervention to be delivered in easily accessible community settings by non-medical professionals, and that a brief intervention can be successful in women who, unlike the populations studied in Chang et al. (1999, 2000, 2005), may not be as adequately connected to supports and services and have as probable a chance of making improvements after intervention.

Motivational interviews (MI) conducted as part of a brief intervention have also shown to be promising in preventing alcohol-exposed pregnancies (AEPs) in at-risk mothers, perhaps because these strategies foster the patient's willingness for change (see Handmaker and Wilbourne, 2001, for a more extensive review). A pilot study conducted by Handmaker et al. (1999) examined the usefulness of a brief MI as a cost-effective way of counseling pregnant drinkers in order to reduce the risk of fetal alcohol effects. Forty-two pregnant women who had reported drinking at least one drink in the last month were recruited from an obstetric clinic and randomly assigned to either the experimental group (a one-hour MI focusing on the health of the client's unborn child and a risk-benefit analysis of the participant's drinking) or the control group (a letter describing the risks related to prenatal alcohol consumption). Participants were also encouraged to conceive of ways to maintain abstinence and alternate options to drinking in high-risk situations. At follow-up, both groups had significantly reduced their alcohol intake, though overall there were not significant differences in drinking reduction between the groups. However, women who had been identified as the heaviest drinkers (highest blood alcohol content) pre-intervention significantly reduced their alcohol intake after the intervention compared to similar controls. This result was particularly encouraging since heavy drinking tends to be most predictive of poor fetal outcomes (Handmaker et al., 1999).

*Selective brief intervention in at-risk non-pregnant women.* As discussed previously, approximately half of women of childbearing age consume alcohol and 1 in 8 binge drink (Floyd and Sidhu, 2004). Since nearly half of all pregnancies in North America are unplanned and the majority of women do not know they are pregnant for the first four to six weeks after conception, a critical period of embryonic development (Floyd et al., 1999), numerous pregnancies may be alcohol-exposed at least initially. As such, interventions that target women of childbearing age who are not currently pregnant but who consume alcohol at risky levels are also critical to the prevention of alcohol-exposed pregnancies.

One of the first randomized clinical trials focusing explicitly on women of childbearing age in primary care in order to prevent alcohol-exposed pregnancies was Project TrEAT (The Trial for Early Alcohol Treatment) (Manwell, Fleming, Mundt, Stauffacher, and Barry, 2000). Two hundred and five women were selected for participation based on their problem drinking, which was defined by consuming >11 drinks per week, more than four drinks per occasion, or a positive score on the CAGE. Participants received follow up interviews at 6, 12, 24, 36, and 48 months. The brief intervention, which consisted of two 15-minute counseling visits with a primary care physician and a workbook, was shown to have long-term treatment effects: after 48 months, there was a 48% reduction in mean alcohol consumption, a decrease in the number of women engaged in binge drinking by 25%, and a 32% reduction in the number of women drinking over 13 drinks per week. Control subjects also reduced their alcohol intake steadily through 48 months, although not as much as the treatment group. Most importantly, women from the intervention group who became pregnant during the follow-up period (21%) had the greatest reduction in alcohol use compared to women in the control group who became pregnant (19%) and to women who did not become pregnant in either group.

Project CHOICES (Changing High-Risk AlcOhol Use and Increasing Contraception Effectiveness Study), a pilot motivational brief intervention, investigated the impact of this community-based intervention in 190 non-pregnant women of childbearing age determined to be at risk for alcohol-exposed pregnancies (The Project CHOICES Intervention Research Group, 2003). Women were considered at-risk based on lack of contraception (while sexually active) and problem drinking, based on results of the AUDIT and reports of drinking >7 drinks per week or one or more binge drinking episodes in the last three months. At baseline, 99.5% reported binge drinking in the last six months, 64.6% reported drinking >7 drinks per week, and 64.2% reported engaging in both behaviors. Participants assigned to the experimental group were given four MI sessions and a contraceptive counseling session; all participants were followed up after six months. Out of the 75% of women who completed the 6-month follow up, 68.5% were no longer considered to be at risk for having an alcohol-exposed pregnancy. Women had either changed their contraceptive use, their alcohol consumption patterns, or both, which highlights the importance of focusing on these two aspects in the prevention of AEPs.

A similar randomized controlled trial conducted by Floyd et al. (2007) examined the effectiveness of a brief motivational intervention on preventing subsequent alcohol-concurrent pregnancies in a larger sample of 830 non-pregnant women (aged 18-44) who were considered at risk for alcohol-exposed pregnancies due to risk-drinking and/or inadequate contraception. The goal of the intervention was to motivate these women to either decrease their risky drinking behaviors, increase their family planning methods, or both. The intervention group received basic information and a brief motivational intervention (four counseling sessions, and one seminar on family planning), and the control group received basic information only. The authors found that a brief motivational intervention decreased the occurrence of the target behaviors (risky drinking and inadequate contraception use), which in turn safeguarded against alcohol-exposed pregnancies. An important implication of this study is that it suggests that high-risk, pre-conceptual women who are not planning to become pregnant, yet are likely to experience unplanned and/or alcohol-exposed pregnancies, can often take measures to prevent either of these outcomes even when provided only basic information about their risks.

In general, selective brief interventions for reducing alcohol consumption in both pregnant and non-pregnant women appear to be promising strategies for promoting alcohol abstinence, but less is known about how these interventions truly impact FASD prevention. Although the merit of many of these studies is bolstered by sound randomized experimental designs, infant outcomes—including the resulting incidence of FASD in study populations—are not typically examined. Additionally, the external validity of the current research base is limited, as the studies overwhelmingly examine the efficacy of these interventions in predominately Caucasian, middle-class, educated populations (e.g. Chang et al., 2000, 2005, 1999). Within these studies, result patterns (e.g. the 'screening effect') have been, in some cases, attributed to motivational effects of pregnancy and the supposition that women who are already well-connected to supports and services will benefit from any type of contact or intervention, regardless of the intervention's scope or intended impact. However, much research has suggested that less educated minority or non-minority women in lower socioeconomic classes are at least equally as vulnerable for having an alcohol-exposed pregnancy. Unlike middle-class study populations, these women are less likely to be connected to services, have a reliable support network, experience 'spontaneous recovery' from any form of treatment, or seek prenatal care where many of these interventions are initiated. These are the women who may need intervention most. In the future, it will be important to consider how established brief interventions will work in these populations, and what, if any, amendments need to be made to intervention techniques and settings, as well as modes of delivery.

*Indicated brief interventions.* Fewer studies have focused exclusively on brief interventions for pregnant women who have the highest risk of having a child with FASD (e.g. those who already have had an affected child, or who have history of drinking during pregnancy). Protecting the Next Pregnancy project was a randomized clinical trial that delivered a brief cognitive-behavioral intervention to women who had reported being heavy drinkers (at least four drinks per week) during their previous (index) pregnancy (Hankin, 2002). The average number of drinks participants consumed at conception of the index pregnancy was over 16 drinks per week. The goal of the study was to examine how the brief intervention would impact drinking during subsequent pregnancies and if birth outcomes would be improved. One month after delivery of the index pregnancy, women were assigned to experimental or control groups; all participants were followed for five years. The experimental group received five intervention sessions over the first year, as well as booster sessions over a five-year follow-up period. The control group simply received a standard warning about prenatal drinking (e.g., You can have a healthier baby if you cut back or stop drinking during pregnancy). Ninety-six of the 300 participants gave birth to one or more children during the follow-up. The group that received the intervention consumed significantly less alcohol during their subsequent pregnancy compared to the control group—a quarter of the women in the control group drank at levels similar to the index pregnancy (i.e. at least four drinks per week), compared to 11% of the experimental group. Further, of the women who continued to drink while pregnant, those who received the intervention consumed half as much alcohol as control participants. Interestingly, women who reported the heaviest drinking prior to their index pregnancy exhibited the greatest reduction in drinking. Perhaps most importantly, the subsequent pregnancies of women who received the intervention resulted in better outcomes, including fewer premature and low-birth rate infants. At 13 months of age, these children also performed better on tests of mental development and psychomotor skills than both the subsequent children of women from the control group, as well as their index pregnancy siblings. Unfortunately, the FASD diagnostic statuses of index or subsequent pregnancy children are not reported; it is not often feasible to follow multiple children to diagnostic age. However, more specific child outcomes (e.g. diagnosis of FASD) are still important factors that must be considered if the ultimate goal of these prevention strategies is to reduce the incidence of FASD.

## Long-Term Indicated Interventions

*Case management.* Case management (CM) is a strategy that usually involves the professional coordination of community, social, personal support, and/or counseling services for clients in need. Although it is considered to be an efficacious intervention for reducing alcohol and drug use during pregnancy and for treating alcohol abuse, not enough research has been done to definitively tie it to FASD prevention (May et al., 2008). However, some studies are beginning to implicate CM as an effective strategy for successfully preventing FASD (Hankin, McCaul, and Heussner, 2000). An early pilot study conducted by Masis and May (1991) followed-up with 32 Native American women 18 months after a CM intervention. The women, who were referred from a prenatal clinic, were determined to be at risk for drinking during pregnancy based on a screening measure for risk-drinking and various health records and assessments. Nine (28%) of the women gave birth to a child with FAS or FAE shortly before beginning the program. The CM was overseen by a member of the Native American community, and involved counseling, detoxification and alcohol treatment with aftercare, and connections to voluntary birth control or tubal ligation (sterilization) services. Eighteen months after CM delivery, 56% of participants were abstinent from alcohol and 12.5% were drinking less. In terms of family planning, 25% of the women were pregnant, 12.5% were using birth control, 18.8% had tubal ligations, and 44% were at risk for another pregnancy. Poorer abstinence outcomes were seen in the nine women who had delivered a child with FAS or FAE; only 33% were abstinent, and 66% were still drinking. Clients who received the CM while pregnant (21) had the highest rate of abstinence:

nearly 86%. From these results, it seems that pregnancy was the most propitious time to offer the CM intervention. Although these results do not seem unanimously positive, the authors felt the program was promising for several reasons. Both the community and nearly all the referred women accepted the program, a success the authors attributed to the presence of trusted community members as program leaders. Additionally, this multifaceted approach addressed several areas of need in at-risk mothers, and also affected general community knowledge of typical and maternal alcohol abuse.

Following this pilot study, May et al. (2008) integrated CM and some strategies of MI to increase the effectiveness of CM and produce greater change in 131 high risk women (women who drink during pregnancy and/or women who have already given birth to a child with an FASD) from four Native American communities in Northern Plains states. After enrollment in the program (the mean length participation was 17.2 months), the authors noted significant reductions in binge drinking and other risky uses of alcohol for the majority of clients. As well, 70% of women who continued to use CM were protected from alcohol-exposed pregnancies, either by abstaining from drinking and/or by using birth control. Pregnancy outcomes also showed positive results – only 2 children born during this time period (out of 149 pregnancies) were suspected of having an FASD.

Although these studies suggest CM may be useful, especially when it is offered in tandem with other approaches, its use as an FASD prevention tool needs to be more rigorously evaluated. Further study in this area may benefit from including more demographically diverse populations and implementing randomized controlled research designs. The next section will discuss an important development in enhanced case management led by paraprofessional advocates: The Seattle Birth to 3 Project, now known as the P-CAP model.

*The P-CAP model.* The Parent-Child Assistance Program (P-CAP) is designed to prevent alcohol and drug exposed births among high-risk mothers (Grant, Streissguth, and Ernst, 2002). Women targeted by P-CAP have a history of abusing drugs or alcohol, are disconnected from community services, and have typically experienced a traumatic upbringing and consequently have a chaotic lifestyle (Grant, Ernst, Streissguth, Phipps, and Gendler, 1996). Most have been born to substance abusing parents, were physically and/or sexually abused as a child, have been jailed more than once, do not use birth control or plan their pregnancies, depend on welfare as their main source of income, and are abused by their current partner. Women identified as high-risk are enrolled in the program, either during pregnancy or by 6 months postpartum on the basis of three criteria: heavy drug/alcohol abuse during pregnancy, inadequate prenatal care, and little or no connection to community services (Grant, Ernst, and Streissguth, 1996). Clients are then matched with highly trained and supervised paraprofessional advocates who share a common history with these women. Advocates spend three years helping each client attend drug and alcohol treatment, remain drug and alcohol free, connect with appropriate community providers, and providing women with much needed support and guidance (Grant, Ernst, and Streissguth, 1996). Key components of the P-CAP model include: establishing a relationship, identifying client goals, establishing links to community services, a written contract defining explicit responsibilities and timelines, role modeling and teaching of basic skills, and evaluating the client's progress (Grant, Ernst, Streissguth, et al., 1996).

The original demonstration of the P-CAP showed remarkable results. After only one year of the program, there were increases in the number of women who were drug and alcohol free for 3 months or more or abstinent for 6 months or more (Grant, Ernst, Streissguth, et al., 1996). More women were regularly using birth control, attending parenting classes, and working in legitimate jobs for pay since the delivery of their child. Moreover, six children were put back in custody of their mother, 98% of infants were receiving well-child health care, and almost half (47%) of target infants were receiving therapeutic services. Grant, Ernst, and Streissguth (1996) reported that after 2 years in the program, 80% of clients were involved in some sort of alcohol or drug treatment, and 48% had been abstinent from alcohol and drugs for at least 6 months. By the end of the program, 85% of P-CAP clients had participated in treatment, 73% were using some form of regular birth control (compared to only 5% at intake), and 69% of target children were in appropriate and safe custody (Ernst, Grant, Streissguth, and Sampson, 1999).

Grant, Ernst, and Streissguth (1999) attribute part of the large success of the program to the employment of paraprofessionals, who are able to bridge the gap and build rapport with clients, partially due to their shared history and extensive involvement with each other. This shared history allows clients to develop and engage in a trusting relationship with advocates, often for the first time in their lives (Grant et al., 2002). Numerous studies have shown that the more time a client spends with her advocate, the more successful the intervention (Ernst et al., 1999; Grant, Ernst, Streissguth, et al., 1996; Grant et al., 2002). Specifically, clients who were the most involved were more likely to be drug and alcohol free for over a year during the intervention, less likely to become pregnant and to have had a subsequent birth during the 3-year intervention (Ernst et al., 1999), and more likely to enter treatment, stay in recovery, and consequently begin to improve other areas of their lives (Grant, Ernst, Streissguth, et al., 1996).

Even after clients exited the P-CAP program, positive effects of the intervention remained (Grant, Ernst, Pagalilauan, and Streissguth, 2003). In a post-program follow up study, Grant et al. (2003) examined outcomes by conducting three interviews: one at program enrollment, one at program exit, and one at the post-program follow-up between 1.6 and 3.6 years later. Upon exit of the program, 31% of women interviewed at all three points had been abstinent for 6 or more months compared with 0% upon enrollment. There was also a decrease in public assistance as a main source of income. Between program exit and follow-up, Grant et al. (2003) documented the following improvements: an increase in abstinence for at least 6 months or more, a decrease in subsequent pregnancies births, an increase in permanent housing, and a decrease in mothers being jailed during the post-program interval. Further, according to maternal self-report, 4 of the 6 children delivered to mothers in the follow-up period were unexposed to drugs or alcohol. Almost half of P-CAP participants attended education or training programs during or after the intervention and when interviewed at follow-up, 6 former clients were attending college. In general, positive program effects from the original demonstration of the P-CAP were maintained and even improved among women located for interviews post-program. Some P-CAP clients experienced cycles of relapse after completing the program; however Grant et al. (2003) found that mothers were maintaining longer periods of abstinence after recuperating from relapses. They also demonstrated that with a supportive, involved relationship, clearly stated goals, connections with community services, and enough time, mothers who were once disconnected and high-risk can attain and maintain productive lives, even several years after exiting the program.

Given the success of the P-CAP program, funding has been provided for multiple replications of the intervention. Grant, Ernst, Streissguth, and Stark (2005) compared outcomes between the original demonstration and two replications: Seattle and Tacoma. Participants from all three projects shared the same background characteristics and faced the same eligibility criteria; however in the replication sites women were enrolled during pregnancy as well as postpartum. Grant et al. (2005) found that a higher proportion of women in both replication projects completed alcohol or drug treatment; maintained longer periods of abstinence for at least one year during the intervention and for one or more years after program exit; and displayed regular (and more dependable) use of birth control than women in the original demonstration. Further, the number of subsequent pregnancies during the program was lower at the Tacoma replication than the original demonstration, and the post-program two-year birth rate remained lower than the average birth rate in Washington State. Among women who gave birth during the intervention, the proportion of unexposed infants at the Seattle and Tacoma sites was double that at the original demonstration (Grant et al., 2005). At both sites, employment as a primary source of income replaced public assistance for 32% of women, fewer target children were in foster homes, and over 3 times as many target children were adopted compared to the original demonstration (Grant et al., 2005). In Canada, a revised replication of PCAP, the First Steps Program, has also been found to be effective at preventing further alcohol-exposed pregnancies in high-risk women, most significantly through increasing regular birth control use and connecting women to community services and supports (Rasmussen et al., in press).

## Conclusions and Future Directions

The literature reviewed supports the contention that there are many effective interventions to prevent alcohol abuse during pregnancy. These interventions range from simple screening tools and brief interventions applied in prenatal primary care or community settings, to longer-term, multifaceted interventions that require much more investment from both the client and the service provider. Many of these interventions are designed to target women who are currently pregnant, but some focus on non-pregnant women who drink heavily and who do not make effective family planning decisions.

Floyd et al. (2009) review recommendations and reviews from the National Task Force on Fetal Alcohol Syndrome and Fetal Alcohol Effects. In their scientific review of current selective interventions for both pregnant and postpartum women, the Task Force found that the literature discussing brief interventions suggests that they are effective in a variety of settings (e.g., community, primary care). Based on this finding, the Task Force recommended the formal establishment of screening and brief intervention initiatives for diverse groups of women, and greater education and training of health professionals to assist in these new programs. For indicated interventions, the Task Force recognized the complexity of implementing these interventions, as well as their many successes. The Task Force advocates for wider access to substance abuse treatment options for pregnant women or women of childbearing age, especially for those with treatment barriers and unique needs (Barry et al., 2009; for a review, see Floyd et al., 2009).

Even though current screening, brief intervention, and long-term intervention techniques are generally supported as being efficacious, many of the studies that examine the interventions are limited in their design or in practical implementation. Screening not only has the ability to identify high-risk pregnant women accurately and efficiently, but it can also often decrease drinking behavior. Despite these benefits, screening is not regularly implemented in primary care settings (see above section on screening). Clearly, there must be changes made around the typical interview protocol for obstetric patients to mandate the use of screening. Additionally, women who do not regularly seek prenatal care must be considered; perhaps future initiatives should examine the use of screening in the community by less highly-trained professionals. Brief interventions are immensely beneficial: they are efficient and produce positive effects in the populations studied. However, more research must be conducted on the use of these interventions in community settings or in women who have a higher risk of being unresponsive to intervention. The feasibility of consistently using brief intervention in primary care must also be examined. Though studies of brief interventions are randomized, the designs of indicated intervention strategies generally lack in this regard and have less sound experimental results. Additionally, few brief intervention and longer-term intervention strategies follow up on infant outcomes. Monitoring outcomes such as diagnostic status and neurobehavioral functioning are paramount in truly understanding if these interventions prevent AEPs and FASD. Future research should endeavor to study the intergenerational effects of prenatal alcohol consumption on offspring, a sentiment that is also supported by the National Task Force.

Although women who drink during pregnancy may be a heterogeneous group, those who drink continually and give birth to children with FASD do have some common characteristics. Astley et al. (2000) examined the profiles of 80 women who had given birth to a child with FASD. The women came from a variety of ethnic, educational, and economic backgrounds; however, common issues experienced by many of the women included having been a victim of physical and/or sexual abuse and having mental health problems. Women who had achieved abstinence had higher incomes, higher IQs, larger social networks, were better connected with mental health services, and more likely to have a religious affiliation than those who were not abstinent. Besides abstinence, another effective way to prevent FASD is the use of regular birth control for sexually active women who still consume alcohol. Key barriers to effective family planning were lack of access to contraceptives, lack of partner support for using birth control, and maternal alcohol and drug use. It is important to further study the characteristics of women who have successful outcomes in various types of FASD prevention programs in order to tailor these programs to address unique needs and build on previous successes.

It is also important to identify barriers that women experience in accomplishing treatment goals (e.g., abstinence, family planning) and accessing substance abuse treatment itself, as these problems exist, despite the positive effects of many FASD prevention programs. As a result, some women never receive treatment. In a study of 36 pregnant and parenting women in a perinatal substance abuse treatment program, Jessup, Humphreys, Brindis, and Lee (2003) found that the majority (34) reported 'fear of punitive actions' as a major barrier to seeking treatment (e.g., fear of arrest or incarceration, loss of child custody). Other barriers included: barriers in the program itself (e.g., there were limits on how many children could attend the program with their mother, resulting in some children having to be placed in foster care for the duration of treatment), partners (domestic violence and substance abuse by partner), participant being opiate-dependent, and status of pregnancy (being currently pregnant at time of treatment created stigma and extra health concerns). Shannon and Walker (2008) state that there are numerous barriers at individual, community, and organization levels for pregnant substance-using women seeking treatment. They call for more research on the barriers to seeking treatment, how to rectify the barriers, and on the perceptions of pregnant substance-using women seeking treatment.

Prevention of alcohol abuse during pregnancy and FASD are significant public health concerns, and fortunately, there is great potential to prevent future alcohol-affected births. With the lifetime cost for each individual with FAS estimated at 2 million (Lupton et al., 2004), preventing FAS in a single individual would have enormous financial, personal, and social implications. The prevention programs reviewed, from screening and brief interventions to longer-term interventions, have the potential to afford many women the opportunity to improve their lives and prevent intergenerational problems, as well as prevent FASD in index and future pregnancies. However, as in any type of prevention research, it is difficult to quantify exactly how many FASD births have been prevented as a result of intervention. Nevertheless, the maintenance and support of such interventions, along with further research on program efficacy, are critical in supporting wider policy and practice related to the prevention of FASD.

## REFERENCES

AADAC. (2004). Estimating the rate of FASD and FAS in Canada. Women and Substance Abuse Information Series.

Alvik, A., Haldorsen, T., and Lindemann, R. (2005). Consistency of reported alcohol use by pregnant women: Anonymous versus confidential questionnaires with item nonresponse differences. *Alcoholism: Clinical and Experimental Research, 29*, 1444–1449.

Arborelius, E., and Damström Thakker, K. (1995). Why is it so difficult for general practitioners to discuss alcohol with patients? *Family Practice, 12*, 419–422.

Astley, S.J., Bailey, D., Talbot, C., and Clarren, S. (2000). Fetal Alcohol Syndrome (FAS) primary prevention through FAS diagnosis: II. A comprehensive profile of 80 birth mothers of children with FAS. *Alcohol and Alcoholism, 35*, 509–519.

Barry, K.L., Caetano, R., Chang, G., DeJoseph, M.C., Miller, L.A., O'Connor, M.J., … Leeks, K. (2009). National Task Force on Fetal Alcohol Syndrome and Fetal Alcohol Effect. Reducing alcohol-exposed pregnancies: A report of the National Task Force on Fetal Alcohol Syndrome and Fetal Alcohol Effect. Atlanta, GA: Centers for Disease Control and Prevention.

Chang, G. (2001). Alcohol-screening instruments for pregnant women. *Alcohol Research and Health, 25,* 204–209.

Chang, G., Behr, H., Goetz, M.A., Hiley, A., and Bigby, J. (1997). Women and alcohol abuse in primary care: Identification and intervention. *American Journal on Addictions, 66*, 183–192.

Chang, G., Goetz, M.A., Wilkins-Haug, L., and Berman, S. (2000). A brief intervention for prenatal alcohol use: An in-depth look. *Journal of Substance Abuse Treatment, 18*, 365–369.

Chang, G., McNamara, T.K., Orav, E.J., Koby, D., Lavigne, A., Ludman, B., … Wilkins-Haug, L. (2005). Brief intervention for prenatal alcohol use: A randomized trial. *Obstetrics and Gynecology, 105*, 991–998.

Chang, G., Wilkins-Haug, L., Berman, S., and Goetz, M.A. (1999). Brief intervention for alcohol use in pregnancy: a randomized trial. *Addiction, 94*, 1499–1508.

Chudley, A.E., Conry, J., Cook, J.L., Loock, C., Rosales, T., and LeBlanc, N. (2005). Fetal Alcohol Spectrum Disorder: Canadian guidelines for diagnosis. *Canadian Medical Association Journal, 172*, S1–S21.

Canadian Paediatric Society, First Nations and Inuit Health Committee. (2002). Fetal Alcohol Syndrome. *Paediatrics and Child Health, 7*, 161–174.

Day, N.L., Cottreau, C.M., and Richardson, G.A. (1993). The epidemiology of alcohol, marijuana, and cocaine use among women of childbearing age and pregnant women. *Clinical Obstetrics and Gynecology, 36*, 232–245.

Denny, C.H., Tsai, J., Floyd, R.L., and Green, P.P. (2009). Alcohol use among pregnant and nonpregnant women of childbearing age – United States, 1991-2005. *Centers for Disease Control and Prevention: Morbidity and Mortality Weekly Report*, 58, 529–532.

Diekman, S.T., Floyd, L., Decoufle, P., Schulkin, J., Ebrahim, S.H., and Sokol, R.J. (2000). A survey of obstetrician-gynecologists on their patient's alcohol use during pregnancy. *Obstetrics and Gynecology, 95*, 756–763.

Ernhart, C., Morrow-Tlucak, M., Sokol, R., Martier, S., and Ager, J. (1989). Underreporting of alcohol use in pregnancy: Relationship to alcohol problem history. *Alcoholism: Clinical and Experimental Research, 13*, 399–401.

Ernst, C.C., Grant, T.M., Streissguth, A.P., and Sampson, P.D. (1999). Intervention with high–risk alcohol and drug–abusing mothers: II. 3–year findings from the Seattle Model of Paraprofessional Advocacy. *Journal of Community Psychology, 27*, 19–38.

Ewing, J.A. (1984). Detecting alcoholism. The CAGE questionnaire. *Journal of the American Medical Association, 252*, 1905–1907.

Floyd, R.L., Decoufle, P., and Hungerford, D.W. (1999). Alcohol use prior to pregnancy recognition. *American Journal of Preventive Medicine, 17*, 101–107.

Floyd, R.L., and Sidhu, J.S. (2004). Monitoring prenatal alcohol exposure. *American Journal of Medical Genetics. Part C, Seminars in Medical Genetics, 127C*, 3–9.

Floyd, R.L., Sobell, M., Velasquez, M.M., Ingersoll K., Nettleman, M., Sobell, L., ... Project CHOICES Efficacy Study Group. (2007). Preventing alcohol-exposed pregnancies: A randomized controlled trial. *American Journal of Preventive Medicine, 32*, 1–10.

Floyd, R.L., Weber, M.K., Denny, C., and O'Connor, M.J. (2009). Prevention of Fetal Alcohol Spectrum Disorders. *Developmental Disabilities Research Review, 15*, 193–199.

Godel, J.C., Pabst, H.F., Hodges, P.E., Johnson, K.E., Froese, G.J., and Joffres, M.R. (1992). Smoking and caffeine and alcohol intake during pregnancy in a northern population: effect on fetal growth. *Canadian Medical Association Journal, 147*, 181–188.

Government of Alberta. August, 2005. Retrieved from http://www.child.gov.ab.ca/whatwedo/fas/page.cfm?pg=Why%20should%20Albertans%20be%20concerned%3F

Grant, T., Ernst, C., Pagalilauan, G., and Streissguth, A. (2003). Post-program follow-up effects of paraprofessional intervention with high-risk women who abused alcohol and drugs during pregnancy. *Journal of Community Psychology, 31*, 211–222.

Grant, T., Ernst, C., and Streissguth, A. (1996). An intervention with high-risk mothers who abuse alcohol and drugs: The Seattle Advocacy Model. *American Journal of Public Health, 86*, 1816–1817.

Grant, T., Ernst, C., and Streissguth, A. (1999). Intervention with high-risk alcohol and drug-abusing mothers: I. Administrative strategies of the Seattle model of paraprofessional advocacy. *Journal of Community Psychology, 27*, 1–18.

Grant, T., Ernst, C., Streissguth, A., Phipps, P., and Gendler, B. (1996). When case management isn't enough: A model of paraprofessional advocacy for drug- and alcohol-abusing mothers. *Journal of Case Management, 5*, 3–11.

Grant, T., Ernst, C., Streissguth, A., and Stark, K. (2005). Preventing alcohol and drug exposed births in Washington State: Intervention findings from three Parent-Child Assistance Program sites. *American Journal of Drug and Alcohol Abuse, 31*, 471–490.

Grant, T., Streissguth, A., and Ernst, C. (2002). Benefits and challenges of paraprofessional advocacy with mothers who abuse alcohol and drugs and their children. *Zero To Three, 23*, 14–20.

Greenfield, T.K., Rehm, J., and Rogers, J.D. (2002). Effects of depression and social integration on the relationship between alcohol consumption and all-cause mortality. *Addiction, 97*, 29–38.

Handmaker, N. S., Miller, W. R, and Manicke, M. (1999). Findings of a pilot study of motivational interviewing with pregnant drinkers. *Journal of Studies on Alcohol, 60*, 285–287.

Handmaker, N.S., and Wilbourne, P. (2001). Motivational interventions in prenatal clinics. *Alcohol Research and Health, 25*, 219–229.

Hankin, J.R. (2002). Fetal Alcohol Syndrome prevention research. *Alcohol Research and Health, 26*, 58–65.

Hankin, J.R., McCaul, M.E., and Heussner, J. (2000). Pregnant, alcohol-abusing women. *Alcoholism: Clinical and Experimental Research, 24*, 1276–1286.

Haynes, G., Dunnagan, T., and Christopher, S. (2003). Determinants of alcohol use in pregnant women at risk for alcohol consumption. *Neurotoxicology and Teratology, 25*, 659–666.

Health Canada (September, 2006). It's your health: Fetal Alcohol Spectrum Disorder. Retrieved from http://www.hc-sc.gc.ca/hl-vs/alt_formats/pacrb-dgapcr/pdf/iyh-vsv/diseases-maladies/fasd-etcaf-eng.pdf

Jacobson, J.L., and Jacobson, S.W. (1994). Prenatal alcohol exposure and neurobehavioral development: Where is the threshold? *Alcohol Health and Research World, 18*, 30–36, 1994.

Jessup, M.A., Humphreys, J.C., Brindis, C.D., and Lee, K.A. (2003). Extrinsic barriers to substance abuse treatment among pregnant drug dependent women. *The Journal of Drug Issues, 33*, 285–304.

Leonardson, G.R., and Loudenburg, R. (2003). Risk factors for alcohol use during pregnancy in a multistate area. *Neurotoxicology and Teratology, 25*, 651–658.

Lupton, C., Burd, L., and Harwood, R. (2004). Cost of Fetal Alcohol Spectrum Disorders. *American Journal of Medical Genetics. Part C, Seminars in Medical Genetics, 127C*, 42–50.

Manwell, L.B., Fleming, M.F., Mundt, M.P., Stauffacher, E.A., and Barry, K.L. (2000). Treatment of problem alcohol use in women of childbearing age: results of a brief intervention trial. *Alcoholism: Clinical and Experimental Research, 24*, 1517–1524.

Masis, K.B., and May, P.A. (1991). A comprehensive local program for the prevention of Fetal Alcohol Syndrome. *Public Health Reports, 106*, 484–489.

May, P.A., and Gossage, J.P. (2001). Estimating the prevalence of Fetal Alcohol Syndrome: A summary. *Alcohol Research and Health, 25*, 159–167.

May, P.A., Hymbaugh, K.J., Aase, J.M., and Samet, J.M. (1983). Epidemiology of Fetal Alcohol Syndrome among American Indians of the Southwest. *Social Biology, 30*, 374–387.

May, P. A., et al. (2008). Enhanced case management to prevent Fetal Alcohol Spectrum Disorders in Northern Plains communities. *Journal of Maternal and Child Health, 12*, 747–759.

Mengel, M.B., Searight, H.R., and Cook, K. (2006). Preventing alcohol-exposed pregnancies. *The Journal of the American Board of Family Medicine, 19*, 494–505.

Nilsen, P. (2009). Brief alcohol intervention to prevent drinking during pregnancy: An overview of research findings. *Current Opinion in Obstetrics and Gynecology, 21,* 496–500.

O'Connor, M.J., and Whaley, S.E. (2007). Brief intervention for alcohol use by pregnant women. *American Journal of Public Health, 97*, 252–258.

Project Choices Research Group (2002). Alcohol-exposed pregnancy: Characteristics associated with risk. *American Journal of Preventive Medicine, 23*, 166–173.

Project CHOICES Intervention Research Group (2003). Reducing the risk of alcohol-exposed pregnancies: A study of a motivational intervention in community settings, *Pediatrics, 111*, 1131–1135.

Rasmussen, C., Kully-Martens, K., Denys, K., Badry, D., Henneveld, D., Wyper, K., Grant, T. (in press). The effectiveness of a community-based intervention program for women at-risk for giving birth to a child with Fetal Alcohol Spectrum Disorder. *Community Mental Health Journal.*

Russell, M. (1994). New assessment tools for risk drinking during pregnancy: T-ACE, TWEAK, and others. *Alcohol Health and Research World, 18*, 55–61.

Russell, M., Martier, S., and Sokol, R. (1996). Detecting risk drinking during pregnancy: A comparison of four screening questionnaires. *American Journal of Public Health, 86,* 1435–1439.

Sampson, P.D., Streissguth, A.P., Bookstein, F.L., Little, R.E., Clarren, S.K., Dehaene, P., … Graham, J. Jr. (1997). Incidence of Fetal Alcohol Syndrome and prevalence of alcohol-related neurodevelopmental disorder. *Teratology, 56*, 317–326.

Serdula, M.K., Williamson, D.F., Kendrick, J.S, Anda, R.F., and Byers, T. (1991). Trends in alcohol consumption by pregnant women: 1985 through 1988. *Journal of the American Medical Association, 265*, 876–879.

Shannon, L., and Walker, R. (2008). Increasing the recognition of barriers for pregnant substance users seeking treatment. *Substance Use and Misuse, 43*, 1266–1267.

Smith, I.E., and Coles, C.D. (1991). Multilevel intervention for prevention of Fetal Alcohol Syndrome and effects of prenatal alcohol exposure. *Recent Developments in Alcoholism, 9*, 165–180.

Smith, I. E., Lancaster, J. S., Moss-Wells, S., Coles, C. D., and Falek, A. (1987). Identifying high-risk pregnant drinkers: Biological and behavioral correlates of continuous heavy drinking during pregnancy. *Journal of Studies on Alcohol, 48*, 304–309.

Sokol, R.J., Martier, S.S., and Ager, J.W. (1989). The T-ACE questions: Practical prenatal detection of risk drinking. *American Journal of Obstetrics and Gynecology, 160*, 863–870.

Stade, B., Ali, A., Bennett, D., Campbell, D., Johnston, M., Lens, C., ... Koren, G. (2009). The burden of prenatal exposure to alcohol: Revised measurement of cost. *Canadian Journal of Clinical Pharmacology, 16*, e91–e102.

Stratton, K.R., Howe, C.J, and Battaglia, F.C., Committee to Study Fetal Alcohol Syndrome, Institute of Medicine (IOM) (Eds.). (1996). *Fetal Alcohol Syndrome: Diagnosis, epidemiology, prevention and treatment.* Washington, DC: National Academy Press.

Substance Abuse and Mental Health Services Administration (SAMHSA), U.S. Department of Health and Human Services. (2002). Prevention of co-occurring disorders: Prevention for children and adolescents. In *Report to Congress on the prevention and treatment of co-occurring substance abuse disorders and mental disorders* (Chapter 3). Retrieved from http://www.samhsa.gov/reports/congress2002/chap3pca.htm

Svikis, D.S., and Reid-Quiñones, K. (2003). Screening and prevention of alcohol and drug use disorders in women. *Obstetrics and Gynecology Clinics of North America, 30*, 447–468.

Thornberry, J., Bhaskar, B., Krulewitch, C.J., Wesley, B., Hubbard, M.L., Das, A., ... Adamson, M. (2002). Audio computerized self-report interview use in prenatal clinics: Audio computer-assisted self interview with touch screen to detect alcohol consumption in pregnant women. Application of a new technology to an old problem. *Computers, Informatics, Nursing, 20*, 46–52.

In: Pregnancy and Alcohol Consumption
Editor: Joshua D. Hoffman, pp. 175-193

ISBN 978-1-61761-122-3


*Chapter 6*

# FETAL ALCOHOL EXPOSURE AND RISK TO THE PREMATURE NEWBORN*

***Theresa W. Gauthier, Sowmya S. Mohan and Lou Ann S. Brown***
Department of Pediatrics,
Division of Neonatal-Perinatal Medicine,
Emory University School of Medicine,
Atlanta, GA, Georgia

## ABSTRACT

Despite its well publicized risks, maternal alcohol use during pregnancy remains a common exposure for the developing neonate. Maternal alcohol use during pregnancy significantly increases the risk of premature delivery, and as such a large number of both term and premature newborns are exposed to this toxic substance in utero. Clinical evidence suggests that fetal alcohol exposure increases the risk of sepsis in both premature and term newborns, but the risks of alcohol exposure on the various morbidities suffered by premature newborns remain under investigation. Alcohol-induced alterations in antioxidant redox defenses occur in both the mother and the developing neonate during pregnancy, placing the premature newborn at particular risk for exaggerated oxidant-induced morbidities. These alcohol-induced redox alterations, particularly in the glutathione system, adversely affect the developing lung and its resident inflammatory cell the alveolar macrophage. This chapter will review the need for detection of the alcohol-exposed newborn, including the premature newborn and explore current biomarkers of fetal alcohol exposure such as fatty acid ethyl esters. Alterations of the glutathione redox system affecting the alcohol-exposed fetal lung are examined using animal models of fetal ethanol exposure. The ethanol-induced oxidant injury to the resident alveolar macrophage of the developing lung deranges immune functioning and increases the risk of pulmonary infection. However, availability of the antioxidant glutathione holds promise as a therapeutic intervention for the at-risk premature lung.

* Supported by National Institutes of Health Grants R01 AA-016348 (T. W. Gauthier), P50 AA-135757 (L. A. S. Brown and T. W. Gauthier), and T32 AA013528 (S. S. Mohan) and the Center for Developmental Lung Biology, Children's Healthcare of Atlanta (L. A. S. Brown).

Continued investigations of in utero alcohol's effects on the risk of adverse outcomes to all vulnerable organs of the developing newborn will allow for a better understanding of in utero alcohol's effects on this high-risk patient population.

## INTRODUCTION

Alcohol use and abuse prior to and during pregnancy contributes to a startling increased risk of extreme premature delivery at an Odds Ratio of ~35 (Sokol et al., 2007). Thus, a significant proportion of both premature and term newborns are alcohol-exposed (Albertsen et al., 2004; Drews et al., 2003; Floyd et al., 2006; Lester et al., 2001). Nearly 50% of pregnancies are unplanned (Finer and Henshaw, 2006) and binge drinking prior to and early in gestation remains a significant problem (Grant et al., 2009). However, the consequences of alcohol exposure during the early stages of pregnancy for the premature baby born before 37 weeks gestation remain poorly understood or undefined. Criteria for the diagnoses of Fetal Alcohol Syndrome (FAS) or Fetal Alcohol Spectrum Disorder (FASD) are based on the full term infants (defined as 37- 40 weeks gestation) and have limited utility in the premature newborn population. Accurately identifying the alcohol-exposed newborn remains a significant challenge and as such the majority of alcohol-exposed infants, whether term or premature, do not have the typical phenotypic characteristics associated with FAS, resulting in a clinical under-identification of the exposed neonate (Little BB, 1990; Mattson et al., 1997).

Clinical and animal-based investigations continue to narrow the gap of knowledge regarding the effects of prenatal exposure to alcohol, accurate identification of the exposed newborn, and the pathophysiological mechanisms underlying alcohol's effects on the at-risk premature newborn. In this chapter, we will discuss the challenges associated with the identification of the newborn exposed to alcohol *in utero*. We will review the effects of prenatal alcohol exposure on the excessive generation of reactive oxygen species in the vulnerable developing newborn and the toxicities of alcohol-induced alterations in redox status. Finally, we will discuss advances made in identifying the association between fetal alcohol exposure and altered immune function in the exposed neonate.

## IDENTIFICATION OF THE ALCOHOL-EXPOSED NEWBORN

The use and abuse of alcohol prior to and during pregnancy is a significant problem in our society despite education regarding the dangers. Contributing to the problem is the uncertainty as to what, if any amount of alcohol is safe to consume during pregnancy. The American College of Obstetricians and Gynecologists (ACOG) has remained strong in its recommendation that alcohol should be avoided entirely during pregnancy or prior to conception because damage can occur in the earliest weeks of pregnancy, even before a woman becomes aware that she is pregnant (ACOG, 2008). Despite conclusive research on the detrimental neurodevelopmental effects of heavy alcohol exposure in the term infant, limited research is available on the short and long term effects of alcohol during pregnancy on the premature infant.

A significant proportion of newborn infants, both premature and term gestations are exposed to alcohol during development (Albertsen et al., 2004; Ebrahim SH, 2003; Lester et al., 2001). In the past, studies of *in utero* exposure have focused on full term infants, with the most publicized consequence of prenatal exposure to heavy alcohol use being Fetal Alcohol Syndrome (FAS). One of the leading forms of preventable mental retardation (Abel EL, 1991), FAS has been characterized by distinctive craniofacial abnormalities (small head circumference, small eye openings, smooth philtrum, thin upper lip), growth retardation, and central nervous system damage (Jones KL, 1973). However, the majority of alcohol-exposed newborns do not have the characteristic phenotypic changes associated with FAS (Little BB, 1990; Mattson et al., 1997). It is estimated that 1% of all newborns are affected by prenatal exposure to alcohol (Sampson PD, 1997) but the inability to recognize those affected results in the majority remaining undiagnosed. In one study, the diagnosis of FAS was missed in 100% of term newborns who were subsequently diagnosed later in childhood (Little BB, 1990). Thus, FAS is recognizable in only a small fraction of exposed term newborns and therefore they often remain undiagnosed (Little BB, 1990; Mattson et al., 1997).

The majority of problems associated with alcohol exposure have been grouped and labeled as Fetal Alcohol Spectrum Disorders (FASD) or Alcohol Related Neurodevelopmental Disorders (ARND). Despite these advances in identifying the spectrum of problems encountered by the alcohol-exposed infant and child, ongoing research continues to unravel the consequences of alcohol exposure on outcomes and therapeutic strategies for those identified as at-risk.

However, limited research has focused on the effects of alcohol exposure on the infant born prematurely with very limited knowledge as to the consequences of similar exposure on the vulnerable and developing preterm newborn. The need for such research was highlighted by a recent study which demonstrated a dramatic increased risk of extreme premature delivery in mothers who drank alcohol during pregnancy (Sokol et al., 2007). We have yet to understand the full spectrum of the effects of prenatal alcohol exposure on common morbidities faced in the premature population such as infection, Chronic Lung Disease, Necrotizing Enterocolitis and Neurodevelopmental Delays.

Comprehensively defining the effects of prenatal alcohol exposure on the premature or term newborn requires accurate identification of the exposed newborn, a process which remains clinically challenging. Studies have assessed maternal blood markers such as carbohydrate-deficient transferring and γ-glutamyl transferase to identify the alcohol using mother during pregnancy, but the specificity and sensitivity of these routine biological tests are lacking (Sarkola et al., 2000; Stoler et al., 1998). Thus, unlike the biomarkers used in the adult population there is no clear biomarker of alcohol exposure that can reliably identify the alcohol-exposed newborn (Bearer et al., 2003). Despite clear evidence that *in utero* alcohol exposure is detrimental to the developing fetus, identifying and appreciating the clinical affects of prenatal alcohol exposure on the newborn often relies on maternal self-reporting of alcohol use during the pregnancy. In non-pregnant adults, determination of alcohol abuse has been standardized using questionnaires such as the Alcohol Use Disorders Identification Test (AUDIT) (Bradley et al., 1998) and the Short Michigan Alcoholism Screening Test (SMAST) (Maisto et al., 1995). Multiple standardized questionnaires have attempted to accurately define alcohol exposure during pregnancy, but the reliability of answers remains a continued concern (Chang et al., 1999; Russell et al., 1996). Ultimately, maternal self reporting continues to underestimate the scope of exposure, allowing exposed newborns to remain undetected. The public awareness of the risks associated with maternal alcohol use during pregnancy has also led to the societal stigma associated with drinking during pregnancy, which heavily contributes to maternal under-reporting the use of alcohol while pregnant.

While researchers continue to look for potential biomarkers that would be a safe, reliable, and accurate marker of prenatal alcohol exposure, Fatty Acid Ethyl Esters (FAEE) have shown promise in this regard. Alcohol is metabolized by both oxidative and non-oxidative pathways (Bearer et al., 2003). FAEE are the product of the non-oxidative pathway where ethanol conjugates to free fatty acids (Lange LG, 1981) in a process mediated by the enzyme Fatty Acid Ethyl Ester Synthase. Unlike alcohol itself or oxidative byproducts of alcohol metabolism, FAEE have a prolonged half-life in tissue and have the potential to accumulate in body fluids and tissue for extended periods of time (Best CA, 2003; Laposata, 1999). FAEE as a biomarker of alcohol abuse in adults has been described, (Kaphalia et al., 2004) while investigations determining the sensitivity and specificity of FAEE as a potential biomarker specifically for fetal alcohol exposure in newborn infants continue.

For the newborn, FAEE accumulate in the infant's first stool also known as meconium. In studies pioneered by Bearer as well as Koren, significantly different levels of FAEE were found in the meconium of term infants exposed to alcohol *in utero* versus those not exposed. In term infants born to mothers who report alcohol use during pregnancy, there was a significant correlation between the accumulation of FAEE in the meconium and alcohol exposure (Bearer CF, 1999). Bearer, et al subsequently demonstrated that *specific* FAEE in the meconium such as ethyl linoleate and ethyl oleate were associated with higher alcohol use when compared to controls who consumed no alcohol (Bearer, 2001). While FAEE were detected in all samples obtained, those obtained from control patients were used to establish standardized cutoff values for this potential biomarker. In contrast, Canadian researchers including Koren, et al showed that there was a significant difference in the *total* accumulated amount of all FAEE in alcohol-exposed infant's meconium compared to controls (Klein J, 1999).

In adults, FAEE accumulated in the extractable hair lipids originating mainly from sebum and from the structural lipids of cell membranes (Refaai MA, 2002; Robbins, 1994) of subjects that abused alcohol when compared to controls, specifically, ethyl palmitate, ethyl stearate, and ethyl oleate (Pargst F, 2000). Similar studies of hair samples from term infants exposed to alcohol showed a significant difference in their FAEE concentration and profile compared to control term newborns (Caprara DL, 2005). Such an approach has expanded the identification of the exposed newborn past the initial hospitalization at the time of birth. This is particularly important given that accumulation of FAEE correlated with alcohol-induced neurodevelopmental disabilities in the newborn (Klein J, 1999; Ursitti F, 1997).

Continued investigations to delineate whether FAEE will be similarly useful and reliable biomarkers of prenatal alcohol exposure in the premature population are essential. Given that alcohol significantly increases the risk of prematurity, the need for validated biomarkers in this already at-risk population is paramount. Without such biomarkers, our understanding of alcohol's effects on adverse outcomes suffered by the premature newborn population remains limited.

Although FAEE were discovered decades ago in different body tissues, research is growing to determine the direct cytotoxic effects of these compounds (Laposata, 1998). In postmortem tissues obtained from patients acutely intoxicated at the time of death, the tissues frequently damaged by alcohol (pancreas, liver, heart, and brain) contained high levels of

FAEE (Laposata EA, 1986). FAEE act as shuttles for fatty acids between cellular fatty acid binding sites and the mitochondria. Once bound to the mitochondria, the FAEE are hydrolyzed and the released free fatty acids uncouple oxidative phosphorylation, impair mitochondrial function and result in cellular death (Laposata EA, 1986). Thus, investigations focusing not only the presence of FAEE as a potential biomarker, but studies aimed at determining the mechanisms of the potential toxicity of FAEE in various organs of the developing newborn are necessary.

## Fetal Alcohol Exposure and Oxidative Stress

As in adults, *in utero* alcohol exposure promotes multiple direct and indirect cascades that culminate in toxicity to developing organs. While it is unlikely that all developing organs respond in a similar manner to alcohol exposure, the excessive generation of highly reactive oxygen species (ROS) appears to play a central role in the pathological processes. Free radicals are small, diffusible molecules that differ from most biological molecules in that they have an unpaired electron. They tend to be reactive and can participate in chain reactions in which a single free radical initiation event can be propagated to damage multiple macromolecules. These ROS include superoxide, peroxides and hydroxyl radicals which are unstable and react with essential components of the cell. With excessive ROS generation, cell functions can be altered because of macromolecule damage such as compromised protein functions because of protein oxidation, compromised membranes because of lipid peroxidation and mutations because of DNA oxidation. In fetal tissues, the increased presence of lipid peroxidation products, proteins containing lipid peroxidation adducts, and increased 8-hydroxy-2'-deoxyguanosine, a DNA oxidation product, demonstrate that ROS are generated in response to *in utero* exposure and that macromolecule damage occurs (Chu et al., 2007; Maffi et al., 2008; Wentzel et al., 2006). When generated, the ROS are normally neutralized through reactions with antioxidants but an imbalance between ROS generation and antioxidant detoxification results in an increasing ROS burden and cell injury. Since developing tissues have poorly developed antioxidant systems, they are particularly vulnerable to the adverse effects of the ROS generated during fetal alcohol exposure.

In addition to the radical oxidants, oxidative stress in biological systems can also generate nonradical oxidants. Within proteins, the amino acids cysteine and methionine contain sulfur groups that can undergo multiple reversible oxidations under biologic conditions. Proteins with active cysteine sites include enzymes, receptors, transporters, transcription factors, structural components, caspases, kinases, phosphatases, and proteases. Therefore, oxidative stress can also occur when these critical cysteine sites become oxidized to disulfides (Jones, 2006; Jones et al., 2004). For example, critical cysteines at the active sites can become chemically altered through adduct formation, thereby turning the protein on or off. Likewise, proteins can become crosslinked through the formation of disulfide bridges at critical thiol sites and subsequently initiate or block signal transduction as well as promote protein aggregates. Alternatively, oxidation at a distal site can change the conformation of a protein resulting in altered enzymatic activity or protein function. A broad range of thiol-dependent regulation can occur because proteins often contain multiple thiol residues that can undergo reversible modifications to intramolecular and intermolecular disulfides, sulfenic acids, sulfonic acid, S-glutathione derivatives, and S-nitroso derivatives. These cysteine sites are also sensitive to adduct formation with acetaldehyde, the primary metabolite of ethanol, as well as lipid peroxidation products such as malonyldialdehyde or hydroxynonenal. Thus, oxidative stress at these critical cysteine sites may occur in the absence of macromolecular damage but affect multiple cellular functions through altered protein conformation, enzyme activity, transporter activity, ligand binding to receptors, protein–protein interactions, protein–DNA interactions, signal transduction, proliferation, transcriptional regulation, cell proliferation, and apoptosis (Kemp et al., 2008).

During development, a role for alcohol-induced oxidative stress in tissue injury has been identified for the placenta (Gundogan et al., 2009), embryo (Dong et al., 2010), liver (Coyle et al., 2009; Ojeda et al., 2009; Wentzel et al., 2006), brain (Cherian et al., 2008; Dong et al., 2008; Sari, 2009; Yan et al., 2010), hippocampus (Green et al., 2006), cerebellum (Grisel and Chen, 2005), and lung (Gauthier et al., 2005b; Gauthier et al., 2009; Sozo et al., 2009). One major source of ROS comes from respiration where the mitochondria continuously release peroxides during oxygen consumption. The ROS generated during normal respiration can be amplified by fetal alcohol exposure as alcohol depletes the antioxidant glutathione within the mitochondria thereby, decreasing the capacity of the mitochondria to detoxify the ROS generated (Green et al., 2006). In a mouse model, fetal ethanol exposure promoted the redistribution of cytochrome C from the mitochondria to the cytosol (Sari, 2009). The loss of cytochrome C from the mitochondrial electron transport chain results in increased mitochondrial-derived ROS. In ethanol-exposed cerebella, the mRNA levels of mitochondrial genes encoding Complexes II-A, IV, and V are depressed resulting in decreased ATP production (Chu et al., 2007), a critical event for developing tissues. In addition to the redistribution of cytochrome C, the compromise in mitochondrial membrane integrity also promotes the translocation of apoptosis inducing factor (AIF) from mitochondria to the nucleus to initiate apoptosis (Cherian et al., 2008). These adverse effects of fetal alcohol exposure are further exacerbated by alcohol-induced increases in expression of the pro-apoptotic proteins Bax and Bak as well as decreases in the anti-apoptotic Bcl-2 protein (Gundogan et al., 2009).

Other ROS are derived from ethanol metabolism. At moderate levels, alcohol is primarily metabolized through alcohol dehydrogenase. Therefore, the enzymatic activity associated with the different polymorphisms will result in different rates of alcohol metabolism and subsequently alter the levels of alcohol exposure for the developing organs (Gemma et al., 2006; Gemma et al., 2007). The by-product of ethanol metabolism by alcohol dehydrogenase is acetaldehyde which promotes oxidative stress and depletion of the antioxidant glutathione. Both the depletion of glutathione and the formation of acetaldehyde-protein adducts can alter the thiol/disulfide of critical cysteine sites in different proteins and subsequently their function (Gemma et al., 2006; Olivares et al., 1997).

Alcohol is also metabolized by mixed function oxidases such cytochrome P450 which use molecular oxygen for detoxification of alcohol but generate ROS. Although cytochrome P450 may minimally contribute to ethanol metabolism at baseline, chronic alcohol exposure increases the activity of cytochrome P450 2E1 (CYP2E1) which is particularly active in generating ROS. The ROS generated by CYP2E1 are hydrogen peroxide, superoxide anion, hydroxyl radicals and substrate-derived radicals (1-hydroxyethyl radical) as by-products. The 1-hydroxyethyl radicals also covalently form protein adducts which can alter protein functions as the thiol/disulfide status of the protein is changed. As with polymorphisms of alcohol dehydrogenase, polymorphisms of CYP2E1 may also contribute to variations in the rate of acetaldehyde generation and subsequent injury that fetal tissues experience with fetal alcohol exposure (Gemma et al., 2006; Gemma et al., 2007). Significant levels of activity and mRNA for CYP2E1 have been detected between gestational days 45 and 53 as organogenesis begins (Brzezinski et al., 1999) increasing the probability that alcohol will be metabolized by CYP2E1 to form acetaldehyde in the fetal tissues. In a mouse model, chronic maternal ethanol administration resulted in increased CYP2E1 expression and activity in both the microsomal and mitochondrial fractions of the fetal liver tissue as observed in adult tissues after chronic ethanol ingestion (Hewitt et al.; Hines and McCarver, 2002; Zakhari, 2006). Acetaldehyde can also be generated in the placenta where the expression of the CYP2E1 protein was related to alcohol consumption (Rasheed et al., 1997). In neuronal tissues, the presence polyunsaturated fatty acid within the membranes makes this organ particularly vulnerable to the acetaldehyde-induced ROS and induction of lipid peroxidation (Gemma et al., 2006; Gemma et al., 2007). Thus, multiple fetal tissues express CYP2E1 resulting in increased generation of acetaldehyde in response to fetal alcohol exposure and are at greater risk for acetaldehyde-induced cellular injury.

ROS can also be generated by NADPH oxidase (NOX), a multi-subunit complex that generates superoxide anions in the one-electron reduction of $O_2$ using the electrons supplied by NADPH (For review see ref (Bedard and Krause, 2007)). Analyses of mRNA expression indicated that ethanol significantly increases mRNA expression of the NOX catalytic subunit Duox-1 (Dong et al., 2010) in addition to NOX1 and 3 (Chu et al., 2007). Ethanol also significantly increased mRNA expression of the NOX regulatory subunits p22phox, p67phox, NOXA1 and NOXO1 as well increased NOX enzyme activity (Dong et al., 2010). A specific role for NOX-derived ROS was demonstrated by the ability of co-treatment with the NOX inhibitor, diphenyleneiodonium to significantly prevent ethanol-induced increases in NOX enzyme activity, ROS generation and oxidative DNA damage in ethanol-exposed embryos. Diphenyleneiodonium treatment also decreased caspase-3 activation and activity as well as apoptosis in the ethanol-exposed embryos. These results suggest that NOX is a critical source of ROS in ethanol-exposed embryos and that it plays an important role in ethanol-induced oxidative stress and pathogenesis.

The availability of the antioxidant glutathione plays a critical role in detoxifying the ROS generated in response to alcohol. However, extended exposure to alcohol and acetaldehyde depletes the glutathione pools. In a rat model, GSH levels were significantly decreased in the fetal brains and livers when the dams received 35% of their calories from ethanol (Reyes et al., 1993). Fetal ethanol exposure also suppressed the enzymes that use glutathione for detoxification (glutathione peroxidase/glutathione reductase) as well as expression of gamma-glutamylcysteine synthetase, the enzyme that performs the rate-limiting step for glutathione synthesis (Siler-Marsiglio et al., 2005). Thus, fetal alcohol exposure depresses the capacity of the tissues to restore the glutathione pools or use glutathione for detoxification. These effects may be secondary to mitochondrial ROS and glutathione availability since treatment with mitochondrially-targeted vitamin E maintained the glutathione-dependent enzymes as well as the glutathione pools. As mentioned above, acetaldehyde treatment of a human fetal hepatic cell line decreased the GSH content by 95% (Olivares et al., 1997) suggesting that acetaldehyde may be the key factor in the depletion of glutathione pools. In the lung, fetal alcohol exposure resulted in decreased glutathione in the fluid lining the alveolar space (Gauthier et al., 2005b). The alveolar macrophages, which reside in the alveolar lining fluid, also had decreased glutathione as well as impaired phagocytosis and increased apoptosis when the pups were exposed to ethanol *in utero* (Gauthier et al., 2005b). Fetal alcohol exposure was also associated with an impaired capacity of the alveolar macrophages to clear *Staph. aureus* or *Group B Strep* (Gauthier et al., 2009; Ping et al., 2007). Addition of the GSH precursor S-adenosyl-methionine (SAM) to the maternal drinking water containing ethanol, prevented glutathione depletion and induction of oxidative stress markers in the lining fluid and in alveolar macrophages. Likewise, SAM treatment prevented the ethanol-induced suppression of alveolar macrophages to internalize infectious particles (Gauthier et al., 2005b; Gauthier et al., 2009; Ping et al., 2007). Furthermore, a central role for ethanol-induced glutathione depletion in impaired macrophage function was demonstrated by the ability of *in vitro* or intra-nasal glutathione treatments to improve macrophage phagocytosis, attenuate lung infections and dissemination of *Group B Strep* (Gauthier et al., 2009). Thus, ethanol-induced glutathione depletion was central to the inability of the fetal lung to clear infectious particles.

However, the heterogeneity of glutathione distribution may mean that not all cell types may be equally susceptible alcohol-induced ROS. Within neuronal populations, the cells have a highly differing sensitivity to ethanol-induced toxicity. One possible explanation could be cellular variations in glutathione homeostasis as evidenced by a striking heterogeneity in glutathione content within cortical neuron populations at baseline (Maffi et al., 2008). When neuron glutathione pools are decreased by treatment with butathione sulfoxamine, the ethanol-mediated enhancement of ROS is exacerbated. When the cells were sorted into high- and low-glutathione populations, the markers of oxidative stress and apoptotic indices were preferentially elevated in the low-glutathione cell populations. Given the link between acetaldehyde concentrations and glutathione depletion, heterogeneity in alcohol dehydrogenase and CYP2E1 expression or polymorphisms would also contribute to heterogeneity in subsequent acetaldehyde generation, glutathione depletion and, ultimately, injury in response to fetal alcohol exposure. Glutathione also pays an important role in detoxification through Glutathione S-transferase which conjugates glutathione to harmful electrophilic compounds to produce a less toxic metabolite that can be excreted. Consequently, the different enzymatic activities associated with different polymorphisms of Glutathione S-transferases may also contribute to the ability of the maternal, placental and fetal tissues to remove the toxic metabolites and ultimately protect against tissue injury (Gemma et al., 2007).

In summary, fetal alcohol exposure promotes several cascades that result in oxidative stress and subsequent injury. Ethanol metabolism, whether through alcohol dehydrogenase or CYP2E1, results in the generation of ROS as well as the oxidant acetaldehyde. Furthermore, the polymorphism profile of the individual would also contribute to the concentrations of acetaldehyde generated in response to the same levels of fetal alcohol exposure. Even moderate alcohol exposure and acetaldehyde generation may promote oxidative stress by promoting acetaldehyde adduct formation at critical cysteine sites of proteins. Additional studies are needed to determine if low levels of fetal alcohol exposure alters protein functions and contributes to subtle injury and/or response to additional stressors, even in the absence of frank tissue injury. ROS can also be derived from poorly coupled mitochondrial respiration or NADPH oxidases. The increases in ROS and acetaldehyde then contribute to glutathione depletion and exacerbate ROS-induced protein oxidation, lipid peroxidation and DNA oxidation. With decreased glutathione availability, there is an inability to restore the thiol/disulfide status of proteins oxidized by acetaldehyde or ROS. Thus, the glutathione concentrations in the different cell types and the extracellular pools serve as important modulators of alcohol-induced changes in critical cysteine sites and subsequent protein function, macromolecular damage, ROS detoxification, and subsequent tissue injury. Quantitative assessment of subtle redox changes in proteins in response to fetal alcohol exposure are needed to understand the nuances of altered protein conformation, enzyme activity, transporter activity, ligand binding to receptors, protein–protein interactions, protein–DNA interactions, signal transduction, proliferation, transcriptional regulation, cell proliferation, and apoptosis.

## FETAL ALCOHOL EXPOSURE AND ALTERED IMMUNE FUNCTION

Despite advances in modern neonatal intensive care, the mortality and morbidity from infections and infection-mediated complications for the newborn infant remain significant, particularly if the child was born prematurely (Alarcon et al., 2004; Benjamin and Stoll, 2006; Cordero et al., 2004; Stoll and Hansen, 2003). Although the use of maternal antibiotics during pregnancy has reduced the incidence of bacterial sepsis for the newborn infant, the risk of infection remains disproportionately elevated in premature newborns and those born within minority groups (Stoll et al., 2002; Stoll et al., 1998)

The occurrence of infection complicates an already tenuous clinical course for the premature neonate residing in the Newborn Intensive Care Unit and significantly prolongs hospital stay. Neonatal infections increase the risk of a variety of adverse outcomes for the premature newborn including patent ductus arteriosus, chronic lung disease (bronchopulmonary dysplasia) and necrotizing enterocolitis (Stoll et al., 2002). Furthermore, infections in the neonatal period significantly increase the risk of adverse neurodevelopmental outcomes in the growing former premature newborn (Adams-Chapman and Stoll, 2006; Stoll et al., 2004).

In addition to bacterial infections, the growing premature newborn is also at risk for increased morbidities from viral respiratory infections. Despite immunization strategies such as palivizumab, which target high risk newborns such as those born prematurely, the growing premature newborn remains at an increased risk for severe and often life threatening respiratory syncytial virus (RSV) infection, particularly in the lower respiratory tract of the lung (2009; Hall et al., 2009). Additionally, former premature newborns remain at high risk for the development of severe influenza infection (Izurieta et al., 2000; Louie et al., 2006).

A limited number of clinical reviews address the risk of infection in infants and children exposed to alcohol *in utero*. Studies suggest that fetal alcohol exposure increases the risk of neonatal bacterial infection in the exposed offspring. Early data of an evaluation of children with diagnosed FAS reported abnormalities in lymphocytes and increased bacterial infections such as meningitis, pneumonia and otitis (Johnson et al., 1981). In the term newborn population, excessive maternal alcohol use of greater than seven drinks per week significantly increased the risk of neonatal infection in the newborn nursery over three fold, particularly if the alcohol use occurred during the second trimester of pregnancy (Gauthier et al., 2005a).

Given the increased risk of prematurity with maternal alcohol use during pregnancy, further clinical data is desperately needed to fully determine the consequences of alcohol exposure *in utero* on neonatal infection for the infant born prematurely. In a small population of very low birth weight premature newborns (birth weight < 1500 grams), maternal alcohol use significantly increased the risk of early onset bacterial sepsis compared to premature newborns without alcohol exposure. Early-onset bacterial sepsis occurred in 10% of the Alcohol group compared to 0.6% of the Control group, significantly increasing the risk of infection with an Odds Ratio approaching 7 (Gauthier et al., 2004).

Multiple studies using animal models of fetal ethanol exposure support these clinical findings and suggest that *in utero* exposure alters multiple arms of the developing fetal immune system. Fetal ethanol exposure at critical periods of gestation delayed both cell-mediated and humoral immunity via alteration in T and B cell development (for review (Zhang et al., 2005))(Biber et al., 1998). By direct effects on the thymus, fetal ethanol exposure disrupted T cell number, development and maturation (Ewald and Frost, 1987; Ewald and Walden, 1988; Taylor et al., 1999), impairing T cell-mediated immunity. Modulation of T cell immunity by T regulatory cells was also altered by fetal ethanol exposure, contributing to impaired immunity in the exposed offspring (Zhang et al., 2005). These disruptions occurred early in gestation, suggesting that premature offspring may be more susceptible to ethanol's effects. The humoral arm of the developing immune system is also damaged by *in utero* ethanol. Within the developing fetal liver, ethanol exposure decreased cell number and delayed maturation of the B cell lineage (Biber et al., 1998). Decreased lymphocyte subpopulations were demonstrated in the ethanol-exposed thymus, spleen, bone marrow and intestine (Basham et al., 1998; Wolcott et al., 1995).

In the developing gut, *in utero* ethanol altered the population of lymphocytes and tissue macrophages in the gut associated lymphoid tissue (GALT) across gestation, suggesting that ethanol exposure deranged gut immunocompetence (Zhu and Seelig, 2000). These effects noted in the immature intestine normalized with advancing age, suggesting that ethanol exposure *in utero* delayed the normal intestinal immune development, but placed the immature intestine at increased risk for immune deficiency. *In utero* ethanol's effects on the developing gut are particularly interesting for premature newborns that are at increased risk for the development of necrotizing enterocolitis. Necrotizing enterocolitis is one of the major causes of death in the premature population. The pathophysiology of necrotizing enterocolitis remains under intense investigation (for review (Lin et al., 2008)) and infectious and immune-mediated deficiencies in the developing gut contribute to the development of this disease (Hunter et al., 2008; Lin et al., 2008). However a potential link between the effects of alcohol exposure *in utero* and the pathophysiology of necrotizing enterocolitis in the premature newborn is unknown and requires investigation.

Understanding *in utero* ethanol's effects on the immune response of the developing neonatal lung has direct implications not only for infection risk but also for the relationship between the inflammatory state of the lung and long term sequelae for the premature newborn such as chronic lung disease. Chronic lung disease has strongly been associated with a persistent influx of inflammatory cells and an elevated and sustained pro-inflammatory environment in the developing lung (Bustani and Kotecha, 2003; De Dooy et al., 2001; Jobe and Ikegami, 1998; Jobe and Ikegami, 2001; Lyon, 2000). A failure to resolve this altered environment in the neonatal lung hallmarks this disease.

As the resident inflammatory cell in the lung, the alveolar macrophage provides the initial defenses against foreign and infectious particles and orchestrates the inflammatory process within the lung (Fels and Cohn, 1986; Standiford et al., 1995). In the premature newborn the baseline function of the alveolar macrophage is impaired (Bellanti and Zeligs, 1995; Hall and Sherman, 1992). Defenses against infectious organisms in the lung such as *Group B streptococcus* is compromised due to reduced number of alveolar macrophage, deficient phagocytosis, chemotaxis and bacterial killing (Kurland et al., 1988). Alveolar macrophage are derived from peripheral circulating blood monocytes which constitutively move into the interstitial space of the lung and are also recruited in response to pro-inflammatory stimuli. These monocytic cells differentiate into mature alveolar macrophage in the alveolar space (Fels and Cohn, 1986; Prieto et al., 1994) in a granulocyte macrophage colony stimulating factor (GMCSF)-dependant process (Bonfield et al., 2003). Modulation of innate immune responses of the fetal monocyte by systemic conditions or exposures during pregnancy may subsequently affect the resident alveolar macrophage population and the inflammatory environment within the newborn lung (Kramer et al., 2004; Kramer et al., 2005).

In addition to the alveolar macrophage, surfactant proteins (collectins) are essential components of the innate immune defenses of the developing lung (Crouch et al., 2000; Kuroki et al., 2007; Wright, 2004). Surfactant protein A (SP-A) and D (SP-D) are cell surface lectins that protect the lung against both bacterial and viral infection (Bruce et al., 2009; LeVine et al., 2004). Collectins provide efficient opsonization of pathogens necessary for effective phagocytosis by alveolar macrophage and modulate dendritic and T cell immunity (Sorensen et al., 2007).

Growing evidence from recent investigations strongly suggest that *in utero* ethanol exposure deranges multiple arms of innate immunity in the developing lung. In sheep models, *in utero* ethanol exposure impaired innate immunity in the developing lung as demonstrated by decreased SP-A and diminished basal pro inflammatory cytokine production (Lazic et al., 2007; Sozo et al., 2009). Furthermore, ethanol decreased surfactant protein B, a marker of lung maturation, suggesting that respiratory distress syndrome of the premature newborn could be increased after *in utero* alcohol exposure (Sozo et al., 2009).

In guinea pig models of fetal ethanol exposure, the function and viability of the developing alveolar macrophage was significantly altered. Premature alveolar macrophage exposed to ethanol *in utero* demonstrated increased oxidant stress and apoptosis and impaired phagocytosis of bacteria *in vitro* (Gauthier et al., 2005b). Ethanol-induced derangements persisted at term gestation, where exposed alveolar macrophage demonstrated impaired phagocytic function *in vitro* and *in vivo* (Ping et al., 2007). These ethanol effects increased the risk of pulmonary and systemic bacterial infection in an experimental *in vivo* model of *group B streptococcus* pneumonia (Gauthier et al., 2009). Adult models of chronic ethanol exposure suggest that ethanol diminished GMCSF receptor expression and signaling in the ethanol-exposed alveolar macrophage (Joshi et al., 2006; Joshi et al., 2005), impairing terminal differentiation of the cell due to ethanol-induced oxidant stress (Brown et al., 2009). Whether fetal ethanol induced oxidant stress impairs the maturation of the developing alveolar macrophage in the premature lung remains under investigation.

As noted, fetal ethanol increases oxidant stress within the developing lung and the alveolar macrophage, in part by diminishing glutathione availability. Strategies to maintain glutathione in the developing lung, via maternal S adenosylmethionine (SAM) ingestion during ethanol ingestion, or via supplemental glutathione to the neonatal animal hold promise to augment immune function in the exposed neonate (Brown et al., 2009; Gauthier et al., 2005b; Gauthier et al., 2009; Ping et al., 2007).

Viral mediated respiratory infections cause substantial injury to the former premature newborn population, particularly RSV and influenza. Emerging data from the growing animal exposed *in utero* to ethanol suggest that ethanol induced a persistent immune dysfunction that persisted into adulthood. Specifically, adult animals demonstrated impaired adaptive immunity and altered B cell responses resulting in increased risk and severity of influenza infection after *in utero* ethanol exposure (McGill et al., 2009). These effects were exacerbated by additional alcohol exposure. Indeed, ethanol *in utero* may alter the hypothalamic-pituitary adrenal axis resulting in augmented stress-induced immunosuppression and increased vulnerability to subsequent infectious illness- a form of fetal programming (Zhang et al., 2005). For the premature newborn and growing former preterm infant, *in utero* alcohol-induced alterations in endocrine function and immune competence remain to be defined.

## Summary/Future Directions

Although alcohol exposure can increase the risk of premature delivery, accurate identification of the premature newborn exposed to alcohol *in utero* remains elusive. Continue advancement in the development and standardization of biomarkers of exposure such as FAEE will enable more accurate surveillance techniques for this at-risk population of newborns. Establishing a reliable biomarker for the detection of prenatal alcohol exposure will allow for the necessary advancement in understanding of the mechanisms of alcohol's systemic effects on the developing newborn. Such early identification will also help target potential clinical interventions to minimize long term sequelae in the effected offspring. *In utero* alcohol-induced alterations in redox homeostasis have broad-reaching implications for multiple organ systems in the developing newborn, particularly newborns at risk for a variety of life threatening oxidant-mediated morbidities due to prematurity. *In utero* alcohol exposure alters multiple arms of the developing immune system and continued research is required to fully identify and understand the full effects of alcohol exposure on infection risk and infectious-mediated morbidities. The antioxidant glutathione holds promise as an important modulator and a potential therapeutic intervention to attenuate alcohol's derangement of redox homeostasis and to preserve cellular functioning.

## References

(2009) From the American Academy of Pediatrics: Policy statements--Modified recommendations for use of palivizumab for prevention of respiratory syncytial virus infections. *Pediatrics* 124(6):1694-701.

Abel EL SR (1991) A revised conservative estimate of the incidence of FAS and its economic impact. *Alcohol. Clin. Exp. Res.* 15:514-24.

ACOG (2008) Alcohol and Pregnancy: Know the Facts, pp American Congress of Obstetricians and Gynecologists News Release.

Adams-Chapman I, Stoll BJ (2006) Neonatal infection and long-term neurodevelopmental outcome in the preterm infant. *Curr. Opin. Infect. Dis.* 19(3):290-7.

Alarcon A, Pena P, Salas S, Sancha M, Omenaca F (2004) Neonatal early onset Escherichia coli sepsis: trends in incidence and antimicrobial resistance in the era of intrapartum antimicrobial prophylaxis. *Pediatr Infect. Dis. J.* 23(4):295-9.

Albertsen K, Andersen AM, Olsen J, Gronbaek M (2004) Alcohol consumption during pregnancy and the risk of preterm delivery. *Am. J. Epidemiol.* 159(2):155-61.

Basham KB, Whitmore SP, Adcock AF, Basta PV (1998) Chronic and acute prenatal and postnatal ethanol exposure on lymphocyte subsets from offspring thymic, splenic, and intestinal intraepithelial sources. *Alcohol. Clin. Exp. Res.* 22(7):1501-8.

Bearer C (2001) Markers to detect drinking during pregnancy. *Alcohol. Res. Health* 25(3):210-8.

Bearer CF, Jacobson JL, Jacobson SW, Barr D, Croxford J, Molteno CD, Viljoen DL, Marais AS, Chiodo LM, Cwik AS (2003) Validation of a new biomarker of fetal exposure to alcohol. *J. Pediatr.* 143(4):463-9.

Bearer CF LS, Savator AE, Minnes S, Swick A, Yamashita T, et al (1999) Ethyl linoleate in meconium: a biomarker for prenatal ethanol exposure. *Alcohol. Clin. Exp. Res.* 23:487-93.

Bedard K, Krause KH (2007) The NOX family of ROS-generating NADPH oxidases: physiology and pathophysiology. Physiol. Rev. 87(1):245-313.

Bellanti JA, Zeligs BJ (1995) Developmental aspects of pulmonary defenses in children. *Pediatr Pulmonol. Suppl.* 11:79-80.

Benjamin DK, Jr., Stoll BJ (2006) Infection in late preterm infants. *Clin. Perinatol.* 33(4):871-82; abstract x.

Best CA LM (2003) Fatty acid ethyl esters: toxi non-oxidative metabolites of ethanol and markers of ethanol intake. *Front Biosci.* 8:e202-217.

Biber KL, Moscatello KM, Dempsey DC, Chervenak R, Wolcott RM (1998) Effects of in utero alcohol exposure on B-cell development in the murine fetal liver. *Alcohol. Clin. Exp. Res.* 22(8):1706-12.

Bonfield TL, Raychaudhuri B, Malur A, Abraham S, Trapnell BC, Kavuru MS, Thomassen MJ (2003) PU.1 regulation of human alveolar macrophage differentiation requires granulocyte-macrophage colony-stimulating factor. *Am. J. Physiol. Lung Cell Mol. Physiol.* 285(5): L1132-6.

Bradley KA, Boyd-Wickizer J, Powell SH, Burman ML (1998) Alcohol screening questionnaires in women: a critical review. *Jama* 280(2):166-71.

Brown SD, Gauthier TW, Brown LA (2009) Impaired terminal differentiation of pulmonary macrophages in a Guinea pig model of chronic ethanol ingestion. *Alcohol. Clin. Exp. Res.* 33(10):1782-93.

Bruce SR, Atkins CL, Colasurdo GN, Alcorn JL (2009) Respiratory syncytial virus infection alters surfactant protein A expression in human pulmonary epithelial cells by reducing translation efficiency. *Am. J. Physiol. Lung Cell Mol. Physiol.* 297(4):L559-67.

Brzezinski MR, Boutelet-Bochan H, Person RE, Fantel AG, Juchau MR (1999) Catalytic activity and quantitation of cytochrome P-450 2E1 in prenatal human brain. *J. Pharmacol. Exp. Ther.* 289(3):1648-53.

Bustani P, Kotecha S (2003) Role of cytokines in hyperoxia mediated inflammation in the developing lung. *Front Biosci.* 8:s694-704.

Caprara DL BJ, Iqbal U, et al (2005) A Guinea Pig Model for the Identification of In utero Alcohol Exposure using Fatty Acid Ethyl Esters in neonatal hair. *Pediatric Research* 58(6):1158-1163.

Chang G, Goetz MA, Wilkins-Haug L, Berman S (1999) Identifying prenatal alcohol use: screening instruments versus clinical predictors. *Am. J. Addict.* 8(2):87-93.

Cherian PP, Schenker S, Henderson GI (2008) Ethanol-mediated DNA damage and PARP-1 apoptotic responses in cultured fetal cortical neurons. *Alcohol. Clin. Exp. Res.* 32(11):1884-92.

Chu J, Tong M, de la Monte SM (2007) Chronic ethanol exposure causes mitochondrial dysfunction and oxidative stress in immature central nervous system neurons. *Acta Neuropathol.* 113(6):659-73.

Cordero L, Rau R, Taylor D, Ayers LW (2004) Enteric gram-negative bacilli bloodstream infections: 17 years' experience in a neonatal intensive care unit. *Am. J. Infect. Control* 32(4):189-95.

Coyle P, Martin SA, Carey LC, Summers BL, Rofe AM (2009) Ethanol-mediated fetal dysmorphology and its relationship to the ontogeny of maternal liver metallothionein. *Alcohol. Clin. Exp. Res.* 33(6):1051-8.

Crouch E, Hartshorn K, Ofek I (2000) Collectins and pulmonary innate immunity. *Immunol. Rev.* 173:52-65.

De Dooy JJ, Mahieu LM, Van Bever HP (2001) The role of inflammation in the development of chronic lung disease in neonates. *Eur. J. Pediatr.* 160(8):457-63.

Dong J, Sulik KK, Chen SY (2008) Nrf2-mediated transcriptional induction of antioxidant response in mouse embryos exposed to ethanol in vivo: implications for the prevention of fetal alcohol spectrum disorders. *Antioxid Redox. Signal* 10(12):2023-33.

Dong J, Sulik KK, Chen SY (2010) The role of NOX enzymes in ethanol-induced oxidative stress and apoptosis in mouse embryos. *Toxicol. Lett.* 193(1):94-100.

Drews CD, Coles CD, Floyd RL, Falek A (2003) Prevalence of prenatal drinking assessed at an urban public hospital and a suburban private hospital. *J. Matern. Fetal. Neonatal. Med.* 13(2):85-93.

Ebrahim SH GJ (2003) Pregnancy-related substance use in the United States during 1996-1998. *Obstet Gynecol.* 101:374-379.

Ewald SJ, Frost WW (1987) Effect of prenatal exposure to ethanol on development of the thymus. *Thymus* 9(4):211-5.

Ewald SJ, Walden SM (1988) Flow cytometric and histological analysis of mouse thymus in fetal alcohol syndrome. *J. Leukoc. Biol.* 44(5):434-40.

Fels AO, Cohn ZA (1986) The alveolar macrophage. *J. Appl. Physiol.* 60(2):353-69.

Finer LB, Henshaw SK (2006) Disparities in rates of unintended pregnancy in the United States, 1994 and 2001. *Perspect Sex Reprod. Health* 38(2):90-6.

Floyd RL, Ebrahim S, Tsai J, O'Connor M, Sokol R (2006) Strategies to reduce alcohol-exposed pregnancies. *Matern Child Health J.* 10(5 Suppl):S149-51.

Gauthier TW, Drews-Botsch C, Falek A, Coles C, Brown LA (2005a) Maternal alcohol abuse and neonatal infection. *Alcohol. Clin. Exp. Res.* 29(6):1035-43.

Gauthier TW, Manar MH, Brown LAS (2004) Is maternal alcohol use a risk factor for early-onset sepsis in the premature newborn? *Alcohol* 33:139-145.

Gauthier TW, Ping XD, Harris FL, Wong M, Elbahesh H, Brown LA (2005b) Fetal alcohol exposure impairs alveolar macrophage function via decreased glutathione availability. *Pediatr Res.* 57(1):76-81.

Gauthier TW, Young PA, Gabelaia L, Tang SM, Ping XD, Harris FL, Brown LA (2009) In utero ethanol exposure impairs defenses against experimental group B streptococcus in the term Guinea pig lung. *Alcohol. Clin. Exp. Res.* 33(2):300-6.

Gemma S, Vichi S, Testai E (2006) Individual susceptibility and alcohol effects:biochemical and genetic aspects. *Ann. Ist Super Sanita* 42(1):8-16.

Gemma S, Vichi S, Testai E (2007) Metabolic and genetic factors contributing to alcohol induced effects and fetal alcohol syndrome. *Neurosci. Biobehav. Rev.* 31(2):221-9.

Grant TM, Huggins JE, Sampson PD, Ernst CC, Barr HM, Streissguth AP (2009) Alcohol use before and during pregnancy in western Washington, 1989-2004: implications for the prevention of fetal alcohol spectrum disorders. *Am. J. Obstet. Gynecol.* 200(3):278 e1-8.

Green CR, Watts LT, Kobus SM, Henderson GI, Reynolds JN, Brien JF (2006) Effects of chronic prenatal ethanol exposure on mitochondrial glutathione and 8-iso-prostaglandin F2alpha concentrations in the hippocampus of the perinatal guinea pig. *Reprod. Fertil. Dev.* 18(5):517-24.

Grisel JJ, Chen WJ (2005) Antioxidant pretreatment does not ameliorate alcohol-induced Purkinje cell loss in the developing rat cerebellum. *Alcohol. Clin. Exp. Res.* 29(7):1223-9.

Gundogan F, Elwood G, Mark P, Feijoo A, Longato L, Tong M, de la Monte SM (2009) Ethanol-Induced Oxidative Stress and Mitochondrial Dysfunction in Rat Placenta: Relevance to Pregnancy Loss. *Alcohol. Clin. Exp. Res.*

Hall CB, Weinberg GA, Iwane MK, Blumkin AK, Edwards KM, Staat MA, Auinger P, Griffin MR, Poehling KA, Erdman D, Grijalva CG, Zhu Y, Szilagyi P (2009) The burden of respiratory syncytial virus infection in young children. *N. Engl. J. Med.* 360(6):588-98.

Hall SL, Sherman MP (1992) Intrapulmonary bacterial clearance of type III group B streptococcus is reduced in preterm compared with term rabbits and occurs independent of antibody. *Am. Rev. Respir. Dis.* 145(5):1172-7.

Hewitt AJ, Walker KR, Kobus SM, Poklewska-Koziell M, Reynolds JN, Brien JF Differential effects of chronic ethanol exposure on cytochrome P450 2E1 and the hypothalamic-pituitary-adrenal axis in the maternal-fetal unit of the guinea pig. *Neurotoxicol. Teratol.* 32(2):164-70.

Hines RN, McCarver DG (2002) The ontogeny of human drug-metabolizing enzymes: phase I oxidative enzymes. *J. Pharmacol. Exp. Ther.* 300(2):355-60.

Hunter CJ, Upperman JS, Ford HR, Camerini V (2008) Understanding the susceptibility of the premature infant to necrotizing enterocolitis (NEC). *Pediatr Res.* 63(2):117-23.

Izurieta HS, Thompson WW, Kramarz P, Shay DK, Davis RL, DeStefano F, Black S, Shinefield H, Fukuda K (2000) Influenza and the rates of hospitalization for respiratory disease among infants and young children. *N. Engl. J. Med.* 342(4):232-9.

Jobe AH, Ikegami M (1998) Mechanisms initiating lung injury in the preterm. *Early Hum. Dev.* 53(1):81-94.

Jobe AH, Ikegami M (2001) Prevention of bronchopulmonary dysplasia. *Curr. Opin. Pediatr* 13(2):124-9.

Johnson S, Knight R, Marmer DJ, Steele RW (1981) Immune deficiency in fetal alcohol syndrome. *Pediatr Res.* 15(6):908-11.

Jones DP (2006) Extracellular redox state: refining the definition of oxidative stress in aging. *Rejuvenation Res*. 9(2):169-81.

Jones DP, Go YM, Anderson CL, Ziegler TR, Kinkade JM, Jr., Kirlin WG (2004) Cysteine/cystine couple is a newly recognized node in the circuitry for biologic redox signaling and control. *Faseb J.* 18(11):1246-8.

Jones KL SD (1973) Recognition of the fetal alcohol syndrome in early infancy. *Lancet* 2:999-1001.

Joshi PC, Applewhite L, Mitchell PO, Fernainy K, Roman J, Eaton DC, Guidot DM (2006) GM-CSF receptor expression and signaling is decreased in lungs of ethanol-fed rats. *Am. J. Physiol. Lung Cell Mol. Physiol.* 291(6):L1150-8.

Joshi PC, Applewhite L, Ritzenthaler JD, Roman J, Fernandez AL, Eaton DC, Brown LA, Guidot DM (2005) Chronic ethanol ingestion in rats decreases granulocyte-macrophage colony-stimulating factor receptor expression and downstream signaling in the alveolar macrophage. *J. Immunol.* 175(10):6837-45.

Kaphalia BS, Cai P, Khan MF, Okorodudu AO, Ansari GA (2004) Fatty acid ethyl esters: markers of alcohol abuse and alcoholism. *Alcohol* 34(2-3):151-8.

Kemp M, Go YM, Jones DP (2008) Nonequilibrium thermodynamics of thiol/disulfide redox systems: a perspective on redox systems biology. *Free Radic. Biol. Med.* 44(6):921-37.

Klein J KT, Korent G (1999) Fatty acid ethyl esters: a novel biologic marker for heavy in utero ethanol exposure: a case report. *The Drug Monit.* 21:644-646.

Kramer BW, Ikegami M, Moss TJ, Nitsos I, Newnham JP, Jobe AH (2004) Antenatal betamethasone changes cord blood monocyte responses to endotoxin in preterm lambs. *Pediatr Res.* 55(5):764-8.

Kramer BW, Ikegami M, Moss TJ, Nitsos I, Newnham JP, Jobe AH (2005) Endotoxin-induced chorioamnionitis modulates innate immunity of monocytes in preterm sheep. *Am. J. Respir. Crit. Care Med.* 171(1):73-7.

Kurland G, Cheung AT, Miller ME, Ayin SA, Cho MM, Ford EW (1988) The ontogeny of pulmonary defenses: alveolar macrophage function in neonatal and juvenile rhesus monkeys. *Pediatr Res*. 23(3):293-7.

Kuroki Y, Takahashi M, Nishitani C (2007) Pulmonary collectins in innate immunity of the lung. *Cell Microbiol*. 9(8):1871-9.

Lange LG BS, Sobel BE (1981) Identification of fatty acid ethyl esters as products of rabbit myocardial ethanol metabolism. *J. Biol. Chem.* 256:12968-73.

Laposata EA LL (1986) Presence of Nonoxidative Ethanol Metabolism in Human Organs Commonly Damaged by Ethanol Abuse. *Science* 231(4737):497-499.

Laposata M (1998) Fatty Acid Ethyl Esters: Ethanol Metabolites which mediate ethanol-induced organ damage and serve as markers of ethanol intake. *Prog. Lipid Res.* 37(5):307-316.

Laposata M (1999) Fatty acid ethyl esters: current facts and speculations. *Prostaglandins Leukot Essent Fatty Acids* 60:313-315.

Lazic T, Wyatt TA, Matic M, Meyerholz DK, Grubor B, Gallup JM, Kersting KW, Imerman PM, Almeida-De-Macedo M, Ackermann MR (2007) Maternal alcohol ingestion reduces surfactant protein A expression by preterm fetal lung epithelia. *Alcohol* 41(5):347-55.

Lester BM, ElSohly M, Wright LL, Smeriglio VL, Verter J, Bauer CR, Shankaran S, Bada HS, Walls HH, Huestis MA, Finnegan LP, Maza PL (2001) The Maternal Lifestyle

Study: drug use by meconium toxicology and maternal self-report. *Pediatrics* 107(2):309-17.

LeVine AM, Elliott J, Whitsett JA, Srikiatkhachorn A, Crouch E, DeSilva N, Korfhagen T (2004) Surfactant protein-d enhances phagocytosis and pulmonary clearance of respiratory syncytial virus. *Am. J. Respir. Cell Mol. Biol.* 31(2):193-9.

Lin PW, Nasr TR, Stoll BJ (2008) Necrotizing enterocolitis: recent scientific advances in pathophysiology and prevention. *Semin. Perinatol.* 32(2):70-82.

Little BB SL, Rosenfeld CR, Gilstrap LC, 3rd, Gant NF (1990) Failure to recognize fetal alcohol syndrome in newborn infants. *Am. J. Dis. Child* 144:1142-1146.

Louie JK, Schechter R, Honarmand S, Guevara HF, Shoemaker TR, Madrigal NY, Woodfill CJ, Backer HD, Glaser CA (2006) Severe pediatric influenza in California, 2003-2005: implications for immunization recommendations. *Pediatrics* 117(4):e610-8.

Lyon A (2000) Chronic lung disease of prematurity. The role of intra-uterine infection. *Eur. J. Pediatr* 159(11):798-802.

Maffi SK, Rathinam ML, Cherian PP, Pate W, Hamby-Mason R, Schenker S, Henderson GI (2008) Glutathione content as a potential mediator of the vulnerability of cultured fetal cortical neurons to ethanol-induced apoptosis. *J. Neurosci. Res.* 86(5):1064-76.

Maisto SA, Connors GJ, Allen JP (1995) Contrasting self-report screens for alcohol problems: a review. *Alcohol. Clin. Exp. Res.* 19(6):1510-6.

Mattson SN, Riley EP, Gramling L, Delis DC, Jones KL (1997) Heavy prenatal alcohol exposure with or without physical features of fetal alcohol syndrome leads to IQ deficits. *J. Pediatr* 131(5):718-21.

McGill J, Meyerholz DK, Edsen-Moore M, Young B, Coleman RA, Schlueter AJ, Waldschmidt TJ, Cook RT, Legge KL (2009) Fetal exposure to ethanol has long-term effects on the severity of influenza virus infections. *J. Immunol.* 182(12):7803-8.

Ojeda ML, Nogales F, Jotty K, Barrero MJ, Murillo ML, Carreras O (2009) Dietary selenium plus folic acid as an antioxidant therapy for ethanol-exposed pups. *Birth Defects Res. B Dev. Reprod. Toxicol.* 86(6):490-5.

Olivares IP, Bucio L, Souza V, Carabez A, Gutierrez-Ruiz MC (1997) Comparative study of the damage produced by acute ethanol and acetaldehyde treatment in a human fetal hepatic cell line. *Toxicology* 120(2):133-44.

Pargst F SK, Sporkert F, Bohnenkamp M (2000) Are there possibilities for the detection of chronically increased alcohol consumption by hair analysis? *Forensic. Sci. int.* 107:201-23.

Ping XD, Harris FL, Brown LA, Gauthier TW (2007) In vivo dysfunction of the term alveolar macrophage after in utero ethanol exposure. *Alcohol. Clin. Exp. Res.* 31(2):308-16.

Prieto J, Eklund A, Patarroyo M (1994) Regulated expression of integrins and other adhesion molecules during differentiation of monocytes into macrophages. *Cell Immunol.* 156(1):191-211.

Rasheed A, Hines RN, McCarver-May DG (1997) Variation in induction of human placental CYP2E1: possible role in susceptibility to fetal alcohol syndrome? *Toxicol. Appl. Pharmacol.* 144(2):396-400.

Refaai MA NP, Steffensen TS, et al (2002) Liver and Adipose Tissue Fatty acid ethyl esters obtained at autopsy are postmortem markers for premortem ethanol intake. *Drug Monitoring and Toxicology* 48(1):77-83.

Reyes E, Ott S, Robinson B (1993) Effects of in utero administration of alcohol on glutathione levels in brain and liver. *Alcohol. Clin. Exp. Res.* 17(4):877-81.

Robbins C (1994) Chemical and physical behavior of humann hair. New York: Springer Verlag 71:79-84.

Russell M, Martier SS, Sokol RJ, Mudar P, Jacobson S, Jacobson J (1996) Detecting risk drinking during pregnancy: a comparison of four screening questionnaires. *Am. J. Public Health* 86(10):1435-9.

Sampson PD SA, Bookstein FL, Little RE, Clarren SK, Dehaene P, et al (1997) Incidence of Fetal Alcohol Syndrome and Prevalence of Alcohol-related neurodevelopmental disorder. *Teratology* 56:317-326.

Sari Y (2009) Activity-dependent neuroprotective protein-derived peptide, NAP, preventing alcohol-induced apoptosis in fetal brain of C57BL/6 mouse. *Neuroscience* 158(4):1426-35.

Sarkola T, Eriksson CJ, Niemela O, Sillanaukee P, Halmesmaki E (2000) Mean cell volume and gamma-glutamyl transferase are superior to carbohydrate-deficient transferrin and hemoglobin-acetaldehyde adducts in the follow-up of pregnant women with alcohol abuse. *Acta Obstet Gynecol. Scand.* 79(5):359-66.

Siler-Marsiglio KI, Pan Q, Paiva M, Madorsky I, Khurana NC, Heaton MB (2005) Mitochondrially targeted vitamin E and vitamin E mitigate ethanol-mediated effects on cerebellar granule cell antioxidant defense systems. *Brain Res.* 1052(2):202-11.

Sokol RJ, Janisse JJ, Louis JM, Bailey BN, Ager J, Jacobson SW, Jacobson JL (2007) Extreme prematurity: an alcohol-related birth effect. *Alcohol. Clin. Exp. Res.* 31(6):1031-7.

Sorensen GL, Husby S, Holmskov U (2007) Surfactant protein A and surfactant protein D variation in pulmonary disease. *Immunobiology* 212(4-5):381-416.

Sozo F, O'Day L, Maritz G, Kenna K, Stacy V, Brew N, Walker D, Bocking A, Brien J, Harding R (2009) Repeated ethanol exposure during late gestation alters the maturation and innate immune status of the ovine fetal lung. *Am. J. Physiol. Lung Cell Mol. Physiol.* 296(3):L510-8.

Standiford TJ, Kunkel SL, Lukacs NW, Greenberger MJ, Danforth JM, Kunkel RG, Strieter RM (1995) Macrophage inflammatory protein-1 alpha mediates lung leukocyte recruitment, lung capillary leak, and early mortality in murine endotoxemia. *J. Immunol.* 155(3):1515-24.

Stoler JM, Huntington KS, Peterson CM, Peterson KP, Daniel P, Aboagye KK, Lieberman E, Ryan L, Holmes LB (1998) The prenatal detection of significant alcohol exposure with maternal blood markers [see comments]. *J. Pediatr.* 133(3):346-52.

Stoll BJ, Hansen N (2003) Infections in VLBW infants: studies from the NICHD Neonatal Research Network. *Semin. Perinatol.* 27(4):293-301.

Stoll BJ, Hansen N, Fanaroff AA, Wright LL, Carlo WA, Ehrenkranz RA, Lemons JA, Donovan EF, Stark AR, Tyson JE, Oh W, Bauer CR, Korones SB, Shankaran S, Laptook AR, Stevenson DK, Papile LA, Poole WK (2002) Late-onset sepsis in very low birth weight neonates: the experience of the NICHD Neonatal Research Network. *Pediatrics* 110(2 Pt 1):285-91.

Stoll BJ, Hansen NI, Adams-Chapman I, Fanaroff AA, Hintz SR, Vohr B, Higgins RD (2004) Neurodevelopmental and growth impairment among extremely low-birth-weight infants with neonatal infection. *JAMA* 292(19):2357-65.

Stoll BJ, Holman RC, Schuchat A (1998) Decline in sepsis-associated neonatal and infant deaths in the United States, 1979 through 1994. *Pediatrics* 102(2):e18.

Taylor AN, Tio DL, Chiappelli F (1999) Thymocyte development in male fetal alcohol-exposed rats. *Alcohol. Clin. Exp. Res.* 23(3):465-70.

Ursitti F KJ, Koren G (1997) Clinical utilization of the neonatal hair test for cocaine: a four-year experience in Toronto. *Biol. Neonate* 72:345-351.

Wentzel P, Rydberg U, Eriksson UJ (2006) Antioxidative treatment diminishes ethanol-induced congenital malformations in the rat. *Alcohol. Clin. Exp. Res.* 30(10):1752-60.

Wolcott RM, Jennings SR, Chervenak R (1995) In utero exposure to ethanol affects postnatal development of T- and B-lymphocytes, but not natural killer cells. *Alcohol. Clin. Exp. Res.* 19(1):170-6.

Wright JR (2004) Host defense functions of pulmonary surfactant. *Biol. Neonate* 85(4): 326-32.

Yan D, Dong J, Sulik KK, Chen SY (2010) Induction of the Nrf2-driven antioxidant response by tert-butylhydroquinone prevents ethanol-induced apoptosis in cranial neural crest cells. *Biochem. Pharmacol.*

Zakhari S (2006) Overview: how is alcohol metabolized by the body? *Alcohol. Res. Health* 29(4):245-54.

Zhang X, Sliwowska JH, Weinberg J (2005) Prenatal alcohol exposure and fetal programming: effects on neuroendocrine and immune function. *Exp. Biol. Med.* (Maywood) 230(6):376-88.

Zhu X, Seelig LL, Jr. (2000) Developmental aspects of intestinal intraepithelial and lamina propria lymphocytes in the rat following placental and lactational exposure to ethanol. *Alcohol. Alcohol.* 35(1):25-30.

In: Pregnancy and Alcohol Consumption
Editor: Joshua D. Hoffman, pp. 195-223

ISBN 978-1-61761-122-3


*Chapter 7*

# ALCOHOL-PREGNANCY AND PLACENTAL HYPOXIA VERSUS FETAL DEVELOPMENT

***Cleofina Bosco[*] and Eugenia Díaz***
Anatomy and Developmental Biology Program, Institute of Biomedical Sciences,
Faculty of Medicine, University of Chile.

## ABSTRACT

Sustained alcohol abuse by pregnant women is clearly on the rise, so their effects on pregnancy outcomes are important public health issues. Alcohol is one of the commonest teratogenic agents and its uncontrolled consumption by pregnant women can give rise to an irreversible condition in the child called Fetal Alcohol Syndrome (FAS). This syndrome is characterized by intrauterine growth restriction (IUGR), craniofacial malformations, physical and mental retardation and cardiac septal defects. However, FAS represents only a part of the spectrum of fetal alcohol effects on pregnancy. Another syndrome expressing a lesser degree of deformities associated to FAS, some times unnoticeable except by close examination, is the Fetal Alcohol Effect (FAE), which only characteristic is a variable degree of mental retardation.

It must be emphasized that all children of mothers who abuse consume of alcohol during pregnancy do not necessarily develop FAS/FAE. This fact suggests that there may be others factors involved, besides the degree of exposure to alcohol, which predisposed the fetus to FAS/FAE syndrome. The potential source of individual variability includes differences in the pattern, frequency and duration of the period of drinking, differences in maternal, fetal and placental metabolism of ethanol/acetaldehyde, as well as genetic factors.

In addition, studies in animal models suggest that acetaldehyde, the primary hepatic oxidative metabolite of ethanol, reaches the fetus either by placental production or placental transference. Acetaldehyde may contribute to alter placental function, which in turn could affect fetal growth and development. The most likely hypothesis regarding the decrease of fetal growth is thought to be via hypoxia and increased oxidative stress,

* Corresponding author: Dr. Cleofina Bosco, Laboratorio de Placenta y Desarrollo Fetal, Programa de Anatomía y Biología del Desarrollo, ICBM, Facultad de Medicina, Universidad de Chile, Independencia 1027, Casilla 70079, Santiago 7, CHILE, Phone : 56-2-6786783, Fax : 56-2-6786264, E-mail : cbosco@med.uchile.cl

which interfere with cellular processes that require oxygen in order to function adequately, e.g. placental transport.

This review summarizes recent findings on placental hypoxia, oxidative stress and fetal development that may play a role in the impairment of the normal transference of essential fetal metabolites that could be related with FAS/FAE syndrome.

## INTRODUCTION

The fetotoxic effects of maternal alcohol consumption have been widely documented for over three decades, but yet the mechanisms underlying this devastating phenomenon remain uncertain. Pregnancy recognition in most women does not occur until 4 to 6 weeks of gestation (Floyd et al., 1999), and thus many women may drink alcohol prior to realizing they are pregnant. Upon recognition of pregnancy, most women spontaneously reduce their alcohol use. Hence, fetal alcohol exposure prior to and after pregnancy outcomes are important public health concerns (Floyd et al., 2009). The wide variety of cellular/biochemical effects of alcohol on fetal tissues is itself a puzzle and strongly suggests that fetotoxic responses to alcohol reflect a multifactorial setting. Many of these responses can be conceptually connected to effects on plasmatic membrane structure and function (Henderson et al., 1999).

Alcohol is one of the commonest teratogenic agents and can give rise to an irreversible condition in the child called Fetal Alcohol Syndrome (FAS). This syndrome, described by Jones and Smith (1973), is mainly characterized by intrauterine growth retardation (IUGR), craniofacial malformations, physical and mental retardation and cardiac septal defects. However, FAS represents only a part of the spectrum of fetal alcohol effects. Another syndrome expressing a lesser degree of the FAS associated deformities, some times unnoticeable except by close examination, is the Fetal Alcohol Effect (FAE), (Chaudhuri, 2000), a term proposed by the Fetal Alcohol Study Group of the Research Society on Alcoholism, which only characteristic is a variable degree of mental retardation (Rosett, 1980).

Maternal ethanol ingestion may cause fetal injury, particularly impaired somatic and brain growth, by at least two mechanisms: i) directly, by fetotoxicity from ethanol and /or acetaldehyde; ii) indirectly, by ethanol induced placental injury and selective fatal malnutrition (Fisher and Karl, 1988).

Accurate information regarding the risks of alcohol consumption during pregnancy is needed for the implementation of programs of health promotion and prevention strategies. Additionally, in order to understand better the teratogenic effects of alcohol, this article review the normal process of placental and human development that can be affected by teratogenic agents.

## DEVELOPMENT PROCESS

The human fetus is formed from the fertilization of the oocyte by the sperm at the oviduct. After fertilization the nuclei of the sperm and oocyte fuse to form a new cell (the zygote). This cell contains 46 chromosomes, 23 from each parent cell. As the zygote travels to the uterus, it divides, forming a cluster of cells (the morula) by about 3 days after fertilization. As the morula enters the uterine cavity, fluid penetrates into it to form the blastocyst. The epithelial outer wall of this structure is the trophoblast, and the inner cell mass is the embryoblast. During implantation, the trophoblast differentiates into two layers, the syncytiotrophoblast and the cytotrophoblast. The former is external and has many nuclei and a continuous cytoplasm forming a syncytium. The cytotrophoblast consists of a layer of ovoid cells immediately under the syncytiotrophoblast. Both structures contribute to the formation of the villi and ultimately the placenta. During placentation, cytotrophoblast cells localized in floating and anchoring villi follow two distinct pathways of differentiation (Cross et al., 1994). Villous cytotrophoblast fuse to form the syncytiotrophoblast layer that contributes to the exchange of gas and nutrient, as well as waste elimination. In anchoring villi, cytotrophoblast generates a multilayered column of highly invasive extravillous trophoblast (EVT) that later migrate into decidua and remodels the endometrial spiral arterioles to produce the low-resistance vascular system that is essential for fetal growth (Aplin, 1991).

Human embryogenesis takes place in a hypoxic environment because the trophoblast shell excludes the entry of maternal blood. This low-oxygen environment is essential for normal embryonic and placental development because the early conceptus has little protection against oxygen-generated free radicals. The first fetal-placental villi develop as trophoblast sprouts. These are invaded by extraembryonic mesoderm to form secondary villi and are transformed, by vasculogenesis, into tertiary villi. The placental barrier to maternal blood is gradually breached between 8-12 weeks of gestation, due to invasion of placental-bed uteroplacental spiral arteries by the EVT, and consequently placental oxygen tension thus rise (Kingdom and Kaufmann, 1999). This developmental period is characterized by an important physiological switch of the oxygen tension at the opening of the intervillous space (Genbacev et al., 1997).

In addition, the embryoblast cells mass give rise to a flat disc-shaped structure, the bilaminar germ disc. This structure consists of two layers of cells, the epiblast and the hypoblast. Further, the primitive streak is formed on the surface of the epiblast. The cells of the epiblast layer migrate towards the primitive streak to form the mesoderm layer between the epiblast layer and the hypoblast layer (gastrulation process) to structure the trilaminar germ disc: ectoderm, mesoderm and endoderm germ layers.

These three germ layers are responsible for the formation of all the body organ systems. The ectodermal germ layer gives rise to the nervous system, the retina of the eye and the epidermal layer of the skin. The mesoderm germ layer gives rise to the cardiovascular system and most part of the musculoskeletal system and the genitourinary system. The endoderm germ layer gives rise to the gastrointestinal system.

Alcohol effects on the described developmental processes probably acts through multiple mechanisms and a range of disabilities has been observed in the absence of dysmorphic features, reflecting variable degrees of damage during fetal development. It is reasonably to assume that timing and degree of exposure are important factors that contribute to this variation (Chudley et al., 2005).

## Placental Functions

The passage of nutrients from the maternal blood to the fetus is mediated by the placenta, an organ that establishes functional connections that are critical for embryonic survival (Cross et al., 1994). It mediates implantation and establishes the interface for nutrient and gas exchange between the maternal and fetal circulation, as well as initiating maternal recognition of pregnancy, altering the immune environment and the maternal cardiovascular and metabolic functions through the production of paracrine and endocrine hormones (Cross, 2006). The placenta transports oxygen, nutrients and antibodies to the fetus by means of the umbilical vein; removes carbon dioxide and metabolic wastes from the fetus by the two umbilical arteries; serves as a protective barrier against harmful effects of certain drugs and microorganisms; acts as a partial barrier between the mother and fetus to prevent fetal and maternal blood from mixing; and produces steroid and peptide hormones essential for maintaining the pregnancy: estrogen, progesterone, and human chorionic gonadotropin (HCG), (Bosco, 2005).

Adequate exchange across the placenta is essential for normal fetal metabolism and growth. The barrier that separates maternal and fetal blood in the human placenta is classified as villous hemomonochorial. It is composed of one layer of trophoblast and the fetal capillary endothelium (Enders, 1965; Bosco , 1994).

One of the earlier review in which the fetal consequences of ethanol-induced disruption of placental transport of nutrients, hypoxia, and calcium-handling mechanisms pinpointed distribution of ethanol onto the lipid membrane of the placental cell as one agent affecting the action of ion channels and proteins (Michaelis, 1990).

Furthermore, the placenta generates reactive oxygen species (ROS) which may contribute to the oxidative stress observed even in normal pregnancy, but this is increased in pregnancies complicated by preeclampsia, IUGR and pregestational diabetes where oxidative stress and nitrative stress are increased (Webster et al., 2008; Myatt, 2010).

In humans, the occurrence of prenatal exposure to ethanol is difficult to validate objectively. In order to assess intrauterine exposure to alcohol, increased concentration of fatty acid ethyl ester (FAEE), nonoxidative ethanol metabolites in the meconium of the newborn has been proposed as a novel screening method (Chan et al., 2004, Brien et al., 2006). Recently, Gareri et al., (2009) demonstrate that identical maternal ethanol exposure levels produced differing levels of fetal exposure in a dizygotic human twin pair. This was also observed in guinea pig littermates through FAEE meconium analysis. The authors concluded that the placenta may have a previously unappreciated role in mediating ethanol induced fetal injury.

## Oxidative Stress in the Fetal Development

Exposure to the developing placenta, embryo or fetus to environmental agents like alcohol or acetaldehyde is known to produce anatomical anomalies leading to *in utero* death or structural birth defects (Gundogan et al., 2008), commonly termed teratogenesis (Wells et al,, 2009). The cellular mechanisms by which ethanol induce damage *in utero* are not well understood, while induction of oxidative stress is believed to be a putative mechanism due to an imbalance in prooxidant and antioxidant levels (Cohen-Kerem and Koren, 2003). Ethanol can induce oxidative stress directly and indirectly. The direct effect is achieved by the formation of free radicals, including hydroxyl and hydroxyethyl groups, which are reacting with various cellular components. Formation of free radicals in the presence of ethanol was demonstrated in cell lines such as rat hepatocytes (Henderson et al,, 1995) and in animals such as rats (Reinke et al,, 1987). The cellular damage caused by free radicals is a consequence of the peroxidation of lipids, nucleic acids and alterations of enzyme activity (Rodrigo et al., 2005). Another direct oxidative stress effect of ethanol is the formation of ROS, (Dong et al., 2010). These are formed as biological products of molecular oxygen reduction (Fridovich, 1978) and they probably play a role in mediating programmed cell death (Jacobson, 1996; Dong et al., 2010).

The formation of ROS induced by cytochrome P-450 2E1 (CYP2E1) is mostly observed in the brain (Montoliu et al,, 1994) and the liver (Morimoto et al,, 1998), organs in which the enzyme is abundant. Formation of ROS is also induced by mitochondria in hepatocytes exposed to ethanol and is probably achieved by reduction in mitochondria-derived components of electron transport (Bailey and Cunningham, 1998).

Oxidative stress mechanism seems to operate in diabetes-induced embryonic damage as well as in the mechanism of teratogenicity caused by hypoxia and alcohol use (Ornoy, 2007). In addition, abnormal placentation may also cause enhanced placental oxidative stress, resulting in embryonic death, preeclampsia or congenital anomalies (Ornoy, 2007). Ethanol can also induce oxidative stress indirectly by reducing intracellular antioxidant capacity, such as the levels of glutathione peroxidase. In rats, chronic ethanol consumption decreased significantly cytosolic and mitochondrial glutathione peroxidase activities by 40% and 30%, respectively, and caused a parallel increase of the oxidative modification of proteins in hepatocytes (Oh et al,, 1998; Bailey et al, 2001). The reason for the reduced activity of glutathione peroxidase might lie in the decreased mitochondrial pool size of glutathione because entry of cytosolic glutathione into mitochondria is impaired (Fernandez-Checa, 1991).

Enhanced production of ROS has also been suggested to be involved in the teratogenic process of ethanol-exposed pregnancy in experimental animals (Kotch et al., 1995; Chen and Sulik, 1996; Henderson et al., 1999; Chen et al., 2000) and pregnant women (Kay et al., 2000).

Developing embryos seem to be very sensitive to high levels of ROS, especially during early organogenesis. High levels of oxygen are toxic to the embryo and fetus, apparently due to the fact that ROS created in such a condition are in excess in relation to the antioxidant capacity of the developing embryos, leading to the production of highly reactive oxygen or nitrogen species and creating oxidative stress and embryonic damage, (Ornoy, 2007).

The effects of ROS and oxidative stress on placental, embryonic and fetal development may adversely alter the development by oxidative damage on the cellular lipids, proteins and DNA, and/or by altering signal transduction. Dysregulation of signal tranduction and/or macromolecular lesions can adversely alter cellular function or trigger apoptotic or necrotic cellular death (Wells et al,, 2009).

ROS such as hydrogen peroxide and hydroxyl radicals are formed via a variety of physiological and pathophysiological reactions, and ROS formation can be enhanced by xenobiotics (Fantel, 1996). To prevent free radical-induced cellular damage, the organism has developed a defence mechanism, the antioxidant system. This system includes antioxidant enzymes such as superoxide dismutase (SOD), catalase (CAT), glutathione peroxidase (GSHPx), and glutathione reductase (GSSGR) and low –molecular antioxidants such as glutathione and plasma proteins (Rodrigo et al, 2005). Although the levels of most antioxidative enzymes, with the exception of glucose-6-phosphate dehydrogenase (G6PD), are low in the embryo, there is some evidence that they nevertheless may provide protection against at least constitutive or physiological levels of ROS, if not drug-enhanced ROS formation. (Wells et al., 2009). In addition to these, Henderson et al (1999) observed that ethanol induced oxidative stress in cultured fetal rat hepatocytes. The authors found that the supplementation with antioxidants or agents that enhance glutathione stores reversed these effects. The oxidative stress is associated with morphological and biochemical signs of mitochondrial damage. Ethanol inhibits activities of the mitochondrial respiratory chain components, a source that increased hydrogen peroxide, hydroxyl radicals, and lipid peroxidation products, along with signs of membrane damage. Additionally, the low antioxidant defences in fetal tissues and accumulation of toxic aldehyde products of lipid peroxidation predispose the fetus to oxidative damage. Wentzel et al., (2006) found that vitamin E treatment of pregnant chronic ethanol consuming rats diminishes fetal malformations. This study was in agreement with the study of Heaton et al., (2000), who blocked the effects of ethanol on Purkinje cells with the use of a very high dose of vitamin E. It seems likely that vitamins C and E could exert a protective effect by the reinforcement of antioxidant defences. An *in vitro* study reported evidence that vitamins C and E protect the strength and integrity of the chorioamnion from ROS-induced damage (Plessinger et al., 2000). However, some authors have not found a clear effect of antioxidant vitamin E supplementation (Tran et al., 2005), thereby raising the issue of the importance of dosage, and variable sensitivity in different tissues towards both, the deleterious effects of ethanol, as well as the beneficial effects of antioxidant vitamin E administration. Furthermore, Henderson et al., (1999) found that supplementation with antioxidants or agents that enhance glutathione stores reversed the oxidative stress induced by ethanol in cultured fetal rat hepatocytes. In addition, Wentzel and Ekiksson (2008) demonstrated in rat embryos (9-11 days of gestation) from 2 different rat strains exposed to 48 hours ethanol in early pregnancy, a role for genetic predisposition, oxidative stress, and apoptosis in ethanol teratogenicity, and suggested that the teratogenic predisposition of the more susceptible rat may reside, at least in part, in the regulation of the ROS scavenging enzymes. Folic acid acts also as an antioxidant, and Cano et al., (2001) studied the effects of folic acid on oxidative stress induced by ethanol. Two groups of pregnant rats were fed chronically with ethanol-supplemented tap water up to a mean of 8.9 ± 0.4g ethanol/kg/day for 3 weeks. Reduction in glutathione reductase was significant in the group that received the high dosage of folic acid. The amount of carbonyl group proteins in the liver and pancreas was also used as an index for oxidative damage. Levels of carbonyl groups were reduced significantly in the liver of offspring supplemented with folic acid but were unchanged in their pancreas. This study showed an association between FAS in an animal model and oxidative stress measurements and mitigation of those measures by using an antioxidant (Oh et al,, 1998; Bailey et al,, 2001). Finally, the study of Nasser et al., (2010) suggested that the antioxidant vitamin C can effectively reduce the severity of ethanol-induced brain injury and growth retardation by the modulation of γ-Aminobutiric acid receptor B ($GABA_B$ R) and protein kinase A-α (PKA) expression during early rat fetal development.

## Oxidative Stress in the Placenta

Placental pathology has long been associated with IUGR and preeclampsia (PE) in humans. However, it is important to note that the specific changes that are observed can be rather variable. The development of the placenta is highly regulated and is therefore quite susceptible to perturbation. Several genetic, epigenetic, nutritional and environmental factors have been identified and are associated with complications in pregnancy outcome, ranging from embryonic lethality to fetal growth restriction (Myllynen et al., 2005; Cross, 2006). Foreign compounds may interfere with placental functions at many levels such as signalling, production and release of hormones and enzymes, transport of nutrients and waste products, implantation, cellular growth and maturation, and finally in the delivery. Placental responses may also be due to alcohol/toxicodynamic responses, e.g. hypoxia (Myllynen et al., 2005). On the other hand, oxidative stress constitutes a unifying mechanism of injury of many types of disease processes. It occurs when there is an imbalance between the production of ROS and the ability of the biological system to readily detoxify these reactive intermediates or easily repair the resulting damage (Rodrigo et al., 2005). ROS such as hydrogen peroxide and hydroxyl radicals are formed via a variety of physiological and pathophysiological reactions, and ROS formation can be enhanced by xenobiotics (Wells et al., 2009). This mechanism seems to operate in alcohol ingest pregnancy (Ornoy, 2007), and Kay et al., (2000) demonstrated that ethanol exposure induces oxidative stress in the human placental villi, which may account for the decreased nitric oxide (NO) release, because NO may be shunted toward scavenging free radicals. The authors concluded that increased endothelial nitric oxide synthase (eNOS) protein expression may be a response to the increased demand for NO. Decreased NO availability could adversely affect placental blood flow regulation, which could, in turn, account for the restriction of growth seen in ethanol-exposed fetuses.

Pregnancy itself is a condition of increased susceptibility to oxidative stress, leading to potential tissue damage (Sies, 1991). Several organs in pregnant women show increased basal oxygen consumption and changes in substrate energy use. The production of ROS within the foetal–placental unit has special relevance due to its highly vascularised nature and since the tissue is rich in mitochondria, there is also an abundance of macrophages. At pregnancy term, the human placenta is hemomonochorial, meaning that only one chorionic trophoblast cell layer exists between maternal and foetal blood (Bosco 1994), which favours the exchange of gases, nutrients, and metabolic products. In turn, oxygen delivery is favoured by the lower partial pressure of oxygen, which raises lactic acid production and lowers pH, within the placental cells and foetal circulation. In addition, as the hypoxic placenta matures, vascularization develops to create an oxygen-rich environment. Moreover, the increasing mitochondrial mass favours the production of ROS (Liochev and Fridovich, 1997). Nitric oxide (NO) is also produced by the placenta (Dotsch et al., 2001), giving rise to another local source of free radicals, likely contributing to endothelial dysfunction.

In addition, the placenta is also rich in macrophages (Hofbauer cells), the local source of production of free radicals, including reactive chlorine species, might also contribute to the development of oxidative stress (Myatt and Cui, 2004). This view is based on the ability of Hofbauer cells to express both inducible nitric oxide synthase (iNOS) activity (Myatt et al., 1997) and NADPH oxidase activity (Matsubara et al., 2001), although studies on xanthine oxidase are still lacking. On the other hand, the defence mechanisms against ROS damage are also enhanced in pregnancy. Thus, a progressive increase in free radical scavengers, such as glutathione and bilirubin, as well as in the activity of antioxidant enzymes in placenta has been reported (Watson et al., 1997, 1998; Qanungo and Mukherjea, 2000).

Gundogan et al., (2010) demonstrated the impact of ethanol-mediated oxidative stress on placental trophoblast function and the potential impact on pregnancy loss. They found that chronic gestation exposure to ethanol suggest that rat placental apoptosis/necrosis are mediated through p21, Bax, and Bak via a p53-independent pathway. Additionally, ethanol mediates its adverse effect on pregnancy maintenance via inhibition of prolactin (PRL) family hormones (placental lactogen 1 and placental lactogen 2). Prolactin receptor (PRLR) is expressed by the uterine decidual cells (Gu et al., 1996) and interacts with PRL hormones to transmit signals that mediated trophoblastic cell functions needed to maintain pregnancy (Soares, 2004).

Finally, ethanol can be placentotoxic, impairing the normal transfer of amino acids, zinc, and glucose, (Fisher and Karl, 1988). Such restriction could occurs regardless of maternal nutritional status, which is known as selective fetal malnutrition (Fisher et al., 1982).

## Peroxynitrite Mediates Lipid Oxidation and Nitration

As the human fetal-placental vasculature lacks autonomic innervation, autocrine and or paracrine agents such as nitric oxide radical ($NO^{\cdot}$) play an important role in the regulation of fetal-placental blood flows (Myatt and Cui, 2004). This has been shown to maintain low-basal tone and attenuate the vasocontrictive effects of thromboxane and endothelin (Myatt et al., 1992, Kossenjan et al., 2000). However, $NO^{\cdot}$ is inactivated by superoxide anion ($O_2^{-\cdot}$), therefore limiting its activity. Conversely, the activity of NO is prolonged by the presence of SOD which removes superoxide. Superoxide is generated in living cells by NADPH oxidase, xantine oxidase, flavin enzymes, and enzymes in the mitochondrial electron transport chain. The reactivity due to the unpaired electron in superoxide then leads to the production of other ROS including the hydroxyl radical and hydrogen peroxide (Myatt et al., 1996; Myatt and Cui, 2004).

The action of superoxide *per se* is limited by its low lipid solubility, limited membrane transport and by its removal by SOD. However, when tissues are induced to simultaneously produce both NO and superoxide in a concentrated and localized manner by inflammatory stimuli, sepsis, and ischemia/reperfusion, NO and superoxide react to produce peroxynitrite anion ($ONOO^{-}$), a powerful oxidant of a variety of biomolecules (Beckman et al., 1990) which has cytotoxic activity and inhibits mitochondrial electron transport resulting in inhibition of cellular respiration (Radi et al., 1994). Under physiological conditions, the production of peroxynitrite will be low and oxidative damage minimized by endogenous antioxidant defences (Radi et al, 2002). The peroxynitrite anion is extremely unstable and consequently it is undetectable and the evidence of its formation *in vivo* has been indirect, via the occurrence of nitrated moieties including nitrated lipids, nitrated nucleotides and nitrotyrosine residues in proteins, (Pacher et al., 2007). Peroxynitrite is a product which reacts with a variety of biomolecules including proteins, lipids and DNA. It can damage DNA by introducing oxidative modifications in both the nucleobases as well as the sugar-phosphate backbone (Burney, 1999). Additionally, is a potent trigger of DNA strand breakage, with subsequent activation of the nuclear enzyme poly-ADP ribosyl synthetase (PARP), with considerable energy depletion and necrosis of the cells (Szabó, 2003). In addition, peroxynitrite cause lipid peroxidation, direct inhibition of the mitochondrial electron transporter system and nitrate tyrosine residues, inactivation of membrane sodium channels, and oxydize sulfhydril groups on proteins, hence altering their activity or disrupting signal transduction pathways (Ischropoulos et al., 1992) and the induction of cell death through both apoptosis and necrosis (Virag et al, 2003). It has been demonstrated that peroxynitrite interacts via direct oxidative reactions or via indirect,—radical-mediated mechanisms (Pacher.et al., 2007). Peroxynitrite may reach mitochondria either from extramitochondrial compartments or may be directly produced within the mitochondria. Indeed, mitochondria can produce both NO, by the activity of a $Ca^{2+}$ -sensitive mitochondrial NOS (mtNOS) (Brookers, 2004), and superoxide, following the partial reduction of oxygen within the mitochondrial matrix due to the natural leak of electron from the respiratory chain. A major physiological function of NO in the mitochondria is to regulate oxygen consumption by reversibly inhibiting cytochrome-*c* oxidase (complex IV of the electron transport chain) via competition with oxygen for the binuclear binding site (Palacios-Callender, 2004). In conditions of high NO production (e.g., during inflammation, reperfusion injury, or neuronal hyperactivation), the interruption of electron transfer at cytochrome oxidase markedly increases the leakage of electrons from the respiratory chain, resulting in enhanced formation of superoxide within the mitochondrial matrix and generation of significant amounts of peroxynitrite (Brown and Borutaite, 1999). The study of MacMillan-Crow and Thompson, (1999) demonstrated that peroxynitrite is the only known biological oxidant competent to inactivate enzymatic activity, nitrate critical tyrosine residues, and induce dityrosine formation in Mn-SOD.

The production of oxidants is a crucial mechanism through which neutrophils and macrophages cause damage or kill microorganisms. When peroxynitrite acts as an oxidant, it produces nitrite and hydroxide ion rather than isomerizing to nitrate. Consequently, the major decomposition products of superoxide and peroxynitrite formation in the phagosome are ultimately hydrogen peroxide and nitrite. Within a neutrophil or macrophage phagolysosome, this serves as a recycling mechanism to reutilize nitrite and hydrogen peroxide to generate more reactive species. These are also substrates for myeloperoxidase and can be a significant source of tyrosine nitration (Burner et al., 2000) due to the fact that myeloperoxidase reacts rapidly and directly with peroxynitrite to produce nitrogen dioxide and efficiently catalyzes tyrosine nitration (Floris et al., 1993). In recent years, it has become common to use nitrotyrosine as a marker of nitrosative stress. Furthermore, nitrotyrosine was first shown to be localized in human atherosclerotic lesions, vascular muscle (Beckmann et al., 1994) and recently in endothelial cells (Dickhout et al., 2005). In addition, Myatt et al., (1998) observed increased expression of nitrotirosine residues in the fetal vasculature and villous stroma of preeclamptic and diabetic placentas.

By other hand, disabling of several cytoskeletal proteins by nitration represents a further major cytotoxic effect attributed to peroxynitrite (Pacher et al., 2007). Tubulin nitration by peroxynitrite or by direct incorporation of free nitrotyrosine has been reported in cell lines derived from intestine (Banan et al., 2000), neurons (Tedeschi, 2005) and muscle (Chang, 2002), resulting in the loss of normal physiological functions. Peroxynitrite also disorganizes actin polymerization through actin nitration, and via the nitration of profiling (Kasina et al, 2005), an important actin-binding protein. These effects have been associated with platelet dysfunction (Kasina et al, 2006), disruption of both intestinal (Banan et al, 2001) and endothelial barrier function (Neumann et al, 2006), as well as impaired migration and phagocytosis of activated polymorphonuclear cells (Clements et al., 2003). It is important to note that the placenta function as intestine to absorb metabolites and it has also been demonstrated that peroxynitrite produce intestinal barrier dysfunction mediate by ethanol-induced microtubule disruption (Banan et al., 2000).

In addition, the placenta is an organ with a large surface to change metabolites, and a major aspect of peroxynitrite-dependent cytotoxicity relies on its ability to trigger lipid peroxidation in membranes (Radi et al., 1993), liposomes, and lipoproteins by removing of an hydrogen atom from polyunsaturated fatty acids (PUFA). Resulting products include lipid hydroperoxyradicals, conjugated dienes, and aldehydes (Denicola, 2005). Such radicals in turn attack neighboring PUFAs, generating additional radicals which propagate free radical reactions and the degeneration of membrane lipids (Radi et al., 1991), causing membrane permeability and fluidity changes with significant biological consequences. Peroxynitrite may play a critical role in inflammatory diseases of the nervous system by initiating peroxidation of myelin lipids, leading to demyelination (Shi, 1999).

Once the level of cellular damage inflicted by peroxynitrite supersedes any possibility of repair, the cell eventually dies via one of the two main pathways of cell demise, necrosis or apoptosis. Necrosis is associated with loss of cellular ATP, leading to membrane disruption, release of noxious cellular debris, and the development of secondary inflammation. In contrast, apoptosis occurs in a well-choreographed sequence of morphological events characterized by nuclear and cytoplasmic condensation with blebbing of the plasma membrane. The dying cell eventually breaks up into membrane-enclosed particles termed apoptotic bodies, which are rapidly ingested and degraded by professional phagocytes or neighboring cells, without inducing any inflammatory response. Apoptosis is orchestrated by the proteolytic activation of cysteine proteases known as caspases, that requires preserved ATP levels to proceed properly, and which may be triggered either by the activation of death receptors (extrinsic pathway) or by the permeabilization of the outer membrane of mitochondria (intrinsic pathway) (Newmeyer and Ferguson-Miller, 2003). Several mechanisms have been proposed to explain the activation of the apoptotic program by peroxynitrite, which appear largely dependent on the cell type studied and the experimental conditions (Virag et al., 2003). However, a common pathway involving the mitochondria and permeabilization of their outer membrane is emerging as a key feature of peroxynitrite-mediated apoptosis. Whereas apoptosis is a typical consequence of low to moderate concentrations of peroxynitrite, exposure of cells to higher concentrations of the oxidant has been associated with necrosis (Bonfoco et al., 1999; Virag et al., 2003). Studies investigating these processes have established that peroxynitrite-dependent cell necrosis is not a purely passive phenomenon, but instead is mediated by a complex process involving DNA damage and activation of the DNA repair enzyme PARP-1 (Szabo et al., 1996).

Olney et al, (2002) demonstrated that a single episode of ethanol intoxication, lasting for several hours, can trigger a massive wave of apoptotic neurodegeneration in the developing rat or mouse brain. The window of vulnerability coincides with the developmental period of synaptogenesis, also known as the brain growth-spurt period, which in rodents is a postnatal event, but in humans extends from the six month of gestation to several years after birth, (Ikonomidou et al., 2000).

Moreover, it has been demonstrated that peroxynitrite also selectively inactivates the prostacyclin receptor in endothelial cells (Zou et al., 1999) and decreases the amount of prostacyclin synthase through a mechanism mediated by nuclear factor kappa-B (NF-κB), (Cooke and Davidge, 2002). NF-κB is a transcription factor involved in the enhancement of the expression of various proinflammatory biochemical markers including cytokines, chemokines and cellular adhesion molecules (Baeuerle and Henkel, 1994; Baldwin, 1996). An inactive form of NF-κB is normally held in the cytoplasm, bound to inhibitory proteins, the I$\kappa$Bs. The first step in this cascade is the activation of cytoplasmic inactive dimmers of NF-κB, which are bound to I-κB. The critical step in NF$\kappa$B activation relies on its dissociation from the I$\kappa$B protein, secondary to phosphorylation and proteasomal degradation of I$\kappa$B. I$\kappa$Bs are phosphorylated by a protein kinase complex, I$\kappa$B kinase (IKK). The classical pathway of NF$\kappa$B activation mainly depends on IKK$\beta$ and triggers transcription of inflammatory and antiapoptotic genes (Chen et al., 2003, Bonizzi et al., 2004). The unbound dimmers so formed are translocated into the nucleus, bind to DNA, and activate inflammatory genes. The alternative pathway, which is dependent on IKK$\alpha$, has been shown to be important for B-cell maturation and lymphoid organ development (Senftleben et al., 2003).

## Placental Apoptosis

The morphological architecture and function of the human placenta depends on an adequate balance of proliferation, differentiation and apoptosis. In placentas from early pregnancy, cell proliferation, especially of cytotrophoblasts, is very high, but this diminishes constantly with the duration of pregnancy (Ishihara et al., 2000). In contrast, the rate of apoptosis is low throughout early pregnancy and only increases shortly before delivery (Smith et al., 1997). The maintenance of the homeostasis of these basic processes in the placenta is necessary for adequate growth and development of the fetus. An imbalance may result in spontaneous abortion, pre-eclampsia, preterm delivery and reduced fetal growth (Myatt, 2002; Crocker et al., 2003). In the last decade Huppertz et al (2006) have characterised the role of the apoptosis cascade in villous trophoblast turnover and syncytium formation. Their observations indicate that the process of syncytial fusion is linked to the ''initiator stages'' of the apoptosis cascade within the cytotrophoblast cells, whereas the extrusion of syncytial knots from the syncytiotrophoblast is the result of the final ''execution stages'' of the apoptosis cascade within the syncytiotrophoblast (Huppertz et al., 1998; Black et al., 2004). The balance between pro- and anti-apoptotic proteins determines whether apoptosis will be triggered or not. The family of caspase proteins includes intracellular proteases that cleave their targets next to an aspartic acid residue, thus termed cysteine aspartases or caspases. On the basis of structural homologies and substrate preferences, the family has been subdivided into subfamilies. All the members of the subfamily of the caspase 3-like caspases (caspases 3, 6, 7, 8, 9, and 10) play central roles in the apoptosis cascade (Huppertz et al., 2006; Miller, 1997). This subfamily is further divided into signalling/initiator caspases 8, 9, and 10 and effector/execution caspases 3, 6, and 7, 12, 13. The major difference between members of the 2 groups is that initiator caspases are active during the early, or reversible, stages of the apoptosis cascade, whereas activation of the so-called effector caspases is a subsequent transition that will ultimately lead to apoptotic cell death. The apoptosis cascade can be divided into three sets of sequential stages: *Initiation stages* include the induction of the cascade, e.g., by ligand-receptor interactions leading to first proteolytic events. *Execution stages* start with the activation of the execution caspases. Their activation is called the 'point of no return' since once activated; these proteases degrade a variety of proteins resulting in irreversible damage of the cell. *Apoptotic death* is the result of a very complex cascade of events that finally leads to the collapse of the nucleus and the cell itself. Even in this final stage the cell does not release intracellular components, thus avoiding inflammatory reactions (Huppertz et al., 1999).

Caspases are synthesized as inactive enzymes that require cleavage to exert their biologic roles. Initiator caspases 8 and 10 are activated in a subset of differentiated cytotrophoblasts, presumably destined for syncytial fusion (Huppertz et al., 2006). By contrast, effector caspases (3, 6, and 7) are expressed only in their inactive forms in the cytotrophoblast layer, (Burton et al., 2003). Activation of the initiator caspase 8 is achieved by ligand-receptor interactions, eg, interactions between tumor necrosis factor-a (TNF-a) and the TNF-receptor 1 (TNF-R1), (Yui et al., 1996; Huppertz et al., 1998). The crucial role of caspase 8 in preparing cytotrophoblasts for syncytial fusion was demonstrated by Black et al., (2004). Caspase 8 activity results in the cleavage of proteins linking the cytoskeleton to the plasma membrane such as alpha-fodrin, and in externalization of phosphatidylserine from the inner to the outer leaflet of the plasma membrane, a prerequisite for syncytial fusion. This is known to be a very early event during the initiation stages of apoptosis (Martin et al., 1995). Externalization of phosphatidylserine is used by cells as a signal for events such as the attraction of macrophages, induction of the coagulation cascade or induction of syncytial fusion (Huppertz et al., 1999). Subsequently initiator caspases cleave and thus activate a second subpopulation of caspases known as the execution caspases. Irreversible progression of the apoptosis cascade commences with activation of the latter. Execution caspase activation is tightly regulated by the bcl-2 family of mitochondrial proteins. The various members of this family promote (bad, bak, bax, bcl-xs, bik, hrk) or inhibit (A1, bcl-2, bcl-w, bcl-xL, bfl-1, brag-1, mcl-1, NR13) cleavage of execution caspases (Hockenberry et al. 1990 ). In general, once a cell has activated the effector caspase pathway, it will die by apoptosis within 24 hours. However, in the villous trophoblast, cytotrophoblast nuclei that enter the syncytiotrophoblast remain intact and viable for a few weeks. Once activated, the execution caspases, either directly or by means of other proteases, cleave a broad array of proteins critical for cell survival. The latter include intermediate filament proteins (such as Cytokeratin 18; Caulin et al., 1997), nuclear envelope proteins (such as lamins A and B; Greidinger et al., 1996), and DFF (DNA fragmentation factor) and other endonucleases resulting in specific fragmentation of DNA (Liu et al., 1997). It has been shown that cytokeratins 18, which is cleaved by caspase 3 or 7, are affected in the early stages of apoptosis (Leers et al., 1997). Additionally, the maintenance of trophoblast structure and specialized function is essential for the provision of adequate oxygen and nutrients to the fetus.

Apoptosis has been observed in placentas of normal human pregnancies, but placentas from women with preeclampsia (PE) or intrauterine growth restriction (IUGR) show enhanced apoptosis as compared to placentas of normal pregnant women (Allaire et al., 2000 ). The typical morphological signs of apoptosis (cellular shrinkage, membrane blebbing, nuclear condensation and fragmentation) are the final results of a complex biochemical cascade of events. The molecular mechanisms leading to apoptosis are complex, and include an ever-expanding list of signalling molecules such as the bcl-2 family of genes, the caspase-3 and NF$\kappa$B (Hetts, 1998).

## Alcohol and Pregnancy Hipertension

It has been demonstrated that pregnancy-induced hypertension contribute to low birth weight and preterm delivery. Although alcohol-associated hypertension is common among women who drink heavily (Asherio, et al., 1996; Seppa, et al., 1996), the effect of alcohol abuse on the course of hypertensive pregnancies has not been studied adequately. However, Mankes, et al., (1985) showed that alcohol administration during pregnancy increased hypertension, caused multiple birth defects, and increased fetal mortality in both normotensive and spontaneously hypertensive rats. In addition, Taylor et al., (1994), found that the pressure effect of ethanol in the isolated perfused human placental lobule may contribute to the pathogenesis of the fetal alcohol syndrome as well as represent an underlying mechanism of ethanol-induced hypertension.

PE is a serius pregnancy complication, affects 5-7% of all pregnancies, and is a leading cause of maternal and perinatal mortality. The placenta plays a pivotal role in the etiology of PE specially the trophoblast cells of the placenta. PE is a two stage disease. In the first stage, a defective implantation and placentation cause a reduction in uteroplacental perfusion and placental ischemia/hypoxia. Placental hypoxia may promote the release of a variety of factors to the maternal circulation. In the second stage, these factors initiate a cascade of cellular and molecular events leading to endothelial and vascular dysfunction (Caniggia et al., 2000). The latter leads to the maternal symptoms of the syndrome: hypertension, proteinuria and edema. The symptoms resolve spontaneously on placental delivery. Fetal complications of PE and IUGR are commonly attributed to clinical conditions that lead to underperperfusion and hypoxia to the placenta (Levy et al., 2002). The pathogenic mechanisms of PE converge on the vascular endothelium and numerous stimuli, including oxidative stress (Aban et al., 2004). Furtheremore, TNF-α and high glucose levels are well known to induce apoptosis in endothelial cells (Muschel et al., 1995).

## Neuroactive Steroid Responses to Hypoxic Stress

Compromised pregnancies can have serious effects on the fetal brain, the nature of which depends, in large part, on the occurring gestation time. Maternal stress, infections or problems with placentation can affect brain development due to changes in the delivery of oxygen and glucose to the brain, or the cytokine environment, leading to acute cell death (Hirst et al., 2009), particularly in vulnerable regions such as periventricular white matter, the hippocampus and the cerebellum (Inder et al., 1999; du Plessis and Volpe, 2002). Certain glial progenitor cells are highly susceptible to such insults. In addition, chronically suboptimal conditions during pregnancy dramatically increase the sensitivity of the fetal brain to further episodes of hypoxia/ischemia around the time of birth and in the immediate neonatal period. The resulting damage can lead to severe neuropathology including intellectual impairment and cerebral palsy (Inder et al., 1999).

The term neurosteroid has been used to refer to steroids synthesized *de novo* from cholesterol in the nervous system or alternatively when the last steps in synthesis take place in the nervous system. In pregnancy, a large proportion of the production of steroids that affect the fetal nervous system are derived from peripheral sources. Therefore, Hirst et al., (2009) used the term neuroactive steroids to refer to steroids that influence fetal or maternal nervous system function and may be synthesized both in the nervous system and/or other peripheral organs. Pregnancy is characterized by elevated neuroactive steroid levels both in the maternal circulation and brain, as well as, importantly, in the fetal brain. The placenta is a source of massive amounts of progesterone that enter not only the maternal circulation, but also the fetal blood and the fetal brain, where it is actively converted into the $GABA_A$ receptor active pregnane steroid, allopregnanolone (Crossley et al.,1997). Allopregnanolone is present in sufficient quantity to effectively raise the threshold for excitotoxicity in the fetal brain, as shown by the fact that severe fetal hypoxia produces greater damage when synthesis of allopregnanolone is suppressed (Yawno et al., 2007). More recent studies suggest that progesterone metabolites may also have a role in development and repair of the fetal brain after exposure to hypoxia and other potential stressors in late pregnancy (Hirst et al., 2009). Evidence from animal studies indicates that elevated neuroactive steroid levels in pregnancy suppress excitability and increase lethargy (Paoletti et al., 2006). This is consistent with the elevated plasma levels of $GABA_AR$ agonist steroids reported in women during pregnancy (Hill et al., 2007). These changes are lost at birth with the removal of the placenta, suggesting that placental progesterone production is mostly responsible for the elevated neuroactive steroid levels in the plasma and their reported effects on mood (Gilbert Evans et al., 2005). Disruption of placental function can cause chronic placental insufficiency and/or low placental perfusion, leading to IUGR. Although not always associated with marked pathology at birth, IUGR can cause severe brain injury and even mild IUGR, and it has been correlated with subtle developmental abnormalities in later life (Hirst et al., 2009). The impact of these complications on the developing brain is dependent upon the gestational age of the fetus at the time of injury and is also dependent on the time when the restriction becomes manifest (Inder and Volpe, 2000; Frisk et al., 2002; Luciana, 2003). If placental function is reduced in early gestation, there is a relatively uniform reduction in body size. In contrast, limitation of placental function later in gestation results in asymmetrical growth restriction where the fetal head and brain are relatively less affected ('spared') compared to the body and somatic organs (Fang, 2005).

In addition, progesterone has been found to act on gene expression in neural cells to promote myelination by interaction with associated Schwann cells. As progesterone receptors were not detectable in Schwann cells, these observations suggest an interaction between neuronal and glial cells to promote myelination (Schumacher et al., 2007).

Children and animals prenatally exposed to alcohol have smaller brain size and thinner cerebral cortex, leading to significant decreases in the total cell number (Miller, 1996; Archibald et al., 2001). Special emphasis was given to the amino acid-activated ion channels of excitation (glutamate) and inhibition (GABA) in prenatal rat brain (Lee et al., 2008; Nasser and Kim, 2010). Additionally, Ikonomidou, (2000) demonstrated that may shed light on how ethanol affects the developing brain is the triggering of widespread neuronal death in the developing rat forebrain by blocking the N-methyl-D-aspartate (NMDA)–glutamate receptor and activating $GABA_A$ receptors.

Neuroactive steroids also reduce NMDA-induced excitotoxicity both *in vitro* (Lockhart et al., 2002) and *in vivo* models of brain injury (Djebaili et al., 2005). These excitatory pathways contribute to brain injury in the neonate following acute hypoxic episodes that may occur around the time of birth. In addition to being at risk of brain damage due to the chronic hypoxia alone, the IUGR fetus is also more susceptible to injury from acute hypoxia/ ischemia-induced cell death at birth (Fang, 2005). Studies show that greater damage is seen in vulnerable brain areas, such as the hippocampus, brainstem and cortex, when asphyxia is encountered by the already IUGR fetus. Burke et al., (2006) found that the dual insult of acute hypoxia in already IUGR fetuses resulted in a marked potentiation of expression of apoptotic marker in the brain of neonatal piglets. Similarly, IUGR human neonates that were exposed to a period of asphyxia due to placental infarction had increased brain injury (Burke and Gobe, 2005).

## Impaired Placentation in Rat Fetal Alcohol Syndrome

Although IUGR is a key feature of FAS, its pathogenesis is still under investigation. Recently, Gundogan et al., (2008; 2010) demonstrated that chronic gestational exposure to ethanol in the rat causes increased fetal resorption, and impairment in placental development and placentation. Since ethanol in maternal blood reaches the fetus and/or the placenta, its toxic effects on the fetus can be mediated either directly or indirectly. Direct effect of ethanol on fetal brain development will be treated below, and indirect effect is related to placental pathology especially within the labyrinthine placental barrier, which is composed by syncytiotrophoblast, chorionic trophoblast, blood vessels and stroma, and is in direct contact with maternal blood. The ischemia or infarction observed in ethanol–exposed placentas reduced thickness of the placenta by an increase in cellular necrosis. Since nutrients exchange between the mother and the fetus occurs within the labyrinthine layer, ethanol induced reductions in the mass of this layer could impair nutrients delivery to the fetus and thereby result in IUGR.

Gundogan et al., (2008; 2010) described that a second major placental abnormality associated with chronic gestational exposure to ethanol was failure of maternal uterine spiral arteries to remodelling from small muscular arteries to the thin-walled, distended, flaccid vessels to produce high-flow, low resistance circulation characteristic of intervillous space. Failure on maternal remodelling of uterine spiral arteries compromises placental blood flow and nutrients exchange (Pijnenborg et al., 1981). Perturbation in this process has been linked to early pregnancy loss, IUGR and /or PE. Therefore, the motile and invasive properties of EVT are critical for establishing and maintaining pregnancy, and ensuring adequate blood and nutrients delivery to the fetus in order to support growth and development (Gundogan et al., 2008).

In addition, insulin-like growth factors (IGF) regulate placentation due to its stimulating effects on extravillous trophoblast (EVT), which are highly motile and invasive (Gundolan et al., 2008). Previously, Gundogan et al., (2007) demonstrated that EVT express high levels of aspartyl-(asparaginyl) β-hydroxylase (AAH), a type 2 transmembrane protein with catalytic activity that hydroxylates epidermal growth factor-like domains of proteins that have a functional role in cell motility and invasion. AAH is regulated by IGF and has a critical role in cell motility and invasion, and recently, Gundolan et al., (2010) demonstrate that ethanol impaired placentation is associated with inhibition of AAH expression in EVT.

## Alcohol Induced Apoptosis of Neural Crest Cells

Exposure to alcohol during gestation can have profound consequences, but not all cells within the embryo are equally affected. Studies in mice and chicks models have demonstrated that alcohol exposure at specific stages of early embryonic development results in significant death among cells destined to give rise to facial structures: cranial neural crest cells (NCC). Alcohol triggers apoptosis in retinoic acid(a type of vitamin A)-deficient cells from the neural crest, and also reduces levels of antioxidant compounds such as free radicals scavengers (Smith, 1997). In addition, Wentzel and Eriksson (2009), demonstrated on NCC of day 10 rat embryo that ethanol causes a shift towards apoptosis in both neural cells from cranial portion (cNCC), and neural cells from trunk portion (tNCC), a shift which is diminished by treatment with the antioxidant N-acetylcysteine. Oxidative defense genes, and genes involved in NCC development are affected differently in cNCC compared to tNCC upon ethanol exposure. cNCC Hox genes are downregulated, whereas tNCC are upregulated. These patterns of ethanol-altered gene expression may be of etiological importance for NCC-associated alterations of development in ethanol-exposed pregnancy.

Normal craniofacial morphology develops as a consequence of interactions between embryonic tissues such as cNCC, mesoderm and ectoderm, and requires precise regulation of cell movement, growth, patterning, and differentiation of craniofacial tissue (Sant´Anna and Tosello, 2006). Gastrulation is a period of intense mitotic activity, particularly in the developing mesoderm in mammalian embryos. Alcohol exposure during this period suppresses rates of cell division in mice embryos (Sulikk, 1984) and the process of migration of mesodermal cells towards the primitive streak (Nakatsuji and Johnsson, 1984). If gastrulation is occurring at the time of alcohol exposure in mammalian embryos (C57B1/6J mice), alcohol suppresses rates of cell division (Sulikk et al., 1984). Gastrulation is a period of intense mitotic activity, particularly in the developing mesoderm. Deficiencies in gastrulating mesodermal cells are responsible for inducing and maintaining neuroepithelial differentiation, an adverse effect on the mesoderm could result in size reduction in the neural plate, which was particularly noticeable in the forebrain region (Sulikk et al., 1984).

Genetics studies have demonstrated the involvement of numerous genes in the craniofacial and dental structures, including genes encoding a variety of transcription factors, growth factors and receptors (Morris-Kay, 1993). The most common facial anomalies associated with FAS include short palpebral fissures, smooth philtrum, thin upper lip, midfacial hypoplasis and/or misaligned teeth (Jones et al., 1973). The craniofacial features include midfacial underdevelopment with gross shortage of bone, cranial base sloping to an extreme degree with backward-facing displacement of the cranio facial base, delayed dental development and enamel anomalies (Jackson and Hussain, 1990).

Although the cNCC contribute to form many tissues, alcohol related research on these cells predominantly focuses on facial bone and cartilage. Alcohol exposure cause cCNN apoptosis only if alcohol is administered before the CNN emigrated from their birthplace in the neuroectoderm. Once the cells began the migration toward the site where the face will develops, CNN cells are resistant to alcohol-induced apoptosis (Cartwright and Smith, 1995). Animal studies have linked the characteristic facial abnormalities in FAS to cell death by apoptosis of cCNN during a very well defined period of vulnerability (gastrulation or neurulation) (Cartwright et al., 1998). One mechanism by which this occurs is thought to be the formation of free radicals (Chen and Sulik, 1996). Others described mechanisms are a deficiency in retinoic acid, altered expression of homeobox genes, intracellular communication and alterations in the activity of growth factors. All of these mechanisms are likely interrelated, since retinoic acid is a key regulator of gene expression, and both free-radical toxicity and altered gene expression can produce apoptosis (Dickman et al., 1997; Smith, 1997).

In addition, the effects of alcohol in the odontogenesis make the tooth a good representative organ model to study developmental toxicity of ethanol (Kattainen et al., 2001). Bowden et al., (1983) shown that ethanol exposure during pregnancy cause retardation of tooth eruption in offspring of macaque monkeys, and Campos and Duranza, (1988) found in mice cellular alterations in the basal layer of the epithelium of the tooth germ in the bud stage and in the inner enamel epithelium.

## FETAL ALCOHOL EXPOSURE SND ALTERATIONS IN BRAIN AND BEHAVIOUR

Although heavy alcohol consumption throughout pregnancy leads to a significant risk of brain injury to the developing fetus, the latter is especially vulnerable to alcohol-induced brain injury during specific stages of brain development, many of which occur early during pregnancy (West, 1987; Ikonomidou et al., 2000). Ethanol exposure during prenatal development causes a wide range of structural and functional brain abnormalities affecting neurogenesis and gliogenesis, resulting in the condition of FAE (Kumada et al., 2007). These authors summarised that the cellular mechanisms by which alcohol affects the migration of immature neurons are $Ca^{+2}$ signalling and cyclic nucleotide signalling. Exposure to alcohol during gastrulation has a negative impact on the developing brain, reducing the neural progenitor pool (Rubert et al., 2006) and causing long-term effects on the forebrain (Ashwell and Zhang, 1996). The cerebral cortex formation as well as the increases in both cortical surface area and neural cell number seems to be critical for the emergence of complex cognitive functions. The neural cell number is in turn dependent on the number of neural progenitor cells, their rate of proliferation and the mitotic cycles that they undergo (Rubert et al., 2006). Ethanol is a toxic compound that can induce microcephaly and deficits in cognitive functions and in the behavioral responses (Mattson and Riley, 1998). A critical period of ethanol induced microcephaly and teratogenesis occurs during early embryogenesis of rat brain development (first 10 day of gestation, first trimester human equivalent) (Maier et al., 1997; Guerri, 2002). During this period, the neural progenitor cells, radial glia (RG,) is generated, and dysfunctions in its proliferation and survival could lead to a reduction in the final number of neural cells.

Radial glia in the development of the central nervous system (CNS) acts both as neural progenitors and as scaffolding that supports neuronal migration. The establishment of RG cells from the neuroepithelium precedes the generation and migration of neurons in the cerebral cortex. During early corticogenesis, RG cells generate neurons and then guide the daughter neurons in their ascent toward the developing cortical plate (Rakic, 1972; Hatten, 1999). Once neuronal migration is completed, most RG disappear by differentiating into astrocytes (Rakic, 1995), the cells that play critical roles in the metabolic processes linked to neuronal activity such as blood flow, energy and glucose utilization (Magistretti, 2006). Furthermore, recent findings demonstrate that RG cells are the predominant form of neural progenitors in the embryonic brain (Malatesta et al., 2000; Noctor et al., 2001 ; Gotz et al., 2002), giving rise to the majority of neurons in all CNS regions (Anthony et al., 2004). In addition, Guerri et al., (2009) suggested that the metabolic anomalies observed in different brain structures of individuals with FAS disorder are consistent with abnormalities in the glial cell pool, rather than in the neurons.

The self-renewal capacity vs. the specification of radial glial into the distinct neuronal and glial fates in the mammalian brain is regulated by intrinsic mechanisms, combined with extracellular temporal gradients of signalling molecules such as Notch (Rubert et al., 2006), and growth factors (e.g., fibroblast growth factor 2, epidermal growth factor); (Temple, 2001). Hence, disruptions in these mechanisms and/or in the gradients of signalling molecules might affect neural progenitor cells and CNS development. The study of Rubert et al., (2006) suggested that the role that RG play as a neuronal progenitor in the embryo may dramatically change the CNS development under normal and pathological conditions, such as those occurring during fetal alcohol exposure. Chu et al., (2007) found that chronic ethanol exposure of pregnant rats causes inhibition of mitochondrial gene expression related with mitochondrial dysfunction, increased expression of pro-apoptotic and pro-oxidant genes with attendant increased DNA damage and lipid peroxidation, and impaired insulin/insulin like growth factor signal transduction. Together, these results point to cerebellar hypoplasia.

Basic animal studies provide evidence of the vulnerability of the CNS to the effects of ethanol, revealing that these effects are not uniform and that some brain areas or cell populations are more vulnerable than others (Guerri 1998, Guerri 2002; Tran and Kelly, 2003). Bonthius et al., (2008) found in cerebellar granule cell cultures that neuronal nitric oxide synthase (nNOS) protects developing neurons against alcohol toxicity by activating the NO-cGMP-PKG signalling and NFkappaB pathway. In addition, Kumar et al., (2010) demonstrated that high-dose ethanol affects the expression and activation of retinoic acid (RA) receptors, which could impair the signalling events and induce harmful effects on the survival and differentiation of cerebellar granule cells. Indeed, it is well established that ethanol is an important toxic substance for the developing fetal brain. In fact, it is one of the leading preventable causes of birth defects and neurobehavioral disorders (American Academy of Pediatrics, 2000).

## EFFECT OF ALCOHOL ON CARDIAC EMBRYO DEVELOPMENT

Cardiac malformations are frequently seen in FAS, the most common being ventricular septal defects. Other associated anomalies are pulmonary artery hypoplasia and interruption of the aortic arch (Terrapon et al, 1977). Atrio-ventricular defects, patent ductus arteriosus and Fallot teratology have been seen to be associated with FAS (Loser et al, 1992). Recently, Dlugos and Rabin, (2010) found that exposure of zebrafish embryos to ethanol during development results in structural and functional changes in the heart that mimic malformations that occur in patients with FAS.

## EFFECT OF ALCOHOL ON LIVER EMBRYO DEVELOPMENT

The liver has also been seen to be affected in FAS. The characteristic deformities are similar to those observed in adult alcoholic liver disease. The features more commonly seen include hepatomegaly and raised serum transaminases. Light microscope revealed increased parenchymal fat with portal and perisinusoidal spaces containing deposits of intermediated and large size collagen fibers, myo-fibroblast and occasional Ito cells as well as subendothelial basement membrane like material (Lefkowitch et al., 1983). The presence of thick sclerotic central veins has also been seen, in conjunction with the simultaneous occurrence of extrahepatic biliary atresia (Daft et al., 1986).

## CONCLUSIONS

In this paper we have reviewed published studies about the principal evidences of the teratogenic effect of prenatal ethanol exposure on placentation, placenta growth, placenta function, and fetal development with emphasis in CNS development. The teratogenic effect was focused with special relevance to the association between hypoxia and oxidative stress, molecular mechanism involved (e.g. apoptosis) and the range of effects. These studies provide a comprehensive picture of the association among structural and functional placenta abnormalities and structural and functional brain abnormalities, in order to identify factors that mediate the relationship between pregnancy alcohol exposure and IUGR and the severity of brain abnormalities and behaviour deficits in individual with FAS/FAE.

## REFERENCES

Aban M, Cinel L, Arslan M, Dilek U, Kapanoglu M, Arpaci R, Dilek S. Expression of nuclear factor-kappa B and placental apoptosis in pregnancies complicated with intrauterine growth restriction and preeclampsia: an immunohistochemical study. *Tohoku J Exp Med*. 2004; 204: 195-202

Allaire A D, Ballenger K A, Wells S R, McMahon M J, Lessey B A. Placental apoptosis in preeclampsia. *Obstet Gynecol*. 2000; 96; 271-276

American Academy of Pedriatics. Committee on Substance Abuse and Committee on Children with Disabilities. Fetal alcohol syndrome and alcohol-related neurodevelopmental disorders. *Pediatrics*. 2000; 106: 358-361

Anthony TE, Klein C, Fishell G, Heintz N. Radial glia serves as neuronal progenitors in all regions of the central nervous system. *Neuron*. 2004; 41: 881-890.

Aplin J D. Implantation, trophoblast differentiation and haemochorial placentation: mechanistic evidence in vivo and in vitro. *J. Cell Sci*. 1991: 99: 681-692

Archibald SL, Fennema-Notestine C, Gamst A, Riley EP, Mattson SN, Jernigan TL. Brain dysmorphology in individuals with severe prenatal alcohol exposure. *Dev Med Child Neurol.* 2001; 43:148-154.

Ascherio A, Hennekens C , Willett WC, Sacks F, Rosner B, Manson J. Witteman J and Stampfer M. Prospective study of nutritional factors, blood pressure, and hypertension among US women. *Hypertension.* 1996; 27, 1065-1072

Bailey S M, Cunningham C C. Acute and chronic ethanol increases reactive oxygen species generation and decreases viability in fresh, isolated rat hepatocytes. *Hepatology* 1998; 28: 1318-1326.

Bailey S M, Patel V B, Young T A, Asayama K, Cunningham C C. Chronic ethanol consumption alters the glutathione/glutathione peroxidase- 1 system and protein oxidation status in rat liver, Alcohol. *Clin Exp Res.* 2001; 25: 726-733.

Banan A, Fields JZ, Decker H, Zhang Y, Keshavarzian A. Nitric oxide and its metabolites mediate ethanol-induced microtubule disruption and intestinal barrier dysfunction. *J Pharmacol Exp Ther.* 2000;294: 997-1008

Banan A, Fields JZ, Zhang Y, Keshavarzian A. iNOS upregulation mediates oxidant-induced disruption of F-actin and barrier of intestinal monolayers. Am J Physiol Gastrointest *Liver Physiol.* 2001;280: G1234-G1246.

Beckman JS, Ye YZ, Anderson PG, Chen J, Accavitti MA, Tarpey MM, White CR. Extensive nitration of protein tyrosines in human atherosclerosis detected by immunohistochemistry. Biol Chem Hoppe Seyler. 1994; 375:81-88.

Black S, Kadyrov M, Kaufmann P, Ugele B, Emans N, Huppertz B. Syncytial fusion of human trophoblast depends on caspase 8. *Cell Death Differ.* 2004; 11: 90-98

Bonfoco E, Krainc D, Ankarcrona M, Nicotera P, Lipton SA. Apoptosis and necrosis: two distinct events induced, respectively, by mild and intense insults with *N*-methyl-D-aspartate or nitric oxide/superoxide in cortical cell cultures. *Proc Natl Acad Sci USA* 1995; 92:7162-7166.

Bonizzi G, Karin M. The two NF-kappaB activation pathways and their role in innate and adaptive immunity. *Trends Immunol.* 2004; 25:280-288.

Bonthius D J, Bonthius N E, Karacay B. The protective effect of neuronal nitric oxide synthase (nNOS) against alcohol toxicity depends upon NO-cGMP-PKG pathway and NF-kappaB. *Neurotoxicology.* 2008; 29: 2080-1091

Bosco C. Morphology of the capillaries in the alpha and beta zone of human term placenta : the relationship between capillary morphology and the trophoblastic layer. *Med Sci Res.* 1994. 22 : 115-117

Bosco C. (2005) Alcohol and Xenobiotics in Placenta Damage. In "Comprehensive Handbook of Alcohol Related Pathology".Ed. Preedy, V.R and Watson, R.R. Elsevier *Science*, London, Vol 2 Chapter 72, pag. 921-935

Bowden D M, Weathersbee P S, Clarren S K, Fahrenbruch C E, Goodlin B L, Caffery S A. A periodic dosing model of fetal alcohol syndrome in the pig-tailed macaque (Macaca nemestrina*). A J Primatol.* 1983; 4: 143-157

Brien J F, Chan D, Green C R, Iqbal U, Gareri J, Kobus S M, McLaughlin B E, Klein J, Rao C, Reynolds J N, Bocking A D, Koren G. Chronic prenatal ethanol exposure and increased concentration of fatty acid ethyl esters in meconium of term fetal Guinea pig. *Ther Drug Monit.* 2006; 28: 345-350

Brookes PS. Mitochondrial nitric oxide synthase. *Mitochondrion* 2004; 3:187-204

Brown GC, Borutaite V. Nitric oxide, cytochrome *c* and mitochondria. *Biochem Soc Symp.* 1999; 66:17-25

Burke C, Gobe G. Pontosubicular apoptosis ('necrosis') in human neonates with intrauterine growth retardation and placental infarction. *Virchows Arch.* 2005; 446: 640-645

Burke C, Sinclair K, Cowin G, Rose S, Pat B, Gobe G, Colditz P. Intrauterine growth restriction due to uteroplacental vascular insufficiency leads to increased hypoxia-induced cerebral apoptosis in newborn piglets. *Brain Res.* 2006; 1098: 19-25

Burner U, Furtmüller PG, Kettle AJ, Koppenol WH, Obinger C. Mechanism of reaction of myeloperoxidase with nitrite. *J Biol Chem.* 2000; 275: 20597-20601

Burney S, Caulfield JL, Niles JC, Wishnok JS, Tannenbaum SR. The chemistry of DNA damage from nitric oxide and peroxynitrite. *Mutat Res.* 1999; 424: 37-49

Burton G L, Skepper J N, Hempstock J, Cindrova T, Jones C J.Jauniaux E. A reppraisal of the contrasting morphological appearances of villous cytotrophoblast cells during early human pregnancy; evidence for both apoptosis and primary necrosis. *Placenta.* 2003 ; 24: 297-305

Campos R M, Duranza M C. Efectos del consumo prolongado de etanol sobre las etapas tempranas del desarrollo dentario en ratones. *Rev Cubana Invest Biome.* 1988; 7: 30-35

Caniggia, I., Winter, J., Lye, S.J. and Post, M. Oxygen and placental development during the first trimester : implications for the pathophysiology of pre-eclampsia. *Placenta.* 2000; 21: S25-S30

Cano M J, Ayala A, Murillo M L, O. Carreras O. Protective effect of folic acid against oxidative stress produced in 21-day postpartum rats by maternal-ethanol chronic consumption during pregnancy and lactation period. *Free Radic. Res.* 2001; 34: 1-8

Caulin C, Salvesen GS, Oshima RG. Caspase cleavage of keratin 18 and reorganization of intermediate filaments during epithelial cell apoptosis. *J Cell Biol.* 1997; 138:1379-1394

Cartwright M M, Smith S M. Increased cell death and reduced neural crest cell numbers in ethanol-exposed embryos: partial basis for the fetal alcohol syndrome phenotype. *Alcohol Clin Exp Res.* 1995; 19: 378-386

Cartwright M M, Tessmer L L, Smith S M. Ethanol induced neural crest apoptosis is coincident with their endogenous death, but is mechanistically distinct. *Alcohol Clin Exp Res.* 1998; 22 : 142-149

Chang W, Webster DR, Salam AA, Gruber D, Prasad A, Eiserich JP, Bulinski JC. Alteration of the C-terminal amino acid of tubulin specifically inhibits myogenic differentiation. *J Biol Chem.* 2002; 277 :30690-30698

Chaudhuri J. Alcohol and the developing fetus- a review. *Med Sci Monit.* 2000; 6 : 1031-1041

Chen S, Sulik K K. Free radicals and ethanol-induced cytotoxicity in neural crest. *Alcohol Clin Exp Res.* 1996; 20: 1071-1076

Chen LW, Egan L, Li ZW, Greten FR, Kagnoff MF, Karin M. The two faces of IKK and NF-kappaB inhibition: prevention of systemic inflammation but increased local injury following intestinal ischemia-reperfusion. *Nat Med.* 2003; 9: 575-581

Chan D, Klein J, Karaskov T, Koren G. Fetal exposure to alcohol as evidence by fatty acid ethyl esters in meconium in the absence of maternal drinking history in pregnancy. *The Drug Monit.* 2004; 26: 474-481

Chu J, Tong M, de la Monte S M. Chronic ethanol exposure causes mitochondrial dysfunction and oxidative stress in immature central nervous system neurons. *Acta Neuropathol.* 2007; 113: 659-673

Chudley AE, Conry J, Cook JL, Look C, Rosales T, LeBlanc N. Fetal alcohol spectrum disorder: Canadian guidelines for diagnosis. *CMAJ.* 2005;172 : S1–S21

Clements MK, Siemsen DW, Swain SD, Hanson AJ, Nelson-Overton LK, Rohn TT, Quinn MT. Inhibition of actin polymerization by peroxynitrite modulates neutrophil functional responses. *J Leukoc Biol.* 2003;73 : 344-355

Cohen-Kerem R, Koren G. Antioxidants and fetal protection against ethanol teratogenicity I. Review of the experimental data and implications to humans. *Neurotoxicology and Teratology.* 2003; 25: 1-9

Cooke, C. L., Davidge, S. T Peroxynitrite increases iNOS through NF-κB and decreases prostacyclin synthase in endothelial cells. *Am J Physiol Cell Physiol.* 2002; 282 : C395-C402

Crocker IP, Cooper S, Ong SC, Baker PN. Differences in apoptotic susceptibility of cytotrophoblasts and syncytiotrophoblasts in normal pregnancy to those complicated with preeclampsia and intrauterine growth restriction. *Am J Pathol.* 2003; 162 : 637-643

Cross C J. Placental function in development and disease. *Reprod Fertil Develop.* 2006; 18 : 71-76

Cross C.J, Werb Z, Fisher S.J. Implantation and the placenta : key pieces of the development puzzle. *Science.* 1994; 26 : 1508-1517

Crossley KJ, Nicol MB, Hirst JJ, Walker DW, Thorburn GD. Suppression of arousal by progesterone in fetal sheep. *Reprod Fertil Dev.* 1997; 9 : 767-773

Daft P A, Johnston M C, Sulik K K. Abnormal heart and great vessel development following acute ethanol exposure in mice. *Teratology.* 1986; 33 : 93-104

Djebaili M, Guo Q, Pettus EH, Hoffman SW, Stein DG. The neurosteroids progesterone and allopregnanolone reduce cell death, gliosis, and functional deficits after traumatic brain injury in rats. *J Neurotrauma.* 2005; 22 : 106-118

Dickhout JG, Hossain GS, Pozza LM, Zhou J, Lhotak S, Austin RC. Peroxynitrite causes endoplasmic reticulum stress and apoptosis in human vascular endothelium: implications in atherogenesis. *Arterioscler Thromb Vasc Biol.* 2005;25 :.2623-2629

Dlugos C A, Rabin R A. Structural and functional effects of developmental exposure to etanol on the zebrafish Heart. *Alcohol Clin Exp Res.* 2010; 34 : 1-9

Dong J, Sulik K K, Chen S Y. The role of NOX enzymes in ethanol-induced oxidative stress and apoptosis in mouse embryos. *Toxicol Lett.* 2010; 193: 94-100

Dotsch, J., Hogen, N., Nyul, Z., Hanze, J., Knerr, I., Kirschbaum, M., Rascher W. Increase of endothelial nitric oxide synthase and endothelin-1 mRNA expression in human placenta during gestation. *Eur J Obstet Gynecol Reprod Biol.* 2001; 97, 163- 167.

du Plessis AJ, Volpe JJ. Perinatal brain injury in the preterm and term newborn. *Curr Opin Neurol.* 2002; 15: 151-157.

Enders A.C. A comparative study of the fine structure of the trophoblast in several hemochorial placentas. *Am. J. Anat.* 1965; 116 : 29-67

Fang S. Management of preterm infants with intrauterine growth restriction. *Early Hum Dev.* 2005; 81: 889-900

Fernandez-Checa J C, Garcia-Ruiz C, Ookhtens M, Kaplowitz N. Impaired uptake of glutathione by hepatic mitochondria from chronic ethanol-fed rats. Tracer kinetic studies in vitro and in vivo and susceptibility to oxidant stress. *J Clin Invest*. 1991; 87: 397- 405

Fisher S E, Atkinson M, Burnap J K, Jacobson S, Sehgal P K, Scott W, Van Thiel D H. Ethanol-associated selective fetal malnutrition : a contributing factor in the fetal alcohol syndrome. *Alcohol Clin Exp Res*. 1982; 6: 197-201

Fisher S E, Karl P I. Maternal ethanol use and selective fetal malnutrition. *Recent Dev Alcohol*. 1988; 6: 277-289

Fridovich I. The biology of oxygen radicals. *Science*. 1978; 201 : 875- 880

Floris R, Piersma SR, Yang G, Jones P, Wever R. Interaction of myeloperoxidase with peroxynitrite. A comparison with lactoperoxidase, horseradish peroxidase and catalase. *Eur J Biochem*. 1993; 215 : 767-775

Floyd R L, Decofle P, Hungerfond D W. Alcohol use prior to pregnancy recognition. *Am J Prev Med*. 1999; 12 : 101-107

Floyd R L, Weber M K, Denny C, O'Connor M J. Prevention of fetal alcohol spectrum disorders. *Dev Disabil Res Rev*. 2009; 15 : 193-199

Frisk V, Amsel R, Whyte HE. The importance of head growth patterns in predicting the cognitive abilities and literacy skills of small-for-gestational-age children. *Dev Neuropsychol*. 2002; 22 : 565–593

Gareri J, Brien J, Reynolds J, Koren G. Potential role of the placenta in fetal alcohol spectrum disorder. *Paediatr Drugs*. 2009; 11 : 26-29

Genbacev O, Zhou Y, Ludlow J W, Fisher S J. Regulation of human placental development by oxygen tension. *Science*. 1997; 27 : 1669-1672

Gilbert Evans SE, Ross LE, Sellers EM, Purdy RH, Romach MK . 3 alpha-reduced neuroactive steroids and their precursors during pregnancy and the postpartum period. *Gynecol Endocrinol*. 2005; 21 : 268–279

Gotz M, Barde YA. 2005. Radial glial cells defined and major intermediates between embryonic stem cells and CNS neurons. *Neuron*. 2005; 46 : 369–372

Gu Y, Srivastava R K, Clarke D L, Linzer D I, Gibori G. The decidual prolactin receptor and its regulation by decidua-derived factors. *Endocrinology*. 1996; 137 : 4878-4885

Guerri C. Neuroanatomical and neurophysiological mechanisms involved in central nervous system dysfunctions induced by prenatal alcohol exposure. *Alcohol Clin. Exp. Res*. 1998; 22 : 304-312

Guerri C. Mechanisms involved in central nervous system dysfunctions induced by prenatal ethanol exposure. *Neurotoxicol Res*. 2002; 4:327– 335

Guerri C, Pascual M, Renau-Piqueras J. Glia and fetal alcohol syndrome. *Neurotoxicology*. 2001; 22 : 593–599

Guerri C, Bazinet A, Riley E P. Foetal alcohol spectrum disorders and alterations in brain and behaviour. *Alcohol & Alcoholism*. 2009; 44 : 108-114

Gundogan F, Elwood G, Greco D, Rubin L P, Pinar H, Carlson RI, Wands J R, de la Monte S M. Role of aspartyl-(asparagyl) beta-hydroxylase in placental implantation : relevance to early pregnancy loss. *Hum Pathol*. 2007; 38 : 50-59

Gundogan F, Elwood G, Longato L, Tong M, Feijoo A, Carlson RI, Wands J R, de la Monte S M. Impaired placentation in fetal alcohol syndrome. *Placenta*. 2008; 29 : 148-157

Gundogan F, Elwood G, Mark P, Feijoo A, Longato L, Tong M, de la Monte S M. Ethanol-induced oxidative stress and mitochondrial dysfunction in rat placenta : relevance to pregnancy loss. *Alcoholism : Clin Exp Res.*2010; 34 : 415-423

Hatten ME. Central nervous system neuronal migration. *Annu Rev Neurosci.* 1999; 22: 511-539.

Heaton M B, Mitchell J J, Paiva M. Amelioration of ethanol induced neurotoxicity in the neonatal rat central nervous system by antioxidant therapy. *Alcohol Clin Exp Res.* 2000; 24 : 512-518

Henderson G I, Devi B G , Perez A, Schenker S. In utero ethanol exposure elicits oxidative stress in the rat fetus, *Alcohol. Clin. Exp. Res.* 1995; 19 : 714- 720.

Henderson G I, Chen J J, Schenker S. Ethanol, oxidative stress, reactive aldehydes, and the fetus. Front Biosci. 1999; 15 : D541-D550

Hetts S W. To die or not to die : an overview of apoptosis and its role in disease. *JAMA.* 1998; 279 : 300-307

Hirst J J, Walker D W, Yawno T, Palliser H K. *Dev Neurosci.* 2009; 31 : 363-377

Hockenberry D, Nunez G, Milliman C, Schreiber RD, Korsmeyer SJ. Bcl-2 is an inner mitochondrial membrane protein that blocks programmed cell death. *Nature.* 1990; 348 : 334-336

Huppertz B, Kadyrov M, Kingdom J C . Apoptosis and its role in the trophoblast. *Am J Obstet Gynecol.* 2005; 195 : 29-39

Huppertz B, Frank H G, Kingdom J C, Reister F, Kaufmann P. Villous cytotrophoblast regulation of the syncytial apoptotic cascade in the human placenta. *Histochem Cell Biol.* 1998; 110 : 495-508

Huppertz B, Frank HG, Kaufmann P. The apoptosis cascade– morphological and immunohistochemical methods for its visualization. *Anat Embryol.* 1999; 200 :1-18

Inder TE, Volpe JJ. Mechanisms of perinatal brain injury. *Semin Neonatol.* 2000; 5 : 3-16

Inder TE, Huppi PS, Warfield S, Kikinis R, Zientara GP, Barnes PD, Jolesz F, Volpe JJ. Periventricular white matter injury in the premature infant is followed by reduced cerebral cortical gray matter volume at term. *Ann Neurol.*1999; 46 : 755-760

Ikonomidou C, Bittigau P, Ishimaru MJ, Wozniak DF, Koch C, Genz K, Price MT, Stefovska V, Hörster F, Tenkova T, Dikranian K, Olney JW. Ethanol-induced apoptotic neurodegeneration and fetal alcohol syndrome. *Science.* 2000; 287 : 1056-1060

Ischiropoulos H, Zhu L, Chen J, Tsai M, Martin J C, Smith C D., and Beckman J S. Peroxynitrite-mediated tyrosine nitration catalyzed by superoxide dismutase. *Arch Biochem Biophys* . 1992; 298 : 431-437

Ishihara N, Matsuo H, Murakoshi H, Laoag-Fernandez J, Samoto T, Maruo T. Changes in proliferative potential, apoptosis and Bcl-2 protein expression in cytotrophoblasts and syncytiotrophoblast in human placenta over the course of pregnancy. *Endocr J.* 2000; 47 : 317-327.

Jackson I T, Hussain K. Craniofacial and oral manifestations of fetal alcohol syndrome. *Plast Reconstr Surg.* 1990; 85 : 505-512

Jacobson M D. Reactive oxygen species and programmed cell death. *Trends Biochem. Sci.* 1996; 21 : 83- 86

Jones KL, Smith DW. Recognition of the fetal alcohol syndrome in early infancy. *Lancet.* 1973; 2 : 999-1001

Jones K L, Smith D W, Ulleland C N, Streissguth A P. Pattern of malformations in offspring of chronic alcoholic mothers. *Lancet*. 1973; 1 : 267-271

Kasina S, Rizwani W, Radhika KV, Singh SS. Nitration of profilin effects its interaction with poly (L-proline) and actin. *J Biochem*. 2005; 138 : 687-695.

Kasina S, Wasia R, Fasim A, Radhika KV, Singh SS. Phorbol ester mediated activation of inducible nitric oxide synthase results in platelet profilin nitration. *Nitric Oxide*. 2006;14 : 65-71.

Kattainen H, Tuukkanen J, Simanainen U, Tuomisto J T, Kovero O, , Lukinmaa P L, Alaluusua S, Tuomisto J, Viluksela M. In utero/lactation 2,3,7,8-tetrachlordibenzo-p-dioxin exposure impairs molar tooth development an rats. *Toxicol Appl Pharmacol*. 2001; 174 : 216-224

Kay, H.H., Grindle, K.M. and Magness, R.R. Ethanol exposure induces oxidative stress and impairs nitric oxide availability in the human placental villi : A possible mechanism of toxicity. *Am J Obstet Gynecol*. 2000; 182 : 682-688

Kingdom J C; Kaufmann P. Oxygen and placental vascular development. . *Adv Exp Med Biol*. 1999; 474 : 259-275

Kossenjans W, Eis A, Sahay R, Brockman D, Myatt L. Role of peroxinitrite in altered fetal-placental vascular reactivity in diabetis or preeclampsia. *Am J Physiol Heart Circ Physiol*. 2000; 278 : H311-H319

Kumada T, Jiang Y, Cameron D B, Komuro H. How does alcohol impair neuronal migration?. *J Neroscience Res*. 2007; 85: 465-470

Kumar A, Singh C K, DiPette D D, Singh U S. Ethanol impairs activation of retinoic acid receptors in cerebellar granule cells in a rodent model of fetal alcohol spectrum disorders. *Alcohol Clin Exp Res*. 2010; 34: 928-937

Leers M P, Kolgen W, Bjorklund T, Tribbick G, Persson B, Bjorklund P, Ramaekers F C, Bjorklund P, Nap M, Jornvall H, Schutte B. Immunocytochemical detection and mapping of a Cytokeratin 18 neo-epitope exposed during early apoptosis. *J Pathol*. 1999; 187 : 567-572

Lefkowitch J H, Rushton A R, Feng-Chen K C. Hepatic fibrosis in fetal alcohol syndrome. Pathologic similarities to adult alcoholic liver disease. *Gastroenterology*. 1983; 85 : 951-957

Levy R, Smith S D, Yusuf K, Huettner P C, Kraus F T, Sadovsky Y, Nelson D M. Trophoblast apoptosis from pregnancies complicated by fetal growth restriction is associated with enhanced p53 expression. *Am J Obstet Gynecol*. 2002; 186 : 1056-1061

Liochev S I, Fridovich I. How does superoxide dismutase protect against tumor necrosis factor: a hypothesis informed by effect of superoxide on ''free'' iron. *Free Radic Biol Med*. 1997; 23 : 668- 671.

Liu X, Zou H, Slaughter C, Wang X. DFF, a heterodimeric protein that functions downstream of caspase-3 to trigger DNA fragmentation during apoptosis. *Cell*. 1997; 89 : 175-184

Lockhart EM, Warner DS, Pearlstein RD, Penning DH, Mehrabani S, Boustany RM. Allopregnanolone attenuates N-methyl- D - aspartate-induced excitotoxicity and apoptosis in the human NT2 cell line in culture. *Neurosci Lett*. 2002; 328 : 33 36.

Loser H, Pgeferkorn J R, Themann H. Alcohol in pregnancy and fetal heart damage. *Klin Padiatr*. 1992; 204 : 235-239

MacMillan-Crow LA, Thompson JA. Tyrosine modifications and inactivation of active site manganese superoxide dismutase mutant (Y34F) by peroxynitrite. *Arch Biochem Biophys.* 1999; 366 : 82-88.

Maier SE, Chen WJ, Miller JA, West JR. Fetal alcohol exposure and temporal vulnerability regional differences in alcohol-induced microencephaly as a function of the timing of binge-like alcohol exposure during rat brain development. *Alcohol Clin Exp Res.* 1997; 21 :1418-1428

Mankes R F, LeFevre R, Fieseher J, Santiago A, Benitz K F, Lyon R. Effects of ethanol on reproduction and arterial hypertension in spontaneously hypertensive and normotensive rats : a preliminary communication. *Alcohol Clin Exp Res.* 1985; 9: 284-290

Malatesta P, Hartfuss E, Gotz M. Isolation of radial glial cells by fluorescent-activated cell sorting reveals a neuronal lineage. *Development.* 2000; 127 : 5253-5263

Martin SJ, Reutelingsperger CP, McGahon AJ, Rader JA, Schie RC van, LaFace DM, Green DR. Early redistribution of plasma membrane phosphatidylserine is a general feature of apoptosis regardless of the initiating stimulus: inhibition by overexpression of Bcl-2 and Abl. *J Exp Med.* 1995; 182 : 1545-1556

Matsubara S, Sato I. Enzyme histochemically detectable NAD(P)H oxidase in human placental trophoblast: normal, preeclamptic, and fetal growth restriction-complicated pregnancy. *Histochem Cell Biol.* 2001; 116 : 1-7

Mattson SN, Riley EP. A review of the neurobehavioral deficits in children with fetal alcohol syndrome or prenatal exposure to alcohol. *Alcohol Clin Exp Res.* 1998; 22 : 279-294

Michaelis E K. Fetal alcohol exposure: cellular toxicity and molecular events involved in toxicity, *Alcohol Clin Exp Res.* 1990; 14 : 819- 826

Miller D K. The role of the caspase family of cysteine proteases in apoptosis. *Semin. Immunol.* 1997; 9 : 35-40

Miller MW, Potempa G. 1990. Numbers of neurons and glia in mature rat somatosensory cortex: effects of prenatal exposure to ethanol. *J Comp Neurol.* 1990; 293 : 92-102

Miller MW. 1996. Effect of early exposure to ethanol on the protein and DNA contents of specific brain regions in the rat. *Brain Res.* 1996; 734 : 286-294

Montoliu C, Sancho-Tello M, Azorin I, Burgal M, Valles S, Renau-Piqueras J, Guerri C. Ethanol increases cytochrome P4502E1 and induces oxidative stress in astrocytes. *J. Neurochem.* 1995; 65 : 2561-2570

Morimoto M, Zern M A, Hagbjork A L, Ingelman-Sundberg M, French S W. Fish oil, alcohol, and liver pathology: role of cytochrome P450 2E1. *Proc Soc Exp Biol Med.* 1994; 207 : 197-205

Morris-Kay G. Retinoic acid and craniofacial development: molecules and morphogenesis. *Bioessay.* 1993; 15 : 9-15

Myatt L. Review: reactive oxygen and nitrogen species and functional adaptation of the placenta. *Placenta.* 2010; 31 : S66-S69

Myatt L . Role of placenta in preeclampsia. *Endocrine.* 2002; 19 : 103-111

Myatt L, Cui X. Oxidative stress in the placenta. *Histochem Cell Biol.* 2004; 122 : 369-382

Myatt L, Brewer A S, Langdon G, and Brockman D E. Attenuation of the vasoconstrictor effect of thromboxane and endothelin by nitric oxide in the human fetal placental circulation. *Am J Obstet Gynecol.* 1992; 16 : 224-230

Myatt L, Rosenfield L D, Eis A L, Brockman D E, Greer E, Lyall F. Nitrotirosine residues in placenta. Evidence of peroxinitrite formation and action. *Hypertension*. 1996; 28 : 488-493

Myatt, L., Eis, A. L., Brockman, D. E., Kossenjans, W., Greer, I., & Lyall, F. Inducible (type II) nitric oxide synthase in human placental villous tissue of normotensive, pre-eclamptic and intrauterine growthrestricted pregnancies. *Placenta*. 1997; 18: 261- 268

Myllynen P, Pasanen M, Pelkonen O. Human placenta. A human organ for developmental toxicology research and biomonitoring. *Placenta* . 2005; 26 : 361-371

Nakatsuji N, Johnsson K E. Effects of ethanol on the primitive streak stage mouse embryo. *Teratology*. 1984; 29 : 269-275

Nasser M I, Lee H I, Kim M O. Neuroprotective effect of vitamin C against the ethanol and nicotine modulation of $GABA_B$ receptor and PKA-α expression in prenatal rat brain. Synapse. 2010; 64 : 467-477

Neumann P, Gertzberg N, Vaughan E, Weisbrot J, Woodburn R, Lambert W, Johnson A. Peroxynitrite mediates TNF-$\alpha$-induced endothelial barrier dysfunction and nitration of actin. *Am J Physiol Lung Cell Mol Physiol.* 2006; 290 : L674-L684

Noctor SC, Flint AC, Weissman TA, Dammerman RS, Kriegstein AR. Neurons derived from radial glial cells establish radial units in neocortex. *Nature*. 2001; 409 : 714-720

Newmeyer DD, Ferguson-Miller S. Mitochondria: releasing power for life and unleashing the machineries of death. *Cell*. 2003;112 : 481-490

Oh S I, Kim C I, Chun H J, Park S C. Chronic ethanol consumption affects glutathione status in rat liver, *J Nutr*. 1998; 128 : 758-763

Olney J W, Wosniak D F, Farber N B, Jevtovic-Todorovic V, Bittigau P, Ikonomidou C. The enigma of fetal alcohol neurotoxicity. *Ann Med.* 2002; 34 : 109-119

Ornoy A. Embryonic oxidative stress as a mechanism of teratogenesis with special emphasis on diabetic embryopathy. *Reproductive Toxicology*. 2007; 24 : 31-41

Pacher P, Beckman J S, Liaudet L. Nitric oxide and peroxynitrite in health and disease. *Physiol Rev*. 2007; 87 : 315-424

Palacios-Callender M, Quintero M, Hollis VS, Springett RJ, Moncada S. Endogenous NO regulates superoxide production at low oxygen concentrations by modifying the redox state of cytochrome *c* oxidase. *Proc Natl Acad Sci USA*. 2004; 101 : 7630–7635

Paoletti AM, Romagnino S, Contu R, Orru MM, Marotto MF, Zedda P, Lello S, Biggio G, Concas A, Melis GB. Observational study on the stability of the psychological status during normal pregnancy and increased blood levels of neuroactive steroids with GABA-A receptor agonist activity. *Psychoneuroendocrinology*. 2006; 31 : 485–492

Plessinger M A, Woods J R, Miller R K. Pretreatment of human amnion-chorion vitamin C and E prevents hypoclorous acid-induced damage. *Am J Obstet Gynecol.* 2000; 183 : 979-985

Qanungo, S., & Mukherjea, M. Ontogenic profile of some antioxidants and lipid peroxidation in human placental and fetal tissues. *Mol Cell Biochem*. 2000; 215 : 11-19

Radi R, Beckman JS, Bush KM, Freeman BA. Peroxynitrite-induced membrane lipid peroxidation: the cytotoxic potential of superoxide and nitric oxide. *Arch Biochem Biophys* 1991; 288 : 481-487

Radi R, Beckman J S, Bush K M, Freeman B A. Inhibition of mitochondrial electron transport by peroxinitrite. *Arch Biochem Biophys*. 1994; 308 : 89-95

Radi R, Cassina A, Hodara R. Nitric oxide and peroxynitrite interactions with mitochondria. *Biol Chem.* 2002; 383 : 401-409

Radi R, Beckman JS, Bush KM, Freeman BA. Peroxynitrite-induced membrane lipid peroxidation: the cytotoxic potential of superoxide and nitric oxide. *Arch Biochem Biophys.* 1991; 288 : 481-487

Rakic P. Mode of cell migration to the superficial layers of fetal monkey neocortex. *J Comp Neurol.* 1972; 145 : 61-83

Rakic P. (1995). In: *Neuroglial cells*. Ketterman H, Ransom BR, editors. New York: Oxford University Press. pag. 746-762

Reinke L A, Lai E K, DuBose C M, McCay B P. Reactive free radical generation in vivo in heart and liver of ethanol-fed rats: correlation with radical formation in vitro, *Proc. Natl. Acad. Sci. USA*. 1987; 84 : 9223-9227

Rodrigo R, Parra M, Bosco C, Fernández V, Barja P, Guajardo J, Messina R. Pathophysiological basis for the prophylaxis of preeclampsia through early supplementation with antioxidant vitamins. *Pharmacol Ther.* 2005;107-: 177-97

Rosset H L. A clinical perspective of the fetal alcohol syndrome. Alcoholism-Clinical and Experimental Research. 1980; 4-:119-122

Rubert G, Miñana R, Pascual M and Guerri C. Ethanol exposure during embryogenesis decreases the radial glial progenitor pool and affects the generation of neurons and astrocytes. *J Neurosc Res*. 2006; 84 : 483-496

Sant´Anna L B, Tosello D O. Fetal alcohol syndrome and developing craniofacial and dental structures-a review. *Orthod Craniofacial Res*. 2006; 9 : 172-185

Schumacher M, Guennoun R, Stein DG, De Nicola AF. Progesterone: therapeutic opportunities for neuroprotection and myelin repair. *Pharmacol Ther*. 2007; 116 : 77-106.

Seppa K., Laippala, P.and Sillanaukee, P. (1996). High diastolic blood pressure : Common among women who are heavy drinkers. *Alcohol Clin. Exp. Res*.1996; 20 : 47-51

Sies, H. (1991). Role of reactive oxygen species in biological processes. *Klin Wochenschr.* 1991; 69 : 965-968

Shi H, Noguchi N, Xu Y, Niki E. Formation of phospholipid hydroperoxides and its inhibition by alpha-tocopherol in rat brain synaptosomes induced by peroxynitrite. *Biochem Biophys Res Commun*. 1999; 257 : 651-656

Senftleben U, Cao Y, Xiao G, Greten FR, Krahn G, Bonizzi G, Chen Y, Hu Y, Fong A, Sun SC, Karin M. Activation by IKKalpha of a second, evolutionary conserved, NF-kappa B signalling pathway. *Science*. 2001; 293 : 1495-1499

Smith SC, Baker PN, Symonds EM. Placental apoptosis in normal human pregnancy. *Am J Obstet Gynecol.* 1997; 177 : 57-65

Smith S M. Alcohol-induced cell death in the embryo. *Alcohol Health Res World*. 1997; 21 : 287-297

Soares M J. The prolactin and growth hormone families : pregnancy-specific hormones/cytokines at the maternal fetal interface. *Reprod Biol Endocrinol*. 2004; 2 : 51-66

Sulik K K. Critical period for alcohol teratogenesis in mice, with special reference to the gastrulation stage of embryogenesis. *Ciba Found Symp*. 1984; 105 : 124-141

Szabo C, Zingarelli B, O'Connor M, Salzman AL. DNA strand breakage, activation of poly (ADPribose) synthetase, cellular energy depletion are involved in the cytotoxicity of macrophages and smooth muscle cells exposed to peroxynitrite. *Proc Natl Acad Sci USA*. 1996; 93 : 1753-1758

Szabó C. Multiple pathways of peroxynitrite cytotoxicity. Toxicol Lett. 2003; 140 : 105-112

Taylor S M, Heron A E, Cannell G R, Florin T H. Pressor effect of ethanol in the isolated perfused human placental lobule. *Eur J Pharmacol*. 1994; 270 : 371-374

Tedeschi G, Cappelletti G, Negri A, Pagliato L, Maggioni MG, Maci R, Ronchi S. Characterization of nitroproteome in neuron-like PC12 cells differentiated with nerve growth factor: identification of two nitration sites in alpha-tubulin. *Proteomics* 2005; 5 : 2422-2432

Temple S. The development of neural stem cells. *Nature*. 2001; 414 : 112-117

Terrapon M, Schneider P, Friedli B, Cox J N. Aortic arch interruption type A with aortopulmonary fenestration in an offspring of chronic alcoholic mother ("fetal alcohol syndrome"). *Helv Pediatr Acta*. 1977; 32 : 141-148

Tran T D, Kelly S J. Critical periods for ethanol-induced cell loss in the hippocampal formation. *Neurotoxicol teratol*. 2003; 25 : 519-528

Tran T D, Jackson H D, Hom K H, Goodleft C R. Vitamin E does not protect against neonatal ethanol-induced cerebellar damage or deficits in eyeblink classical conditioning in rats. *Alcohol Clin Exp Res*. 2005; 29 : 117-129

Virag L, Szabo E, Gergely P, Szabo C. Peroxynitrite-induced cytotoxicity: mechanism and opportunities for intervention. *Toxicol Lett*. 2003; 140 :113-124

Watson, A. L., Palmer, M. E., Jauniaux, E., & Burton, G. J. (1997). Variations in expression of copper/zinc superoxide dismutase in villous trophoblast of the human placenta with gestational age. *Placenta*. 1997; 18 : 295-299

Webster RP, Roberts VH, Myatt L. Protein nitration in placenta : functional significance. *Placenta*. 2008; 29 : 985-994

Well PG, Ma Callum GP, Chen CS, Henderson J T, Lee CLL , Perstin J, Preston T J, Wiley MJ, and Wong AW. Oxidative stress in developmental origins of disease : teratogenesis, neurodevelopmental deficits, and cancer. *Toxicological Sciences*. 2009; 108 : 4-18

Wentzel P, Eriksson U J. Genetic influence on dysmorphogenesis in embryos from different rat strains exposed to ethanol in vivo and in vitro. *Alcohol Clin Exp Res*. 2008; 32 : 874-887

Wentzel P, Eriksson U J. Altered gen expression in neural crest cells exposed to ethanol in vitro. *Brain Res*. 2009; 1305 : S50-S60

Wentzel P, Rydberg U, Eriksson U J. Antioxidative treatment diminishes ethanol-induced congenital malformations in the rat. *Alcohol Clin Exp Res*. 2006; 30 : 1732-1760

Yawno T, Yan EB, Walker DW, Hirst JJ. Inhibition of neurosteroid synthesis increases asphyxia-induced brain injury in the late gestation fetal sheep. *Neuroscience*. 2009; 146: 1726-1733

Yui J, Hemmings D, Garcia-Lloret M, Guilbert LJ. Expression of the human p55 and p75 tumor necrosis factor receptors in primary villous trophoblasts and their role in cytotoxic signal transduction. *Biol Reprod*. 1996; 55 : 400 409

Zou, M. H., Leist, M., & Ullrich, V. Selective nitration of prostacyclin synthase and defective vasorelaxation in atherosclerosic bovine coronary arteries. *Am J Pathol*. 1999; 54 : 1359-1365

In: Pregnancy and Alcohol Consumption
Editor: Joshua D. Hoffman, pp. 225-244

ISBN 978-1-61761-122-3


*Chapter 8*

# THE TIMING OF ALCOHOL CONSUMPTION DURING PREGNANCY AND FETAL ALCOHOL-INDUCED BRAIN DAMAGE

***Susan E. Maier***[1,1] ***and Wei-Jung A. Chen***[2,2]

1. Office of Initiative Development,
National Institute of Allergy and Infectious Diseases,
National Institutes of Health, Bethesda, Maryland
2. Neuroscience and Experimental Therapeutics,
Texas A&M Health Science Center College of Medicine

## ABSTRACT

One of the most challenging goals in fetal alcohol research is to identify the risk factors and mechanisms that influence the outcomes of alcohol exposure during pregnancy since not every woman who drinks alcohol during pregnancy will deliver an offspring with fetal alcohol spectrum disorder or fetal alcohol syndrome. Various key risk factors have been studied that can account for some of the variability in the severity of fetal alcohol-induced damage observed among the affected offspring, and the timing of alcohol exposure during gestation relative to specific developmental events appears to play a significant role affecting the variability in offspring deficits. Although the clinical research on this risk factor is sparse due to the difficulty in partitioning timing, duration and amount of alcohol consumed during pregnancy, considerable pre-clinical research shows a distinct pattern of offspring deficits when the timing of alcohol exposure is well-controlled in laboratory settings. This review outlines the effects of timing of alcohol exposure during gestation in various animal model systems and draws parallels between the effects observed in laboratory settings with those from clinical outcomes.

---

[1] Office of Initiative Development, National Institute of Allergy and Infectious Diseases, National Institutes of Health, 6700B Rockledge Drive, Suite 2156, Bethesda MD 20892-7610, 301-594-7198, 301-402-1063 (fax). E-mail: maiers@niaid.nih.gov.

[2] Neuroscience and Experimental Therapeutics, Texas A&M Health Science Center College of Medicine, College Station, TX 77843-1114. 979-845-5940, 979-845-0790 (fax). E-mail: wchen@medicine.tamhsc.edu.

## INTRODUCTION

The phrase "timing is everything" within the context of developmental biology describes the nature of development from conception through birth, and additionally captures the essence of outcome upon exposure to a teratogen during development. The developmental biology literature is filled with examples of well-choreographed molecular and cellular events that result in successful embryonic and fetal development, whereas the teratology literature presents examples of the adverse effects on the developing fetus – ranging from mild to severe – resulting from exposure to a teratogen. At what stage the conceptus is exposed to a teratogen will have a tremendous impact on its development, from subtle change undetectable at birth but revealed through specific behavioral or cognitive tests later in life to observable abnormalities at birth. Through its ubiquitous nature, alcohol is a teratogen that results in a range of offspring outcomes when consumed during pregnancy. The most severe consequence of heavy maternal drinking during pregnancy is fetal alcohol syndrome (FAS). FAS is defined by four criteria: maternal drinking during pregnancy, a characteristic pattern of facial abnormalities, growth retardation, and brain damage (manifest as behavioral or cognitive difficulties); signs of brain damage in the absence of other indicators of FAS is termed alcohol related neurodevelopmental disorder (Stratton et al., 1996). Not all children born to mothers who drank alcohol during pregnancy will have FAS. The entire spectrum of deficits resulting from prenatal alcohol exposure is captured under the term fetal alcohol spectrum disorder (FASD). FASD includes individuals diagnosed with FAS (the most severe consequence of maternal alcohol consumption), neurobehavioral disorders, isolated birth defects, and/or cognitive dysfunction resulting from confirmed gestational alcohol exposure (Bertrand et al., 2004).

A significant amount of experimental evidence using research animals ties prenatal alcohol exposure to adverse development of fetal and postnatal brain. Researchers have utilized a number of animal model systems to investigate the underlying disruption of brain development following alcohol exposure at various doses and critical periods of brain development. On the other hand, there are far fewer studies in the clinical literature showing the effects of timing of alcohol exposure and adverse brain development in human subjects, and much of that literature is derived from autopsy materials from severe cases of FAS infants and children. Therefore, the results from animal studies are important to demonstrate a causal relationship between adverse neuroanatomical outcome and controlled variables, such as the timing of alcohol exposure during critical stages of brain development. The results from these well-controlled animal studies will drive the future direction of human studies in this particular research area.

The goal of this chapter is to provide an overview of the clinical (human) and experimental (animal) data related to the timing of alcohol exposure and aberrant brain development.

## RISK FACTORS FOR FAS OR FASD

Not all women who drink alcohol during pregnancy will deliver babies with hallmark features of FAS or with deficits associated with FASD. Research during the past three decades has been performed to explore the difference in outcome related to this question. Through such research efforts, several important risk factors have been identified that may account for the differential outcome of prenatal alcohol exposure. The discussion of risk factors in this review are the ones that impact the developing brain tissues leading to abnormal brain development, such as small brain volume or agenesis of corpus callosum. It is particularly important to make a distinction between "risk factor" and "mechanism" for prenatal alcohol-induced brain injury. Although alcohol may exert its injurious action through the same mechanisms, risk factors may work individually or in concert to modulate the extent of brain damage (induced by the same mechanisms). Although the focus of this chapter is on the effect of timing of alcohol exposure during gestation as a risk factor influencing the severity and the specificity of developmental brain injury, in the following paragraphs, brief summaries of other risk factors are discussed within the context of how they affect the nature and severity of prenatal alcohol-induced brain damage.

The nature and severity of brain injury observed in FAS or FASD is not determined solely by the total amount of alcohol consumed during any drinking episode. It is the blood alcohol concentration that plays a more significant role in predicting the severity of developmental brain injury (Bonthius and West, 1988). In essence, the achievement of a higher blood alcohol concentration results in more severe brain damage. Thus, factors capable of influencing the level of blood alcohol concentration, such as the pattern of drinking, the combined use of alcohol and other drugs, and the genetic makeup of an individual are also risk factors that may account for the nature and severity of brain damage following prenatal alcohol exposure. In order to achieve a better understanding of this concept, three potential risk factors, pattern of alcohol drinking, polydrug use and genetic variation, are described to demonstrate how they interact with alcohol metabolism to elevate the circulating alcohol in the bloodstream.

*Pattern of Alcohol Drinking (Binge Drinking).* The drinking pattern that significantly raises the blood alcohol concentration is binge drinking. According to a publication from the National Institute on Alcohol Abuse and Alcoholism (NIAAA, 2004), binge drinking is defined as having five or more standard drinks (one standard drink: one 12-oz. beer, one 6-oz. wine or one 1.5-oz distilled spirit) in males, or four or more drinks in females within a 2-hour period. Binge drinking leads to higher blood alcohol concentration (Donovan, 2009; Read et al., 2008) and binge drinking has been modeled in animal subjects in order to examine the effects of gestational alcohol exposure on neural development and functions in the offspring (Helfer et al., 2009; Lee et al., 2008; Ramadoss et al., 2007; Watari et al., 2006). The elevated blood alcohol concentration in binge drinking is closely related to the rate of alcohol metabolism and elimination. Alcohol dehydrogenase (ADH), a family of several isozymes (isoenzymes; a group of enzymes share the same function, but differ in physical structures and efficacy), is capable of metabolizing alcohol in liver, and the ADH metabolic pathway is readily saturated following consumption of only a few drinks (Fujimiya et al., 1989). Moreover, the rate of alcohol elimination follows zero-order kinetics, which means that the elimination of alcohol from the body is independent of the level of alcohol in the physiological system (Jones, 2010). Combining the quick saturation of ADH metabolism pathway and the zero-order elimination rate, a high blood alcohol concentration would be the most direct consequence of the pharmacokinetic model if an individual continues to drink alcohol over a short period of time. Although it has been suggested that non-ADH pathways may be involved in the elimination of alcohol at higher blood concentrations (Norberg et al.,

2003; Zakhari, 2006), it does not change the fact that the high blood alcohol concentration has already been achieved from the binge drinking episode and the detrimental effects on organ tissues are most likely inevitable

*Polydrug Use.* The use of alcohol and other drugs simultaneously (polydrug use) is common among a subset of the population in our society (NIAAA, 2008), including women of reproductive age (SAMHSA, 2008). The serious dangers associated with polydrug use are the unpredictable pharmacokinetic interactions among drugs that may alter the bioavailability of alcohol or other drugs in the blood. Results from the literature suggest that the combination of alcohol with some over-the-counter (OTC) drugs may lead to an elevation of blood alcohol concentration by interfering with the metabolism of alcohol. For example, cimetidine (Tagamet®) and ranitidine (Zantac®), two drugs that are used to relieve heartburn, may inhibit the gastric ADH activity if used simultaneously with alcohol, which allows more alcohol to be absorbed by the small intestine leading to a higher blood alcohol concentration (Fraser, 1998; Gentry et al., 1999). Thus, an unpredictable increase in the blood alcohol concentration is a result of consuming alcohol and some OTC medications at the same time. Another example of the potential for deleterious effects of polydrug use is related to the production of another toxic compound in the physiological system by way of a drug-drug interaction. The interaction between alcohol and cocaine is a common example used to demonstrate how the concurrent use of these two drugs is more injurious than the use of each drug individually. The liver enzyme carboxylesterase is able to convert cocaine into a pharmacologically active and toxic compound cocaethylene in the presence of ethyl alcohol (ethanol) (Brzezinski et al., 1994). The toxicity of cocaethylene is far greater than the toxicity of either alcohol or cocaine, and place individuals at risk for increased tissue damage, including the developing fetus (Farooq et al., 2009; Tacker and Okorodudu, 2004; Wilson et al., 2009). Interestingly, recent data have suggested that the increased toxicity following the concurrent use of alcohol and cocaine is due to an alcohol-induced delay in cocaine metabolism and elimination leading to the prolonged action of cocaine on tissue (Parker and Laizure, 2010). Regardless of the underlying mechanism for the additive effects of concurrent alcohol and cocaine use, polydrug use has the potential to be a significant risk factor for FASD or FAS.

*Genetic Variation.* Genetic variation may affect the severity of alcohol-induced brain damage through multiple means, however, differences in the genes encoding ADH enzymes may have an impact on the level of blood alcohol achieved based on the efficiency of the enzymes to metabolize alcohol. Humans have several ADH isozymes (Edenberg, 2007) but they vary in their distribution among different ethnic groups. For example, $\beta_3$-ADH, encoded by *ADH1B*3* gene, capable of eliminating alcohol at a higher rate is found in about 22% of the African-American population, but only less than 5% of European-American population (Warren and Li, 2005). Similar ethnic diversity is found in the *ADH1B*2* genes encoded for $\beta_2$-ADH. This *ADH1B*2* gene is more prevalent in the Chinese and Japanese populations, but much less in the Indian population (Eng et al., 2007). Since ADH isozymes do not have an identical efficiency in the metabolism of alcohol and not all ethnic groups share the same distribution of ADH isozymes, the assumption is that alcohol may exert a detrimental effect differentially among various ethnic populations depending on how fast alcohol is metabolized by ADH. Recent data suggest that the developing fetus is protected from prenatal alcohol if its mother has higher frequencies of *ADH1B*2* or *ADH1B*3* genes (for reviews see Jacobson et al., 2006; Warren and Li, 2005).

Taken together, there is evidence to support the role of certain risk factors, such as drinking pattern, polydrug use and genetic differences, in the variability of outcome in individuals with FAS or FASD. Obviously there are other risk factors, such as maternal nutrition, maternal age, lack of prenatal care, parity, and preconception alcohol exposure that may play an important role in explaining the variation in outcomes, however, those and other risk factors are not discussed in this chapter, but are important in the consideration of normal and abnormal fetal brain development.

## Comparative Aspect of Brain Development

In order to make comparisons of the findings between animals and humans as will be done in this chapter, it is important to consider species differences in the timing of various developmental stages. While all mammals pass through the same stages of brain development, those stages differ relative to parturition. For example in humans, the most dynamic period of brain development including a significant increase in brain mass and acceleration in synaptogenesis and neuronal proliferation begins during early pregnancy, peaks near birth and continues into the early postnatal period. This stage of brain development is known in the literature as the brain growth spurt. In the rat and mouse models, the most commonly used animal model, the brain growth spurt occurs entirely postnatally (Dobbing and Sands,1979), but in the guinea pig, sheep and non-human primate models, the brain growth spurt occurs entirely before parturition, thus alcohol exposure must stop prior to the end of pregnancy in these species. Thus, it is critically important to consider this difference in the timing of brain development when making comparisons across species with regard to the alcohol-induced effects related to specific periods of exposure. Given the specificity of the terms used to describe the temporal developmental window of alcohol exposure in animal models, the term "trimester equivalent" will be used in the discussion of the three stages of gestation in the animal models.

## Evidence for Temporal Vulnerability: Clinical Evidence from Humans

Since FAS was defined in 1973 (Jones and Smith, 1973), researchers have learned a significant amount about the behavioral, cognitive, and physical features of FAS, FASD, and related diagnoses. A significant body of research in human infants, children and adults points to neuroanatomical alterations resulting from heavy prenatal alcohol exposure, including changes in brain microstructure derived from autopsy material (Clarren et al., 1978; Coulter et al., 1993; Ferrer and Galofre, 1987), volumetric whole brain and regional brain abnormalities from MRI in living subjects (reviewed by Roebuck et al., 1998), and detailed regional and microstructural brain alterations in CNS with correlations to cognitive function (e.g., Bookstein et al., 2002a, 2002b; Lebel et al., 2008; 2010; see review by Norman et al., 2009). Unfortunately, much of the clinical research was conducted without consideration of or knowledge about the timing of the alcohol exposure for each case of brain malformation observed. Therefore, the majority of the knowledge regarding the effects of alcohol exposure on brain development during various stages of pregnancy is derived from research using animal models. In this section, we provide an overview of the clinical evidence in humans to show how the timing of alcohol exposure affects human brain development.

Most of the clinical evidence for the timing of alcohol exposure risk factor comes from studies using a retrospective study design. In general, affected infants or children are identified and their mothers are asked to provide information about their alcohol consumption habits during their index pregnancy. Their answers to questions such as "when during your pregnancy did you consume alcohol?" and "how much alcohol did you consume each time you drank?" are used to reflect the timing, amount and frequency of alcohol consumption. Although the data from these retrospective studies are valuable, more accurate data might be collected through the use of a prospective study design to capture the incidence of drinking closer to the time point at which it occurred.

A small body of literature shows that the cessation of alcohol consumption during specific stages of pregnancy is beneficial for the growth and later development of offspring. The measurements that are common to these studies involve birth weight and head circumference. Head circumference has been the surrogate measurement for brain size, while birth weight and body weight reflect overall growth. Smith and colleagues (1986) reported that women who stopped drinking at midgestation (before the end of the second trimester) had babies that were no different in terms of birth weight and head circumference from infants of women who never drank during their pregnancy. Women who were identified as heavy drinkers, but who reduced their drinking during the third trimester, gave birth to infants who were similar in birth weight and head circumference to infants born to women who never drank during their pregnancy (Rosett et al., 1983). Furthermore, Jacobson and coworkers (1994) reported a significant, yet negative, correlation between measures of birth weight and head circumference with alcohol consumption during the last half of gestation, however, these significant correlations no longer existed at follow-up (at 13 months of age). Similarly, Coles (1994) described results from offspring of three groups of mothers: those who never drank during pregnancy, those who stopped drinking during the second trimester, and those who drank continuously throughout their pregnancy. On measures of birth weight and head circumference (measured at birth and again at 5-7 years of age), there was a significant benefit for the offspring from mothers who stopped drinking during the second trimester. The measurement of birth weight and head circumference was significantly worse in the offspring born to mothers who drank throughout their pregnancy. However, when measured at follow-up (5-7 years of age), the group differences in body weight were no longer detected, but the head circumference remained robustly smaller in offspring from those who never stopped drinking during pregnancy.

One of the goals in the fetal alcohol research field is to identify individuals affected by prenatal alcohol exposure as early as possible in order to give them access to treatments or potential therapies that can assist with their postnatal development. Given this goal, several researchers have used *in utero* and early postnatal ultrasound imaging of fetal or neonatal brain in order to identify affected fetuses and babies, respectively. One of the earliest studies to show an effect of timing of alcohol exposure on the developing fetus was performed by Handmaker and colleagues (2006). Using ultrasound imaging techniques, they took measurements of fetal size using bony landmarks (biparietal diameter, frontooccipital diameter, head circumference, femur length), soft tissue (abdominal circumference), and brain structure (transcerebellar diameter, lateral ventricular atrial diameter, cisterna magna) from fetuses between 18 and 41 weeks of development. At the time of ultrasound, pregnant women were screened for alcohol consumption and grouped into three groups of women: those who continued to drink throughout their pregnancy, those who stopped drinking after they found out about their pregnancy, and those who did not drink during their pregnancy. Women from all groups became aware of their pregnancy around five weeks gestation. After controlling for several variables, fetal head circumference (relative to abdominal circumference) and fetal cerebellar growth (measured by transcerebellar diameter) were reduced in fetuses of women who continued to drink after learning of their pregnancy relative to those measurements from fetuses of women in the other two groups. There were no significant differences observed on any variable in the fetuses from women who stopped drinking after pregnancy recognition and those from women who did not drink during pregnancy. The authors concluded that the cessation of alcohol consumption alleviated some of the increased damage associated with continued gestational alcohol exposure and support the use of fetal biometrics for the assessment of alcohol-induced damage.

The clinical evidence in humans for adverse offspring outcome as a function of differential timing of alcohol exposure during pregnancy is very sparse. However, it is important to recognize that the clinical studies were not designed to address the question of temporal vulnerability. The findings from the few studies show quite convincingly that both brain growth (measured by head circumference) and body growth are inhibited by the continued consumption of alcohol throughout pregnancy, and that the cessation of alcohol consumption prior to the third trimester can ameliorate some of the growth deficits. This suggests that the third trimester is a period of vulnerability for brain and body growth. Given the limitations for manipulating alcohol exposure in pregnant women, research using animal subjects will produce results that may guide future clinical prospective studies to include variables related to timing in the study design.

## Evidence For Temporal Vulnerability: Experimental Evidence from Animals

Given the significant gap in the clinical literature with regard to the effect of timing of alcohol exposure and offspring outcome, experimental studies using animals have played a more integral role in exploring the nature of timing of alcohol exposure during gestation on brain development. For several decades, researchers using animal models have shown that the timing of alcohol exposure during fetal brain development is an important variable in predicting the nature of the outcome observed in offspring.

The clinical evidence for temporal vulnerability has commonly focused on microcephaly (head circumference representing brain size/growth) and body growth (birth weight and body weight) as primary dependent variables and the results show that these variables may be linked to the third trimester. There is a robust experimental literature using animal models comparing the effects of alcohol exposure during various trimesters equivalent to the equivalent times of human pregnancy. Maier et al. (1997) measured brain and body growth in offspring from separate groups of pregnant rats given alcohol during the first trimester equivalent, the second trimester equivalent, the third trimester equivalent, all three trimesters equivalent (the first two trimesters via the mother, the third trimester via artificial rearing), and appropriate corresponding controls. The results indicate that exposure to alcohol during all three trimesters equivalent results in significant body growth deficits; that the third trimester in particular is a period of unique susceptibility for volume-based reductions in whole brain, forebrain, cerebellum and brainstem. These results are consistent with the conclusion reached by Coles (1994) and the results from Handmaker et al. (2006) that the third trimester in human is a sensitive period for alcohol-induced body growth restrictions and expand that conclusion to include brain growth restrictions as vulnerable to the third trimester alcohol exposure.

While the above example is interesting, far more comprehensive information can be obtained from animal subjects. Changes resulting from alcohol exposure during various stages of brain development can be measured at the gross level (e.g., brain weight; morphology), microscopic level (e.g., neuronal number; cellular structure or function of the neuron), genomic level (e.g., methylation; regulatory microRNA) and molecular level (e.g., protein content; signaling pathways). In each of the following paragraphs, alcohol-induced changes in brain morphology are summarized based on findings following exposure during the first trimester equivalent, second trimester equivalent or third trimester equivalent relative to controls. In Table 1, a more complete presentation of outcomes related to the timing of alcohol exposure in animal studies is presented, since not all experimental findings will be discussed in the text below. These data are taken from studies employing animal model systems including mouse, rat, guinea pig, sheep, and non-human primate. It is important to note the consistent theme across all studies is the measurement or estimation of blood alcohol concentration, given the importance of this risk factor and the comparison of effects across species and differential timing of alcohol exposure (temporal windows).

The cerebellum is highly vulnerable to alcohol-induced changes following exposure during the third trimester equivalent or in cases where the exposure overlaps the third trimester equivalent. This effect holds regardless of animal model (rat, mouse, sheep) or nature of the parameters measured (cerebellum weight, number of Purkinje cells, blood flow, or gene expression). Furthermore, the results are consistently in the same direction. For example, the number of Purkinje cells is significantly reduced in alcohol exposed sheep and rats from third, but not second trimester equivalent exposure. While the Purkinje cells may be depleted in number by alcohol exposure during the first or third trimester equivalent, the abundant granule cells are not reduced in number in any species of alcohol-exposed subject. Furthermore, the results from gene expression and cell loss are consistent insofar as there is an increase in proapoptotic gene expression during the third trimester equivalent similar to the consistent loss of Purkinje cells. Thus, the results from the animal studies provide a wealth of detailed information regarding the structural, cellular and molecular events that occur in the developing cerebellum resulting from alcohol exposure at a level that the clinical MRI studies cannot accomplish.

The brainstem is composed of a multitude of fiber tracts and nuclei important for the integration of many critical homeostatic functions; and the axons of many nuclei located in the brainstem project to the thalamus, the major relay structure for many afferent inputs. The brain develops in a general caudal to rostral pattern, thus brainstem structures develop earlier than, for example, cortical structures. Experimental evidence from animal models supports the tenet of teratology that structures during their most rapid period of development are most vulnerable to a teratogen, given that first and second trimester equivalent alcohol exposure has more impact on brainstem development than does third trimester equivalent alcohol exposure. Within the brainstem, neurons of specific nuclei are vulnerable to alcohol-induced depletion following first (trigeminal, facial and hypoglossal nuclei) or second (ventrolateral nucleus of the thalamus) trimester equivalent exposure, but not third trimester equivalent exposure. Also, the gross brainstem weight is markedly reduced following first trimester equivalent alcohol exposure relative to exposure during second or third trimester equivalent.

The hippocampus is an extensively studied brain structure due to its unique and important role in learning and memory. Any errors in neural circuitry or loss of specific neuronal populations within hippocampus will interfere with learning new tasks and retrieving stored memories. Hippocampus integrity has been measured using several techniques from counting neurons, measuring functional aspects of neurons, to assessing blood flow to the hippocampus. Alcohol exposure during the third trimester equivalent seems to have the greatest impact on cell loss (pyramidal cells in CA1, possibly CA3 and granule cells of the dentate gyrus) compared with cell loss from alcohol exposure during the first or second trimester equivalent, even though the results from a study by Byrnes and colleagues (2003) showed no effects of third trimester equivalent alcohol exposure on these neuronal populations in a guinea pig model. Other measurements, such as hippocampal glutamatergic transmission and blood flow, appeared to be significantly affected by the third trimester equivalent alcohol exposure. It is interesting to note, but beyond a complete discussion in this chapter, that many behavioral studies have shown learning and memory-related deficits following third trimester equivalent alcohol exposure with concomitant loss of pyramidal cells in hippocampal CA1 field. Thus, the evidence from structural and functional studies suggests that third trimester equivalent alcohol exposure appears to be a vulnerable period for the development of hippocampus.

The olfactory bulb has been a region of interest because of its unique cellular organization and function (other than olfaction) since it provides neurotrophic support to the basal forebrain (Jezierski and Sohrabji, 2003). Compromise to the integrity of the neural structures of the olfactory bulb will disrupt olfactory function and other forebrain regions that depend on olfactory bulb neurons for neurotrophic support. Alcohol exposure during brain development does significantly reduce the primary output neurons, the mitral cells, but only when the exposure period is restricted to the third trimester equivalent. Similar to the granule cells in the hippocampus, the granule cells of the olfactory bulb are much less vulnerable to alcohol exposure during the third trimester equivalent. In addition, alcohol exposure during the first or second trimester equivalent does not affect the number of mitral or granule cells. One clinically relevant question that needs to be explored is whether the inadequate social skills or emotional disturbance seen in FAS patients is a result of compromised olfactory integrity, given the complex nature of human olfaction (Stevenson, 2010; Yeshurun and Sobel, 2010) and its interaction with brain regions that regulate emotion and social activities.

The cerebral cortex is the center of integration for multifaceted sensory input and the command center for the execution of motor output. All higher cognitive functions are coordinated in the cerebral cortex within each cortical hemisphere through short and long intrahemisphere longitudinal fasciculi, and between the two hemispheres through the corpus callosum and anterior commissure. One of the most striking features from autopsy cases of FAS is the complete absence of the corpus callosum. Using MRI techniques, corpus callosum volume, shape and size has been demonstrated in living FAS subjects, however the extent of the alcohol-induced damage to the corpus callosum in FAS subjects cannot be related to the timing of the alcohol exposure (Norman et al., 2009; Wozniak et al., 2009).

**Table 1. Effects of alcohol exposure during specific developmental windows (first trimester, second trimester, third trimester) and brain region or structure (whole brain, cerebellum, brainstem, hippocampus, olfactory bulb, cortex and basal ganglia)**

| | First Trimester | Second Trimester | Third Trimester |
|---|---|---|---|
| Whole brain | ↔ brain/body weight ratio<br>*Maier et al., 1997* | ↔ brain/body weight ratio<br>*Maier et al., 1997*<br>*Qiang et al., 2002* | ↓ brain/body weight ratio<br>*Goodlett et al., 1989*<br>*Maier et al., 1997* |
| | | ↓ blood flow under hypoxia (in supratentorial tissue)<br>*Mayock et al., 2007* | |
| Cerebellum | ↓ number of Purkinje cells<br>*Ramadoss et al., 2007* | ↔ number of Purkinje cells<br>*Maier et al., 1999*<br>*Maier and West, 2003**<br>*Marcussen et al., 1994** | ↓ number of Purkinje cells<br>*Goodlett et al., 1990***<br>*Goodlett and Lundahl, 1996**<br>*Goodlett and Eilers, 1997**<br>*Hamre and West, 1993**<br>*Karaçay et al., 2008**<br>*Maier et al., 1999*<br>*Marcussen et al., 1994*<br>*Miki et al., 1999**<br>*Parnell et al., 2007*<br>*Ramadoss et al., 2007*<br>*Thomas et al., 1998* |
| | ↔ number of Purkinje cells<br>*Maier et al., 1999* | ↔ cerebellum/body weight ratio<br>*Maier et al., 1997* | ↓ cerebellum/body weight ratio<br>*Goodlett et al., 1989*<br>*Goodlett et al., 1990***<br>*Maier et al., 1997* |
| | ↔ cerebellum/body weight ratio<br>*Maier et al., 1997* | ↔ number of granule cells<br>*Maier et al., 1999* | ↔ number of granule cells<br>*Maier et al., 1999* |
| | ↔ number of granule cells<br>*Maier et al., 1999* | | ↑ blood flow to cerebellum<br>*Parnell et al., 2007* |
| | | | ↑ proapoptotic gene expression<br>*Heaton et al., 2003a** |
| | | | ↓ number of cells in deep cerebellar nuclei<br>*Green et al., 2006* |
| | | | ↓ expression of bcl2, bad<br>*Ge et al., 2004** |

| | First Trimester | Second Trimester | Third Trimester |
|---|---|---|---|
| Brainstem | ↓ brainstem/body weight ratio<br>*Maier et al., 1997* | ↔ brainstem/body weight ratio<br>*Maier et al., 1997* | ↔ brainstem/body weight ratio<br>*Maier et al., 1997* |
| | ↔ number of cells in ventrolateral nucleus of thalamus<br>*Livy et al., 2001* | ↔ number of cells in ventrolateral nucleus of thalamus<br>*Livy et al., 2001* | ↔ number of cells in ventrolateral nucleus of thalamus<br>*Livy et al., 2001* |
| | ↓ number of cells in trigeminal (motor and sensory), facial and hypoglossal nuclei<br>*Mooney and Miller, 2007** | ↓ number of cells in ventrolateral nucleus of thalamus<br>*Livy et al., 2001** | |
| | ↓ length of rostral hindbrain<br>*Dunty et al., 2002** | ↓ number of cells in locus coeruleus<br>*Maier and West, 2003** | |
| | | ↔ number of cells in inferior olive nucleus<br>*Maier and West, 2003** | |
| Hippocampus | ↔ number of CA1, CA3 pyramidal cells and DG granule cells<br>*Tran and Kelly, 2003* | ↔ number of CA1, CA3 pyramidal cells and DG granule cells<br>*Livy et al., 2003*<br>*Tran and Kelly, 2003* | ↓ number of CA1 pyramidal cells<br>*Livy et al., 2003*<br>*Tran and Kelly, 2003* |
| | ↔ density total glutamate receptor binding<br>*Savage et al., 1992* | ↔ number of CA1, CA3 pyramidal cells<br>*Livy et al., 2003** | ↓ number of CA3 pyramidal cells and DG granule cells<br>*Livy et al., 2003* |
| | | ↓ density total glutamate receptor binding<br>*Savage et al., 1992** | ↔ CA3 pyramidal cells and DG granule cells<br>*Tran and Kelly, 2003* |
| | | | ↔ CA1 field fEPSP amplitude<br>*Byrnes et al., 2004* |
| | | | ↔ density total glutamate receptor binding<br>*Savage et al., 1992* |
| | | | ↔ blood flow to hippocampus<br>↔ number of CA1, CA3 pyramidal cells<br>*Parnell et al., 2007* |
| Olfactory bulb | ↔ number of mitral cells<br>*Maier et al., 1999* | ↔ number of mitral cells<br>*Maier et al., 1999* | ↓ number of mitral cells<br>*Maier et al., 1999* |
| | ↔ number of granule cells<br>*Maier et al., 1999* | ↔ number of granule cells<br>*Maier et al., 1999* | ↔ number of granule cells<br>*Maier et al., 1999* |
| | | | ↔ blood flow to olfactory bulb<br>↔ number of mitral cells<br>*Parnell et al., 2007* |

**Table 1. Effects of alcohol exposure during specific developmental windows (first trimester, second trimester, third trimester) and brain region or structure (whole brain, cerebellum, brainstem, hippocampus, olfactory bulb, cortex and basal ganglia) (Continued)**

| | First Trimester | Second Trimester | Third Trimester |
|---|---|---|---|
| Cortex and Basal Ganglia | ↑ midsagittal area of corpus callosum and number of corpus callosum axons<br>*Miller et al., 1999* | ↑ number and length of apical and basilar dendritic branches of corpus callosum cells<br>*Qiang et al., 2002* | ↓ area corresponding to barrel field cortex<br>*Oladehin et al., 2007* |
| | ↓ area (forebrain) and density of cells corresponding to somatosensory area<br>*Miller, 2007* | ↔ density in cerebral microvessels (forebrain)<br>*Simon et al., 2008* | ↑ proapoptotic gene expression<br>*Heaton et al., 2003c** |
| | ↓ density in VIP-stained cells (forebrain)<br>*Anderson et al., 2008* | ↔ reactivity of cerebral arterioles (forebrain) to endogenous vasoactive mediators<br>*Mayock et al., 2008* | ↓ expression of GDNF and Akt phosphorylation<br>*Tsuji et al., 2008** |
| | ↔ density in neu-N stained cells (forebrain)<br>*Anderson et al., 2008* | | ↔ expression of BDNF, PMAPK, -p70S6K (decrease equivalent on all PD exposure days)<br>*Tsuji et al., 2008** |
| | | | ↑ proapoptotic gene expression (striatum)<br>*Heaton et al., 2003b** |
| | | | ↓ $GABA_AR$ response (septum)<br>*Hsiao et al., 2004** |
| | | | ↓ CREB phosphorylation<br>*Krahe et al., 2009* |
| | | | ↓ forebrain/body weight ratio<br>*Maier et al., 1997* |
| | | | ↓ number of cells in frontal lobe<br>*Burke et al., 2009* |
| Other | ↑ intensity of stain for macrophage activity (white matter tracts)<br>*Watari et al., 2006* | | |

Direction or type of effect: ↑ - increase, ↓ - decrease, ↔ - no change.

* effect related to limited days of alcohol exposure within a specific trimester equivalent period (e.g., postnatal day 4 within the period of third trimester equivalent).

** under conditions of high blood alcohol concentration (BAC) relative to lower BACs achieved by similarly-treated groups in the same study.

Experimental evidence from animal studies supports the notion that the corpus callosum is affected by prenatal alcohol exposure, but expands on that by showing alterations related to the timing of alcohol exposure. While first trimester equivalent alcohol exposure increases the mid-sagittal area and number of cells within the corpus callosum, second trimester equivalent alcohol exposure increases the number and length of dendritic branches of callosal neurons. In addition, regional cortical areas connected by the corpus callosum are differentially affected by first (decreased in density of neurons in somatosensory cortex) and third (decrease in areas of barrel field cortex) trimester equivalent alcohol exposure. Finally, comparisons of genomic or molecular changes, for example, an increase in pro-apoptotic gene expression, and a decrease in the expression of GDNF and CREB phosphorylation have been reported in the cortex following alcohol exposure during the third trimester equivalent.

The discussion of the experimental animal studies has not been exhaustive, but serves as a starting point for the discussion of the available literature comparing brain structure and neuronal function from animal subjects exposed to alcohol during various stages of brain development. Undeniably, the experimental evidence offers a more in-depth understanding of how timing of alcohol exposure affects brain development. However, at the same time, these findings point out a critical need to employ better designed experiments that include comparisons of all trimesters equivalent on the same dependent variables in a study. The results from such studies will be the key to comprehensively answer questions related to temporal vulnerability and the most dynamic periods of brain development.

## CONCLUSION

Drinking alcohol during pregnancy can cause changes in offspring brain development. Based on the available clinical (human) and experimental (animal) literature presented in this chapter, there is considerable risk for variability in outcome based on the timing of alcohol exposure during pregnancy. To date, there is no formula for predicting the nature and extent of offspring brain injury following alcohol exposure during a specific period of brain development. It will be important to identify reliably the outcome from alcohol exposure at different times of brain development in order to provide services for those children who manifest deleterious changes in brain anatomy as unexplained behavioral dysfunction. One immediate goal of clinical research could be the early identification of alcohol exposed fetuses and research of this nature has already shown that brain injury can be identified early in clinical populations (Bookstein et al., 2005; Handmaker et al., 2006; Kfir et al., 2009). Although this research will not ameliorate the neuroanatomical damage, the early identification of affected fetuses will improve their chance of receiving specialized care and attention during postnatal life that might lessen the behavioral impact of the brain injury.

For each grossly defined developmental period, first, second or third trimester, there is evidence of vulnerability to alcohol-induced brain damage, and the nature of such damage is brain region and neuronal specific. At various stages in the life of a neuron or its connections, programmed molecular changes signaling an upcoming role in crafting the various elements that constitute brain occur in rapid sequence. Therefore, not only is brain development a moving target, its well choreographed developmental events are not necessarily linear, making its fate in response to external influences (e.g., drugs or environmental toxins) not entirely predictable. Nonetheless, several statements about the effect of alcohol on brain development are supported by the evidence presented in this chapter.

First, regardless of experimental animal model, there are similar alcohol-induced effects, even given the broad range of species and the nature of equivalent brain development during pre- or post-natal life. Although there are advantages and disadvantages to all the animal models, the consistencies among them in alcohol-induced brain damage are remarkable, and support the further use of appropriate animal models to address research questions that are not appropriately addressed in humans.

Second, the effects of alcohol on brain injury appear to be related to higher alcohol doses or higher BAC achieved regardless of differential developmental period. For example, the Purkinje cells of the cerebellum can be depleted following alcohol exposure during the first or third trimester equivalent, however, the BACs must reach a certain level for this to occur.

Third, the third trimester (or third trimester equivalent in experimental alcohol models) is uniquely vulnerable to the effects of alcohol exposure, even though there may be trimester-specific brain damage depending on the critical developmental events within each trimester. Much of the experimental animal literature confirms what was concluded from the clinical human studies that alcohol exposure during the third trimester uniquely affects the brain development of the offspring. However, some caution needs to be taken in assuming that the third trimester is more vulnerable that the first or second, because much of what is known about alcohol and brain development has been conducted in animals during the third trimester equivalent. Considerably less attention has been focused on discovering the variation in effects from alcohol exposure restricted to only the first or second trimester equivalent and comparing those outcomes to third trimester equivalent exposure using the same dependent variables.

There is one important caveat to using animal models. While animal models have been optimal to address temporal windows of vulnerability associated with prenatal alcohol exposure, many of the current animal models do not take into account the human condition. Women do not begin drinking at the beginning of their pregnancy (or at a critical period of their pregnancy), yet almost all of the experimental studies using animals begin alcohol exposure at the developmental period of interest. The results from experimental studies on the timing of alcohol exposure may be different if the research was conducted to more closely parallel the human condition. Furthermore, research in this area might provide insight into other aspects of alcohol on reproduction in general, including fertility, fecundity, and perhaps fetal origins of adult disease. Clearly, the consideration of alcohol consumption prior to pregnancy will be an important improvement to the animal models to closely mimic human condition of alcohol-exposed pregnancy, and in addition, may provide additional information on the effects of alcohol on reproduction in general.

## References

Anderson, D.J., Mondares, R.L., Born, D.E. and Gleason, C.A. (2008). The effect of binge fetal alcohol exposure on the number of vasoactive intestinal peptide-producing neurons in fetal sheep brain. *Developmental Neuroscience* 30, 276-284.

Bertrand, J., Floyd, R.L., Weber, M.K., Weber, M.K., O'Connor, M.J., Riley, E., Johnson, K.A., and Cohen, D.E. (2004). Fetal alcohol syndrome: guidelines for referral and diagnosis. Atlanta, GA: US Department of Health and Human Services, Centers for Disease Control and Prevention.

Bonthius, D.J. and West, J.R. (1988). Blood alcohol concentration and microencephaly: a dose-response study in the neonatal rat. *Teratology* 37, 223-231.

Bookstein, F.L., Sampson, P.D., Connor, P.D. and Streissguth, A.P. (2002a). Midline corpus callosum is a neuroanatomical focus of fetal alcohol damage. *The Anatomical Record* 269, 162–174.

Bookstein, F.L., Streissguth, A.P., Sampson, P.D., Connor, P.D. and Barr, H.M. (2002b). Corpus callosum shape and neuropsychological deficits in adult males with heavy fetal alcohol exposure. *NeuroImage* 15, 233–251.

Bookstein, F.L., Connor, P.D., Covell, K.D., Barr, H.M., Gleason, C.A., Sze, R.W., McBroom, J.A. and Streissguth, A.P. (2005). Preliminary evidence that prenatal alcohol damage may be visible in averaged ultrasound images of the neonatal human corpus callosum. *Alcohol* 36, 151-160.

Brzezinski, M.R., Abraham, T.L., Stone, C.L., Dean, R.A. and Bosron, W.F. (1994). Purification and characterization of a human liver cocaine carboxylesterase that catalyzes the production of benzoylecgonine and the formation of cocaethylene from alcohol and cocaine. *Biochemical Pharmacology* 48, 1747-1755.

Burke, M.W., Palmour, R.M., Ervin, F.R. and Ptito, M. (2009). Neuronal reduction in frontal cortex of primates after prenatal alcohol exposure. *NeuroReport* 20, 13-17.

Byrnes, M.L., Reynolds, J.N. and Brien, J.F. (2003). Brain growth spurt – prenatal ethanol exposure and the guinea pig hippocampal glutamate signaling system. *Neurotoxicology and Teratology* 25, 303-310.

Byrnes, M.L., Richardson, D.P., Brien, J.F., Reynolds, J.N. and Dringenberg, H.C. (2004). Spatial acquisition in the Morris water maze and hippocampal long-term potentiation in the adult guinea pig following brain growth spurt-prenatal ethanol exposure. *Neurotoxicology and Teratology* 26, 543-551.

Clarren, S.K., Alvord Jr., E.C., Sumi, S.M., Streissguth, A.P. and Smith, D.W. (1978). Brain malformations related to prenatal exposure to ethanol. Journal of Pediatrics. 92, 64-67.

Coles, C. (1994). Critical periods of prenatal alcohol exposure: evidence from animal and human studies. *Alcohol Health Research World* 18, 22-29.

Coulter, C.L., Leech, R.W., Schaefer, G.B., Scheithauer, B.W. and Brumback, R.A. (1993). Midline cerebral dysgenesis, dysfunction of the hypothalamic-pituitary axis, and fetal alcohol effects. *Archives of Neurology* 50, 771–775.

Dobbing, J. and Sands, J. (1979). Comparative aspects of the brain growth spurt. *Early Human Development* 3, 79-83.

Donovan, J.E. (2009). Estimated blood alcohol concentrations for child and adolescent drinking and their implications for screening instruments. *Pediatrics* 123, e975-e981.

Dunty Jr., W.C., Zucker, R.M., Sulik, K.K. (2002). Hindbrain and cranial nerve dysmorphogenesis result from acute maternal ethanol administration. *Developmental Neuroscience* 24, 328-342.

Edenberg, H.J. (2007). The genetics of alcohol metabolism: Role of alcohol dehydrogenase and aldehyde dehydrogenase variants. *Alcohol Research and Health* 30, 5-13.

Eng, M.Y., Luczak, S.E., and Wall, T.L. (2007). ALDH2, ADH1B, and ADH1C genotypes in Asians: A literature review. *Alcohol Research and Health* 30, 22-27.

Farooq, M.U., Bhatt, A. and Patel, M. (2009). Neurotoxic and cardiotoxic effects of cocaine and ethanol. *Journal of Medical Toxicology* 5, 134-138.

Ferrer, I., and Galofre, E. (1987). Dendritic spine anomalies in fetal alcohol syndrome. *Neuropediatrics* 18, 161–163.

Fraser, A.G. (1998). Is there an interaction between H2-antagonists and alcohol? *Drug Metabolism and Drug Interactions* 14, 123-145.

Fujimiya, T., Yamaoka, K. and Fukui, Y. (1989). Parallel first-order and Michaelis-Menten elimination kinetics of ethanol. Respective role of alcohol dehydrogenase (ADH), non-ADH and first-order pathways. *Journal of Pharmacology and Experimental Therapeutics* 249, 311-317.

Ge, Y., Belcher, S.M., Pierce, D.R. and Light, K.E. (2004). Altered expression of bcl2, Bad and Bax mRNA occurs in the rat cerebellum within hours after ethanol exposure on postnatal day 4 but not on postnatal day 9. *Brain Research Molecular Brain Research* 129, 124-134.

Gentry, R.T., Baraona, E., Amir, I., Roine, R., Chayes, Z.W., Shjarma, R. and Lieber, C.S. (1999). Mechanism of the aspirin-induced rise in blood alcohol levels. *Life Sciences* 65, 2505-2512.

Goodlett, C.R. and Eilers, A.T. (1997). Alcohol-induced Purkinje cell loss with a single binge exposure in neonatal rats: a stereological study of temporal windows of vulnerability. *Alcoholism: Clinical and Experimental Research* 21, 738-744.

Goodlett, C.R. and Lundahl, K.R. (1996). Temporal determinants of neonatal alcohol-induced cerebellar damage and motor performance deficits. *Pharmacology, Biochemistry and Behavior* 55, 531-540.

Goodlett, C.R., Mahoney, J. and West, J.R. (1989). Brain growth deficits following a single day of alcohol exposure in the neonatal rat. *Alcohol.* 6, 121-126.

Goodlett, C.R., Marcussen, B.L. and West, J.R. (1990). A single day of alcohol exposure during the brain growth spurt induces brain weight restriction and cerebellar Purkinje cell loss. *Alcohol.* 7, 107-114.

Green, J.T., Arenos, J.D. and Dillon, C.J. (2006). The effects of moderate neonatal ethanol exposure on eyeblink conditioning and deep cerebellar nuclei neuron numbers in the rat. *Alcohol.* 39, 135-150.

Handmaker, N.S., Rayburn, W.F., Meng, C., Bell, J.B., Rayburn, B.B. and Rappaport, V.J. (2006). Impact of alcohol exposure after pregnancy recognition on ultrasonographic fetal growth measures. *Alcoholism: Clinical and Experimental Research* 30, 892-898.

Hamre, K.M. and West, J.R. (1993). The effects of the timing of ethanol exposure during the brain growth spurt on the number of cerebellar Purkinje and granule cell nuclear profiles. *Alcoholism: Clinical and Experimental Research* 17, 610-622.

Heaton, M.B., Moore, D.B., Paiva, M., Madorsky, I., Mayer, J. and Shaw, G. (2003a). The role of neurotrophic factors, apoptosis-related proteins, and endogenous antioxidants in the differential temporal vulnerability of neonatal cerebellum to ethanol. *Alcoholism: Clinical and Experimental Research* 27, 657-669.

Heaton, M.B., Paiva, M., Madorsky, I., Mayer, J. and Moore, D.B. (2003b). Effects of ethanol on neurotrophic factors, apoptosis-related proteins, endogenous antioxidants, and reactive oxygen species in neonatal striatum: relationship to periods of vulnerability. *Developmental Brain Research* 140, 237-252.

Heaton, M.B., Paiva, M., Madorsky, I. and Shaw, G. (2003c). Ethanol effects on neonatal rat cortex: comparative analyses of neurotrophic factors, apoptosis-related proteins, and oxidative processes during vulnerable and resistant periods. *Developmental Brain Research* 145, 249-262.

Helfer, J.L., Goodlett, C.R., Greenough, W.T. and Klintsova, A.Y. (2009). The effects of exercise on adolescent hippocampal neurogenesis in a rat model of binge alcohol exposure during the brain growth spurt. *Brain Research* 1294, 1-11.

Hsiao, S., DuBois, D., Miranda, R. and Frye, G. (2004). Critically timed ethanol exposure reduced GABAAR function on septal neurons developing in vivo but not in vitro. *Brain Research* 1008, 69-80.

Jacobson, S.W., Carr, L.G., Croxford, J., Sokol, R.J., Li, T.-K. and Jacobson, J.L. (2006). Protective effects of the alcohol dehydrogenase-ADH1B allele in children exposed to alcohol during pregnancy. *The Journal of Pediatrics* 148, 30-37.

Jacobson, J.L., Jacobson, S.W. and Sokol, R.J. (1994). Effects of prenatal exposure to alcohol, smoking, and illicit drugs on postpartum somatic growth. *Alcoholism: Clinical and Experimental Research* 18, 317-323.

Jezierski, M.K. and Sohrabji, F. (2003). Estrogen enhances retrograde transport of brain-derived neurotrophic factor in the rodent forebrain. *Endocrinology* 144, 5022-5029.

Jones, A. W. (2010). Evidence-based survey of the elimination rates of ethanol from blood with applications in forensic casework. Forensic Science International. doi:10.1016/ j.forsciint.2010.02.021.

Jones, K.L. and Smith, D.W. (1973). Recognition of the fetal alcohol syndrome in early infancy. *Lancet* 2, 999-1001.

Karaçay, B., Li, S. and Bonthius, D.J. (2008). Maturation-dependent alcohol resistance in the developing mouse: cerebellar neuronal loss and gene expression during alcohol-vulnerable and –resistant periods. *Alcoholism: Clinical and Experimental Research* 32, 1439-1450.

Kfir, M., Yevtushok, L., Onishchenko, S., Wertelecki, W., Bakhireva, L., Chambers, C.D., Jones, K.L. and Hull, A.D. (2009). Can prenatal ultrasound detect the effects of in-utero alcohol exposure? A pilot study. Ultrasound in Obstetrics and Gynecology. 33, 683-689.

Krahe, T.E., Wang, W. and Medina, A.E. (2009). Phosphodiesterase inhibition increases CREB phosphorylation and restores orientation selectivity in a model of fetal alcohol spectrum disorders. *PLoS One* 4, e6643.

Lebel, C., Rasmussen, C., Wyper, K., Walker, L., Andrew, G., Yager, J. and Beaulieu, C. (2008). Brain diffusion abnormalities in children with fetal alcohol spectrum disorder. *Alcoholism: Clinical and Experimental Research* 32, 1732-1740.

Lebel, C., Rasmussen, C., Wyper, K., Andrew, G. and Beaulieu, C. (2010). Brain microstructure is related to math ability in children with fetal alcohol spectrum disorder. *Alcoholism: Clinical and Experimental Research* 34, 354-363.

Lee, Y., Rowe, J., Eskue, K., West, J.R. and Maier, S.E. (2008). Alcohol exposure on postnatal day 5 induces Purkinje cell loss and evidence of Purkinje cell degradation in lobule I of rat cerebellum. *Alcohol.* 42, 295-302.

Livy, D.J., Maier, S.E. and West, J.R. (2001). Fetal alcohol exposure and temporal vulnerability: effects of binge-like alcohol exposure on the ventrolateral nucleus of the thalamus. *Alcoholism: Clinical and Experimental Research* 25, 774-780.

Livy, D.J., Miller, E.K., Maier, S.E. and West, J.R. (2003). Fetal alcohol exposure and temporal vulnerability: effects of binge-like alcohol exposure on developing rat hippocampus. *Neurotoxicology and Teratology* 25, 447-458.

Maier, S.E., Chen, W.-J.A., Miller, J.A. and West, J.R. (1997). Fetal alcohol exposure and temporal vulnerability: regional differences in alcohol-induced microencephaly as a function of the timing of binge-like alcohol exposure during rat brain development. *Alcoholism: Clinical and Experimental Research* 21, 1418-1428.

Maier, S.E., Miller, J.A., Blackwell, J.M. and West, J.R. (1999). Fetal alcohol exposure and temporal vulnerability: regional differences in cell loss as a function of the timing of binge-like alcohol exposure during brain development. *Alcoholism: Clinical and Experimental Research* 23, 726-734.

Maier, S.E. and West, J.R. (2003). Alcohol and nutritional control treatments during neurogenesis in rat brain reduce total neuron number in locus coeruleus, but not in cerebellum or inferior olive. *Alcohol* 30, 67-74.

Marcussen, B.L., Goodlett, C.R., Mahoney, J. and West, J.R. (1994). Developing rat Purkinje cells are more vulnerable to alcohol-induced depletion during differentiation than during neurogenesis. Alcohol. 2, 147-156.

Mayock, D.E., Ness, D., Mondares, R.L. and Gleason, C.A. (2007). Binge alcohol exposure in the second trimester attenuates fetal cerebral blood flow response to hypoxia. *Journal of Applied Physiology* 102, 972-977.

Mayock, D.E., Ngai, A.C., Mondares, R.L. and Gleason, C.A. (2008). Effects of binge alcohol exposure in the second trimester on intracerebral arteriolar function in third trimester fetal sheep. *Brain Research* 226, 111-115.

Miki, T., Harris, S., Wilce, P., Takeuchi, Y. and Bedi, K. (1999). The effect of timing of ethanol exposure during early postnatal life on total number of Purkinje cells in rat cerebellum. *Journal of Anatomy* 194, 423-431.

Miller, M.W., Astley, S.J. and Clarren, S.K. (1999). Number of axons in the corpus callosum of the mature Macaca nemestrina: increases caused by prenatal exposure to ethanol. *Journal of Comparative Neurology* 412, 123-131.

Miller, M.W. (2007). Exposure to ethanol during gastrulation alters somatosensory-motor cortex and the underlying white matter in the macaque. *Cerebral Cortex*. 17, 2961-2971.

Mooney, S.M. and Miller, M.W. (2007). Time-specific effects of ethanol exposure on cranial nerve nuclei: gastrulation and neurogenesis. *Experimental Neurology* 205, 56-63.

National Institute on Alcohol Abuse and Alcoholism (2004). NIAAA Newsletter. Number 3.

National Institute on Alcohol Abuse and Alcoholism (2008). Alcohol and Other Drugs. Alcohol Alert (No 76). US Department of Health and Human Services.

Norberg, A., Jones, A.W., Hahn, R.G. and Gabrielsson, J.L. (2003). Role of variability in explaining ethanol pharmacokinetics: research and forensic applications. *Clinical Pharmacokinetics* 42, 1-31.

Norman, A.L., Crocker, N., Mattson, S.N. and Riley, E.P. (2009). Neuroimaging and fetal alcohol spectrum disorders. *Developmental Disabilities Research Reviews* 15, 209-217.

Oladehin, A., Margret, C.P., Maier, S.E., Li, C.X., Jan, T.A., Chappell, T.D. and Waters, R.S. (2007). Early postnatal alcohol exposure reduced the size of vibrissal barrel field in rat somatosensory cortex (SI) but did not disrupt barrel field organization. *Alcohol.* 41, 253-261.

Parker, R.B. and Laizure, S.C. (2010). The effect of ethanol on oral cocaine pharmacokinetics reveals an unrecognized class of ethanol-mediated drug interactions. *Drug Metabolism and Disposition* 38, 317-322.

Parnell, S.E., Ramadoss, J., Delp, M., Ramsey, M., Chen, W.-J.A., West, J.R. and Cudd, T.A. (2007). Chronic ethanol increases fetal cerebral blood flow specific to the ethanol-sensitive cerebellum under normoxaemic, hypercapnic and acidaemic conditions: ovine model. *Experimental Physiology* 92, 933-943.

Qiang, M., Wang, W. and Elberger, A. (2002). Second trimester prenatal alcohol exposure alters development of rat corpus callosum. *Neurotoxicology and Teratology* 24, 719-732.

Ramadoss, J., Lunde, E.R., Chen, W.-J.A., West, J.R. and Cudd, T.A. (2007a). Temporal vulnerability of fetal cerebral Purkinje cells to chronic binge alcohol exposure: ovine model. *Alcoholism: Clinical and Experimental Research* 31, 1738-1745.

Read, J.P., Beattie, M., Chamberlain, R. and Merrill, J.E. (2008). Beyond the "binge" threshold: Heavy drinking patterns and their association with alcohol involvement indices in college students. *Addictive Behaviors* 33, 225-234.

Roebuck, T.M., Mattson, S.N. and Riley, E.P. (1998). A review of the neuroanatomical findings in children with fetal alcohol syndrome or prenatal exposure to alcohol. *Alcoholism: Clinical and Experimental Research* 22, 339-344.

Rosett, H.L., Weiner, L., Lee, A., Zuckerman, B., Dooling, E. and Oppenheimer, E. (1983). Patterns of alcohol consumption and fetal development. *Obstetrics and Gynecology* 61, 539-546.

Savage, D.D., Queen, S.A., Sanchez, C.F., Paxton, L.L., Mahoney, J.C., Goodlett, C.R. and West, J.R. (1992). Prenatal ethanol exposure during the last third of gestation in rat reduces hippocampal NMDA agonist binding site density in 45-day-old offspring. *Alcohol* 9, 37-41.

Simon, K.E., Mondares, R.L., Born, D.E. and Gleason, C.A. (2008). The effects of binge alcohol exposure in the 2nd trimester on the estimated density of cerebral microvessels in near-term fetal sheep. *Brain Research* 231, 75-80.

Smith, L.E., Coles, C.D., Lancaster, J., Fernhoff, P.M. and Falek, A. (1986). The effect of volume and duration of prenatal ethanol exposure on neonatal physical and behavioral development. *Neurobehavioral Toxicology and Teratology* 8, 375-381.

Stevenson, R.J. (2010). An initial evaluation of the function of human olfaction. *Chemical Senses* 35, 3-20.

Stratton, K., Howe, C. and Battaglia, F. (1996). Fetal Alcohol Syndrome: Diagnosis, Epidemiology, Prevention, and Treatment. Washington, DC: National Academy Press.

Substance Abuse and Mental Health Services Administration, Office of Applied Studies. (2008). Treatment Episode Data Set (TEDS): 1996-2006. National Admissions to Substance Abuse Treatment Services, DASIS Series:S-43, DHHS Publication (SMA) 08-4347.

Tacker, D.H. and Okorodudu, A.O. (2004). Evidence for injurious effect of cocaethylene in human microvascular endothelial cells. *Clinica Chimica Acta* 345, 69-77.

Thomas, J.D., Goodlett, C.R. and West, J.R. (1998). Alcohol-induced Purkinje cell loss depends on developmental timing of alcohol exposure and correlates with motor performance. *Development Brain Research* 105, 159-166.

Tran, T.D. and Kelly, S.J. (2003). Critical periods for ethanol-induced cell loss in the hippocampal formation. *Neurotoxicology and Teratology* 25, 519-528.

Tsuji, R., Fattori, V., Abe, S., Costa, L. and Kobayashi, K. (2008). Effects of postnatal ethanol exposure at different developmental phases on neurotrophic factors and phosphorylated proteins on signal transductions in rat brain. *Neurotoxicology and Teratology* 30, 228-236.

Warren, K.R. and Li, T.-K. (2005). Genetic polymorphisms: Impact on the risk of fetal alcohol spectrum disorders. *Birth Defects Research* (Part A). 73, 195-203.

Watari, H., Born, D.E. and Gleason, C.A. (2006). Effects of first trimester binge alcohol exposure on developing white matter in fetal sheep. *Pediatric Research* 59, 560-564.

Wilson, L.D., Malik, M. and Wilson, H. (2009). Cocaine and ethanol: combined effects on coronary artery blood flow and myocardial function in dogs. *Academic Emergency Medicine* 16, 646-655.

Wozniak, J.R., Muetzel, R.L., Mueller, B.A., McGee, C.L., Freeks, M.A., Ward, E.E., Nelson, M.L., Chang, P.N. and Lim, K.O. (2009). Microstructural corpus callosum anomalies in children with prenatal alcohol exposure: an extension of previous diffusion tensor imaging findings. *Alcoholism: Clinical and Experimental Research* 33, 1825-1835.

Yeshurun, Y. and Sobel, N. (2010). An odor is not worth a thousand words: from multidimensional odors to unidirectional odor objects. *Annual Review of Psychology* 61, 219-241.

Zakhari, S. (2006). Overview: How is alcohol metabolized by the body. *Alcohol Research and Health* 29, 245-257.

In: Pregnancy and Alcohol Consumption
Editor: Joshua D. Hoffman, pp. 245-261
ISBN 978-1-61761-122-3


*Chapter 9*

# THE FRENCH PARADOX: FORBIDDING ALCOHOL DURING PREGNANCY, BUT MAKING AN EXCEPTION FOR WINE!

***Agnès Dumas[1], Stéphanie Toutain[1] and Laurence Simmat-Durand[1]***

1. CERMES3 (Centre de Recherche Médecine, Sciences, Santé, Santé Mentale et Société), Université Paris Descartes, CNRS UMR 8211, INSERM U988, Paris, France

## ABSTRACT

France was the second country in the world to adopt a radical position with regard to the consumption of alcohol during pregnancy, with a campaign recommending "zero alcohol during pregnancy", and compulsory labelling of all containers of alcoholic beverages (even Champagne). This position is surprising in view of the fact that no updated prevalence data is available nationally whether on consumption by pregnant women or on the numbers of infants affected by neonate alcohol syndrome. In addition, until recently, advice to pregnant women allowed one to two glasses of wine a day, good for the heart, and the consumption of beer was even recommended to facilitate breast feeding. Generally speaking, pressure from lobbies to have red wine recognised as a foodstuff and not as alcohol, or the famous "French paradox" reputed to prove that life expectancy increases with regular moderate consumption of red wine, seemed to leave very little chance for the message to be adopted in France.

After the issue was avoided for some twenty years, giving as pretext this French paradox, it suddenly came into the limelight in the media in 2004, the state fearing legal action against it (by women giving birth to children with foetal alcohol syndrome and considering they had not been informed of the risk) and this led to legislation that made the warning labels on alcoholic beverages compulsory in 2004.

Although no risk threshold has been defined in the international medical literature, this radical position was justified by what was viewed as the simplicity of the message, despite the fact that it is quite inadequate in a country where total abstinence is still far from standard. Even if surveys on knowledge about the dangers of alcohol during pregnancy reflect better levels of information in the general population, health professionals as individuals and women generally feel they are not really concerned, and view the danger as being related drinking strong alcohols or concerning alcoholics.

This chapter, in addition to a review of the literature, of the French debate and of the surveys available, sets out to provide original results from the prevalence surveys at present underway.

## INTRODUCTION

While the intuition that alcohol has damaging effects on the foetus dates back to Antiquity, it was only in the 20$^{th}$ century that medical research provided evidence (Armstrong 2003). The foetal alcohol syndrome (FAS), first described in 1968 by a French physician, Lemoine (1968), and rediscovered in 1973 by American researchers, Jones and Smith (1973), affects infants whose mothers have daily or occasionally consumed large quantities of alcohol. Following this, the discovery of incomplete or partial forms led to the definition of Foetal Alcohol Spectrum Disorder (FASD), which may occur with only moderate daily use, or binge drinking (five or more drinks on a single occasion). Nevertheless, not all the infants of alcohol-using women are affected by these disorders, since the effects of alcohol on the foetus are obviously determined not only by the quantities of alcohol consumed daily or occasionally, but also by genetic, nutritional and environmental factors. The failure to set a risk threshold below which alcohol can be consumed without harming the foetus has therefore resulted in a recommendation for complete abstinence from alcohol during pregnancy.

In France, alcohol consumption occurs in a specific cultural environment as it is deeply rooted in interpersonal sociability and in French society generally. When the work by Lemoine involving 127 children born from "alcoholic parents" was published in *L'Ouest Médical*[1] in 1968 (Lemoine 1968), it was not taken seriously by anyone, and the research went unnoticed. Even if France can claim the discovery of FAS, a complete vacuum, both political and scientific, followed on this work. Apart from a few isolated local initiatives from health professionals practising in the areas most affected by alcohol, for 40 years the French did not hear about drinking during pregnancy. And then suddenly in 2004 legislation was passed compelling alcohol producers to label their beverages with a warning about the dangers of alcohol during pregnancy.

In contrast, when in 1973 Jones and Smith published an article in *The Lancet* reporting the same conclusions as Lemoine on the basis of 8 cases (Jones and Smith 1973), they met with very considerable interest. The American discovery was very soon followed by political consequences, and the first warnings about the dangers of alcohol during pregnancy were issued in 1977 by the NIAAA (National Institute on Alcohol Abuse and Alcoholism). In 1981, the Surgeon General recommended abstinence during pregnancy, and set up health education measures targeting the general public. Since 1989 all alcoholic beverage containers have been labelled with a health advisory warning stating that: "women should not drink alcoholic beverages during pregnancy because of the risk of birth defects".

Before considering the adoption of this warning label policy in France, this chapter proposes an overview of French data about drinking during pregnancy, even though it should be noted that in France there are almost no quantitative or qualitative surveys on that

[1] French local medical journal.

particular subject. However, research has recently been carried out to understand representations entertained by the general public and by pregnant women in particular.

## A. Prevalence

Very little is known to date about the incidence of FAS and the prevalence of prenatal exposure to alcohol in France. No systematic diagnosis is performed at birth, and there is no national data collection of the numbers of cases among newborn infants, whether for FAS or FASD. An experiment was attempted involving the establishment of a national register of children presenting these disorders, but the initiative ran up against methodological difficulties and resistance from hospitals. This experiment was conducted in five French administrative areas for the years 2006 to 2008, but it enabled the detection of only 12 infants with FAS and 17 doubtful cases, or cases more likely to be FASD (Bloch et al. 2009) thus generating underestimations of prevalence rates for these areas. The lack of diagnosis of alcohol-related effects at birth is patent, in the absence of biological or radiological criteria (Hoyme et al. 2005). As a result the only other remaining possibility is to question women on their alcohol use. But there are very little data on these issues of consumption prevalence in France, whether at national or local level. Before presenting the data that does exist, it is worth broaching the methodological difficulties that are specific to the assessment of alcohol-related behaviours during pregnancy.

### Frequency, Quantity, Standard Drink, Time Scale, Mean Behaviour, Data Collection Tools: So Many Possible Biases

In general, alcohol drinking patterns vary widely, both in terms of frequency – occasional or regular – and in terms of quantity – people can drink large amounts of alcohol infrequently, as in binge drinking. Also, alcohol-use terminology is complex: the ICD-10 World Health Organization classification uses a qualitative definition, "harmful use" or "dependence", while the NIAAA sets risk thresholds based on the number of drinks per day or per occasion. There is consequently a wide diversity in methods for assessing alcohol consumption, based on frequency, quantity or qualitative risk thresholds. Numerous questionnaires on alcohol consumption have been developed to assess the qualitative risk thresholds (AUDIT, CAGE, etc), some being specifically adapted to assessing harmful drinking during pregnancy (T-ACE, TWEAK). The former have been adapted and validated in French, but not the latter.

Unlike studies aiming at screening at-risk populations, the challenge to any research exploring the prevalence of drinking patterns is that it requires very precise questions to be asked on the frequency of consumption, the number of drinks per occasion, the particular type of beverage, or even the trade mark (the percentage of alcohol may be different from one beer to another for instance). Indeed, international comparisons are biased by the varying definitions of the "standard" glass of alcohol. For instance the International Center for Alcohol Policies (ICAP) considers that in the UK a standard drink contains 8g of pure alcohol, compared to 14g in Portugal or in the US. In the US, according to the NIAAA, a standard drink equals one 12-ounce bottle of beer (5%), one 5-ounce glass of wine (12%), or

1.5 oz of distilled spirits (40%). In France a standard glass corresponds to about one 8.5 oz glass of beer (5% alcohol), one 4.2 oz glass of wine (12%), one 1.2 oz glass of distilled spirit (40%), and corresponds to around 10g of pure alcohol (Beck et al. 2007). Of course these are general standards, and wines at 14% or beers at 8.5% can be purchased.

But above all the determining element in this type of data collection is probably the time scale used in the questions: do items refer to consumption in the last month? The last week? The previous day? The shorter the time scale, the more accurate the memory is likely to be; but at the same time, the shorter the time scale the less likely is the report to be representative of actual consumption for occasional and binge drinkers. This question of the time scale is all the more delicate for alcohol consumption during pregnancy, because of the change in behaviours throughout pregnancy. There is no "average pregnant woman": women have time to change their habits in the course of the nine months. A woman may not know that she is pregnant at the beginning of her pregnancy, and her drinking patterns are likely to differ from those of a woman who is 8 months pregnant, and who may have received advice on the dangers of alcohol during her pregnancy. That is why using a mean consumption over nine months is not very meaningful. If women are interviewed at the time of childbirth, problems of recall are unavoidable, unless assessing only the third semester, when the prevalence of alcohol use is likely to be the lowest. On the other hand, if women are interviewed in the course of their pregnancy, the results might combine widely different consumption patterns, unless the pregnancy semesters are pinpointed. Yet often studies deal with "drinking during pregnancy" without any regard for the semesters. Further to this, the women receiving little or inadequate follow-up during pregnancy are likely to be missed in this type of survey, as are those who leave the maternity hospital early. In pregnancy, inadequate follow-up of the expectant mother has been identified as a marker for substance use, in particular multiple drug use, and this is all the more true because women using alcohol or opiates often become aware of their pregnancy at a late stage (Edwards and Werler 2006).

Another bias is the method used, whether a self-administered questionnaire or a face-to-face interview, with the health professional in charge of the follow-up of the pregnancy or with a complete stranger: obviously there is a methodological effect, as in all surveys involving a social desirability component, such as those about drug use. Whatever the method used, there is probably under-report, because alcohol consumption is less well accepted among women (Beck et al. 2006; Berthelot et al. 1984), as is the case for other psychoactive substances (Simmat-Durand 2009a), and even more so for pregnant women (Simmat-Durand 2009b).

Finally French research often diverges in the methods implemented, with variations in the data collection tools used and the criteria for defining risk-prone behaviours, so that data are not readily comparable from one study to another. There is however partial data available from national and local statistics and this will be detailed below.

## National Data

National data are incomplete: on the one hand surveys dealing with substance use in the general population provide little specific information on women of childbearing age, and mostly do not ask questions about pregnancy. On the other hand surveys that do cover the perinatal period give very little information on consumption, with the possible exception of tobacco, and they often lack precision on frequencies and quantities.

The periodic French national survey known as the "Health barometer" (*Baromètre Santé*) implemented in 2005 on a representative general population sample of 30 00 individuals was the first edition to include a variable relating to pregnancy. The detailed data acquired from the inclusion of this variable has not yet been published, except for an indication that "in the 15-49 year age group, 11% of the responding women reported having consumed alcohol in the week preceding the survey, as compared to 38% of the other women" (Guillemont et al. 2006).

Surveys covering the perinatal period have been conducted in a medical environment at the time of childbirth. The most recent data derived from the *National perinatal survey ("Enquête nationale périnatale"*[2]*)* on alcohol use dates back to 1998, because the question was removed from later editions of the survey. Indeed, the survey designers considered that under-report was too great for the relevant item, and that the resulting prevalence was too low. In 1998, 3.9% of the women responding in maternity hospitals following childbirth reported consuming at least one glass of alcoholic beverage a day during pregnancy (Blondel et al. 1999). For the third trimester, on average, 19.4% of the women reported drinking 1 to 6 glasses, 3.1% from 7 to 13 glasses, 0.6% reported a consumption of 14 to 20 glasses and 0.2% 21 glasses or more per week (Blondel et al. 1999). The national survey planned for October 2009 was postponed on account of the flu epidemic, and was planned for March 2010.

There is also a multicentre study conducted periodically on around 7 500 births, using data from obstetric files (i.e. reports made by women to professionals in the setting of prenatal consultations). Maternity wards participate on a voluntary basis, and while these facilities are spread over the French territory as a whole, recruitment is not exhaustive (Bouyer et al. 2004). So far the results are similar to those derived from the *National perinatal survey*: in 2003, 0.2% of the women reported a level of consumption of more than three drinks a day during pregnancy (Mamelle 2004).

## Local Data

At local level, data are available from some years back from a maternity department located in northern France, which is a region where alcohol consumption is higher than in the rest of the country, on account of a precarious socioeconomic environment: in 1985-1986, 15% of women in the region were drinking at least two glasses a day, in 1990-1991 the figure was only 10% and in 1992 4% (INSERM 2001).

Seven studies have been conducted more recently in French maternity departments. Most implemented the AUDIT questionnaire, either in part or as a whole, (de Chazeron et al. 2008; Hillaire et al. 2002; Senn et al. 2005) two studies used the T-ACE questionnaire (Varescon et al. 2007; Villet et al. 2008), and two used self-reported consumption (Dumas et al. 2008; Houet et al. 2005). Table 1 presents prevalence data on alcohol consumption during pregnancy derived from these seven studies on the basis of two indicators: presence of

[2] A survey on a national representative sample of around 15,000 births, amounting to about 2% of yearly births in France.

alcohol consumption during pregnancy, without taking account of frequency or quantity (*any use*), and the proportion of women reporting regular consumption (4 to 6 times a week, in reference to the first item in the AUDIT questionnaire). In view of the abovementioned national data, the studies conducted after 2000 all show a fall in consumption, the only point of comparison here being daily intake. This could first of all be related to a tendency towards reduction in consumption that has also been observed in the general population (Beck et al. 2007), but it could also be attributable to prevention policies.

With regard to binge drinking (defined according to studies as drinking 4 to 6 glasses on a single occasion) the studies presented in Table 1 also reported the following prevalence rates:

- consumption of 4 drinks (at least one time): 2.4% during the first trimester of pregnancy, and 0.4% during the second and third trimesters, this report referring to the preceding month (Dumas et al. 2008).
- consumption of 5 glasses (during pregnancy, at least one time): 5.3% (Houet et al. 2005), 6.6% (Senn et al. 2005), and 7.2% (de Chazeron et al. 2008). Another study was conducted in the same area, at the same time than the latter one and the percentage reported was only 0.5% (Malet et al. 2006), but without specifying whether the question referred to the whole pregnancy or not.
- consumption of 6 glasses (during pregnancy): 0.4% (Villet et al. 2008) and 4.4% (Hillaire et al. 2009).

These results show notable variations, which may be partly attributable to the fact that alcohol consumption may be more or less culturally established in the locations where the surveys were implemented. But these contrasted results are also probably the result of methodological divergences: questions sometimes refer to the whole pregnancy (and use a mean value) for women who gave birth, or sometimes they refer to precise periods (the previous month) for women who were pregnant at the time of the survey.

**Table 1. Drinking during pregnancy in France, recent local data**

| Study | 1 | 2 | 3 | 4 | 5 | 6 | 7 |
|---|---|---|---|---|---|---|---|
| *N* | 1361 | 923 | 837 | 403 | 245 | 150 | 115 |
| Intervie-wed at childbirth or during pregnancy | Pre--gnancy | Child--birth | Child--birth | Child--birth | Pre--gnancy | Both | Pre--gnancy |
| Multicentre study | Yes | Yes | Yes | No | No | No | No |
| Any use during pregnancy | - | 12,2 | 52.2 | 48.0 | 25,3 | 43.0 | 17,4 |
| 4-6 times weekly during pregnancy | - | 0,0 | 0,3 | 0,5 | - | - | - |

Legend: 1 (Hillaire et al. 2009) ; 2 (Villet et al. 2008) ; 3 (de Chazeron et al. 2008) ; 4 (Senn et al. 2005) ; 5 (Dumas et al. 2008); 6 (Houet et al. 2005) ; 7 (Varescon et al. 2007).

This overview of data on consumption rates in France nevertheless gives a rough idea of reported consumption patterns during pregnancy in France. Although alcohol is rooted in French culture, daily consumption during pregnancy appears fairly rare, at not more than 1% for these studies overall. Binge drinking appears more frequent, but extremely variable (ranging from 0.4% for Villet et al. to 7.2% for De Chazeron et al.). This variation may arise from the wordings of the questions, which can take on two forms (the exact wording of items is rarely quoted in articles): 1) it may be the first item of the AUDIT questionnaire that is used, i.e. "how many glasses do you drink on a typical day on which you drink alcohol?", or 2) the respondent may be asked if there has been an episode of binge drinking during pregnancy – have you drunk 5 glasses or more on a single occasion since you have been pregnant? In the first instance the information gathered is a mean figure, which can have a levelling effect on results and provide low values, while in the second instance there is a likelihood of obtaining higher values, in particular if women are interviewed in the first trimester of pregnancy.

But this overview above all shows how little interest the risks of alcohol in pregnancy have raised in the scientific community: the majority of publications on FAS and FASD are from physicians who are confronted head on with these issues in their clinical practice, on account of the fact that they are practising in French regions that are particularly affected by alcohol abuse and addiction. In 2005 a review of the number of articles published on the general subject of alcohol in pregnancy showed absence of media coverage, whether in the scientific literature or in the printed media addressed to the general public: apart from a book by a paediatrician entirely devoted to the subject that was published in the 1990s (Dehaene 1995), in the scientific press there are only about ten articles in the 1980s, about 30 in the 1990s and around 50 in the years 2000 to 2004. In the general press media, there was only one article in the 1990s, and five between 2000 and 2004 (Dassonville 2005). In contrast, after 2004, and the adoption of legislation on the labelling of alcoholic beverages, the number of articles in the general-interest press literally exploded, while in the scientific literature the rise was far more moderate (a quick search using a meta-motor including several medical databases such as Medline or Pascal, with the key words "alcohol and pregnancy" in French language provides a result of 20 articles for the years 2004 to 2010).

If little is happening on the French research scene regarding the risks of alcohol in pregnancy, on the political scene the year 2004 heralded a very marked change. In December 2004 the French parliament passed legislation making it compulsory to include a message on the dangers of alcohol in pregnancy on labels of all alcoholic drink containers. This was completely unexpected in view of the absence of any scientific or society debate on the subject. When the legislation was passed, the form that the message should take was not specified (written message or pictogram), and it was finally a pictogram that appeared on October 1st 2007.

## B. French Policy[3]

In 2001, the national research body INSERM (*Institut National de la Santé et de la Recherche Médicale*) published an expert report on the dangers of alcohol for health, and a chapter was devoted to prenatal exposure to alcohol (INSERM 2001). Following this publication, in 2002, French health agencies issued the first recommendations for abstinence during pregnancy. In March 2004, the national Academy of Medicine published a text stating the dangers of the use of alcohol, tobacco or cannabis during pregnancy. Among the academy's five recommendations, one recommended that information on the dangers of alcohol during pregnancy should be included on labelling of alcoholic beverages (Nordmann 2004). However no national campaign was launched to back up this information, which was ignored by the media, so that these recommendations went largely unnoticed.

If the issue of FAS, and more generally the risk of alcohol in pregnancy, arrived on the political scene, it did not come from health watchdog institutions, but above all from the initiative of one woman, Anne-Marie Payet, a Senator belonging to a centrist political party. She is from Reunion island, a French overseas territory not far from Madagascar, where the incidence of FAS is higher than in metropolitan France – estimated at around 5 to 6‰ on the island compared to 1 to 2‰ in metropolitan France (INSERM 2001). Elected to the Senate in 2001, she first encountered children affected by FAS in 2002 on the occasion of a mission on the subject of ill treatment of disabled individuals. It was on this occasion that health professionals mentioned the container labelling directed towards pregnant women that is compulsory in the USA. In January 2004, Ms Payet proposed an amendment in the Senate (the second decisional chamber in France) modelled on the American provision.

### The French Paradox

In the course of the parliamentary debate in the Senate, members from wine-growing regions spoke up to oppose the labelling measures. None really talked about the subject of the amendment, that is to say the prevention of alcohol-related risks in pregnancy. Nor was it the "aesthetic" argument, or that of the cost that a change in labelling would generate for the sector, that were brought to the fore. The fact that producers were already being forced to alter labelling for export to the USA was not mentioned in the debate either. All the interventions focused on economic and political arguments: the Senators recalled that wine was not only a "part of French civilisation", but above all a "cultural and economic reality". There were numerous more or less covert references to the fragile economic situation of the

[3] The sources used for section B are interviews conducted with political players, physicians and legal professionals implicated in the adoption of the legislation on labelling. In addition, the complete debates in the French Senate and National Assembly were also used; they are available on the websites of the two institutions.

For the debates relating to the proposed legislation on public health policy (see Article 17) refer to the Senate website (complete minutes of public debate of 13th, 14th, 15th and 19th January 2004 http://www.senat.fr /dossierleg/pjl03-019.html

For the debate on the proposed legislation for equal opportunities, participation and citizenship for disabled individuals (see additional articles following Article 1) refer to National Assembly website (second sitting 20th December 2004)http://www.assembleenationale.fr/12/dossiers/handicapes.asp and the Senate website (complete minutes of the public debate of the 19th, 20th and 21st October 2004) http://www.senat.fr/ dossierleg/pjl03-183.html

wine-growing sector, and the need to avoid giving it another "hit on the head", since there was already a crisis. Indeed, the daily consumption of wine has been decreasing for several decades. Today it is mainly people over 50 that drink wine regularly, while the younger age groups prefer beer (Beck et al. 2007). But for the wine-growing lobby, if the sector was experiencing a crisis, it was also a result of health policies targeting alcoholism and alcohol abuse, which were seen as damaging the image of wine. The Senators speaking in the debate thus denounced campaigns that were "confusing" wine and alcohol. This view may seem improbable in the eyes of readers unfamiliar with the countries of southern Europe, since everyone is aware that wine, which is fermented grape juice, contains alcohol (one bottle generally contains 12 to 14° of alcohol).

Indeed, one of the major issues for the wine-growing lobby is to get the idea across that wine "is not alcohol". Wine professionals and the interest groups that support them set out to distinguish wine from "hard" alcohols, on the grounds that wine possesses "therapeutic virtues". In this respect, reference is made to the "French paradox", which arose from the following contradictory observation: despite the large number of risk factors such as tobacco use, cholesterol and hypertension, mortality from coronary and vascular pathologies in France is the lowest of all industrialised countries. However, this phenomenon, which concerns only red wine, is still widely disputed in scientific fields. Health professionals and alcohol specialists object to what they call a "scientific counter-truth" and a "mystification". For several years, they have repeatedly recalled that a glass of wine contains the same degree of alcohol as a standard glass of beer or a standard glass of distilled spirit, and that consequently it is liable to harm the health of excessive consumers.

Naturally, in a society where we are increasingly required to take care of ourselves and our physical and mental well-being, scope for communicating on the notion that wine can also be beneficial for health could be an enormous advantage for the wine sector. The real problem with the alcohol warning label for pregnant women is indeed that it suggested that wine could be a danger to health, which is just what the champions of the wine-growers were trying to deny by all means, bringing to the fore the "therapeutic virtues" of wine. One of the "pro-wine" Senators thus stated that the labelling amendment "wrongly lumps together wine and strong alcohols, and contradicts all the scientific research showing the health benefits of moderate consumption of wine". Likewise, another claimed that the warning label policies "systematically sully our products with a negative connotation".

At the end of this first debate, the amendment on labelling was rejected by 228 votes against 14. Things might have remained as such, but a parallel legal action by three women whose children had FAS was to precipitate events.

## The Fear of Legal Liability

Alongside the action by the Senator Anne-Marie Payet, in 2003 three women whose infants presented FAS launched into legal proceedings because they considered that they had not been made aware of the risks of alcohol-related damage to the foetus. They were represented by a lawyer who is also the son of Maurice Titran, a paediatrician well known in the past for his commitment to combating FAS in France. After a first failure with an administrative court, the affair was filed in a local penal court. In April 2004 the deputy prosecutor of this court decided to open a penal enquiry on the grounds of failure to inform on the dangers of alcohol for the foetus, extending to the accusations of endangering life and unintended injury. There was no plaintiff, and the prosecutor decided to conduct the enquiry on his own initiative. On August 3rd, the lawyer was interviewed by a local newspaper, and he mentioned the penal enquiry. The very next day the AFP (French press agency) took up the story, and the following day all the French press was covering the affair.

Subsequently events occurred fast: on August 5th the Minister of health stated that he was ready to "legislate before the end of the year" on labelling –"using the first appropriate legislative framework"[4]. On the same day, he announced that campaigns would be organised and published in the press from December. It is in this setting that the first communication campaign for the prevention of FAS was launched in France. It was published in the press addressed to women in December 2004 (with the slogan "Zero alcohol during pregnancy") and in February and March 2005 in women's magazines, television periodicals, and popular news magazines.

## The Information Campaigns

The law was passed in December 2004, and came into force in October 2007. Instead of the "health message mentioning the dangers of excessive consumption of alcohol, and recommending abstinence for pregnant women" planned in the legal draft, it was finally a pictogram that appeared on the containers of alcoholic beverages. In fact the Ministry had allowed the alcohol industry to choose between a pictogram and a written message. Yet a poll conducted by a private polling agency in November and December 2004 on the choice between pictogram and message derived the following results: 73% of women agreed to a written message and 92% approved a pictogram; 87% of the pregnant women responding and 72% of general public respondents stated they were in favour of a pictogram accompanied by a written message, against 15% of pregnant women and 18% of the general public who preferred a pictogram on its own[5].

As the size and colour of the pictogram are not specified, each manufacturer is free to adapt the colours to the container, and the size is sometime so small (0.3 cm) that it can be confused with the pictogram concerning the recycling of the packaging, which is the only other compulsory pictogram on alcoholic beverage labels. An amendment should be submitted this year concerning the size of the pictogram, to make it "readable". It was therefore to give emphasis and "give increased visibility" to the pictogram printed on alcohol containers that a communication campaign was organised in September and October 2007 in the written press and on the radio (but not on television) with the message "Zero alcohol during pregnancy". The information on the risks incurred was given solely on postcard-size flyers. These were issued to health facilities generally receiving pregnant women: GPs, gynaecologists in private practice (these practitioners post the messages as they think appropriate), hospitals (via the no-smoking-in-pregnancy network) and social centres (of the mother and infant care type). In addition, the INPES website[6] issued two posters "9 months / 0 alcohol / 0 tobacco" and "Zero alcohol during pregnancy".

[4] "Journal du Dimanche" 08/07/2004.

[5] Source: internal documents from the Ministry of solidarity, health and the family, 2005.

[6] "Institut National de Prevention et d'Education à la Santé", a national agency devoted to health prevention.

# C. Knowledge and Representations

## Advice Given to Pregnant Women

In child-rearing manuals, recommendations on the subject of alcohol consumption during pregnancy are more or less categorical, as can be seen from the following two examples.

In the book by Laurence Pernoud "*J'attends un enfant*" *(Nine Months to Motherhood)*, expecting mothers are advised "to drink as little alcohol as possible, or none at all… alcohol enters the baby's blood because the placenta does not stop it". This book also recommends the banning of "strong alcoholic drinks" but notes that "drinking a glass of champagne on occasion cannot do any harm" (Pernoud 2003 (1st édition 1956)). In contrast, the recommendations given in the book by Marie-Claude Delahaye are considerably less ambivalent: "…if you drink just one glass of wine or an aperitif, which represent only a small quantity of alcohol for a woman of around 110 pounds, it is an enormous amount for an embryo of a few grams who is unable to break it down. So you should abstain completely from alcohol. Your baby is worth this small sacrifice" (Delahaye 2002). She also paints a very dark picture of the irreversible consequences of "*alcoholism… which is responsible for malnutrition, delayed development, serious malformations, in particular cardiac, and a particular facial appearance*" (Delahaye 2002). These consequences are not broached at all in the work by Laurence Pernoud, despite the fact that the book has been a reference in child-rearing since the sixties.

As for generalist websites devoted to pregnancy such as "*Doctissimo", "Santé médecine",* or *"Santé au feminin",* they give very clear messages regarding the drinking during pregnancy: "daily consumption of alcohol, even at low levels, during pregnancy can lead to complications"; "the fetus prefers abstinence"; "the baby does not tolerate alcohol". Finally, the information delivered by specialised websites such as that of INPES states that the "precautionary principle" requires abstinence during pregnancy: the two posters aimed at the general public, "9 months / 0 alcohol / 0 tobacco" and "Zero alcohol during pregnancy" can be downloaded from the website.

## Professionals and Their Training

The majority of health care professionals seem rather ill-at-ease when approaching the subject of alcohol consumption with a pregnant woman (Dumas et al. 2006). These difficulties can be explained, for the older practitioners, by the virtual absence of this issue in the medical teaching curriculum before the 1990s, and for the younger practitioners by teaching programmes that are inadequately oriented towards broaching this subject with pregnant women, a subject that is still taboo in French society (Toutain 2009). French health care professionals are also hostile overall towards any form of record system or black-listing of alcohol-abusing women, although certain hospitals do not hesitate to resort to biological tests or reporting to child protection agencies for unborn infants, a practice that also exists in other countries (Armstrong 2003). Nevertheless, in recent years, health care professionals interested in these issues have been able to complete their initial training by voluntary continuing-education courses, for which the offer is expanding.

Indeed, certain members of the medical profession from regions such as Normandie, Nord-Pas-de-Calais, or Reunion Island, particularly affected by alcohol consumption among pregnant women and FAS, have been active in associations promoting, among other things, continuing education for professionals (Chabrolle and Chabrolle 2005; Lejeune 2001). In 1997 an association was created in Reunion island under the name REUNISAF, presided by Denis Lamblin (paediatrician), aiming to raise public awareness on the harmful effects of alcohol during pregnancy. Reunion Island is particularly affected by chronic alcohol abuse in the population, linked to historical factors (slavery, sugar cane plantations for the production of rum, etc) and also to geographical factors (overseas area, isolated volcanic island with problems of accessibility). Since January 2007, REUNISAF has been recognised as a training body, and it offers health medical professionals training modules on the issues of alcohol, such as "Foetal Alcohol Syndrome, a consequence of perinatal alcohol use", "Alcohol, pregnancy and women's health", or "Talking about alcohol and women" (REUNISAF website).

In the same period, in metropolitan France, another association, *"Groupe d'Etudes Grossesse et Addictions"* (GEGA, study group on pregnancy and addictions) presided by Professor Claude Lejeune was created in 2000. This association aims to improve the competence of professionals involved in the care of pregnant women who are substance abusers, in particular alcohol abusers. The association also offers health professionals who are interested one-day training sessions on these issues three or four times a year. Since January 2008, health medical professionals have been able to extend the knowledge they have acquired in GEGA training sessions by enlisting for a university diploma "*Périnatalité et Addictions*", a course that has been specifically designed, and headed by the president of GEGA (Paris 7 University). This course is intended in particular for different professionals in the medical field who, in their practice, encounter psychoactive substance use (which includes alcohol) during pregnancy and its consequences.

The year 2008, during which there were numerous events relating to these issues, also saw the creation of the association "FAS France" presided by Denis Lamblin. This association aims to promote information, training, research, care provision, support, and prevention of FAS and FASD. Health professionals interested in these issues were able to complement their knowledge by way of a first international conference organised by SAF France in September 2009 entitled "*Alcool et grossesse: qu'en penser en 2009?"* (*Alcohol and pregnancy – what should our attitudes be in 2009?*).

## The General Population

The question of knowledge and representations of alcohol consumption during pregnancy has not been widely explored in France. Two surveys on the theme can be mentioned, the first with a quantitative approach and the second with a qualitative approach.

The first, a quantitative study on a representative sample of the French general population aged 15 years and over, was a telephone survey conducted in 2004 (Guillemont et al. 2006), i.e. during the parliamentary debate about alcohol warning label for pregnant women. This survey aimed to measure knowledge in the French population on the subject of the risks of alcohol consumption during pregnancy. The results showed that the vast majority of the French respondents (82%) knew about both the recommendation not to drink alcohol during pregnancy, and the risks of prenatal exposure to alcohol. However the results showed that in 2004 the knowledge about these risks in terms of levels and period of consumption, or about the different types of alcoholic products, was inaccurate. More specifically, for 33% the recommendation "Zero alcohol during pregnancy" was not perceived as being absolute. For 50% the first trimester of pregnancy was viewed as being the only period of risk, and 33% thought that only strong alcohol was to be banned during pregnancy. To measure the impact of the "zero alcohol during pregnancy" prevention campaigns, the effects of the alcohol warning label on alcoholic beverages and the evolution of knowledge in the French general population regarding these issues, the quantitative study conducted in 2004 was reiterated in 2007 (Guillemont and Léon 2008). The results showed a noticeable improvement in awareness in the French population regarding the recommendation of abstinence from alcohol during pregnancy (87%) and the periods related to risk (45%). However, the distinction between "mild alcoholic drinks" (such as wine or beer) and "strong alcoholic drinks" (distilled alcohols) persisted. This survey also showed widely differing results according to gender, where the better knowledge observed among women can be explained by the fact that pregnancy is of course a very "feminine" issue.

The second survey, which was qualitative, aimed to focus on representations concerning alcohol consumption among pregnant women (Toutain 2009). This survey involved the collection and content analysis of discussions involving 42 pregnant women at different stages in their pregnancies on internet chat groups. This is a recent communication tool and thus constitutes an original corpus. The women gave their opinions on the theme "Alcohol and pregnancy" accessed via "Food and pregnancy". Three forums mainly targeting women were consulted in 2007. The data corpus included 250 messages characterised by pseudonyms, among which 110 were accompanied by a profile when authorised by the contributor, giving age, profession and number of children. The discussion content was analysed using Nvivo 8 (QSR International).

The results of this qualitative survey tended to back up those of the quantitative survey. They confirmed that the recommendation of abstinence, with the exception of women in medical professions and abstaining subjects, was not well understood, insofar as it was not perceived as being absolute: "*A few sips of wine from time to time would not shock me* (Emmanuelle, estate agent, aged 29). The dominant representations of these internet users did not relate to abstinence[7] but rather to tolerance[8] of a few indulgences from time to time, for pleasure and relaxation (Toutain 2009). This observation was particularly true for women with higher and secondary education, with children, and/or whose mothers had consumed alcohol during their pregnancies. In addition, these women also distinguished the tolerated "milder" alcoholic beverages (like beer) from alcoholic beverages to be banned, "strong alcohols" (distilled alcohol). These women considered that the different types of alcoholic beverage did not have the same effects on the unborn child: "*Strong alcohol can really have serious consequences on the baby's development... a glass of wine is good for the heart*" (Nathalie, primary school teacher, aged 23). Regarding the periods in which alcohol is consumed, the first trimester was viewed as being the only period of potential risk: "*because it is during this time that the organs are formed*" (Caroline, aged 20).

[7] Abstinence during the last year.

[8] Occasional use (once or twice a month) during the last year.

The sources of knowledge on alcohol consumption for these internet users were various: scientific publications for the most highly qualified, television or websites for the others, and also government prevention campaigns. The information received from health professionals in the course of prenatal consultations was very prominent in what these women had to say (Toutain 2009). They also saw their gynaecologists as providing contradictory information: "*There isn't one [gynaecologist] who says the same thing as the other*" (Geraldine, aged 31).

These women, and in particular those with a secondary level of education, widely referred to their mothers' experiences, and therefore minimised the dangers of alcohol: they were providing a concrete demonstration *via* their own family history that alcohol consumption does not necessarily have damaging effects on the foetus. "*My mother continued drinking two glasses a day throughout her pregnancies, and we're all normal*" (Erika, aged 25, managerial assistant). The mother, with her accounts of her experience, appeared as the person whose opinion on alcohol consumption carried the most weight, in comparison with other family members who appear very little in the discussions among these internet users (Toutain 2009).

## Conclusion

In 2004 France was the second country to instate a mandatory warning on *every* container of alcoholic beverages (at the time, labelling requirements intended for pregnant women were also partially in force in several Canadian states and in South Korea). The ICAP regularly reviews health warning label policies all over the world. To date, health warning labels about drinking during pregnancy have also been made mandatory in Russia and in South Africa. In Japan and China alcohol producers can use this labelling, but on a voluntary basis. Since January 2007 bottles of wine, vodka and other spirits sold in Russia must be labelled with a warning stating that *"Alcohol is not for children and teenagers up to age 18, pregnant and nursing women, or for persons with diseases of the central nervous system, kidneys, liver and other digestive organs"* (ICAP 2010). In South Africa and in South Korea there are several health warning labels (on drinking during pregnancy, cirrhosis risk, car accident, etc): at least one of them must be placed on the alcoholic beverages. One of the South Korean warnings states: *"Excessive consumption of alcohol may cause liver cirrhosis or liver cancer, and especially, women who drink while they are pregnant increase the risk of congenital anomalies"* (ICAP 1997). Since August 2007, South African warning labels have included *"Drinking during pregnancy can be harmful to your unborn baby"* (ICAP 2010). A Canadian bill requiring warning labels on alcoholic beverages about drinking during pregnancy (among other things) was rejected in 2006, so that it is mandatory only in a few states. Finally, very little is known about Europe: there is almost no national or European data available about the prevalence of drinking during pregnancy, neither have we known about any literature about policies or debates on drinking during pregnancy. According to the ICAP, abstinence is recommended in Ireland, Spain and the Netherlands, while "one to two units of alcohol once or twice a week" or "one glass per day, not everyday", are considered as safe in the UK and in Switzerland respectively (ICAP 2009).

Even if France, the second country to adopt measures for the labelling of alcoholic beverages, has taken serious steps towards the prevention of the alcoholic risk during pregnancy, there is still nevertheless a considerable need for progress in the area of training of health professionals. It is urgent that the health-care professionals should all agree and recommend total abstinence during pregnancy in order to avoid irreversible consequences on the unborn babies. Awareness campaigns should be implemented to impress and educate the general public, putting an end to dangerous misconceptions and replacing them by messages aimed at encouraging prevention and safety.

## REFERENCES


Armstrong, E. M. (2003). *Conceiving Risk, Bearing Responsibility: Fetal Alcohol Syndrome and the Diagnosis of Moral Disorder*. Baltimore: Johns Hopkins University Press.

Beck, F., Guilbert, P., & Gautier, A. (2007). Baromètre santé 2005 In INPES (Ed.) (pp. 593). Saint-Denis: Editions INPES.

Beck, F., Legleye, S., & de Peretti, G. (2006). L'alcool donne-t-il un genre ? *Travail, genre et sociétés*, 15, 141-160.

Berthelot, J., Clement, S., Druhle, M., Forne, J., & Membrado, M. (1984). Les alcoolismes féminins. *Cahiers du centre de recherches sociologiques*, 1, 1-285.

Bloch, J., Cans, C., De Vigan, C., de Brosses, L., Doray, B., Larroque, B., & Perthus, I. (2009). Faisabilité de la surveillance du syndrome d'alcoolisation foetale, France, 2006-2008. *Bulletin Epidémiologique Hebdomadaire*, 102-104.

Blondel, B., Norton, J., & Du Mazaubrun, C. (1999). Enquête nationale périnatale 1998 (pp. 51). Paris INSERM.

Bouyer, J., Bréart, G., De la Rochebrochard, E., & Sarlon, E. (2004). Surveillance dans le domaine de la reproduction et de la périnatalité (pp. 83). Paris: INSERM-InVS.

Chabrolle, J., & Chabrolle, R. (2005). Alcool et grossesse : Dépistage et prise en charge des enfants exposés in utero à l'alcool, *XXXVème journées de la Société Française de Médecine Périnatale*. Paris

Dassonville, A. (2005). La diffusion de l'information sur le Syndrome d'alcoolisation foetale dans la presse. In L. Dupont, A. Dassonville & G. Cresson (Eds.), *Alcool, grossesse et santé des femmes*. Lille: ANPAA 59.

de Chazeron, I., Llorca, P. M., Ughetto, S., Vendittelli, F., Boussiron, D., Sapin, V., Coudore, F., & Lemery, D. (2008). Is pregnancy the time to change alcohol consumption habits in France? *Alcohol Clin Exp Res*, 32, 868-73.

Dehaene, P. (1995). *La grossesse et l'alcool*. Paris: PUF.

Delahaye, M. (2002). *Le livre de bord de la future maman*. Paris: Marabout.

Dumas, A., Lejeune, C., Simmat-Durand, L., Bonnaire, C., Michaud, P., Hillaire, S., & GEGA (2006). Prévention du Syndrome d'Alcoolisation Foetale (SAF). Pratiques et représentations des professionnels de la périnatalité. *Alcoologie et Addictologie*, 28, 311-317.

Dumas, A., Lejeune, C., Simmat-Durand, L., Crenn-Hébert, C., & Mandelbrot, L. (2008). Grossesse et substances psychoactives : étude de prévalence de la consommation déclarée. *Journal de gynecologie obstetrique et biologie de la reproduction*, 37, 770-778.

Edwards, E. M., & Werler, M. M. (2006). Alcohol consumption and time to recognition of pregnancy. *Maternal and Child Health Journal*.

Guillemont, J., & Léon, C. ( 2008). Alcool et grossesse : connaissances du grand public en 2007 et évolutions en trois ans. *Évolutions*, 15.

Guillemont, J., Rosilio, T., David, M., Léon, C., & Arwidson, P. (2006). Connaissance des Français sur les risques liés à la consommation d'alcool pendant la grossesse. *Evolutions*, 3.

Hillaire, S., Lejeune, C., Michaud, P., Simmat-Durand, L., & Toutain, S. (2009). Enquête de prévalence des consommations de tabac et d'alcool dans quatre hôpitaux de la région parisienne. In L. Simmat-Durand (Ed.), *Grossesses avec drogues. Entre médecine et sciences sociales* (pp. 37-47). Paris: L'Harmattan.

Hillaire, S., Simonpoli, A. M., Lejeune, C., Simmat-Durand, L., & Michaud, P. (2002). Prévalence de l'alcoolisation à risque chez les femmes enceintes et utilisation du questionnaire AUDIT pour le repérage. *Alcoologie et Addictologie*, 24, 7-8.

Houet, T., Vabret, M., Herlicoviez, M., & Dreyfus, M. (2005). Comparaison de la consommation d'alcool avant et pendant la grossesse. A partir d'une série prospective de 150 femmes. *Journal de gynecologie obstetrique et biologie de la reproduction*, 34, 687-693.

Hoyme, H., May, P., & Kalberg, W. (2005). A practical clinical approach to diagnosis of fetal alcohol spectrum disorders: clarification of the 1996 Institute of Medicine criteria. *Pediatrics*, 115, 39-47.

ICAP (1997). Health Warning Labels, *ICAP Reports*: Washington: International Center for Alcohol Policies.

— (2009). Policy Table: International Guidelines on Drinking during Pregnancy. Washington: International Center for Alcohol Policies.

— (2010). Health Warning Labels. Washington: International Center for Alcohol Policies.

INSERM (2001). *Alcool : Effets sur la santé*. Paris: INSERM.

Jones, K., & Smith, A. (1973). Recognition of the fetal alcohol syndrome in early infancy. *Lancet*, 3, 999-1001.

Lejeune, C. (2001). Syndrome d'alcoolisation foetale. *Médecins thérapeutique Pédiatrie*, 4, 173-186.

Lemoine, P. (1968). Les enfants de parents alcooliques : Anomalies observées à propos de 127 cas. *Ouest Médical*, 25 476-82.

Malet, L., de Chazeron, I., Llorca, P. M., & Lemery, D. (2006). Alcohol consumption during pregnancy: a urge to increase prevention and screening. *Eur J Epidemiol*, 21, 787-8.

Mamelle, N. (2004). La santé périnatale en 2002-2003 : évaluation des pratiques médicales (pp. 40). Lyon: Association des Utilisateurs de Dossiers Informatisés en Périnatalogie Obstétrique et Gynécologie (AUDIPOG).

Nordmann, R. (2004). Au nom de la Commission V (Troubles mentaux Toxicomanies). Consommation d'alcool, de tabac ou de cannabis au cours de la grossesse. *Journal de Pédiatrie et de Puériculture*, 17, 349-50.

Pernoud, L. (2003 (1st édition 1956)). J'attends un enfant (pp. 475). Paris Horay.

Senn, M., Straub, D., Pellet, J., & Boussiron, D. (2005). Etude portant sur la consommation d'alcool pendant la grossesse. *Alcoologie et Addictologie*, 27, 181-190.

Simmat-Durand, L. (2009a). Femmes et addictions dans la littérature internationale : sexe, genre et risques. *Bulletin Epidémiologique Hebdomadaire*, 86-89.

— (2009b). *Grossesses avec drogues. Entre médecine et sciences sociales*. Paris: L'Harmattan.

Toutain, S. (2009). Abstinence pendant la grossesse. Ce qu'en disent les femmes en France. *Alcoologie et Addictologie*, 31, 107-114.

Varescon, I., Gaugue, J., & Wendland, J. (2007). Alcool et grossesse : Première utilisation du questionnaire de dépistage T-ACE dans une population française. *Alcoologie et Addictologie*, 29, 221-226.

Villet, H., Lefebvre, A., Flamand, M., & Yon, A. (2008). Étude "grossesse et alcool". Enquête auprès des femmes en maternité (pp. 127). Rouen: Observatoire Régional de la Santé de Haute Normandie.

In: Pregnancy and Alcohol Consumption
Editor: Joshua D. Hoffman, pp. 263-279

ISBN 978-1-61761-122-3


*Chapter 10*

# MEDICOLEGAL CONSIDERATIONS CONCERNING FETAL ALCOHOL SPECTRUM DISORDERS

***Christos I. Evaggelakos, Stavroula A. Papadodima and Chara A. Spiliopoulou***
Department of Forensic Medicine and Toxicology,
School of Medicine,
University of Athens, Greece

## ABSTRACT

Prenatal, intrauterine exposure to alcohol can cause life-long physical, neurological, and psychological impairments, totally named FASD (Fetal Alcohol Spectrum Disorders). The neurological and psychological impairments, including learning disabilities, impulsivity, hyperactivity, social ineptness, and poor judgment, can increase susceptibility to victimization and involvement in the criminal justice system (CJS) , and consequently, their disabilities must be considered at all stages in the legal process. Whether people with FASD appear in court as complainant, witness or accused, their testimony should be taken under great consideration and doubt. Even in case of illegal or criminal behaviour, this category of people requires special treatment. They must be punished with increased lenity and incarceration is not always an ideal solution for them. In principles, people with FASD should be helped to understand the court rules and their legal rights, which is sometimes very difficult for them to achieve. Of course, FASD should be officially diagnosed by experts, such as general practitioners, psychiatrists and medical examiners. Judges and lawyers need to be advised and informed by these kinds of professionals on the impacts FASD have induced on every individual patient, assessing how decisive this syndrome is for his/her behavior.

## 1. INTRODUCTION

Originally, fetal alcohol syndrome (FAS) identified those children who displayed the full phenotype, whether *fetal alcohol effects* (FAE) applied to individuals demonstrating some, but not all of the features of FAS (Steinhausen *et al.* 2003). Fetal Alcohol Syndrome (FAS) is characterized by unique facial features, growth retardation, and developmental delays. FAS represents one end of a spectrum disorder (fetal alcohol spectrum disorder or FASD), and more specifically the most severe form of clinical presentation. The National Organization on FAS (NOFAS 2004), defined fetal alcohol spectrum disorders as the range of effects that can occur in a person whose mother drank alcohol during pregnancy, including physical, mental, behavioral, and learning disabilities, with possible lifelong implications. As this definition implies, multiple diagnostic categories - *e.g.* fetal alcohol syndrome (FAS), partial fetal alcohol syndrome (partial FAS), alcohol-related neurodevelopment disorder (ARND), and alcohol-related birth defects (ARBD) are subsumed under the term FASD.

## 2. ABOUT FAS AND FASD

Since FAS was first described in 1973, (Jones and Smith, 1973) it has become apparent that it is complex; affected people exhibit a wide range of expression, from severe growth restriction, intellectual disability, birth defects and characteristic dysmorphic facial features to normal growth, facial features and intellectual abilities, but with lifelong deficits in several domains of brain function. Less severe findings are known as fetal alcohol spectrum disorders which includes a range of developmental outcomes, such as learning deficits and neurobehavioral abnormalities (Sokol *et al.*,2003).

A substantial body of evidence has emerged for the devastating consequences of prenatal alcohol exposure on the developing CNS, allowing a clearer appreciation of the specific brain regions affected, mechanisms involved and the range of effects. In their initial report, Jones and Smith (1973) noted widespread damage in the brain of an infant with FAS, including microcephaly, agenesis of the corpus callosum (CC) and anterior commissure, errors in migration, and anomalies in the cerebellum and brainstem. Subsequent reports confirmed these findings and added ventricular abnormalities, CNS disorganization, and abnormalities in the basal ganglia, hippocampus, pituitary gland and optic nerve (Jones and Smith, 1975; Clarren *et al.*, 1978; Clarren, 1986; Coulter *et al.*, 1993). The cerebellum has also been identified as particularly vulnerable to prenatal alcohol exposure. Specifically, individuals with FASD show reduced cerebellar volume (Mattson *et al.*, 1994; Archibald *et al.*, 2001) and surface area (Autti-R¨am¨o *et al.*, 2002) as well as reduced volume and displacement of the anterior vermis of the cerebellum (Sowell *et al.*, 1996; Autti- R¨am¨o *et al.*, 2002; O'Hare *et al.*, 2005).

Given that the cerebellum is responsible for the execution of motor behavior such as posture, balance and coordination, the structural abnormalities observed may help to explain motor deficits often seen in individuals with FASD (Roebuck *et al.*, 1998; Roebuck-Spencer and Mattson, 2004). The cerebellum is also involved in other functions, such as attention regulation (Akshoomoff *et al.*, 1997) and classical conditioning (Woodruff-Pak *et al.*, 2000). In accordance with this, deficits in classically conditioned eyeblink responses are noted in children with FAS (Coffin *et al.*, 2005) and cerebellar vermis displacement is negatively correlated with verbal learning and memory in FASD (O'Hare *et al.*, 2005).

Heavy prenatal alcohol exposure has been associated with widespread neuropsychological deficits across several domains, including general intelligence, memory, language, attention, learning, visuospatial abilities, executive functioning, fine and gross motor skills, and social and adaptive functioning (Mattson and Riley, 1998; Guerri, *et al.* 2009). The mean IQ of children with FAS is estimated in the low 70s (Mattson and Riley, 1998), and FAS is the leading preventable cause of mental retardation (Abel and Sokol, 1987). However, the majority of children with FAS are not mentally retarded, and IQ scores show a wide range (Mattson and Riley, 1998).

The mechanism by which prenatal alcohol exposure affects brain development is multifactorial. The teratogenic consequences of ethanol exposure during the preimplantation period partly depend on an interaction with the maternal system (e.g., through production of toxic metabolites, such as acetaldehyde) (Haycock 2009). Ethanol is a known inhibitor of one-carbon metabolism and DNA methyltransferase, and it interferes with various epigenetic factors, including DNA methylation, histone modifications, and small ncRNAs. The correlation between major periods of epigenetic reprogramming and critical periods of teratogenesis suggests that an epigenetic perspective is able to explain a large number of phenomena associated with ethanol exposure (Fukui and Sakata-Haga, 2009). The main, however CNS, (neurobehavioral) effects are very likely triggered in the third trimester by a transmitter disruption mechanism, a mechanism that is only operative when synaptic connections are being established and which, therefore, could not possibly be operative in the first trimester (Archibald *et al.*, 2001; Sowell *et al.*, 2001a, 2002a). Ethanol exposure causes neuronal cell loss in both the hippocampus and cerebellum (Goodlett and Lundahl, 1996; Dikranian *et al.*, 2005), alters synaptogenesis and glial development (Guerri and Renau-Piqueras, 1997).

The number of drinks consumed per day prenatally which have been found to produce developmental delays in children is, in fact, quite low, ranging from 1 to 4 drinks (Jacobson, *et al.,* 1993). Furthermore, deficits in body growth have been recorded with as little as two drinks per day (Hanson *et al.,* 1978). Moreover, the degrees to which people with FASD are impaired differ from person to person. Factors contributing to this variation include maternal drinking pattern, difference in maternal metabolism of alcohol, difference in genetic susceptibility, timing of the alcohol consumption during pregnancy, variations in the vulnerability of different brain regions, maternal nutrition, maternal age, socioeconomic status and synergistic reactions with other drugs. Among these factors, the levels of alcohol reaching the fetal brain and the duration of exposure markedly influence the type and the extent of the damage (Maier *et al.*, 1996).

Ethanol is considered to be one of the most common substances that impact the developing brain, and prenatal alcohol exposure is a leading preventable cause of birth defects, mental retardation and neurodevelopment disorders (American Academy of Pediatrics, 2000). Approximately 4 million infants are born each year with prenatal alcohol exposure, and an estimated 1,000–6,000 are born with FAS. Women bearing children with FAS or other diagnoses within the Fetal Alcohol Spectrum Disorders (FASD) are generally very heavy drinkers. Many of them continue to drink, usually bingeing throughout all trimesters. Therefore, they present a substantial challenge to maternal and child health professionals. Such behavior is usually quite entrenched and reinforced by many social and economic factors, and therefore, change is difficult (Nayak R.B., Murthy P, 2008). In spite of the fact that prevention of FASD is theoretically very simple (it is 100% preventable), behavioral change for an alcohol abusing woman is difficult. Recent data from the Behavioral Risk Factors Surveillance System indicate that an estimated 12% - 13% of U.S. women aged 18--44 years are sexually active, do not use contraception effectively, and drink alcohol frequently or binge drink, thereby putting them at risk for an alcohol-exposed pregnancy (Ebrahim *et al.*, 1999). Because data are available for all subpopulations, prevalence might be greater than these data indicate (Brimacombe *et al.* 2008).

## 3. Diagnosis

The diagnosis of FASD is complex and guidelines are warranted. One of the most important works on the matter is that of the Canadian Public Health Agency of Canada's National Advisory Committee on Fetal Alcohol Spectrum Disorder (Chudley *et al.* 2005). The above committee reviewed, analyzed and integrated current approaches to diagnosis to reach agreement on a standard in Canada. The guidelines were based on widespread consultation of expert practitioners and partners in the field (Goh *et al.*2008). The guidelines are organized into 7 categories: screening and referral; the physical examination and differential diagnosis; the neurobehavioral assessment; and treatment and follow-up; maternal alcohol history in pregnancy; diagnostic criteria for fetal alcohol syndrome (FAS), partial FAS and alcohol-related neurodevelopment disorder; and harmonization of Institute of Medicine and 4-Digit Diagnostic Code approaches. The criteria for the diagnosis of fetal alcohol syndrome according to the above guidelines, after excluding other diagnoses, are shown in the table 1.

**Table 1. Criteria for the diagnosis of fetal alcohol syndrome**

| |
|---|
| A. Evidence of prenatal or postnatal growth impairment, as in at least 1 of the following:<br><br>a. Birth weight or birth length at or below the 10th percentile for gestational age.<br>b. Height or weight at or below the 10th percentile for age.<br>c. Disproportionately low weight-to-height ratio (= 10th percentile). |
| B. Simultaneous presentation of all 3 of the following facial anomalies at any age:<br><br>a. Short palpebral fissure length (2 or more standard deviations below the mean).<br>b. Smooth or flattened philtrum (rank 4 or 5 on the lip-philtrum guide).<br>c. Thin upper lip (rank 4 or 5 on the lip-philtrum guide).<br>C. Evidence of impairment in 3 or more of the following central nervous system domains: hard and soft neurologic signs; brain structure; cognition; communication; academic achievement; memory; executive functioning and abstract reasoning; attention deficit/hyperactivity; adaptive behaviour, social skills, social communication. |
| D. Confirmed (or unconfirmed) maternal alcohol exposure. |

In the wide array of FASDs, facial dysmorphology is often absent and, in the final analysis, has little importance compared with the impact of prenatal alcohol exposure on brain function. However, it is important to note that the facial phenotype is a midline defect that is the most sensitive and specific marker for alcohol-related brain damage (Bertrand *et al.* 2005). The purpose of dysmorphology assessment is to identify those with features related to prenatal alcohol exposure and also to identify children with dysmorphic features due to other causes (Spohr *et al.* 2007). Three facial features (reduced palpebral fissure length/inner canthal distance ratio, smooth philtrum, and thin upper lip) are the cluster of features that differentiate individuals with and without FAS with 100% accuracy (Astley and Clarren, 1996). Other facial features which can be present are short upturned nose, depressed nasal bridge, hypo plastic maxilla, ear anomalies (low set ears, malformed ears, "Railroad track" ear), palmar crease anomalies and micrognathia. All the above mentioned features and additionally some other associated physical features (abnormalities such as midface hypoplasia, abnormal position or formation of the ears, high arched palate, hypertelorism, epicanthic folds, limb and palmar crease abnormalities and short-upturned nose) should be recorded but do not contribute to establishing the diagnosis. Occasionally, children with prenatal alcohol effects may have another genetic syndrome as comorbidity. When in doubt and if feasible, a genetic dysmorphology assesment is advisable (Nayak and Murthy, 2008) .

Children affected by prenatal alcohol exposure may have prenatal or postnatal growth deficits. They can be small for gestational age in utero and remain below average throughout their lives with respect to head circumference, weight and height. Growth should be monitored to detect deficiency. Presence of pre- or post-natal growth deficiency should be recorded, defined as height or weight at or below the 10th percentile (1.5 standard deviations below the mean) or a disproportionately low weight-to-height ratio (at or below the $10^{th}$ percentile) using appropriate norms. To determine, however, that a child is growth deficient requires taking into consideration confounding variables such as parental size, genetic potential and associated conditions (e.g., gestational diabetes, nutritional status, illness). Gestational diabetes can lead to increased fetal size, which can mask the effects of growth retardation from prenatal alcohol exposure. Furthermore, if the infant is born into a family or a community where "normal" size is above the average for the general population, growth impairment may be masked if the child is compared with standard growth parameters rather than community norms Growth deficiencies may not persist with age, and infant growth records may not be available for adults coming in for assessment for the first time. Finally, if there is no alcohol exposure in the third trimester, the growth parameters can be normal (Square, 1997).

The physical features of people with FASD are most recognizable in childhood, and diagnosis is more difficult in newborns, adolescents, and adults. In a follow-up study by Spohr et al., only 10% of the original diagnosed group continued to have the recognizable features of FAS or FAE. Facial features should be measured in all age groups, although some people can show 'evidence of central nervous system neurodevelopment abnormalities' without growth deficiencies or craniofacial anomalies. If a patient's facial features change with age, the diagnosis of the facial features should be based on the point in time when the features were most severely expressed. When diagnosing adults, it can be helpful to view childhood photographs (Stratton *et al,* 1996).

Though physical features are essential to make the diagnosis of FAS, it is important to note that neurocognitive and behavioral deficits can be present in the absence of physical features (alcohol related neurodevelopment disorder or ARND). Research has shown that the brain dysfunction associated with FASD can be extreme and pervasive. Identifying CNS abnormalities resulting from prenatal alcohol exposure can be the most difficult aspect of a FAS diagnosis because of the heterogeneity of expression for these deficits across persons. Approximately one fourth of persons who receive a diagnosis of FAS perform at two standard deviations below the mean (which approaches substantial impairment [i.e., mental retardation]) on standardized measures of cognition (Streissguth *et al.,* 1996). To capture the full spectrum of effects adequately, two levels of functional deficits are consistent with the criteria for a CNS abnormality: 1) performance below the third percentile (i.e., two standard deviations below the mean) on a measure of global cognitive functioning or 2) performance <16th percentile (i.e., one standard deviation below the mean) on standardized measures of three functional domains. Thus, persons scoring below the normal range on a global measure of intelligence or development and persons scoring in the below-average range on standardized measures of three specific functional domains would be consistent with the criteria for functional CNS abnormality for diagnostic purposes (Chudley *et al.,* 2005).

A psychological assessment for the brain damage caused by prenatal exposure to alcohol is not different from an assessment for acquired brain injury. The domains of cognitive performance are the same. These include: IQ, memory, perception, language, motor skills, and adaptive functioning. Attention deficits are frequently cited in the FASD population (Coles *et al.*, 2002; Mattson *et al.*, 2006). Several studies have reported executive functioning deficits in individuals with FASD, including problems with response inhibition, set shifting, planning and concept formation, and verbal and nonverbal fluency (Kodituwakku *et al.*, 1995; Mattson *et al.*, 1999). Finally, motor dysfunction such as tremors, weak grasp, poor hand/eye coordination, and gait and balance difficulties were described in early reports of FAS (Jones and Smith, 1973) and supported in later studies (Mattson *et al.*, 1998; Roebuck *et* 98*al.*, 19). Motor deficits may also exist and they persist into adulthood in heavily exposed populations (Connor *et al.*, 2006).

People with FASD are also in high risk for psychiatric disorders, trouble with the law, alcohol and other drug abuse, and other maladaptive behaviors. They suffer from poor socialization and communication skills and are less likely to be living independently. They are more likely than non-alcohol exposed children to be rated as hyperactive, disruptive, impulsive, or delinquent. The assessment of the above characteristics is also very difficult. Only a few questions relate to the dangerously impulsive behaviors and poor decision making that put themselves and others at risk. Some questions relate to specific activities of daily living such as cooking, cleaning, and laundry but do not include the problems, for example, that people with FASDs have in preventing unwanted friends from entering their places of residence, stealing their belongings, and creating chaos resulting in their evictions (Fast and Conry, 2004).

## 4. Differential Diagnosis

Establishing the diagnosis of FASD may be a major challenge. Other diagnoses with similar physical and behavioral features exist and they also need to be considered. Information from multiple sources (e.g., school records, hospital records, social services, previous assessments) should be obtained; this might involve meetings with relevant professionals who know the patient (e.g., teachers, physicians, social workers, psychologists). Other relevant documentation would include birth and pregnancy records, medical and hospital records, adoption records, academic records, achievement tests, developmental assessments, psychological and psychometric assessments, legal reports and documentation of the family history. The comprehensive assessment by the diagnostic team provides important information about the individual's unique needs and allows interventions to be tailored to his or her strengths and challenges. The post-diagnostic report should state the basis for the diagnosis by including the history of alcohol use, the physical criteria and the psychological data that support it (Bertrand *et. Al.,*2005).

FAS with confirmed prenatal alcohol exposure requires documentation of the alcohol consumption patterns of the birth mother during the index pregnancy on the basis of clinical observation; self-reports; reports of heavy alcohol use during pregnancy by a reliable informant; medical records documenting positive blood alcohol levels or alcohol treatment; or other social, legal, or medical problems related to drinking during the index pregnancy. Clinicians, however, often have to evaluate a child or adult for FAS without definitive information regarding the mother's use of alcohol during pregnancy. This situation occurs frequently for children in foster and adoptive homes. In such cases, every effort should be made to obtain the necessary information, but lack of confirmation of alcohol use during pregnancy should not preclude a diagnosis of FAS if all other criteria are present. In rare instances, absence of exposure will be confirmed. Documentation that the birth mother did not drink any amount of alcohol from conception through birth would indicate that a FAS diagnosis is not appropriate. This finding typically implies either that the birth mother knew the date of conception (e.g., a planned pregnancy) and did not consume alcohol from that day forward or that she was prevented from drinking for a certain reason (e.g., incarceration)(Chudley *et al.,* 2005).

Certain syndromes have single overlapping features with FAS. With the exception of toluene embryopathy, no other known syndrome has the full constellation of small palpebral fissures, thin vermillion border, and smooth philtrum. However, for certain syndromes (e.g., Williams syndrome, Dubowitz syndrome, or fetal dilantin syndrome), the overall constellation of features (primary, occasional features, or both) is similar to FAS, and these syndromes should be considered in particular when completing the differential diagnosis (Bertrand *et. Al.,*2005).

CNS abnormalities resulting from environmental influences (e.g., abuse or neglect, disruptive homes, and lack of opportunities) are harder to differentiate. To assist with differential diagnosis between FAS and environmental causes for CNS abnormalities, clinicians should obtain a complete, detailed history from the person and family members.

The face of FAS is the result of a specific effect of ethanol teratogenesis altering growth of the midface and brain. Those exposed to other embryotoxic agents may display a similar, but not identical, phenotypic facial development, impaired growth, a higher frequency of anomalies and developmental and behavioural abnormalities [for a review, see Chudley and Longstaffe(Square, 1997)]. However, because FAS facial criteria have been restricted to short palpebral fissures, smooth philtrum and thin upper lip, there is far less overlap with the facial phenotypes associated with other syndromes. Knowledge of exposure history will decrease the possibility of misdiagnosing FASD.

Finally, in addition to ruling out other causes for CNS abnormalities, a complete diagnosis should identify and specify other disorders that can coexist with FAS (e.g., autism, conduct disorder, or oppositional defiant disorder). A particular person might have a conduct disorder in addition to FAS; however, not all persons with FAS have conduct disorders, and not all persons with conduct disorders have FAS (Bertrand *et. Al.,*2005).

## 5. Criminal Justice System

The life-long neurological impairments found in people with fetal alcohol spectrum disorders (FASDs), including learning disabilities, impulsivity, hyperactivity, social ineptness, and poor judgment, can increase susceptibility to victimization and involvement in the criminal justice system (CJS). Individuals with FASDs become involved in the Criminal Justice System as complainants, witnesses, and accused. Their disabilities, resulting from the prenatal alcohol exposure, must be considered at all stages in the legal process (Fast and Conry, 2009).

In one follow-up study (Streissguth *et al.,* 2004), trouble with the law (defined as ever charged, arrested, convicted, or otherwise in trouble with the law) was reported for 60% of the adolescents and adults with FASDs examined. The most frequent category was crimes against persons (45%). Among those in trouble with the law, the percentage who were actually charged, arrested, and/or convicted was 67% for adolescents and 87% for adults. Conry and Lane [2009] found that, when screening included adverse social histories, problematic behaviors, and some suspicion of prenatal alcohol exposure, the percentage ultimately receiving an alcohol-related diagnosis could be large: 86% in youth referred by their probation officers for an FASD assessment.

The cognitive and behavioral disabilities found in people with FASDs in the Criminal Justice System are described as including problems that spell the mnemonic 'ALARM': Adaptive behavior, Language, Attention, Reasoning, and Memory.

The term impaired adaptive (or maladaptive) functioning/behavior has been used to describe a broad range of problematic behaviors and difficulties in life that bring children and adults to the attention of professionals. Adaptive behavior refers to the effectiveness with which a person meets the standards of personal independence and social responsibility expected of an individual of the same age and cultural group. People with FASD have impaired adaptive behavior; they may struggle with basic requirements of day-to-day living, such as maintaining appropriate self-care, managing money, getting and maintaining employment, and using leisure time in healthy and acceptable ways (Fast and Conry, 2009).

There is very little research on the language development of individuals with FASDs. Many have been described as "chatty." When standardized measures of expressive and receptive language are compared youth with FASDs are shown to have impairments in both their understanding of spoken language and their ability to produce language forms at the level expected for their age (Conry and Lane, 2009). Language deficits have important implications for individuals with FASDs in the legal system in understanding the proceedings, understanding questions, and providing answers. Also, their superficial talkativeness may lead others (e.g., judges, lawyers) to overestimate their competence and level of understanding.

Attention deficit was described in 60% of the youth and adults (Streissguth *et al.* 1996) and in 70% of the youth in trouble with the law (Conry and Lane, 2009). For the diagnosis of attention deficit people need to have impairments in some or all of the areas of attention, impulsivity, and hyperactivity. Individuals with attention deficit seem more likely to develop conduct disorder (Biederman *et al.*, 1993; Antshel and Barkley, 2009). It appears that having additional comorbid disorders, such as conduct disorder and substance use disorder, can increase the risk for trouble with the law in people with attention deficit. (Bukstein *et al.*, 1989; Washburn *et al.,* 2008) and with ADHD and FASDs (Streissguth *et al.*, 1996; Conry *et al.*, 1997).

The area of reasoning encompasses abstract thinking, executive functioning, and other higher level cognitive processes. This is a broadly defined area and usually a battery of tests is used for the assessment (Mattson *et al.*, 1999). In the review by Rasmussen [2005], it was noted that people with FASDs have been found to have impaired executive functioning, with deficits in the areas of cognitive flexibility, planning and strategy use, verbal reasoning, some aspects of inhibition, set shifting, verbal fluency, working memory, and emotional regulation. These impairments can contribute to difficulties in social functioning (Schonfeld *et al.*, 2006).

People with FASD can have sporadic memory recall, which can be influenced by suggestion. They can confabulate, confusing details of a specific event with previous and subsequent real events and with fictional events. They may have poor concepts of time and sequence. Working memory deficits have been found in children (Streissguth *et al.,* 1990), in adults (Kerns *et al.,* 1997), and in most of youth justice clients (Conry and Lane, 2009) with FASDs.

A combination of memory deficits and language deficits can produce confused and seemingly unreliable testimony in court (Conry and Fast, 2000). People with poor memories may also confabulate, i.e., they may reconstruct events with ''grains of truth'' combined with inaccurate recollections based on unrelated past and fictional events. This tendency to confabulate may compromise the reliability of the witness' testimony. In addition, since people with FASDs have difficulty learning from experience and planning for the future, they may not be deterred by traditional punishments of the CJS (Fast and Conry, 2004).

Moreover, the significant problem behaviors noted in youth with FAS or FASDs are being socially inept/inappropriate and having poor understanding of personal boundaries. An example of this is the inappropriate sexual behavior shown by some individuals with FASDs (Streissguth *et al.,* 2004). Schonfeld et al. [2005] found that, for both youth with prenatal alcohol exposure and controls, the overall level of moral maturity was correlated with Verbal IQ on intelligence tests. Deficits in relations with family and friends, however, were specific to the group with prenatal alcohol exposure and were not simply due to their lower Verbal IQ; this may help explain their higher rates of delinquent behavior.

Individuals with FASD often come from dysfunctional backgrounds and may have mental illnesses and substance use disorders. The complex interactions among the brain damage caused by prenatal alcohol exposure, genetics, and the environment are difficult to disentangle and become more complex the older the individual is. Within the home environments of alcoholics in general, abuse or neglect of children, violence, poverty and chaotic disorganization are common. (Lund and Landsman-Dwyer, 1979; Nylander I., 1960; Tarter *et al.*, 1984; Woodside M., 1983; Carmichael-Olson H., 2002). In the study by Conry et al., 73.1% of the youth with FASD reported experiencing some form of abuse (emotional, physical, and/or sexual). As they get older, their own substance abuse problems may play a role in their criminal behavior (Fast and Conry, 2009).

The current abuse of drugs and alcohol is associated with a significant number of crimes. Statistics from both the Canadian Centre on Substance Abuse and the US Department of Justice indicate that over half of jail inmates were under the influence of alcohol and drugs at the time of the offense. The offense may also be committed to support the addiction. Anecdotal reports suggest that when people committing offenses have FASD, they are likely to be influenced by others, and having a substance use disorder further compromises the person with FASD. The combination of vulnerability or poor judgment relating to the brain damage caused by FASD and the influence of drugs and/or alcohol creates a situation that perpetuates the cycle of involvement with the legal system.

A comprehensive medical – legal report, prepared by a professional experienced with FASD, can help judges and lawyers understand how complex the interactions are among brain damage, genetics, and the environment. The person with FASD can be misunderstood in court, victimized in jails, and mismanaged in the transition back to the community, unless those working with the individual are aware of FASD and its implications (Fast and Conry, 2009).

## 6. Imputation

People with FASD can appear in court as complainant, witness, or accused and care must be taken to ensure that their statements are accurate. Clare and Gudjonsson (1993) found that people with mild learning disabilities or mild mental handicap were more suggestible and thus more unreliable than their average-ability counterparts, agreeing with leading questions and changing answers in response to negative feedback. They are vulnerable to making false confessions. They may misunderstand basic legal terms such as ''guilty'' and ''not guilty'' and may presume that a false confession can be retracted (Clare and Murphy, 1998).

Perske has studied why individuals with mental disabilities might confess to a crime they did not commit. Some of his relevant points, which also apply to people with FASD, include a desire to please people in authority, an inability to understand abstract concepts, confabulating, taking blame quickly to 'get out of the situation and go home', and being victimized by the plea bargaining of an accomplice, watching for clues from the interrogator to guess what the person wants to hear (or sometimes simply agreeing when not understanding what is being asked), an inability to understand abstract concepts, confabulating (distorting or fabricating story elements to hide real memory gaps), an inability to understand court proceedings, appearing too pleasant or defiant, taking blame or confessing too quickly, bargaining of an accomplice, and having cooccurring mental disorders. People with FASDs may eventually become exhausted, break down, and confess to what is being asked. They may also be confused by the way the question is worded, and may also appear too pleasant or defiant (Clarren and Astley., 2001).

These concerns must be considered by police taking statements at the scene of the crime, and by legal counsel talking to clients. People with FASD may not understand concepts such as waiving rights to counsel, lawyer – client privilege, and the implications of their plea. They may not appreciate when they are free to speak and when they should remain silent. Because of their language and other disabilities, care must be taken to corroborate information and to not assume that their statements are accurate. They may not be purposefully ''lying'' but explaining what happened as they understand it (Fast and Conry, 2004).

Individuals with FASD with a normal IQ (above the range of mental handicap) may have significant deficits in these areas. The courts often understand only the importance of low IQ as a mitigating factor. However, most individuals with FASD do not have IQs in the range of mental handicap (IQ less than 70), and in those cases it is more difficult to convince the court that the individual may not have appreciated the severity of the offence committed nor the resulting consequences. A comprehensive medical – legal report can assist the judge and others involved with the individual with FASD, as he or she navigates the legal process. The report can describe the disabilities of the offender and implications for sentencing. Only professionals who are recognized as being experienced in assessing people suspected of having FASD should prepare the medical – legal reports, psychological assessments, and social histories. The report should clearly document the evidence supporting FAS or a related diagnosis. Assessments can be prepared before or after sentencing, and should describe the disabilities of the offender and implications for sentencing. The psychological report should include findings from assessments of intelligence, language, memory, reasoning, executive function, and adaptive skills (Streissguth *et al.*, 1996).

The person with FASD often has difficulties in comprehension and recall, and it is critical not to use the person being assessed as the sole informant. Information contained in previous reports cannot be taken at face value without verification. Often the most difficult part is obtaining a confirmed history of prenatal alcohol exposure. Since people with FASDs have difficulties in comprehension and recall, it is critical that they are not the only informants. Birth parents, adoptive parents, foster parents, and other caregivers have an important role when their child with FASD becomes involved with the legal system, whether that person is chronologically a child or an adult. The parents may be the only ones who have experienced the impact of the person's disabilities, and how those disabilities could perpetuate misunderstanding. If permitted, they can help the person with FASD navigate the legal system, and aid communication between the courts and the custodial system (Steinhausen *et al.,* 2003)

In general, when people with FASD are found unfit to stand trial, they may be institutionalized and treated until such time as they are found fit to stand trial. For individuals with FASDs, who have permanent brain damage, this could be never.

## 7. Sentencing

The fundamental purpose of sentencing is to denounce unlawful conduct, to deter the offender and other persons from committing offences, to assist in rehabilitating the offender, and to protect society. The gravity of the offense and the degree of responsibility of the offender must be considered. The principles of sentencing are based on cognitive functioning and reasoning abilities that may not be present in a person with FASD. The concepts of 'consequences', 'rehabilitation', and 'deterrence', when used at a sentencing hearing, may not apply. The time between the offence and the sentencing may be long, and people with FASDs may not connect the consequence with the act. Also, if other offences are committed before the trial or before sentencing, people with FASDs may not understand which events are connected, especially if some offences are more serious than others.

Moreover, incarceration has the potential for victimization (physically, sexually, and emotionally). Although there is structure and routine in jail, people with FASDs may have trouble "getting" the rules and their actions may be misinterpreted by staff who do not understand about FASDs. People with FASDs may then have lengthy periods in solitary confinement due to their behavior being seen as willfully noncompliant. Individuals with FASD can be negatively influenced by their peers or become scapegoats. The person with FASD can also be influenced negatively by their peers because they want to 'fit in' and be liked (Fast and Conry, 2004).

The most effective sentences for people with FASDs may be those that aim to change their living or social situation, rather than their behavior. Accomplishing this may be difficult, as the judge's power does not extend to individuals other than the accused (Conry and Fast, 2000). Some individuals with FASDs may be undiagnosed and already be involved in the legal system, having lengthy criminal records. Once a diagnosis is made, a judge will need to decide whether to base the sentence on the criminal record, which would imply harsher sentences consistent with repeat offences, or on the disabilities associated with FASD, which would consider whether the individual would be deterred or rehabilitated by incarceration.

Alternatives to incarceration can include conditional sentences, diversion, or sentencing circles. Sentencing circles have been used in First Nations and American Indian communities. In this approach community members express to the offender how they have been affected and how they will support the offender, who assumes responsibility for the offence and seeks forgiveness and reconciliation with the community. The community thus becomes more actively involved and assumes greater responsibility for resolving conflicts involving one of its members (Fast and Conry, 2004).

Conditional sentences allow offenders to serve time in an alternative setting such as their homes. The goal is to prevent the negative outcomes of incarceration while establishing a more productive life (going to school and/ or holding a job). However, some people with FASD will require custodial sentences for the protection of the community. People with FASD who receive conditional sentences will need intense supervision, which may require being supervised by a responsible adult for 24 h a day.

Probation orders for individuals with FASD need to be written clearly and in simple, concrete language. People with FASDs may be able to repeat the probation orders and even explain what they mean, but without constant supervision will be unable to follow them when in the community, continuing the cycle of trouble with the law (Fast and Conry, 2004).

In the legal system, the disabilities of people with FASD need to be accommodated. Once involved with the legal system, people with FASD face many difficulties with incarceration. Offenders with FASD return to the community after release. They should not return worse off than when they left, due to misunderstanding, victimization, and mismanagement of their disabilities. Their mental illnesses and substance use disorders need to be recognized and treated. Planning the transition from jail to the community requires input from corrections, caregivers, the community, and the individual with FASD. There needs to be ongoing education of professionals to develop skills in recognition and referral for diagnosis. Recognition of the disability, particularly early recognition, may reduce the over-representation of this group in the criminal justice system (Fast and Conry, 2004).

## 8. Conclusion

The learning and life skills affected by prenatal alcohol exposure vary among persons, depending on the amount, timing, and pattern of exposure and on each person's current and past environment (Abel, 1998; Davis, 1994). As a result, services needed for persons with FAS and their families vary according to the parts of the brain affected, the person's age or level of maturation, the health or functioning of the family, and the person's overall living environment (May *et al.* 2008, Incerti *et al.* 2010). Thus, the service needs of affected persons and their families should be individualized (Briesmeister and Schaefer, 1998). Early recognition of the disabilities of people with FASDs may reduce the over representation of this group in the criminal Justice System and better understanding of FASD should lead to improved support and fair treatment of individuals with FASD. Understanding of the disorder should be increased among law enforcement personnel, and other professionals who might become involved with the affected person.

## References

Abel EL Fetal alcohol abuse syndrome and fetal alcohol effects. 1998.

Abel EL, Sokol RJ Incidence of fetal alcohol syndrome and economic impact of FAS-related anomalies. *Drug Alcohol Depend* 1987; 19: 51–70.

Akshoomoff NA, Courchesne E, Townsend J. Attention coordination and anticipatory control. *International review of neurobiology* 1997; 41: 575-598.

Antshel KM, Barkley R Developmental and behavioral disorders grown up: attention deficit hyperactivity disorder *Journal of developmental and behavioral pediatrics* 2009; 30(1): 81-90.

Archibald SL, Fennema-Notestine C, Gamst A, Riley EP, Mattson SN, Jernigan TL Brain dysmorphology in individuals with severe prenatal alcohol exposure. *Developmental medicine and child neurology* 2001; 43(7): 504.

Astley SJ, Clarren SK A case definition and photographic screening tool for the facial phenotype of fetal alcohol syndrome. *The Journal of Pediatrics* 1996; 129: 33-41.

Autti-R¨am¨o I, Autti T, Korkman M *et al.* MRI findings in children with school problems who had been exposed prenatally to alcohol. *Developmental medicine and child neurology* 2002; 44: 98–106.

Bertrand J, Floyd LL, Weber MK Fetal Alcohol Syndrome Prevention Team, Division of Birth Defects and Developmental Disabilities, National Center on Birth Defects and Developmental Disabilities, Centers for Disease Control and Prevention (CDC). Guidelines for Identifying and Referring Persons with Fetal Alcohol Syndrome. *Morbidity and Mortality Weekly Report. Recommendations and Reports* 2005; 54:1-14.

Biederman J, Faraone SV, Milberger S, Doyle A Diagnoses of attention-deficit hyperactivity disorder from parent reports predict diagnoses based on teacher reports. *Journal of the American Academy of Child and Adolescent Psychiatry.* 1993; 32(2): 315-317.

Briesmeister JM, Schaefer CE (ed). Handbook of parent training: parents as co-therapists for children's behavior problems. 2nd ed. *New York, NY: John Wiley and Sons,* Inc. 1998.

Brimacombe M, Nayeem A, Adubato S, DeJoseph M, Zimmerman-Bier B Fetal Alcohol Syndrome Related Knowledge Assessment and Comparison in New Jersey Health Professional Groups *The Canadian Journal of Clinical Pharmacology* 2008; 15 (1): 57-65

Bukstein OG, Brent DA, Kaminer Y Comorbidity of substance abuse and other psychiatric disorders in adolescents. *The American Journal of Psychiatry* 1989; 146: 1131-1141.

Carmichael-Olson H Helping individuals with fetal alcohol syndrome and related conditions: a clinician's overview. *The effects of parental dysfunction on children*. 2002; 147-177.

Chudley AE, Conry J, Cook JL, Loock C, Rosales T, LeBlanc N Fetal Alcohol Spectrum Disorder: Canadian Guidelines for Diagnosis *Canadian Medical Association journal,* 2005; 172 (5 suppl)

Clare ICH, Murphy GH Working with offenders or alleged offenders with intellectual disabilities. *Clinical psychology and people with intellectual disabilities*. 1998; 154-176.

Clarren SK Neuropathology in fetal alcohol syndrome. *Alcohol and Brain Development* 1986; 158–166.

Clarren SK, Alvord EC Jr, Sumi SM *et al.* Brain malfunctions related to prenatal exposure to alcohol. *Journal of Pediatrics* 1978; 92: 64–67.

Clarren SK, Astley SJ Fetal alcohol syndrome. *Management of genetic syndromes*. 2001; 151 – 64.

Coffin JM, Baroody S, Schneider K *et al.* Impaired cerebellar learning in children with prenatal alcohol exposure: a comparative study of eyeblink conditioning in children with ADHD and dyslexia. *Cortex* 2005; 41: 389–398.

Coles CD, Platzman KA, Lynch ME *et al.* Auditory and visual sustained attention in adolescents prenatally exposed to alcohol. *Alcoholism, clinical and experimental research* 2002; 26: 263-271.

Connor PD, Sampson PD, Streissguth AP *et al.* Effects of prenatal alcohol exposure on fine motor coordination and balance: a study of two adult samples. *Neuropsychologia* 2006; 44: 744-751.

Conry J, Fast DK Fetal alcohol syndrome and the criminal justice system. *Vancouver: British Columbia Fetal Alcohol Syndrome Resource Society* 2000.

Conry JL, Fast DK, Loock CA. Youth in thecriminal justice system: identifying FAS and other developmental disabilities. *Vancouver, BC: Final Report to the Ministry of the Attorney General* 1997.

Conry JL, Lane KA Characteristics of youth with FASD on adjudicated probation orders. *Final report to the Department of Justice Canada and British Columbia Ministry of Children and Family Development* 2009.

Coulter CL, Leech RW, Schafer B *et al.* Midline cerebral dysgenesis, dysfunction of the hypothalamic pituitary axis, and fetal alcohol effects. *Archives of Neurology* 1993; 50: 771–775.

Davis D Reaching out to children with FAS/FAE: a handbook for teachers, counselors, and parents who work with children affected by fetal alcohol syndrome and fetal alcohol effects. *West Nyack, NY: The Center for Applied Research in Education* 1994.

Dikranian K, Qin YQ, Labruyere J *et al.* Ethanol-induced neuroapoptosis in the developing rodent cerebellum and related brain stem structures. *Brain research. Developmental brain research* 2005; 155: 1-13.

Ebrahim SH, Anderson AK, Floyd RL Alcohol consumption by reproductive-aged women in the USA: an update on assessment, burden and prevention in the 1990s. *Prenatal and Neonatal Medicine* 1999; 4: 419-430.

Fast DK, Conry J Fetal Alcohol Spectrum Disorders and the Criminal Justice System *Developmental Disabilities Research Reviews* 2009; 15: 250 – 257

Fast DK, Conry J The Challenge of Fetal Alcohol Syndrome in the Criminal Legal System *Addiction Biology* 2004; 9: 161 – 166

Fukui Y, Sakata-Haga H Intrauterine Environment-Genome Interaction and Childrens Development: Ethonol: A Teratogen in Developing Brain *The Journal of Toxicological Sciences* 2009; 34:273-278

Goh YI, Chudley AE, Clarren SK, Koren G, Orrbine E, Rosales T, Rosenbaum C Development of Canadian Screening Tools for Fetal Alcohol Spectrum Disorders *The Canadian Journal of Clinical Pharmacology* 2008; 15 (2): 344-366

Goodlett CR, Lundahl KR Temporal determinants of neonatal alcohol-induced cerebellar damage and motor performance deficits. *Pharmacology, biochemistry, and behavior* 1996; 55: 531–540.

Guerri C, Bazinet A, Riley EP Foetal Alcohol Spectrum Disorders and Alterations in Brain and Behaviour *Alcohol and Alcoholism* 2009; 44(2): 108–114

Guerri C, Renau-Piqueras J Alcohol, astroglia, and brain development. *Molecular Neurobiology* 1997; 15: 65–81.

HansonJW, Streissguth AP, Smith DW The effects of moderate alcohol consumption during pregnancy on fetal growth and morphogenesis. *Journal of Pediatrics* 1978; 92: 457–460.

Haycock PC (*Division of Human Genetics, University of the Witwatersrand and National Health Laboratory Service,Johannesburg, South Africa)* Fetal Alcohol Spectrum Disorders: The Epigenetic Perspective *Biology of Reproduction 81,*2009; 607–617

Incerti M, MD, Vink J, MD, Roberson R, Wood L, Abebe D, Spong CY, MD Reversal of Alcohol-Induced Learning Deficits in the Young Adult in a Model of Fetal Alcohol Syndrome *Obstetrics and Gynecology* 2010; 115:350–356

Jacobson, JL, et al. Teratogenic effects of alcohol on infant development. *Alcoholism, Clinical and Experimental Research.* 1993; 17: 174–183.

Jones KL, Smith DW Recognition of the fetal alcohol syndrome in early infancy. *Lancet* 1973; 2(7836):999-1001.

Jones KL, Smith DW The fetal alcohol syndrome. *Teratology* 1975; 12(1): 1-10.

Kerns KA, Don A, Mateer CA, Streissguth AP. Cognitive deficits in nonretarded adults with fetal alcohol syndrome. *Journal of learning disabilities* 1997; 30(6): 685-693.

Kodituwakku PW, Handmaker NS, Cutler SK *et al.* Specific impairments in self-regulation in children exposed to alcohol prenatally. *Alcoholism, clinical and experimental research* 1995; 19: 1558–1564.

Lund C, Landsman-Dwyer S Pre-delinquents and disturbed adolescents: the role of parental alcoholism. *Currents in alcoholism* 1979; 5: 339 – 348.

Maier SE, Chen W, West JR The effects of timing and duration of alcohol exposure on development of the fetal brain. *Fetal Alcohol Syndrome: From Mechanism to Prevention,* 1996; 27–50.

Mattson SN, Calarco KE, Lang AR Focused and shifting attention in children with heavy prenatal alcohol exposure. *Neuropsychology* 2006; 20: 361-369.

Mattson SN, Goodman AM, Caine C, et al. Executive functioning in children with heavy prenatal alcohol exposure. *Alcoholism, clinical and experimental research* 1999; 23: 1808-1815.

Mattson SN, Riley EP, Gramling LJ *et al.* Neuropsychological comparison of alcohol-exposed children with or without physical features of fetal alcohol syndrome. *Neuropsychology* 1998; 12: 146-153.

Mattson SN, Riley EP, Jernigan TL *et al.* A decrease in the size of the basal ganglia following prenatal alcohol exposure: a preliminary report. *Neurotoxicology and teratology* 1993; 16: 283–289.

Mattson SN, Riley EP. A review of the neurobehavioral deficits in children with Fetal Alcohol Syndrome or prenatal exposure to alcohol. *Alcoholism, clinical and experimental research* 1998; 22: 279-292.

May PA, Miller JH, Goodhart KA, Maestas OR, Buckley D, Trujillo PM, Gossage JP Enhanced Case Management to Prevent Fetal Alcohol Spectrum Disorders in Northern Plains Communities *Maternal and Child Health Journal* 2008; 12:747–759

Nayak RB, Murthy P Fetal Alcohol Spectrum Disorder (Review Article) *Indian Pedriatrics* 2008; 45

Nylander I Children of alcoholic fathers. *Acta Paediatrica Scandinavica* 1960; 49(suppl): 121.

O'Hare ED, Kan E, Yoshii J *et al.* Mapping cerebellar vermal morphology and cognitive correlates in prenatal alcohol exposure. *NeuroReport* 2005; 16: 1285-1290

Roebuck TM, Simmons RW, Richardson C, Mattson SN, Riley EP. Neuromuscular responses to disturbance of balance in children with prenatal exposure to alcohol. *Alcoholism, clinical and experimental research* 1998; 22(9): 1992-1997.

Roebuck-Spencer TM, Mattson SN Implicit strategy affects learning in children with heavy prenatal alcohol exposure. *Alcoholism, clinical and experimental research* 2004; 28: 1424-1431.

Schonfeld AM, Paley B, Frankel F, O'Connor MJ Executive functioning predicts social skills following prenatal alcohol exposure. *Child neuropsychology : a journal on normal and abnormal development in childhood and adolescence* 2006; 12(6): 439-452.

Sokol RJ, Delaney-Black V, Nordstrom B Fetal alcohol spectrum disorder. *The Journal of the American Medical Association.* 2003; 290: 2996–2999.

Sowell ER, Jernigan TL, Mattson SN *et al.* Abnormal development of the cerebellar vermis in children prenatally exposed to alcohol: size reduction in lobules I-V. *Alcoholism, clinical and experimental research* 1996; 20: 31-34.

Sowell ER, Thompson PM, Mattson SN *et al.* Regional brain shape abnormalities persist into adolescence after heavy prenatal alcohol exposure. *Cerebral Cortex* 2002a; 12: 856-865.

Sowell ER, Thompson PM, Mattson SN *et al.* Voxel-based morphometric analyses of the brain in children and adolescents prenatally exposed to alcohol. *Neuro Report* 2001a; 12: 515-523.

Spohr HL, MD, Willms J, MD, and Steinhausen HC, MD, PHD Fetal Alcohol Spectrum Disorders in Young Adulthood *The Journal of Pedriatrics* 2007;150:175-179

Square D Fetal alcohol syndrome epidemic on Manitoba reserve. *Canadian Medical Association Journal* 1997; 157(1): 59-60.

Steinhausen HC, Winkler Metzke C, Spohr HL, Behavioural phenotype in fetal alcohol syndrome and fetal alcohol effects. *Developmental medicine and child neurology* 2003; 45:179-182.

Stratton K, Howe C, Battaglia FC Fetal alcohol syndrome: diagnosis, epidemiology,prevention, and treatment. *Washington: Institute of Medicine and National Academy Press;* 1996. Available: www.nap.edu/books/0309052920/html/ index .html (accessed 2004 Oct 29).

Streissguth AP, Barr HM, Kogan J, Bookstein FL Understanding the occurrence of secondary disabilities in clients with fetal alcohol syndrome (FAS) and fetal alcohol effects (FAE): final report. *Seattle, WA: University of Washington Publication Services* 1996.

Streissguth AP, Barr HM, Sampson PD Moderate prenatal alcohol exposure: Effects on child IQ and learning problems at age 7½ years. *Alcoholism, Clinical and Experimental Research* 1990; 14: 662-669.

Streissguth AP, Bookstein FL, Barr HM, Sampson PD, O'Malley K, Young JK. Risk factors for adverse life outcomes in fetal alcohol syndrome and fetal alcohol effects. *Journal of developmental and behavioral pediatrics* 2004; 25(4): 228-238.

Tarter R, Hegedus A, Goldstein G, Shelly C, Alterman A Adolescent sons of alcoholics: neuropsychological and personality characteristics. *Alcoholism, clinical and experimental research* 1984; 8: 216-222.

Washburn JJ, Teplin LA, Voss LS, et al. Psychiatric disorders among detained youths: a comparison of youths processed in juvenile court and adult criminal court. *Psychiatric Services* 2008; 59: 965–973.

Woodruff-Pak DS, Goldenberg G, Downey-Lamb MM *et al.* Cerebellar volume in humans related to magnitude of classical conditioning. *Neuro Report* 2000; 11: 609-615.

Woodside M Children of alcoholic parents: inherited and psychosocial influences. *Journal of psychiatric treatment and evaluation* 1983; 5: 531-537.

In: Pregnancy and Alcohol Consumption
Editors: Joshua D. Hoffman, pp. 281-298
ISBN: 978-1-61761-122-3


*Chapter 11*

# FETAL ALCOHOL SYNDROME IN URBAN SCHOOLS

***Giorgie Petković and Ingeborg Barišić***
Children's University Hospital Zagreb, Zagreb, Croatia

## ABSTRACT

Learning disabilities are frequent and important cause of poor school performance. One of the most frequent causes of mental and learning problems in children is fetal alcohol syndrome (FAS). The syndrome is caused by maternal alcohol consumption during pregnancy which causes facial anomalies, growth retardation and neurological manifestations in children. One of the hallmarks of FAS is an impaired neurological function with attention deficiency, speech, reasoning, and learning disabilities. Dyscalculia is the most frequent learning problem present in these children. Later-life complications include poor academic performance, low income, and unemployment, which lead to other undesirable social consequences.

Estimated FAS prevalence is highly variable, and ranges from 3.1 to 74.2 per 1000 schoolchildren. A high variability of FAS prevalence is attributed to the differences between races, ethnic groups, socioeconomic status, educational level, and alcohol consumption habits. Most studies performed so far, have focused on rural high-risk populations of low socioeconomic status. However, recent studies have revealed important changes in lifestyle and alcohol consumption habits among women. These studies have suggested that urban, employed women with higher income and higher educational level represent another high-risk population when it comes to drinking during pregnancy. However, FAS studies in urban schoolchildren populations are rare.

In this work we have reviewed drinking habits reported in women, together with risk factors and pregnancy drinking habits. These habits pose a risk factor for the development of FAS in children. We have also reviewed clinical characteristics and estimated FAS prevalence of FAS in general schoolchildren population, with a special emphasis put on urban population.

FAS is one of the most common congenital but preventable causes of neurological deficits in children. Epidemiologic studies have contributed to the degree of awareness on this problem among healthcare professionals, and have improved the primary prevention in terms of reducing alcohol intake among women of the childbearing age. It is necessary to further increase the awareness of school personnel in order to enhance secondary prevention of later-life complications by adequate scholastic interventions carried out among these children. These interventions should help the children with their scholastic curriculum so as to become productive members of society.

## INTRODUCTION

Fetal alcohol syndrome (FAS) is one of the common causes of developmental delays, behavioural problems, and unsatisfactory school performance. It is characterised by permanent congenital impairments caused by maternal alcohol consumption during pregnancy. The syndrome manifests itself with growth retardation, combination of characteristic dysmorphic features, impairment and dysfunction of the central nervous system (CNS) and possible presence of other anatomic and/or functional disorders [1].

Alcohol consumption during pregnancy causes a spectrum of anomalies included under the common denominator "Fetal Alcohol Spectrum Disorders" (FASD) [2, 3]. FASD embraces several clinical categories, as follows: 1. Fetal Alcohol Syndrome (FAS); 2. Partial Fetal Alcohol Syndrome (PFAS); 3. Alcohol-Related Neurodevelopmental Disorder (ARND); and 4. Alcohol-Related Birth Defects (ARBD). FAS is clinically the most severe of mentioned categories.

## PATHOGENESIS

Fetal alcohol syndrome is caused by alcohol consumption during pregnancy. Alcohol exerts an embryotoxic (lunar weeks 5-12) and fetotoxic effect (from lunar week 12 on). Alcohol toxicity is attributed to direct noxious impact of ethanol or its metabolites; nevertheless, the exact mechanism of alcohol-induced teratogenesis during intrauterine development has not been fully clarified yet. The research carried out so far has suggested that clinical consequences arising from the noxious alcohol impact are the result of a complex interplay between genetic and environmental factors, and depend on pregnancy stage, the amount and frequency of alcohol consumption [4-9].

## CLINICAL PRESENTATION

Clinical consequences arising from alcohol consumption during pregnancy are highly variable and range from mild to severe, the outermost severity being represented by fetal death. Alcohol consumption during pregnancy contributes to miscarriage and stillbirth rates, as well as to perinatal mortality [10-12]. In proof of the foregoing, the risk of having a spontaneous miscarriage registered among alcohol-consuming pregnant women is 2-3 folds higher as compared to general population, while the perinatal mortality registered among children delivered by heavily drinking mothers, rises up to 17%. The overall mortality rate encountered among those diagnosed with FAS in early childhood is 6%.

**Table 1. Clinical manifestations of FAS**

| System | Defects |
|---|---|
| Pregnancy complications | Abortion<br>Stillbirth<br>High perinatal mortality |
| Growth | Low birth weight<br>Low birth length<br>Low weight<br>Low height |
| Face | Short palpebral fissure length<br>Epicantal folds<br>Hypertelorism<br>Smooth philtrum<br>Thin upper lip<br>Broad and flat nasal bridge<br>Anteverted nostrils<br>Low set ears<br>"Railroad track" ears<br>Micrognathia |
| Ocular | Strabismus<br>Ptosis<br>Optic nerve hypoplasia<br>Refractive anomalies<br>Retinal vascular anomalies |
| Auditory | Conductive / sensory hypoacusia |
| Cardiovascular | Atrial septal defects<br>Ventricular septal defects<br>Great vessels anomalies<br>Conotruncal heart defects<br>Tetralogy of Fallot |
| Urogenital | Aplastic / hypoplastic / dysplastic kidneys<br>Horseshoe kidney<br>Ureteral duplications |
| Musculosceletal | Pectus carinatum / excavatum<br>Radioulnar synostosis<br>Klippel-Feil syndrome<br>Scoliosis<br>Haemivertebrae |
| Extremities | "Hockey stick" palmar crease<br>Hypoplastic nails<br>Camptodactilia<br>Clinodactilia |
| CNS | Microcephaly<br>Structural brain anomalies<br>Neurologic deficiencies<br>Functional deficits |
| Secondary complication | Intellectual disability<br>Unemployment<br>Behavioral problems<br>Antisocial behavior<br>Alcoholism and drug abuse<br>Unable of independent living |

From the clinical standpoint, FAS is featured by low birth body mass and length, accompanied by tiny constitution and postnatal growth retardation (Table 1) [13]. Facial dysmorphia is characterised by short palpebral fissures, hypertelorism, epicanthus, broad and flat nasal bridge, anteverted nostrils, mid-face hypoplasia, low-set and malformed ears ("railroad track ears"), smooth and elongated philtrum, and thin upper lip [14]. The palms of the hands usually present with hockey stick-like palmar crease, campto or clinodactyly and hypoplastic nails can be seen as well [13-15]. It should be pointed out, though, that facial anomalies develop gradually. In newborns, certain features otherwise typical of the syndrome are blurred, while a number of them disappear after puberty. The research carried out so far has indicated that dysmorphic features typical of FAS are most striking starting from the age of 3 until the age of 12 [2, 16].

Individuals with FAS have been reported to have malformations of inner organs, e.g cardiac and vascular malformations (atrial and/or ventricular septal defects, tetralogy of Fallot, large vessel anomalies), renal malformations (aplastic or hypoplastic kidneys, ureteral duplications, hydronephrosis, horseshoe-like kidney), bone malformations (radio-ulnar synostosis, Klippel-Feil anomaly, hemi-vertebra, scoliosis), ophthalmologic disorders (strabismus, refractive anomalies, amblyopia, coloboma, blepharoptosis, anomalies of the ocular fundus blood vessels, microphtalmia), and hearing defects (conductive and perceptive hearing loss) [14, 17, 18].

Alcohol exposure has an adverse impact on CNS development. Microcephalia at birth is a result of diminished brain volume [19]. The latter is consequential to the reduction of white and grey matter volume. CNS diagnostic imaging reveals a number of structural anomalies, such as the impairments of the cingulate gyrus, basal ganglia, corpus callosum, cerebellum and hippocampus, as well as polymicrogyria and volumetric reduction of frontal and parietal lobes [20-22].

In addition to structural brain defects, functional impairments can be seen as well, in terms of a lower IQ, more common left-handedness, slower executive functioning and data processing, learning disorders, dyscalculia, slower speech development, impaired social interaction, and higher risk of febrile convulsions and seizure disorder [23-31]. Attention Deficit Hyperactivity Disorder (ADHD) is more common in FASD children, and FAS children are more deeply cognitively involved in their everyday activities [25, 32]. Throughout infancy, troubles falling asleep, as well as impaired sleeping and feeding patterns can be encountered.

FAS children are hospitalised more frequent than children from general population. The most common indications for such hospitalisations are mid-ear inflammation, pneumonia, bronchitis, anaemia, growth retardation, child abuse, feeding difficulties, and gastroenteritis [33].

Secondary complications, arising on the grounds of an unrecognised disorder and/or badly-tailored and poorly-managed interventional programme and implementation of adequate preventative measures, are of the outermost importance for FAS patients [1, 34]. Latter in life, inadequate rehabilitation of FAS children may lead to unemployment, mental health disorders, especially depression and anxiety, violent behaviour, unacceptable and risky sexual behaviour, alcoholism, drug abuse, poor academic performance, and inability to lead an independent life [35]. When it comes to FAS patients, a special attention should be paid to their family members. A higher frequency of FASD has been encountered in siblings of FAS patients, while in adult family members heavier alcohol consumption is common [36 37].

## ESTABLISHING A DIAGNOSE

Despite the fact that FAS clinical presentation has been known for forty years now, the identification of FAS patients and the establishment of a precise diagnosis represent diagnostic challenge. Diagnosing is difficult due to the fact that specific laboratory tests capable of corroborating the existence of fetal alcohol syndrome in a given child are non-existent. The diagnosing process calls for data on alcohol consumption during pregnancy and a detailed clinical examination of the child, the latter serving the purpose of detecting the FAS features held to be of diagnostic relevance. Therefore, the establishment of precise, standardised, and universally-adopted clinical diagnostic criteria is necessary (1). The criteria currently in place are based on the investigations of Jones and Smith, dating back to 1973 (38). The authors performed the first systematic investigation of clinical symptoms of fetal alcohol syndrome and proposed diagnostic criteria that still represent the basics of FAS diagnostics (39). In line with the suggestions given by Jones and Smith, diagnostic criteria include a verified alcohol consumption during pregnancy, as well as clinical signs falling into three basic groups, as follows: 1. prenatal and postnatal growth retardation; 2. specific facial anomalies (short palpebral fissures, smooth philtrum and thin upper lip); and 3. CNS anomalies. A wide variety of clinical consequences arising from alcohol consumption during pregnancy has imposed the need for classification and standardisation of individual clinical categories embraced by FASD. In 1996, the Institute of Medicine (IOM) operating under the wing of the National Academy of Sciences, proposed the following five FASD diagnostic categories: 1. FAS with and without confirmed maternal alcohol consumption during pregnancy; 2. PFAS (Partial Foetal Alcohol Syndrome) with confirmed maternal alcohol consumption during pregnancy; 3. Alcohol-Related Neurodevelopmental Disorder (ARND); and 4. Alcohol-Related Birth Defect (ARBD) (2). However, the proposed classification failed to clearly define individual diagnostic criteria, thus restricting the possibility of their practical implementation. Four years later, Astley and Clarren proposed a novel quantitative approach to the classification in reference, the 4-Digit Diagnostic Code or the Washington criteria (40). The Washington criteria are underpinned by four basic, widely adopted diagnostic parameters, as well as by ranking of these parameters into four ranks and the total (4-digit) score reflecting the share of individual diagnostic parameters taken into account with FAS diagnostics. The proposed classification embraces a total of 22 different diagnostic categories (or 9, should the grading of the consumed amount of alcohol be excluded). The Washington system is very precise, but the vast number of different diagnostic categories renders its routine clinical implementation difficult. In 2004, the US Centre for Disease Control (CDC) published novel directives and guidelines for FAS diagnostics, but, unlike its predecessors, took the stand that definite data and studies providing for the establishment of diagnostic criteria applicable to the remainder of FASD spectrum disorders are lacking (1). In 2005, Chudley et al. proposed new directives and guidelines for FASD diagnostics that unite IOM recommendations and Washington criteria (41). In the very same year, Hoyme et al. published the supplement to 1996 IOM diagnostic FASD classification (13). According to the new, revised classification, FASD comprises a total of 6 diagnostic categories (Table 2). In order to uncover FAS and PFAS patients, the authors pay special attention to the clinical examination and the detection of specific cranial and facial anomalies and dysmorphic features including microcephalia, palpebral fissure length, and facial midline hypoplasia (13).

**Table 2. Revised IOM diagnostic categories and diagnostic criteria of FASD (Hoyme et al. 2005)**

| Diagnostic categories | Diagnostic criteria |
|---|---|
| 1 FAS with confirmed maternal drinking during pregnancy | 1. Confirmed maternal drinking during pregnancy<br>2. Minor facial anomalies (including ≥2 of features):<br>Short palpebral fissures (≤ $10^{th}$ percentile)<br>Thin vermilion border of the upper lip (score 4-5 lip/philtrum guide)<br>Smooth philtrum (score 4-5 lip/ philtrum guide)<br>3. Prenatal and/or postnatal growth retardation (including ≥1 of following):<br>High ≤ $10^{th}$ percentile<br>Weight ≤ $10^{th}$ percentile<br>4. Deficient brain growth or abnormal morphogenesis (including ≥1 of following):<br>Head circumference ≤ $10^{th}$ percentile<br>Structural brain abnormalities |
| 2 FAS without confirmed maternal drinking during pregnancy | 1. Minor facial anomalies (including ≥2 of features):<br>Short palpebral fissures (≤ $10^{th}$ percentile)<br>Thin vermilion border of the upper lip (score 4-5 lip/philtrum guide)<br>Smooth philtrum (score 4-5 lip/ philtrum guide)<br>2. Prenatal and/or postnatal growth retardation (including ≥1 of following):<br>High ≤ $10^{th}$ percentile<br>Weight ≤ $10^{th}$ percentile<br>3. Deficient brain growth or abnormal morphogenesis (including ≥1 of following):<br>Head circumference ≤ $10^{th}$ percentile<br>Structural brain abnormalities |
| 3 PFAS with confirmed maternal drinking during pregnancy | 1. Confirmed maternal drinking during pregnancy<br>2. Minor facial anomalies (including ≥2 of features):<br>Short palpebral fissures (≤ $10^{th}$ percentile)<br>Thin vermilion border of the upper lip (score 4-5 lip/philtrum guide)<br>Smooth philtrum (score 4-5 lip/ philtrum guide)<br>3. One of following characteristics:<br>Prenatal and/or postnatal growth retardation (including ≥1 of following):<br>-High ≤ $10^{th}$ percentile<br>-Weight ≤ $10^{th}$ percentile<br>Deficient brain growth or abnormal morphogenesis (including ≥1 of following):<br>-Head circumference ≤ $10^{th}$ percentile<br>-Structural brain abnormalities<br>Evidence of behavioral or cognitive abnormalities:<br>-Impairment in the performance of complex tasks<br>-Receptive and expressive language deficit<br>-Behavioral problems |

| Diagnostic categories | Diagnostic criteria |
|---|---|
| 4 FAS without confirmed maternal drinking during pregnancy | 1.Minor facial anomalies (including ≥2 of features):<br>Short palpebral fissures (≤ $10^{th}$ percentile)<br>Thin vermilion border of the upper lip (score 4-5 lip/philtrum guide)<br>Smooth philtrum (score 4-5 lip/ philtrum guide)<br>2. One of following characteristics:<br>Prenatal and/or postnatal growth retardation (including ≥1 of following):<br>-High ≤ $10^{th}$ percentile<br>-Weight ≤ $10^{th}$ percentile<br>Deficient brain growth or abnormal morphogenesis (including ≥1 of following):<br>-Head circumference ≤ $10^{th}$ percentile<br>-Structural brain abnormalities<br>Evidence of behavioral or cognitive abnormalities<br>-Impairment in the performance of complex tasks<br>-Receptive and expressive language deficit<br>-Behavioral problems |
| 5 ARBD | 1. Confirmed maternal drinking<br>2. Minor facial anomalies (including ≥2 of features):<br>Short palpebral fissures (≤ $10^{th}$ percentile)<br>Thin vermilion border of the upper lip (score 4-5 lip/philtrum guide)<br>Smooth philtrum (score 4-5 lip/ philtrum guide)<br>3. Congenital structural defects including one of the following:<br>Including ≥1 malformations and dysplasias of following organs: cardiac, skeletal, renal, eyes, ears<br>If the patient displays minor anomalies only ≥2 anomalies must be present: hypoplastic nails, short fifth finger, clino/ camptodactyly, hockey stick palmar crease, railroad track ears, refractive errors, pectus carinatum or excavatum |
| 6 ARND | 1. Confirmed maternal drinking during pregnancy<br>2. At least one if the following:<br>Deficient brain growth or abnormal morphogenesis (including ≥1 of following)<br>-Head circumference ≤ $10^{th}$ percentile<br>-Structural brain abnormalities<br>Evidence of behavioral or cognitive abnormalities:<br>-Impairment in the performance of complex tasks<br>-Receptive and expressive language deficit<br>-Behavioral problems |

The novel classification and newly proposed diagnostic criteria are useful and handy, and have been successfully put in use in several FASD frequency studies.

## Making a Differential Diagnosis of FAS

The differential diagnosis of FAS includes a number of syndromes: Aarskog syndrome, Cornelia deLange syndrome, Dubowitz syndrome, Williams's syndrome, Opitz syndrome,

Miller-Dieker syndrome, DiGeorge syndrome, velo-cardio-facial syndrome, Noonan syndrome, fetal valproate syndrome, toluene embryopathy, and trisomy 18 (1). Due to the lack of laboratory methods capable of precisely diagnosing FAS, the differential diagnosis of FAS is difficult to make. Therefore, clearly defined and specific diagnostic criteria are mandatory. In 1996, Astley and Clarren had analysed anomalies present in FAS patients (42). They discovered a group of anomalies constituting the FAS phenotype and embracing a short palpebral fissure, smooth philtrum and thin upper lip. The combination of these three dysmorphic features bears a 100% FAS specificity and sensitivity (43). The photographic screening method makes use of the combination of three facial anomalies and has a sensitivity of 100%, a specificity of 99.8%, a positive predictive value of 85.7%, and a negative predictive value of 100% (44). The combination of the three features is not seen in any other entity accounted for in differential diagnosis. Therefore, the FAS phenotype combined with growth impairments and neurological anomalies represents a distinctive, specific, and sensitive criterion both when it comes to FAS screening and FAS diagnosing in paediatric population (43, 44).

## FAS Prevention

It should be emphasised that alcohol consumption witnessed during intrauterine development leads to permanent damages beyond treatment, hence causing lifelong problems not only to the diseased, but also to his/her family and social community in broader terms. It should also be pointed out that FAS and its associated conditions may be successfully prevented, so that special attention should be paid on prevention.

The sole measure capable of preventing the development of fetal alcohol syndrome is the refraining from alcohol consumption during pregnancy (45, 46). Successful prevention of alcohol consumption during pregnancy calls for familiarisation with customary alcohol consumption patterns in general female and pregnant women population, as well as for the recognition of risk factors and the definition of measures to be taken to the effect of identifying women and pregnant women at higher risk of becoming alcoholics. Women and pregnant women prone to alcohol consumption should be screened, informed of, and instructed on noxious impact of alcohol exposure during pregnancy, as well as on FAS clinical presentation and consequences. The ultimate goal of all these activities is timely restrain of alcohol consumption when planning to conceive. Nevertheless, the cessation of alcohol consumption at any given point during the course of pregnancy has a beneficial effect on fetal development.

Secondary FAS prevention calls for early recognition and early diagnostics of this condition. The prevention of secondary disorders embraces early habilitation planning, the development of an adequately-tailored interventional programme oriented towards risk elimination and reinforcement of protective factors capable of preventing secondary complications, as well as an appropriate patient education and training programmes developing independent living skills (45, 47). Therefore, it is imperative to recognise FAS at the youngest age possible.

## EPIDEMIOLOGY OF FEMALE ALCOHOL CONSUMPTION

The research done so far has revealed that alcohol consumption is a common habit in the female population. In Italy, alcohol is consumed by 62.1% of non-pregnant women, 22% of Israeli women are occasional drinkers, while around 54% of US women of reproductive age consume alcohol on a regular basis, out of those 15% are heavy and 13% are binge drinkers (1, 48-50).

Studies performed so far have indicated a high rate of alcohol consumption during pregnancy. Alcohol intake in US pregnant women has been estimated at 12.4-13.8%; among this drinking population, 3.4-4.6% of women are binge or heavy drinkers, 7-9 % of them drink throughout the entire pregnancy, while 75% have at least one alcoholic beverage while pregnant (51, 52). According to a more recent analysis carried out by the CDC, 12.2% of women confessed to alcohol consumption during pregnancy; 1.9% of the interviewed pregnant women are binge drinkers (53). Alcohol consumption and occasional drinking issues were more pronounced in elder, more educated, employed and single pregnant women. In Australia, alcohol is consumed by as many as 58.7% of pregnant women (54). A Danish study has demonstrated that 44.8% of pregnant women drink at least ½ an alcoholic beverage a week, as well as that 26% of them have at least one binge drinking episode; alcohol consumption during pregnancy was proven to be associated with a higher educational level and concurrent smoking (31). In France, at least one drink is consumed by 52.2% of pregnant women, while 13.7% confessed to at least one binge episode (55). In Ireland, alcohol is consumed by 53.9% of pregnant women, out of which 6.1% confess to the intake of 5-10 alcoholic beverages a week, and 2.2% to more than 10 alcoholic beverages a week (56). Alcohol is consumed by 52.6% of Italian pregnant women, out of which even 11.7% drink on a frequent basis (48).

A number of contributions published so far, have reported on several risk factors held responsible for the alcohol intake during pregnancy. Among those, age, educational background, socioeconomic status, employment status, rural or urban residency, marital status, alcohol consumption while not pregnant, and cigarette smoking have been listed (31, 57, 58).

The results of the research carried so far, have suggested that women are not appropriately informed on the noxious impact of alcohol exposure during pregnancy. In proof of that, only 21.5% of Italian women decided to cut down or cease drinking while pregnant; at the same time, even 68.4% of them reduced or stopped smoking (59). Women's stand on the impact of alcohol on pregnancy outcome is well-illustrated by a New Zealand study reporting that only 44% of women believe that any alcohol intake is harmful to pregnancy outcome (60). US had witnessed a slight drop in alcohol consumption rate registered in pregnant women (from 12.2% registered in 1991-2005 period to 11.2% registered in 2001-2005 period); at the same time, alcohol consumption in non-pregnant women remained unchanged (53). As opposed to the data quoted above, as many as 97% of Croatian women perceive alcohol consumption during pregnancy as harmful (61). Nevertheless, despite of such a high level of awareness on noxious fetal impact of alcohol exposure, both drinking and smoking still come as common habits of Croatian pregnant women. In proof of that, a survey carried out among urban population of 656 mothers of lower grade pupils, uncovered the facts that 89

(13.56%) of them had consumed alcohol during pregnancy on a regular basis, 18 (2.74%) had at least one binge episode, while 105 (15.83%) of them used to smoke while pregnant (62).

## FAS Epidemiology

Studies aimed at revealing FAS frequency are of special clinical and scientific interest. However, studies carried out are low in number, and data collected are unsatisfactory. The majority of the available data refers to the US, while European studies devoted to the topic are scarce. Three different approaches are used in FAS frequency research, as follows (63):

1. Passive surveillance system.
2. Clinically based study.
3. Active case ascertainment method.

Each method listed above has its strong points and downsides. Passive observation method makes use of the existent registries such as hospital registries, or registries keeping track on children suffering from developmental disorders or congenital anomalies (63). The strong side of this method lies within the easiness of data accessibility, while the downside is represented by either questionable or inappropriate data quality. The method is capable of revealing solely the frequency of already recognised FAS cases, while those undisclosed remain unregistered, significantly contributing to the bias in terms of underestimation of the disorder frequency.

The method most commonly used in FAS frequency estimation is the in-hospital research (63). It is carried out in form of pre-planned prospective studies often performed in maternity wards. Such study includes surveys on alcohol consumption during pregnancy carried out among mothers, as well as clinical examinations of their children. The advantage of such an approach lies within the possibility of research planning, inclusion of a high number of examinees, collection of data on pregnant women, and the possibility of clinical examination of their children. The downside, however, is the inability to precisely diagnose FAS, since in newborns dysmorphic facial features tend to be blurred. The prevailing opinion is that FAS can be most precisely diagnosed starting from the age of 3, and until the age of 12 (2, 16, 64).

The method of active FAS detection is of special interest, and represents the method of choice when it comes to studies aiming at the disorder frequency (63). The method in reference enables for the screening of children of the most appropriate age for the precise FAS diagnostics. It also allows for the detection of the diseased across general population, lowers the selection bias, and provides for the precise estimation of FAS frequency in the studied group. The investigation may embrace mothers as well, and enable for the collection of valuable information on risk factors responsible for the proneness to alcohol intake during pregnancy. However, these investigations have a number of difficulties. Such a research is time-consuming, and calls for extensive preparations and well-established collaboration with non-medical staff, so as to be able to gain access to study populations; it also requires a well-established collaboration with parents, mothers and children (14). It should be borne in mind that, when it comes to studies bearing a high risk of stigmatisation, as is the case with FAS-devoted studies and studies investigating the issue of alcohol consumption during pregnancy, good collaboration is often hard to establish (65).

Data on FAS frequency gathered so far, have pointed towards huge differences between study outcomes (14). These inconsistencies may have arisen on the grounds of racial, ethnic, geographical, social, economic and religious differences, as well as on the grounds of differences in alcohol consumption traditions and habits observed across female population; last but not least, they may have arisen on the grounds of research methodology. For instance, US studies have revealed a higher FAS frequency among African (0.48/1000 children) and American Indian populations as compared to Caucasians (0.29/1000 children) (66, 67). According to literature sources, US FAS frequency equals to 2.8-4.6/1000 deliveries, and that of FASD to 9.1/1000 deliveries (68). As opposed to America, FAS frequency estimated in Europe is far less, and equals to 0.08/1000 deliveries (69). May et al. have demonstrated that the identification of FAS patients and the estimation of FAS frequency are strongly dependent on the applied research methodology. Passive observational method yields the lowest FAS frequency rates (0.85/1000) compared to in-hospital research (1.8/1000) and the method of active FAS patients' detection across general population (15.6/1000) (65).

## FAS EPIDEMIOLOGY IN SCHOOLCHILDREN

A distinctive form of an active detection of FAS is the investigation carried out among schoolchildren (65). This approach is of special interest for the estimation of FAS frequency, since schoolchildren pose as the representatives of the entire local population, and are of age in which the dysmorphic facial features are apparent, making the FAS diagnosis more accurate. The research carried out so far is scarce, while the estimated FAS frequency markedly varies. According to literature sources, a total of ten studies have been completed, aiming at the estimation of FAS prevalence in schoolchildren. The majority of these studies (6/10) have made use of the clinical criteria proposed by the revised IOM classification, the criteria in reference being clearly defined and allowing for the simple and precise investigation among a larger group of children (13).

A special attention has been paid to high-risk rural populations. Two studies have been undertaken in the USA. Clarren et al. reported a study aimed at evaluating the feasibility of FAS screening within a school system (16). The authors used the 4-Digit Diagnostic Code criteria with the active and passive system of informed consent; the study was carried out in two counties of the Washington State. The active system of informed consent yielded poor participation rates, so that the FAS prevalence could not be calculated in one of the counties. By contrast, in the second county the passive system of informed consent yielded high participation rates, with the estimated FAS prevalence of 3.1 per 1000 children. In 2003, Poitra et al. used the 32-item FAS screening tool in order to investigate the FAS prevalence in the population of kindergarten children coming from North Dakota (70). Over a 9-year period, 1384 students had been screened, and the prevalence of FAS was estimated at 1 per 230 students or 4.4 per 1000 (70). A higher prevalence of FAS was observed in South Africa. Over a seven-year period, three studies have been performed in the Western Cape Province of South Africa, and the remarkable differences in FAS prevalence have been observed. In 2000, May et al. investigated a sample of 992 first-grade schoolchildren aged 5 to 9 years, and came up with the estimated FAS rate of 40.5-46.4 per 1000 students (71). Out of 46 children diagnosed with FAS, 39% (18/46) originated from urban, and 61% (28/46) from rural school settings. A higher FAS rate (65.2-74.2 per 1000 children) was observed in the second study undertaken a few years later on a sample of 863 children (72). The increased FAS prevalence was attributed to social changes and changes in maternal drinking habits. In the third study, the estimated rate of FAS/PFAS was 68.9-89.2 per 1000 first-grade schoolchildren (73). As with the previous analysis, the mothers of FASD children were more likely to be farm workers and were more likely to be living in rural areas at the time of gestation. The fourth study was undertaken among first-grade students in the rural Northern Cape Province of South Africa; the study in reference included a total of 1835 children and observed FAS prevalence of 67.2, and PFAS prevalence of 20.8 per 1000 students (74). Epidemiological investigations of FAS carried out in Europe are rare; so far only two studies have been performed (75, 76). The first European study was undertaken in Italian schools of the Lazio region including small towns and rural areas (75). The estimated FAS prevalence was 3.7-7.4 per 1000 children, and that of FASD 20.3-40.5 per 1000 pupils.

**Table 3. Survey of FASD prevalence rate in sample of urban schoolchildren reported in literature.**

| Author | Location (population) | No. of enrolled children | No. of screened children | Participation rate | Type of consent | Rate per 1000 children | | |
|---|---|---|---|---|---|---|---|---|
| | | | | | | FAS | PFAS | FASD |
| May et al. 2009. (70) | Western USA (urban, suburban) | Not reported | Not reported | 55% | Active consent | 1.4-2.5 | 8.1-14.9 | 9.5-17.4 |
| May et al. 2009. (70) | Western USA (urban, suburban) | Not reported | Not reported | 56% | Active consent | 6.4-11.3 | 7.7-13.5 | 14.1-24.8 |
| Petković & Barišić, 2010. (76) | Croatia (urban) | 912 | 466 | 51% | Passive consent | 6.44 | 34.33 | 40.77 |

The second European study was performed in Croatia (76). The aim of the investigation was to determine the FAS prevalence rate in the population of students enrolled in urban schools. Investigations of FAS prevalence in urban schools are rare; so far only three such studies have been reported (Table 3). Two pilot studies were undertaken in small city urban and suburban schools of the Western United States in two different years (65). The investigations were carried out on the samples of first-grade schoolchildren, and had used the active informed consent method. The overall prevalence of FASD estimated in the first study was 9.5-17.4 and that in the second study 14.1-24.8 per 1000 schoolchildren. The observed difference in FASD prevalence was attributed to the variations in maternal drinking habits during pregnancy, and to the selection bias arising from participation consent. The third study was performed on a sample of urban Croatian schoolchildren (76). The research included 912 first- to fourth-grade elementary schoolchildren. Observed FAS prevalence was 3 children, and of PFAS was 16 children per 466 examined students. The estimated prevalence of FASD was 40.77 per 1000 children, and was higher as compared to that observed in the USA. The higher prevalence of FASD in Croatia may be attributed to the higher PFAS rate seen in the investigated cohort (Table 3). The observed difference in PFAS prevalence between the USA and the Croatian studies may be attributed to the variations in the drinking habits, or to the differences in maternal risk factors. These data therefore impose the need for additional investigation of the prevalence of these conditions in urban schoolchildren.

## Conclusion

FAS is an important and frequent cause of neurological functional impairments seen in children. The prevalence estimated in schoolchildren varies across different studies, and ranges from 3.5 to 74.2 per 1000 children. In the recent years, new data on FAS risk factors in children have become available. Recent studies have identified urban women of higher socioeconomic and educational level as high-risk population when it comes to alcohol consumption. These data suggest a higher risk of alcohol consumption during pregnancy, and a higher risk of FAS onset in urban children. However, the investigations of FAS prevalence in urban school settings are rare. Limited data from the USA and Europe indicate that the FAS rate range from 1.4 to 11.3 per 1000 children and that of PFAS from 7.7 to 34.3 per 1000 pupils. The available data thus indicate that FASD represent a serious medical and social issue. These studies have shown that FASD may be frequent among schoolchildren of urban residence, with the resulting neurological functional impairments such as dyscalculia, learning difficulties, memory and language problems, dysfunctional organization and planning, lower IQ, ADHD, and other lifelong disabilities. Data published so far have pointed towards the importance of early FASD diagnosis providing for the possibility of learning and behavioural deficits' management by school practitioners, as well as for the prevention of secondary complications of this condition.

As of now, our knowledge on the prevalence and clinical effects of various quantities of alcohol intake, as well as on the drinking habits during gestational period, is limited. Therefore, the effective FASD prevention calls for additional investigations of the prevalence rates and for the studies of the association between the maternal drinking patterns observed during pregnancy and clinical disabilities seen in children. These studies will contribute to primary prevention which leads to reduced alcohol consumption in pregnancy and FAS prevalence, and secondary prevention which reduces risk factors in FAS patients and enhances independent living and working skills.

## References

[1] Fetal Alcohol Syndrome: Guidelines for Referral and Diagnosis. *CDC* July 2004.

[2] Stratton KR, Howe CJ, Battaglia FC. (Eds.), *Fetal alcohol syndrome: diagnosis, epidemiology, prevention and treatment.* Washington DC: National Academy Press 1996.

[3] Barr HM, Streissguth AP. Identifying maternal self-reported alcohol use associated with fetal alcohol spectrum disorders. *Alcohol Clin Exp Res* 2001; 25: 283-287.

[4] Chaudhuri JD. Alcohol and the developing fetus – a review. *Med Sci Monit* 2000; 6: 1031-1041.

[5] Mattson SN, Scoenfeld AM, Riley EP. Teratogenic effects of alcohol on brain and behavior. *Alcohol Res Health* 2001; 25: 185-191.

[6] Gemma S, Vichi S, Testai E. Individual susceptibility and alcohol effects: bichemical and genetic aspects. *Ann Ist Super Sanita* 2006; 42: 8-16.

[7] Gemma S, Vichi S, Testai E. Metabolic and genetic factors contibuting to alcohol induced effects and fetal alcohol syndrome. *Neurosci Biobehav Rev* 2007; 31: 221-229.

[8] Henderson J, Kesmodel U, Gray R. Systematic review of the fetal effects of prenatal binge-drinking. *J Epidemiol Community Health* 2007; 61: 1069-1073.

[9] Haycock PC. Fetal Alcohol Spectrum Disorders: The Epigenetic Perspective. *Biol Reprod* 2009; 81: 607-617.

[10] Henriksen TB, Hjollund NH, Jensen TK, Bonde JP, Andersson AM, Kolstad H, Ernst E, Giwercman A, Skakkebaek NE, Olsen J. Alcohol consumption at the time of conception and spontaneous abortion. *Am J Epodemio* 2004; 160: 661-667.

[11] Strandberg-Larsen K, Nielsen NR, Gronbaek M, Andersen PK, Olsen J, Andersen AM. Binge drinking in pregnancy and risk of fetal death. *Obstet Gynecol* 2008; 111: 602-609.

[12] Burd L, Klug M, Martsolf J. Increased sibling mortality in children with fetal alcohol syndrome. *Addict Biol* 2004; 9: 179-186.

[13] Hoyme HE, May PA, Kalberg WO, Kodituwakku P, Gossage PJ, Trujillo PM, Buckley DG, Miller JH, Aragon AS, Khaole N, Viljoen DL, Jones KL, Robinson LK. A practical clinical approach to diagnosis of fetal alcohol spectrum disorders: Clarification of the 1996 Institute of Medicine Criteria. *Pediatrics* 2005; 115: 39-47.

[14] Nayak BR, Murthy P. Fetal alcohol spectrum disorder. *Indian Pediatr* 2008; 45: 977-983.

[15] Manning MA, Hoyme HE. Fetal alcohol spectrum disorders: A practical clinical approach to diagnosis. *Neurosci Biobehav Rev* 2007; 31: 230-238.

[16] Clarren SK, Randels SP, Sanderson M, Fineman RM. Screening for fetal alcohol syndrome in primary school: a feasibility study. *Teratology* 2001; 63: 3-10.

[17] Bruce BB, Biousse V, Dean AL, Newman NJ. Neurologic and ophthalmic manifestation of fetal alcohol syndrome. *Rev Neurol Dis* 2009; 6: 13-20.

[18] Abdelrahman A, Conn R. Eye abnormalities in fetal alcohol syndrome. *Ulster Med J* 2009; 78: 164-165.

[19] Riley EP, McGee CL, Sowell ER. Teratogenic effects of alcohol: A decade of brain imaging. *Am J Med Genet* 2004; 127C: 35-41.

[20] Bjorkquist OA, Fryer SL, Reiss AL, Mattson SN, Riley EP. Cingulate gyrus morphology in children and adolescent with fetal alcohol spectrum disorders. *Psychiatry Res* 2010; 181: 101-107.

[21] Swayze II VW, Johnson VP, Hanson JW, Piven J, Sato Y, Giedd JN, Mosnik D, Andreasen NC. Magnetic resonance imaging of brain anomalies in fetal alcohol syndrome. *Pediatrics* 1997; 99: 232-240.

[22] Reinhardt K, Mohr A, Gartner J, Spohr HL, Brockmann K. Polymicrogyria in fetal alcohol syndrome. *Birth Defects Res A Clin Mol Teratol* 2009; Sep 17 (Epub ahead of print).

[23] Dalen K, Bruaroy S Wentzel-Larsen T, Laegreid LM. Cognitive functioning in children prenatally exposed to alcohol and psychotropic drugs. *Neuropediatrics* 2009; 40: 162-167.

[24] Domellof E, Ronnqvist L, Titran M, Esseily R, Fagard J. Atypical functional lateralization in children with fetal alcohol syndrome. *Dev Psychobiol* 2009; 51: 696-705.

[25] Burden MJ, Andrew C, Saint-Amour D, Meintjes EM, Molteno CD, Hoyme HE, Robinson LK, Khaole N, Nelson CA, Jacobson JL, Jacobson SW. The effects of fetal alcohol syndrome on response execution and inhibition: an event-related potential study. *Alcohol Clin Exp Res* 2009; 33: 1994-2004.

[26] Willford JA, Leech SL, Day NL. Moderate prenatal alcohol exposure and cognitive status of children at age 10. *Alcohol Clin Exp Res* 2006; 30: 1051-1059.

[27] Lebel C, Rasmussen C, Wyper K, Andrew G, Beaulieu C. Brain microstructure is related to math ability in children with fetal alcohol spectrum disorder. *Alcohol Clin Exp Res* 2010; 34: 354-363.

[28] Cassano PA, Koepsell TD, Farwell JR. Risk of febrile seizures in childhood in relation to prenatal maternal cigarette smoking and alcohol intake. *Am J Epidemiol* 1990; 132: 462-473.

[29] Vahidnia F, Eskenazi B, Jewell N. Maternal smoking, alcohol drinking and febrile convulsion. *Seizure* 2008; 17: 320-326.

[30] O'Mally KD, Barr H. Fetal alcohol syndrome and seizure disorder. *Can J Psychiatry* 1998; 43: 1051.

[31] Sun Y, Standberg-Larsen K, Vestergaard M, Christensen J, Nybo Andersen AM, Gronbaek M, Olsen J. Binge drinking during pregnancy and risk of seizures in childhood: a study based on the Danish national birth cohort. *Am J Epidemiol* 2009; 169: 313-322.

[32] Burd L, Carlson C, Kerbeshian J. Fetal alcohol spectrum disorders and mental illness. Special issue on neuropsychological effects of alcohol use and misuse. *Int J Disabil Human Dev* 2007; 6: 383-396.

[33] Kvigne VL, Leonardson GR, Borzelleca J, Neff-Smith M, Welty TK. *Hospitalization of children who have fetal alcohol syndrome or incomplete fetal alcohol syndrome.* SD Med 2009; 62: 101-103.

[34] Kodituwakku PW. A neurodevelopmental framework for the development of interventions for children with fetal alcohol spectrum disorders. *Alcohol* 2009; doi: 10.1016/j.alcohol.2009.10.009 (Epub ahead of print).

[35] Hellemans KG, Verma P, Yoon E, Yu WK, Young AH, Weinberg J. Prenatal alcohol exposure and chronic mild stress differentially alter depressive- and anxiety-like behaviors in male and female offspring. *Alcohol Clin Exp Res* 2010; doi: 10.1111/j.1530-0277.2009.01132.x (Epub ahead of print).

[36] Kvigne VL, Leonardson GR, Borzelleca J, Neff-Smith M, Welty TK. Characteristics of children whose siblings have fetal alcohol syndrome or incomplete fetal alcohol syndrome. *Pediatrics* 2009; 123: e526-533.

[37] Kvigne VL, Gary LR, Borzelleca J, Welty TK. Characteristics of grandmothers who have grandchildren with fetal alcohol syndrome or incomplete fetal alcohol syndrome. *Matern Child Health J* 2008; 12: 760-765.

[38] Jones KL, Smith DW. Recognition of the fetal alcohol syndrome in early infancy. *Lancet* 1973; 2: 999-1001.

[39] Calhoun F, Warren K. Fetal alcohol syndrome: historical prospectives. *Neurosci Biobehav Rev* 2007; 31: 168-171.

[40] Astley SJ, Clarren SK. Diagnosing the full spectrum of fetal alcohol-exposed individuals: introducing the 4-digit diagnostic code. *Alcohol Alcohol* 2000; 35: 400-410.

[41] Chudley AE, Conry J, Cook JL, Loock C, Rosales T, LeBlanc N. Fetal alcohol spectrum disorder: Canadian guidelines for diagnosis. *CMAJ* 2005; 172, S1-S21.

[42] Astley SJ, Clarren SK. A case definition and photographic screening tool for the facial phenotype of fetal alcohol syndrome. J Pediatr 1996; 129: 33-41.

[43] Astley SJ, Clarren SK. Measuring the facial phenotype of individuals with prenatal alcohol exposure: correlations with brain dysfunction. *Alcohol Alcohol* 2001; 36: 147-159.

[44] Astley SJ, Stachowiak J, Clarren SK, Clausen C. Application of the fetal alcohol syndrome facial photographic screening tool in a foster care population. *J Pediatr* 2002; 141: 712-717.

[45] Tough S, Clarke M, Clarren S. Preventing fetal alcohol spectrum disorders. *Can Fam Physician* 2005; 51: 1199-1201.

[46] Awopetu O, Brimacombe M, Cohen D. Fetal alcohol syndrome disorder pilot media intervention in New Jersey. *Can j Clin Parmacol* 2008; 15: e124-e131.

[47] Kalberg WO, Buckley D. Educational planning for children with fetal alcohol syndrome. *Ann Ist Super Sanita* 2006; 42: 58-59.

[48] Fiorentino D, Coriale G, Spagnolo PA, Prastaro A, Attilia ML, Mancinelli R, Ceccanti M. Fetal alcohol syndrome disorders: experience on the field. The Lazio study preliminary report. *Ann Ist Super Sanita* 2006; 42: 53-57.

[49] Bar-Hamburger R, Ezraci Y, Steinberg D. Israel illegal use of drugs and alcohol in the sixth national epidemiological survey, 2005. *National Anti-Drug and Anti-Alcohol Authority of Israel.*

[50] Senechy Y, Inbar D, Diamond G, Basel-Vanagaite L, Rigler S. Fetal alcohol spectrum disorder in Israel. *IMAJ* 2009; 11: 619-622.

[51] Floyd RL, Sidhu JS. Fetal Alcohol Syndrome. *Am J Med Gen* 2004; 127C: 4-9.

[52] Tough S, Tofflemire K, Clarke M, Newburn-Cook C. Do women change their drinking behaviors while trying to conceive? An opportunity for preconception counseling. *CM&R* 2006; 2: 97-105.

[53] Center for disease control and prevention: Alcohol Use among pregnant and nonpregnant woman of childbearing age. United States, 1991-2005. 2004. *(www.cdc.gov/ncbddd/fas/documents/).*

[54] Colvin L, Payne J, Parsons D. Alcohol consumption during pregnancy in nonindigenous west Australian women. *Alcohol Clin Exp Res* 2007; 31: 276-284.

[55] Chazeron I, Llorca PM, Ughetto S, Vendittelli F, Boussiron D, Sapin V, Coudore F, Lemerey D. Is pregnancy the time to change alcohol consumption habits in France. *Alcohol Clin Exp Res* 2008; 32: 868-873.

[56] Donnelly JC, Cooley SM, Walsh TA, Sarkar R, Durnea U, Geary MP. Illegal drug use, smoking and alcohol consumption in a low-risk Irish primigravid population. *J Perinatal Med* 2008; 36: 70-72.

[57] Mengel MB, Searight HR, Cook K. Preventing alcohol-exposed pregnancies. *JABFM* 2006; 19: 494-505.

[58] Morojele NK, London L, Olorunju SA, Matjila MJ, Davids AS, Rendall-Mkosi KM. Predictors of risk of alcohol-exposed pregnancies among women in an urban and a rural area of South Africa. *Soc Sci Med* 2009; doi:10.1016/j.socimed.2009.10.040.

[59] Ceccanti M, Spagnolo PA, Tarni L, Attilia ML, Chessa L, Mancinelli R, Stegagno M, Sasso GF, Romeo M, Jones KL, Robinson LK, del Campo M, Gossage JP, May PA, Hoyme HE. Clinical delineation of fetal alcohol spectrum disorders (FASD) in Italian children: comparisson and contrast with other racial/ ethnic groups and implication for diagnosis and prevention. *Neurosci Biobehav Rev* 2007; 31: 270-277.

[60] Parackal SM, Parackal MK, Harraway JA, Ferguson EL. Opinions of non-pregnant New zeland women aged 16-40 years about the safety of alcohol consumption during pregnancy. *Drug Alcohol Rev* 2009; 28: 135-141.

[61] Petković G, Barišić I. Konzumacija alkohola u populaciji hrvatskih trudnica. *Paediatria Croatica* 2007; 51 (suppl 1): 137.

[62] Petković G, Barišić I. Alcohol drinking and smoking habits during pregnancy in a sample of Croatian urban mothers. *Paediatria Croatica* 2009; 53 (suppl 2): 13.

[63] May PA, Gossage JP. Estimating the prevalence of fetal alcohol syndrome: *A summary. Alcohol Res Health* 2001; 25: 159-167.

[64] Aase JM. Clinical recognition of FAS: difficulties of detection and diagnosis. *Alcohol Health Res World* 1994; 18: 5-9

[65] May PA, Gossage JP, Kalberg WO, Robinson LK, Buckley D, Manning M, Hoyme HE. Prevalence and epidemiologic characteristics of FASD from various research methods with an emphasis on recent in-school studies. *Dev Disabil Res Rev* 2009; 15: 176-192. .

[66] Abel EL, Sokol RJ. A revised conservative estimate of the incidence of FAS and its economic impact. *Alcohol Clin Exp Res* 1991; 15: 514-524.

[67] May PA, McCloskey J, Gossage JP. *Fetal alcohol syndrome among American indians: epidemiology, isssues and research review*. NIAAA monograph 37, Bethesda, MD: US Departament of Health and Human Services. 2002.

[68] Sampson PD, Streissguth AP, Bookstein FL, Little RE, Clarren SK, Dehaene P. Incidence of fetal alcohol syndrome and prevalence of alcohol-related neurodevelopmental disorder. *Tetralogy* 1997; 56 : 317-326.

[69] Mukherjee RA, Turk J. Fetal alcohol syndrome. *Lancet* 2004; 363: 1556.

[70] Poitra BA, Marion S, Dionne M, Wilkie E, Dauphinais P, Wilkie-Pepion M, Martsolf JT, Klug MG, Burd L. A school-based screening program for fetal alcohol syndrome. *Neurotoxico Teratol* 2003; 25: 725-729.

[71] May PA, Booke L, Gossage PJ, Croxford J, Adnams C, Jones KL, Robinson L, Viljoen D. Epidemiology of fetal alcohol syndrome in a South African Community in the Western Cape Province. *Am J Public Health* 2000; 90: 1905-1912.

[72] Viljoen DL, Gossage PJ, Brooke L, Adnams CM, Jones KL, Robinson LK, Hoyme HE, Snell C, Khaole NCO, Kodituwakku P, Assante KO, Findlay R, Quinton B, Marais AS, Kalberg WO, May PA. Fetal alcohol syndrome epidemiology in a South African

community: a second study of a very high prevalence area. *J Stud Alcohol* 2005; 66: 593-604.

[73] May PA, Gossage PJ, Marais AS, Adnams CM, Hoyme HE, Jones KL, Robinson LK, Khaole NCO, Snell C, Kalberg WO, Hendricks L, Brooke L, Stellavato C, Viljoen DL. The epidemiology of fetal alcohol syndrome and partial FAS in a South African community. *Drug Alcohol Depend* 2007; 88: 259-271.

[74] Urban M, Chersich MF, Fourie LA, Chetty C, Olivier L, Viljoen D. Fetal alcohol syndrome among grade 1 schoolchildren in Northern Cape province. *S Afr Med J* 2008; 98: 877-882.

[75] May PA, Fiorentino D, Gossage JP, Kalberg WO, Hoyme HE, Robinson LK, Coriale G, Jones KL, del Campo M, Tarani L, Romeo M, Kodituwakku PW, Deiana L, Buckley D, Ceccanti M. Epidemiology of FASD in a province in Italy: Prevalence and characteristics of children in a random sample of schools. *Alcohol Clin Exp Res* 2006; 30: 1562-1575.

[76] Petković G, Barišić I. FAS prevalence in a sample of urban schoolchildren in Croatia. *Reprod Toxicol* 2010; 29: 237-241.

In: Pregnancy and Alcohol Consumption
Editor: Joshua D. Hoffman, pp. 299-313
ISBN 978-1-61761-122-3


*Chapter 12*

# LIFE AS AN ADULT WITH FOETAL ALCOHOL SYNDROME

***Stéphanie Toutain***
Université Paris Descartes, Cnrs, Inserm, France

## INTRODUCTION

For more than fifty years, it was supposed that Maria had inherited the slight mental handicap of her mother and her half sister. In reality, she is a victim of her mother's alcoholism and was born with foetal alcohol syndrome (FAS). Besides the physical handicaps (dysmorphy, deformations), this syndrome provokes deficiencies of the central nervous system, mild to moderate mental retardation, social and professional difficulties as well as dysfunctional families (Danel, Karila and Mezerete, 2007). FAS children are clearly handicapped by their syndrome and their future is further jeopardized by the absence of suitable care programmes for them. The follow-up of a cohort of American children (Streissguth and al., 1991) shows that 43 % of the children exposed to alcohol in utero were later excluded from the school system, 70 % interrupted their education, 60 % spent some time in prison and 30% in psychiatric hospitals, 65% presented sexual deviances and 80% faced endemic problems with finding and keeping a job or a secure place to live. The relation of cause and effect between FAS and social problems thus seems rather undeniable. At its most serious, the syndrome results in the association of characteristics which tend to become less conspicuous with age: small heads, slanty eyes, thin superior lips, smooth-grooved upper lips, some abnormal internal organs, a slower growth ante and postnatal and some confusion in their neurological development (small intelligence quotients). If the physical characteristics of this syndrome tend to become less obvious with age, the abnormalities of the central nervous system remain irreversible. At its least severe form, the syndrome becomes "foetal alcohol spectrum disorders" (FASD). In this case, facial dysmorphy is not necessarily visible. Maria's story, from birth to adulthood (she is now 58) is that of a typical FAS victim. It is extremely useful in throwing light on the difficulties FAS victims face in our society.

## The Story of Maria's Parents and of Her Siblings

Maria's parents had been drinking excessively for many years before her birth, in December 1951. Compared to the average age for the first maternity which was lower than 25 at the time, her parents could be said to be relatively old: her father was nearly fifty and her mother in her early 40's. The age of her mother was an aggravating factor, indeed, the older the mothers, the more likely they are to give birth to FAS babies (Dorris, 1989); (Société Française d'Alcoologie, 2003); (Dehaene and al., 1981); (Jacobson and al., 1993). Maria is the only child of a reconstituted family, and the fourth and last child of her mother. When her mother died, her father looked after her. After his death, she was brought up by her two half brothers. To this day, on of them is her legal guardian.

Her father was a skilled worker in an iron factory, making spare parts for aeroplanes. His alcoholism led to numerous health problems. He was very often out of work, in which case he was confined to his home. Her mother was a housewife; she stayed at home to bring up her children with the occasional odd jobs to make ends meet. Almost immediately after the death of her first husband in 1950, she started a relationship with the man who was to become Maria's father. Her mother's excessive drinking was made worse by the death of her first husband and her new alcoholic boyfriend. Her mother presumably used alcohol as a kind of self medication, in order to anesthetize her pain at the loss of members of her family. Both her parents, widowers with children, got married in haste, in September 1951, when they became aware that Maria's mother was pregnant. Children born out of wedlock were frown upon in France at the time.

Her half brothers and half sister, on her mother's side, were brought up by their biological parents until their father's death in 1950. Only her younger half brother seems to have been spared by the syndrome. He had a normal school life, albeit hindered by health problems with his lungs which meant that he had to go to hospital on many occasions. Her elder half brother was taken away from main stream education and sent to a school for children with special needs where the children were made "to drawn all day long" according to him: today, he would be diagnosed as having "foetal alcohol spectrum disorders" (FASD), judging by his behavioural symptoms. Her half brothers lived alternatively at home and with their maternal grandmother. Last, according to the statements of her aunts, her half sister probably had, like Maria, foetal alcohol syndrome (FAS). At the age of 9, her half sister was sent to a convent school for social and financial reasons. She died of meningitis in 1954, at the age of 11.

The family life was marked by financial precariousness, alcoholism and conjugal violence. Maria lived in a dysfunctional environment as do most children touched by this syndrome. The regular purchase of alcohol and the excessive time spent in "cafés" seriously reduced the household budget and forced the family to live on child benefit and various other allowances. Generally, FAS seems to touch the working classes more than the upper classes in spite of comparable alcohol consumption (Société Française d'Alcoologie, 2003); (Bignol and al., 1987); (Abel, 1995); (Dehaene, 1991). It is however justifiable to question the reliability of the results, since they are given by social workers who are more likely to be in contact with working class families.

At the time, Maria's father had already been to detoxification centres (Beaujon hospital near Paris and in Chartes). The rehabilitation programmes proved to be useless. One of her half brothers remembers the role of his mother in making the programme fail in Beaujon Hospital: "when we arrived on the 9th floor of the hospital, before we got to my step-father's room, I saw my mother take a small bottle of alcohol out of her bag. She gave the bottle to my step-father who swallowed it in the space of seconds! I understood then that he was far from being sober!" When the father was away on these rehabilitation programmes, the mother brought up her three children on her own. She was depressed because she had lost many people in her family. Nevertheless, the family life was better, because there were fewer financial difficulties and no conjugal violence. Maria's mother died in 1964, when she was 52. Her half brothers had already left home. The cause of her death, cirrhosis, remains a taboo in the family to his day. Maria's mother is an example of the so called "bad mother" (Simmat-Durand, 2005). Her father looked after her until he died, two years later in March 1966, of the same disease. Maria was then an orphan. The remaining family: her half brothers, her aunts and uncles legally trusted her younger half brother with her supervision.

## MARIA'S CHILDHOOD

Life during Maria's mother's pregnancy was marked by an excessive consumption of alcohol and episodes of drunkenness. Judging by Maria's symptoms, her mother is bound to have been drinking throughout her pregnancy even toward the end. Medical advice was twisted and used as an excuse to drink, to help with her anaemia, or breast feeding, for example (Gaugue, Varascon and Wendland, 2006). Furthermore, pregnancy is a vulnerable period when women's fears are made worse, which can contribute to an increase in alcohol consumption (Titran, 1991).

Maria was born one month before term, in December 1951 in Beaujon hospital near Paris, which interestingly has a department for alcohol related diseases. As her first daughter was already put in care by social services, her mother gave up the medical follow-up of her pregnancy for fear that her new born baby should also be taken away from her.(Simmat-Durand, 2005). At birth, Maria was a small baby. She was underweight with a weight of 2.4 kg, and measured only 41 centimetres. Her small size was attributed to heredity: her father and her mother were respectively 1,55 m and 1,48 m tall. Even if foetal alcohol syndrome (FAS) was not diagnosed at the time, the attentive examination of family photos led, at posteriori, to the conclusion that she had facial dysmorphy.

After her birth, Maria was taken home. Although she was the only child brought up at home, and her family and socio cultural environment did little for her intellectual development. Her family life was marked by crises, bouts of alcoholism and violence, which disrupted her development (Olson, O' Connor and Fitzgerald, 2001). The flat was filthy and degraded: the window panes were broken, and the heating never worked for lack of money. The social situation of the parents was always precarious and the risk of Maria being put in care always real. The parents fearing that Maria be taken away from them, vaccinated their daughter more than was necessary. Indeed, vaccines were the only legal medical obligation for the parents, and the medical visits could not be missed without alerting social services. As she grew, the physical characteristics of foetal alcohol syndrome became less visible. Maria remained small, scraggy, with a small upturned nose, a smooth-grooved upper lip and a chin at the same time massive and striking.

After one year at nursery school, she was sent to a class for children with special needs, which did not help her reduce her handicaps (Dorris, 1989). Her cognitive difficulties were a major obstacle to her learning, judging by her school results. From her first year at school, she was failing, and her difficulties were seen as the consequence of her premature birth and her family situation: "*she does not apply herself*", "*she never does her homework*", and "her parents do not bring her up correctly Her written work was slow and laborious; her letters were badly formed. She found it extremely difficult to concentrate especially on abstract notions. Her oral expression and her lack of ease in answering even the simplest questions were blatant. She managed to learn how to read with extreme difficulty, but even then, she could never understand what she read. Because of her dyscalculia, she could never do maths. Every year, she had to begin learning right from the beginning, and she could never move up to the next class (Dorris, 1989). To her reduced capacities in maths, were added confusions in reasoning and spatial vision. Even in her class for children with special needs, she underwent the mockery of her peers. This shook the little confidence she had. She preferred to stay at home, far from the gibes of the peers. Her father endorsed her numerous absences. The vicious circle of exclusion had begun, the older she got, the bigger the distance with the children of her age. The gap between her and the other children widened. She withdrew within herself and took fewer and fewer risks. Her younger half brother remembers: "*I knew that she had a problem but, I thought that she would overcome it, that she had fallen behind because of her lack of stimulation and her numerous absences from school, as her father preferred that she should stay with him, keep him company rather than go to school* ". Furthermore, Maria felt no curiosity, no motivation which would have urged her to look around her and learn (Dorris, 1989).

## MARIA'S ADOLESCENCE

After her mother's death and from the age of 13, she stayed at home most of her time with her father, during his long illness. Her father did not realize, or refused to see his daughter's mental handicap. Maria adored staying at home with her very accommodating father, who asked very little to her. She worshiped her father, a bohemian, who enjoyed doing magic tricks. On the other hand, she rejected her second half brother because he asked her to make some efforts. For example, at the age of twelve, he tried in vain to teach her multiplication tables. She could obviously memorize no lesson and had to learn everything all over again at the beginning of every lesson. She could never build from what she had learnt the day before. Her young brother did not know that she could not learn and put a lot of effort into teaching her mathematics: *"I was mad, I was incensed. Every time was the same; what came in through one ear came out immediately through the other one, she remembered nothing. I lost faith and gave up, it was hopeless. At the time, I thought that she was somewhat behind but that she would be able reduce her handicap. This never happened"*.

After the death of her father in 1966, Maria became an orphan. Her younger half brother become her legal guardian, he says: "*I then understood that Maria could not improve, that it would be unreasonable to expect any progress. I gave up hope for a normal life for her, with a job, a family and children. She would be a burden for me for the rest of my life. I thank her father and my step-father, for giving me such a precious gift !*"

If her younger half brother understood the situation, his elder half brother continued to blame Maria's father: "*If Maria is behind today, it's my step-father's fault. He never sent her to school*". Furthermore, as all children affected by this syndrome, Maria gave the impression of being more capable, than she really was "(Forbes, 1984). A social worker got her a place at a boarding school for children with special needs in a "Classe de perfectionnement" near Paris. She seemed to adapt suitably well to this new life, even if she was considered "*too naive, too accommodating and too spontaneous*" by her teachers. Besides, her school reports give evidence of her attitude: she "*was polite, always smiling, and affectionate but too sensitive*", and she also liked to be useful (Streissguth and LaDue, on 1985).

At the age of 15, her achievements were characteristic of children with this syndrome. Her level in maths was non existent. Her spelling and reading was comparable to those of primary school children's. She confuses words, such as "lower" and "superior", "heavy" and "light", "young" and "old", "early" and "late". Her student reports highlight her "willingness" to do well, but also her weak possibilities, her failing memory, her inability to understand and answer questions. Her intelligence quotient was estimated at 56, against 68 on average for the children with foetal alcohol syndrome in the United States (Streissguth and al., 1991). This explains her mental confusion, as it is the case for 90 % of FAS's children (Deschamps-Frosio, 1998). With an intelligence quotient lower than 75, she is thus considered a FAS victim (Picherot, 2005). The weakness of her intelligence quotient and her limited manual abilities did not bode well for her future. The mediocrity of her results and her relatively young age meant that another type of institution had to be found for her. Hence, from the age of 17, Maria went from institution to institution, nobody seemed to want to keep her. She integrated a new school for students with special needs in the Somme. Teaching in French, maths, physical education were aimed at facilitating her autonomy in her everyday life. Nevertheless, she still found it most difficult to read, and still did not understand what she read. Her vocabulary remained extremely poor and her speech was "childish" and "not really correct". The mechanisms of maths remained a mystery for her, as did all mathematical problems. These difficulties were the result of her bad memory, reduced potential for abstractions and difficulties in solving mathematical problems (Streissguth and LaDue, 1985). In physical education, as all the children with this syndrome, she suffered from confused motricity and poor coordination (Titran and Gratias, 2005). According to her school reports, she was "*very nervous*", did not know how to "*control her movements* ", "*did not measure her strength*". In the various workshops, her willingness and her desire to do well could not compensate her weakness. Whether it was sewing, ironing or doing laundery, her capacity for memorization and attention was extremely weak: "*she does not remember what we tell her*"; "*she thinks of other things rather than her work*", "*she forgets the advice given for the execution of the tasks*", "*she daydreams*". As all the children with this syndrome, her lack of concentration can be partly accounted for by her sensitivity to visual or sound stimuli, which catch her attention and disturb her (Titran and Gratias, 2005). Finally, her relations in professional situations are childish, as shown in her reports for professional training courses; only small responsibilities were attributed to her within the framework of teamwork because of her "naïve, childish, easily influenced and gullible" character. The written conclusions of the manager as she left his establishment reveal all her difficulties: "*Maria is a nice girl, but I am afraid that, in life, she will be exploited and taken advantage of because of her extreme innocence. In spite of her age, she is not ready to work* ". She became too old for school. However, the heaviness of the handicap meant that she could not fend to herself and had to be put in institutional care as 15 to 20 % of the children with this syndrome (Lemoine and Lemoine, 1992). The search for a suitable institution was still devolved to the family: "*it was a pain, they did not want her any more at school, they did not want to keep her any more. One fine day, they said that we had to find a solution, that after such a date, they did not want her any more, and that for lack of better solution, we had to take her home with us because she could not live alone. She was incapable of managing her money, organizing her time, making decisions. She needed help. It was naturally impossible to have her live with us because our house was too small, and also because, we did not want her at home. It was mission impossible; it would have ended up in a divorce!"*, her sister-in-law remembers. For lack of a place in an institution specialized and adapted to her handicap, she temporarily integrated a convent school for the deaf where she stayed for two years. Sewing, learning the language of the deaf and praying occupied her days: "*life in this institution seemed very austere but it was very structuring for Maria. We were never able to visit her room, or the dining hall. The convent school was forbidden to us, but Maria did not complain* ". She could visit her half brothers one weekend every three weeks, and her family could visit her on Sundays: "*we would go and see her for two hours on Sunday afternoons, we often went for a walk in the park, she was happy to see us and proud to show us what she could say in sign language. For the first time in her life, she had achieved something special. However, this annoyed her half brothers who considered that it stigmatized their half sister even more. I remember that really annoyed them*" her sister-in-law remembers.

## Her Adult Life

When Maria reached 18, she could no longer stay in the convent school. As her family did not have the facilities for a handicapped person at home, they looked for a specialized institution for adults with a light mental handicap. Her sister-in-law remembers "*My mother advised us to find a place for her in the country, where she could work in the fields or in a farm. She said that it would be suitable for this slightly simple-minded girl. The country air would be good for her. Fortunately, we did not listen to her. She was incapable of coping on her own, outside an institution. I realized that it was impossible, that she needed constant supervision*". For example, the risk of sexual abuse was always a real possibility, as analyzed by Dehaene (Dehaene, 2002): "in brief, the newborns of alcoholic mothers, brought up in families intellectually and morally deficient are easy preys for pimps. On the other hand, those who have been lucky enough to live in stable homes, stimulated by competent social workers or who were placed or adopted by warm and gratifying families have a totally different life, similar to that of Down syndrome children. Maria is in this second scenario, thanks to her caring family.

A social worker found a place for Maria in the country, in a boarding school for severely mentally handicapped people. Contrary to the convent school, the family was invited to a preliminary visit with Maria. "*It was a vast rehabilitated farm building, with a dining room, dormitories of two or three beds, workhops for bindin or, needle work. It was full of Down syndrome, and crazy people, some even had three hands. They were monsters. I cried when I left*", her sister-in-law remembers. As for Maria, she was indifferent during the visit and resigned herself to live there, without the slightest reserve.

This indifference towards her surroundings is characteristic of children with this syndrome (Dorris, 1989). She integrated this institution at the end of 1972 : " Admittedly, *the institution was far from her brother's home. Compared to the others she appeared almost normal or at least she seemed to manage her handicap suitably well. She was top of the range, there!. But, we had no choice. It was the only institution willing to take her. Furthermore, we hoped to get a place in a more suitable institution which the headmaster was planning to build soon. We were thus encouraged by the prospect of a better situation in the future*". Maria worked for the first time in an adult training centre (CAT) and received a salary. Her leisure activities consisted essentially of walks in the country. "*It was already much better than the convent school, she was more stimulated and she worked a little. She was also a much valued member of the community because intellectually, she was sharper than the other residents and that helped to boost her self-confidence*" one of the half brothers remembers. She was also allowed to go home one weekend every three weeks: "*she used to take the bus to Saint-Cloud on Friday evenings at about 6 pm. My husband, her half brother, used to fetch her after work. She'd spend the weekend with us and we'd drive her back to the same bus stop on Sundays at about 4 pm* ". Her expenses were partially covered by Maria's family: "*400 francs a month shared between the two half brothers. At the time, it was a fair amount of money, and we also had to pay for her bedding in particular for her mattress*". This placement, once again, was supposed to be temporary but continued, contrary to all expectations, for nine years, until 1981. This stresses the necessity of a follow-up in the lives of FAS people, which she never had before.

The headmaster eventually placed Maria in a new institution more suited to her needs, near Paris, in 1981. She was then 30 and finally had a room of her own, because her mental handicap was comparatively light. She was almost autonomous and could cope with most difficulties and constraints: "*when I left for the weekend, I had to return to school between 5:30 and 6:30 on Sundays. That wasted the afternoon, time seemed to fly*". She pursued her professional activities, in CAT, which she combined with new more elaborate leisure activities such as horse riding and yoga. "*I used to make things for the Tagada sweet factory. Loads of things, fun things, taps. I used to put it all under the machine. And that was it. It was always the same, on and on, and on...*" she remembers. So, she gradually became more self-confident, to the point that she even made plans to get married to a resident of the home in 1983. The marriage was subject to the authorization of her guardian. Her younger half brother considered the potential difficulties and added responsibilities more than he did, the happiness of his half sister: "*We did not want her to get married, unless it was with a bright guy, which would have been quite surprising. We preferred for her to concentrate on herself. We had already had enough of a difficult life because of her. Furthermore, what was the point of her getting married ?*". The headmaster of the institution encouraged them to meet her boyfriend. "*We met him at a station in Paris. He was really a very, very thick guy, incapable of doing anything on his own. We told Maria to forget it. It was simply not possible, and she resigned herself without any resistance*". Professionally, her protected employment at a printing office provided her with regular incomes. She complained however about the repetitive tasks: "*I drilled holes in sheets to be put in files, it was always the same thing, on and on. It was always the same, I went round and round in circles*".

In 1988, at the age of 37, she shared a flat with a resident of the institution, who like herself had a light mental handicap. This proved how much she had improved, and how much more self-sufficient she had become. An educator helped with her paper work (accounts, health insurances, holiday allowances, sports activities). She remained however unstable in her professional life and changed employment repeatedly while staying in the flat. "*She complained endlessly. Her colleagues did not like her, the customers were not kind, the pots were too heavy, and the dishwater gave her eczema. We stopped listening. In fact, she easily gets tired of things. She gets tired of everything*". In 2000 her endless complaints lead her employer to place Maria in a job, away from anyone else, as a cleaner. However, she complained even more. "*The customers were very dirty, they took her for a skiwv, and they did not respect her. It was true that her tasks were thankless. She should have kept her previous job which was nicer. She argued with everybody*". The working relations with her colleagues and the people in charge were often tense, conflicted and difficult, which seems rather characteristic of adults with this syndrome. Her leisure activities changed as rapidly as her jobs. She could never settle down with anything. "*At first, she rode horses once a week, she went by bus, and then walked the remaining distance to the riding school. She had a good laugh because she always rode round in circles; then, she gave it up because the lessons finished too late. She also did yoga; then started gymnastics which she stopped because the movements were too repetitive. She also tried judo, but it was too dangerous. She took evening classes to improve her maths but that proved a losing battle. I believe what she likes most is to stay at home and watch television, it is less effort*". Nothing seemed to interest her in long run, she was apathetic and lacked motivation (Streissguth and al., 1991). In order to give her as normal a life as possible, she was sent on package tours in Egypt and Greece. She seemed neither enthusiastic, nor disappointed by this new experience. But, because she felt stigmatized by the other tourists, and had no interest in the visits of historic sites, Maria stopped going on such trips.

In 2000, at the age of 49, she met her current companion, which motivated her to find a flat of her own, all the more so as, she fell out with her flat mate. "*We lived on top of one another, many times, many times we lived on top of one another with her. And one day, she left Viener Street, she now lives at the Stadium. We were too much together. After it did not work, there were storms. When she left the other day, I was upset*". Since then, Maria has had her own flat and lived with her boyfriend. She still works in a protected environment and she was even given a medal for good services in 2004. This reward, her biggest pride, is the symbol of her achievements as a citizen in her own right. She seems to have reached her peak.

## The Everyday Life of a Person with SAF

Her everyday life is very structured and repetitive, to make up for her failing memory. Indeed, she cannot remember the chronological chain of events or movements in her working day. She gets confused "can't make head or tail of things" she keeps saying. For example, about her working mornings, she says: "*I get up at about seven, quarter to seven, every morning. Later at 8:30, I leave home, I go straight to work. I have a thing to store my "cloth", my "pants". At 9, I go downstairs to clean, to clean the floor, and so on. At 11, we eat. We have a break at 11:30. At noon, we go to serve the others who work below in the workshops and we serve them* ". Her year is also regulated, by visits to her younger half brother who lives near Paris every other month, and to her elder half brother who lives in the country twice a year, and during the summer holidays she visits her boyfriend's parents. She has no memory or notion of time, yet she shows great ingenuity in finding ways to make up for it, in her everyday life. In order to keep in touch, she has a telephone address book, and she sends standard messages which she copies on postcards. The two postcards below sent in 1998 and 2006, eight years apart, show the same message (personal archives):

These gimmicks cannot totally make up to her lack of control of time, which is in evidence both in her leisure activities and at work: "*at half past two, quarter to three, I finish my work and I have to wait for a little while, we have to come down at 5, and if we go down before 5, we get caught by the boss*". To call a wait of two hours and a half, "of a little while", is very revealing of her lack of appreciation of the passing of time.

Her rudimentary vocabulary is associated with her simplistic syntax, problems of delivery and difficulty in understanding simple questions. Hence when, questioned about the composition of her lunch, she answers: "*It is the Sannois service which gives us trays to put in ovens*". Furthermore, her ability to synthesize is non-existent. She lingers over minor details with a childish vision. For example, giving a brief description of her professional activity proves impossible: "*I serve meals, I serve high class customers who rent rooms. I serve breakfast. Later I go downstairs again, I serve people in the dining room. I return. And then later, when people have finished eating, I am free. I clean with a product to clean tables. After I have cleaned tables, I use the "pitch, pitch". Later I leave the tables like that. There is another colleague who puts the chairs on the tables. And then after when the tables are ready, I take a duster with a special broom, I make a heap of dust. And then I add more dust and that makes a big heap. Later, I collect the dust, I put it in the garbage can. And later, I take a bucket and a special thing, a disinfectant, I wash the ground* ". Her capacity for generalization is also rather weak: "*on the weekend, sometimes, I go to see a friend, at noon. On Saturday, at midday, I eat with my friend Josette because she is alone and nice, I eat with her. From time to time I go to see her sometimes, she is happy and sometimes she is unhappy. I go to see her to see if she is well and everything. I watch TV a little, she cannot go out because she has water in her feet. And then, she has tests to know where that comes from. The doctors, they made blood tests, urine tests in a jar and they found nothing that's the matter with her*". In fact, she has a very limited capacity for reflection, and understands concepts and the general ideas with the greatest difficulty.

Any calculation of distances, time, weight, size, enumeration … is a mystery to her (Titran and Gratias, 2005), "*division and multiplication, I cannot do*" she says. She finds ways to make up for these difficulties too.

August $8^{th}$, 1998
Dear everyone,
I am writing this card to tell
how I am. I am well. I think you
are having nice holidays.
Love to everyone.

August $16^{th}$, 2006
Dear X and Dear Y,
I am writing this card to *telle* how
I am. I am well. I think you are
having nice… in Toulouse.
Love.

Figure 1. Two postcards.

Her evaluation of distances is almost non existent and she answers systematically that "*it is not too far* ", or by giving names of streets or places :"*my friend Martine, she lives on the Maréchal Joffre Street; the gym, it is in Victor Hugo school* ". Concerning the estimation of workforce or measurements, she answers: "*We are many of us*", "*I am not too heavy*", "*I am small* ". She can tell the time with great difficulty. Her estimation of durations is even more problematic: her gym lesson is from 6:30 to 8:30 pm every week but she cannot infer that it is a two hour lesson. Money means as much to her as it would a 6- or 7-year-old child. She does not distinguish five euros from fifty and can never give the correct change. She cannot organize her various possessions into a hierarchy, be it a "baguette" or her car or even her house. As a consequence, her management of money is limited to the basics. She cannot manage a bank account. So, when fifty euros are assigned to her every week to do her shopping, she comments: " I have 55 *oros* a week, 30 *oros* for food and 20 for fun".

Maria generally resists changes (Titran and Gratias, 2005) as soon as they affect her routine. She seems most comfortable when she has to deal with a familiar situation, and is very disrupted if she has to face a new situation (Dorris, 1989). For example, for her, August is the month of her holidays and agrees very reluctantly to organise her holidays on any other month. That causes tension with her colleagues and her boss. But, these tensions do not teach her anything, she clings to her ways, year after year. Her reluctance to adapt is particularly obvious on public transportation. She cannot find an alternative solution in an unexpected situation such as a strike on the underground, or the momentary stop of a train: "*when I realized that she was completely lost, I took the decision to go and fetch her, which doesn't help her become more autonomous*" her younger half brother admits. Her spatial memory is particularly deficient, which explains that she cannot pass her driving licence. She cannot find her way on a map, or tell the difference between where she lives and where she goes on holidays. Moreover, she is not interested in knowing about these differences. Nevertheless, her survival instinct warns her of danger. But to accept a change, even in dire circumstances remains problematic. For example, the violence of his companion led her to call the police on many occasions. One of her sisters in law recalls: "*she told me that he used to knock her about, that she had to call the cops, but that he had stopped, that it was a thing of the past. She said that she was not seeing him any longer. I told her that she should not see him ever again. As usual, she agreed with me. Then later, she returned to him. I make fun of her and asked her whether she enjoyed being beaten up like her mother. But, it's up to her, it's her life after all. We can do nothing about it*. Even if she somewhat reproduces her mother's story with her companion, she seems to have integrated that conjugal violence is unacceptable.

To all this is added her lack of judgment, the most prevalent symptom in FAS (Streissguth and al., 1991). Her lack of judgment explains her incapacity to measure the consequences of her actions, or establish a chain of causality between events. She never sees the connection between the amount she eats and the fact that she's overweight, between her having a free travel card and her handicap (more exactly, that her rate of incapacity is superior to 80 %); between her lack of employment and her limited consuming power. She has however the capacity to use her emotions to deal with conflicts. Foetal alcohol syndrome seems to prevent the development of analytical and intellectual intelligence. Conversely her impulsiveness and irritability are very developed (Titran and Gratias, 2005): she can take a decision on a whim, and leave her employment without thinking of the consequences. She cannot think for herself, present her point of view, argue or make the right decision in a rational way. Maria never learns from her mistakes. She has a very weak tolerance level and is very highly strung: "*when I'm cross, you mustn't annoy me, when I'm cross, don't even think about it"*.

Finally, she knows that she needs to rely on other people, such as her educators or her family, therefore we can wonder whether she is not somehow, at least partly aware, of her failing memory, her bad control of money, her weak capacity for adaptation and her difficulties in doing most things. Her educators organise her life, her short or long-term objectives, her decisions. Someone comes regularly to her flat to deal with her administrative tasks and medical follow up and to manage her budget. However, she appears to be in denial of her own difficulties: "*no, no, there is no educator, I manage on my own, I go to the bank, I go every Tuesday, to remove from my allowance. For the doctor also I phone the doctor, or I go alone to the doctor* ". She is also in denial when she says that she buys her own train ticket to visit her half brother living in the country: "*I phone to ask for schedules and for everything and when I have the schedules, I go to the station, to show the schedules and everything, I phone my other brother to say at what time I come* ". This denial betrays her desire for emancipation but also brings to light her short comings. She has however a capacity to find tactics and parades in spite of her certain intellectual deficiencies. So, she seems to have understood that she can disguise reality when she thinks others cannot double check. When she thinks that reality can be double checked, she refrains from transforming it. She does not hide that she cannot choose clothes alone: "*Someone has to go with me to see if it is good or not, because I was conned before, and I do not want that. Well, I took the clothes, I notice problems and then when I return I cannot exchange even with the receipt. I don't remember, I tried it in the shop and everything, the woman said to me "yes, yes, it suits you", I believed the woman, I bought it and when I came home, it didn't suit me, not at all* ". Moreover, she does not take a good care of her physical appearance; she does not know how to match colours and choose colours which suit her complexion. She also often wears inappropriate[2] clothes for the season.

She must be partly aware of her mental handicap, and she seems to have learnt what is advisable to say or to do in order to appear "normal". Her answers are made of standard phrases. For example, she gives the impression that she is fussy about hygiene and cleanliness. However, force is to notice that, as half of the people with this syndrome (Streissguth and LaDue, 1985), she has difficulty in keeping her place neat and tidy, as her niece remarks: "*everything is untidy, there is the hairdryer in the dining room, dirty dishes everywhere, the table is so cluttered that you can't use it. She has no notion of what it is to tidy up"*. As for television and her musical preferences, she also seems to have integrated what is socially acceptable: "*I watch TV, the news, I like the figures skating and also things to do with ri,ri, riding. I like the classical music, Vivaldi, Rossini, lot of others*". This does not exclude the possibility that she might actually like what she describes, but it is difficult to know for sure.

In her relationships with others, she oscillates between two opposite attitudes: she is either excessively friendly or, totally aloof. In the presence of her familiar circle of acquaintances, she answers without restraint, explains her daily concerns in a repetitive way, like a child but never asks any questions. When given advice, she always agrees, whatever she really thinks. Her actions, however show that she has not really taking into account any advice or anything she has learnt from past experience. This perhaps shows a certain degree of autonomy, but also a lack of analysis, or capacity to take advantage and make the most of given advice. On the other hand, in the presence of strangers, as she does not know them or how they will react, she prefers to play dumb and observe. She makes herself discreet when she is afraid to appear ridiculous because of her expressions and her mental handicap. Maria dreads the judgment of others. She gives the impression that she does not differentiate the way she relates to animals to her relationship with her members of her family: "*everybody is on the same plan*" (Dorris, 1989), while she will turn to the persons or things which will not cause her any problem. So, she worries more about the health of her pets more than about that of the members of her family.

## Conclusion

It is fundamental to understand that FAS is not hereditary, to prevent any exclusion or eugenism. Maria has never had a child because her mental handicap was supposed to be incompatible with bringing up a child, but also because her syndrome was supposed to be hereditary. So she avoided passing the syndrome on to a new generation. The child of a mother with this syndrome will not inherit it, unless she drinks during her pregnancy. If it is generally thought that the carriers of this syndrome have more chances to become excessive consumers of alcohol (Streissguth and al., 1991); (Dorris, 1989), Maria seems to be an exception because she is extremely sensitive to alcohol consumption. Her excessive physiological reaction may be explained by the destruction of her defences in utero. Even if Maria finally leads an almost normal life thanks to the care of her family and institution, her story was full of pitfalls as are most of the lives of the carriers of this syndrome. Her well established routine will presumable continue until she retires. However, her retirement will need to be supervised, in view of her foreseeable diminishing capacities with old age and her special needs.

In view of FAS people's difficulties in adapting to life in society and the necessary human and material investments throughout their lives, abstinence during pregnancy must be recommended in order to avoid any risk to generate a pathology for which there is no treatment, solution or educational method. Let us note however that progress can be realized in early childhood with re education or sessions of psychomotricity, orthophony and available in the centres for early medical and social action (Dehaene, 1991).

## References

Abel, E. (1995). An update on incidence of FAS: FAS is not an equal opportunity of birth defect. *Neurotoxicology and Teratology, 17*, 437-443.

Bignol, N., Schuster, C., Fuchs, M., Iosub, S., Turner, G., Stone, R.K., and Gromisch, D.S. (1987). The influence of socioeconomic factors on the occurence of foetal alcohol syndrome. *Advances in Alcohol* and *Substance Abuse, 6*, 105-118.

Danel, T., Karila, L., and Mezerete, C., (2007). Syndrome dysexécutif et addiction. *Alcoologie et Addictologie, 29,* 27-32.

Dehaene, P., (1991). Boire et avoir un enfant. *Sciences Sociales et Santé, 9*, 25-30.

Dehaene, P., Crepin, G., Delahousse, G., Querleu, D., Welbaum, R., Titran, M. and Samaille-Villette C. (1981). Aspects épidémiologiques du syndrome d'alcoolisation foetal, 45 observations en trois ans. La *Nouvelle Presse Medicale, 10*, 2639-2643.

Deschamps-Frosio, D. (1998). Alcoolisme et maternité. Le syndrome d'alcoolisation foetale : données historiques épidémiologiques statistiques regionales. *Profession Sage-Femme, 52*, 21-22.

Doris M. (1989). *L'enfant brisé*. Paris : Denoel.

Forbes, R. (1984). Alcohol-related Birth Defected. *Public Health, 98*, 239-240.

Gaugue, J., Varascon, I., and Wendland, J. (2006). "Le syndrome d'alcoolisation foetale : état de la question " *Psychotropes, 12*, 113-124.

Jacobson, J.L., Jacobson, S.W., Sokol, R.J., Martier, S.S., Ager, J.W and Kaplan-Estrin, M.G. (1993). Teratogenic effects of alcohol on infant development. *Alcoholism Clinical Experimental Research, 17*, 174-183.

Lemoine, P., and Lemoine, H. (1992). Avenir des enfants de mères alcooliques et quelques constatations d'ordre prophylactique. *Annales de pédiatrie, 39,* 229-235.

Olson, H.C., O'Connor, M.J., and Fitzgerald, H. (2001). Lessons learned from study of developmental impact of parental alcohol use. *Infant Mental Health Journal, 22*, 271-290.

Picherot, G. (2005). Le syndrome d'alcoolisation foetal : le point de vue du pédiatre. *Le Courrier des addictions, 4,* 131-132.

Simmat-Durand, L. (2005). *Maternité à risques : signalements et placements des enfants de mère toxicomane*. Habilitation à dirigés des recherches en Sociologie, Saint-Quentin en Yvelines.

Société Française d'Alcoologie. (2003). Etat de connaissances actuelles sur, d'une part, la consommation d'alcool et ses effets durant la grossesse et, d'autre part, les répercussions de cette consommation sur l'enfant à venir. *Alcoologie et Addictologie*, *2*, 74S-81S.

Streissguth, A.P., Aase, J.M., Clarren, S.K., Randels, S.P., LaDue, R.A, and Smith DF. (1991). Fetal alcohol syndrome in adolescents and adults. *Journal of the American Medical Association, 265*, 1961-1967.

Streissguth, A.P., and LaDue R.A. (1985). Psychological and behavioral effects in children prenatally exposed to alcohol. *Alcohol, Health and Research World 10*, 6-12.

Titran, M. (1991). L'intervention médico-sociale précoce dans le cadre de l'alcoolisme foetal. L'expérience du centre de Roubaix. *Sciences Sociales et Santé, 9*, 31-34.

Titran, M., and Gratias, L. (2005). *A sa santé*. Paris : Albin Michel.

# APPENDICES

**Table 1. Synthesis of Maria's story**

| Period | Institutions | Schooling and employment |
|---|---|---|
| 1951 | NHS hospital | |
| 1951-1966 | Parents' home | Class for special needs children |
| 1966-1967 | Boarding school in Val d'Oise | Class for special needs children |
| 1967-1970 | Boarding school in the Somme | Class for special needs children |
| 1970-1972 | Convent school in Hauts-de-Seine | helped the nuns |
| 1972-1981 | Medical educational institution in Eure et Loire | Job for CAT (Adult training centre) |
| 1981- 1986 | Medical educational institution in Hauts-de-Seine | Job in a protected employment |
| 1987-2000 | Supervised apartments in Hauts-de-Seine with a flat mate | Job in a protected employment |
| 2000-2006 | Apartments under the supervision of the IME in Hauts-de-Seine with her companion | Job in a protected employment |

**Table 2. Maria's school reports when she was 18 (personal archives)**

| National education Minister |
|---|
| Class for special needs children |
| *Student information*<br>Name of candidate: |
| First name: Maria |
| Date of birth: |
| Address: |
| School: |
| Class: Class for special needs children |
| *School level*<br>Reading: Second grade |
| Spelling: First grade |
| Math: First grade |
| Comments: A lot of good will but no potential whatsoever |
| *Mental age*<br>Real age: 18 years and 2 months |
| Terman K individual test: MA : 7 years IQ : 56 |
| *Manual skills* |
| When she does a very simplistic task, she can focus and enjoy her work. |
| *Behaviour* |
| Docile, very naïve, spontaneous. She does not understand even simple questions and her answers are always beside the point. |

| National education Minister |
|---|
| *Remarks* |
| She is small but strong, never ill. |
| *Class* |
| Maths: Weak results. She does not understand much. She cannot do simple calculation. |
| Reading: Slow, hesitant, shaky reading |
| Talking: Poor vocabulary. Childish talk. |
| Behaviour: Not very interesting in her work. No improvement. |
| *Workshops* |
| Cooking: Some good will but very little potential |
| Sewing: Cannot remember what she is told. Daydreams. Doesn't pay attention to her work. Chats. No improvement |
| Ironing: Keeps forgetting the instructions. |
| Washing: No initiatives |
| Physical education: Nervous pupil. Cannot control her movement. |
| *Work experience* |
| Naïve, childish, shy pupil. Very sensitive to peer pressure. |

Conclusion: Maria is good natured but I fear that in life people will exploit her and take advantage of her. In spite of her age, she is far from ready to be able to work or to have a job.

In: Pregnancy and Alcohol Consumption
Editor: Joshua D. Hoffman, pp. 315-329
ISBN 978-1-61761-122-3


*Chapter 13*

# FACTORS ASSOCIATED WITH ALCOHOL ABUSE AMONG WOMEN OF CHILD-BEARING AGE

***Sanna J. Thompson and Jina Jun***
University of Texas at Austin, School of Social Work,
Substance Abuse Research Development Program,
Austin, Texas, USA

It is estimated that of the 15.1 million alcohol-abusing or alcohol-dependent individuals in the United States, nearly one-third (5,277,000) are women. Drinking behavior differs with age, life role, and marital status among women. In general, the incidence of alcohol dependence is greater among women of child-bearing age and the development of consequences associated with alcohol use may be accelerated. Women are more sensitive to alcohol, become addicted quicker, develop alcohol-related problems sooner, and die at a younger age than men with similar drinking problems. Equal proportions of black and white women drink heavily; however, African American women report fewer alcohol-related personal and social problems than white women, but a greater proportion of black women experience alcohol-related health problems.

The National Health Interview Survey (Center for Disease Control and Prevention, 2009) provides rates of current drinking status among individuals in the United States. Specifically, in 2008 more than half of women (58.3%) drank alcohol and the number of females who never drink is decreasing. Among females, 45.1% are light drinkers or those who drink three or fewer drinks per week during the past year. 8.3% were moderate drinkers (those who average 3-6 drinks per week during past year) and 5% were heavy drinkers (consume more than one drink per day during the past year). When race/ethnicity considered, 2.7% of Hispanic female drinkers, 2.8% of black female drinkers, and 6% of white female drinkers were heavy drinkers who defined as more than 1 drink per day in the past year (Center for Disease Control and Prevention, 2009).

Problem drinking levels that are considered an addiction are defined as abuse and dependency.

*Alcohol abuse* is defined in the Diagnostic and Statistical Manual- IV by the American Psychiatric Association as:

1. Recurrent substance use resulting in a failure to fulfill major role obligations at work, school, or home (such as repeated absences or poor work performance related to substance use; substance-related absences, suspensions, or expulsions from school; or neglect of children or household).
2. Recurrent substance use in situations in which it is physically hazardous (such as driving an automobile or operating a machine when impaired by substance use)
3. Recurrent substance-related legal problems (such as arrests for substance related disorderly conduct)
4. Continued substance use despite having persistent or recurrent social or interpersonal problems caused or exacerbated by the effects of the substance (for example, arguments with spouse about consequences of intoxication and physical fights)

*Alcohol dependency* is defined as a maladaptive pattern of substance use leading to clinically significant impairment or distress, as manifested by three (or more) of the following, occurring any time in the same 12-month period:

1. Tolerance, as defined by either of the following:

(a) A need for markedly increased amounts of the substance to achieve intoxication or the desired effect

*or*

(b) Markedly diminished effect with continued use of the same amount of the substance.

2. Withdrawal, as manifested by either of the following:

(a) The characteristic withdrawal syndrome for the substance

*or*

(b) The same (or closely related) substance is taken to relieve or avoid withdrawal symptoms.

3. The substance is often taken in larger amounts or over a longer period than intended.
4. There is a persistent desire or unsuccessful efforts to cut down or control substance use.
5. A great deal of time is spent in activities necessary to obtain the substance, use the substance, or recover from its effects.
6. Important social, occupational, or recreational activities are given up or reduced because of substance use.
7. The substance use is continued despite knowledge of having a persistent physical or psychological problem that is likely to have been caused or exacerbated by the substance (for example, continued drinking despite recognition that an ulcerwas made worse by alcohol consumption).

The National Institute on Alcohol Abuse and Alcoholism (National Epidemiologic Survey on Alcohol and Related Conditions (NESARC) (Grant et al., 2004) provides some recent statistics related to the prevalence of alcohol dependence and abuse in women. When only alcohol dependence was considered, the prevalence rate was 2.3% (approximately 2,515,000 women). 84% of these women were in child-bearing age (18-44 years old). In terms of race, 72% of female alcohol dependents are white, 12% are black, 9% are Hispanic, 4% are Native American, and 2.5% are Asian. Drawing upon these same data, 2.5% women (2,762,000) met criteria for alcohol abuse. 77% of them were between 18 to 44 years of age. Among these female alcohol abusers, 81% were white, 6.6% were black, 6% were Hispanic, 3.5% were Native American, and 2% were Asian. Thus, it appears that women's drinking during child-bearing age and during pregnancy has increased substantially.

Although it is clear that alcohol abuse and dependency among women has become a concern, the heavy drinking and drinking problems among women are most alarming among younger age groups who are of child-bearing age (approximately 18-45 years of age). Trend analyses of the Behavioral Risk Factor Surveillance System between 1991 and 1999 indicated that alcohol use by both pregnant women and non-pregnant women of child-bearing age increased (Caetano, Ramisetty-Mikler, Floyd, and McGrath, 2006). The rates of any alcohol use among pregnant women increased nearly 4% from 1991 to 1995 (CDC, 2002b). The rates of binge drinking reported by pregnant women were approximately 2.9% and frequent alcohol use rates were 3.5% in 1995 (CDC, 2002b); these rates have changed little during past decade.

Some research suggests that alcohol use declines during pregnancy (Higgins, Clough, Frank, and Wallerstedt, 1995; Lohr, Gillmore, Gilchrist, and Butler, 1992). However, at the same time, many studies suggest that women still drink alcohol during their pregnancy (Abma and Mott, 1991; Merrick, 1993; Pagliaro and Pagliaro, 2000) and the extent of their drinking was related to various demographic characteristics (e.g., age and marital status) (Wilsnack and Cheloha, 1987; Wilsnack, Klassen, Schur, and Wilsnack, 1991), socioeconomic status (e.g., race, education, employment, and income) (Droomers, Schrijvers, Stronks, Mheen, and Mackenback, 1999; Gomberg, 1994; NIAAA, 2002; Schmidt, Klee, and Ames, 1990), adverse experiences in childhood (Nolen-Hoeksema, 2004; Salomon, Bassuk, and Huntington, 2002), adverse experiences in adult (Clum, Nishith, and Calhoun, 2002; Kaysen, Neighbors, Martell, Fossos, and Larimer, 2006; Ullman and Najdowski, 2009), and interrelationship problems (Abbey, Smith, and Scott, 1993; Covington and Surrey, 1997; NIAAA, 2008; Olenick and Chalmers, 1991). Therefore, it is necessary to review relationships between these characteristics and alcohol use among child-bearing aged women.

## DEMOGRAPHIC CHARACTERISTICS OF WOMEN AND DRINKING

Various characteristics has been studied to more fully understand and explain women's drinking, including age, race/ethnicity, and marital status (Caetano et al., 2006; Salomon et al., 2002; Wilsnack and Cheloha, 1987; Wilsnack et al., 1991). With regard to age, Caetano et al. (2006) studied women of childbearing age to investigate predictors of heavy drinking among pregnant and non-pregnant women. Results of this study noted that binge drinking, alcohol abuse and/or dependence were higher in younger pregnant and non-pregnant women, particularly those less than 30 years of age. Similarly, Wilsnack and Cheloha (1987) studied the relationship between women's problem drinking and social roles across the life span. They found that younger women 21 to 34 were more likely to be problem drinkers compared to other women.

With regard to women's marital status, research that has investigated the relationship between marital status and women's drinking has shown inconsistent results. Some studies report that women who have never married or who cohabitate are at increased risk for problem drinking (Wilsnack and Cheloha, 1987; Wilsnack et al., 1991). Specifically, Wisnack and Cheloha (1987) reported unstable marital status, especially among women aged 21 to 34, was significantly related to problem drinking. Similarly, Wilsnack et al., (1991) reported that marital status was an important factor to predict the incidence of problem drinking and the persistent use of alcohol. Specifically, cohabiting was a predictor of problem drinking and not being married was a predictor of persistent problem drinking. In contrast, Salomon et al (2002) reported different results, suggesting that impoverished women who had been never been married were less likely to report alcohol use than similarly situated women who had been married.

In addition to marital status and age, prior research has also noted that individual socioeconomic status is associated with women's drinking. Having lower education level (Droomers et al., 1999; Lantz et al., 1998), having a part-time job(Wilsnack et al., 1991), having a male dominant job and lower job satisfaction (Nakken, 2002), and having higher income (Caetano et al., 2006; Lantz et al., 1998) were related to women's drinking. With regard to education, Droomers et al. (1999) studied 756 women drinkers and 1006 men drinkers to examine the relationship between educational differences in excessive alcohol consumption, the amount of stress experienced, and stress-moderating factors. Results of this study suggested that excessive alcohol use was more common among groups with lower educational achievement. Material stressors, such as financial problems, deprivation, and income were related to part of the educational gradient in excessive alcohol use.

Lantz et al. (1998) conducted a similar study of 3617 adults to investigate the degree of four behavioral risk factors on alcohol consumption. In terms of alcohol use, the result of the study was that fewer years of education were related to heavy drinking (an average of 90 drinks in the past month). With regard to work status, Wilsnack et al. (1991) also reported that women who had part-time jobs were more likely to have persistent problem drinking. Similarly, Nakken (2002) reviewed studies that examined the relationship between women's socioeconomic status and problems associated with alcohol consumption. They found that women who work in male dominant jobs had higher rates of heavy drinking. In addition, women who were not satisfied with their work were more likely to be heavy drinkers. Finally, with regard to income, Caetano et al. (2006) examined the predictors of heavy drinking among child-bearing aged women. They reported that women with income levels over $ 40,000 were at higher risk for heavy drinking. Other found similar results. For example, Lantz et al (1998) found that women with incomes over $30,000 were more likely to be heavy drinkers; Nakken (2002) found similar results among women who had over $75,000 in income.

## ISSUES OF RACE AND ETHNICITY AMONG WOMEN AND DRINKING

Demographics related to race and/or ethnicity must be included in any discussion of women's drinking behaviors due to the different cultural experiences of these women. Overwhelmingly, studies have consistently demonstrated that white women are more likely to drink than other ethnic groups (Caetano and Kaskutas, 1995; Grant et al., 2004; NIAAA, 2002; Schmidt et al., 1990). However, alcohol abuse and dependence rates were relatively similar in all racial/ethnic groups (Caetano et al., 2006). Although little research exists concerning alcohol use among minority women, a little more research is available on alcohol use of African-American and Hispanic women. Studies have noted that the lower socioeconomic status for African-American women (Gray and Littlefield, 2002; Hanson, 1995; Ward and Beck, 1990) and acculturation stress for Hispanic women (Mora, 2002; Rey, 1995) are associated with drinking alcohol. However, there is little agreement on predictors of alcohol use among Asian-American and American-Indian women. This knowledge gap impedes understandings of reasons women drink and thus development of culturally competent services are scarce. Therefore, it is necessary to review what research is available to understand predictors of women's alcohol use as it relates to their race and ethnicity.

*African American Women.* Compared to other ethnic groups, African American women are either abstainers or heavy drinkers (Gray and Littlefield, 2002; Jasinski, Williams, and Siegel, 2000). However, Black women are more likely to experience more serious health consequences due to their alcohol use than white women (Pagliaro and Pagliaro, 2000). Research has suggested that lower SES levels among black women (Gray and Littlefield, 2002; Lillie-Blanton, MacKenzie, and Anthony, 1991) and those who experience violence (Caetano, Cunradi, Clark, and Schafer, 2000) have increased alcohol use. Lillie-Blanton et al (1991) studied 809 black women and 1291 white women to examine the relationship between individual socioeconomic status and heavy drinking. They found that black women with 12 or more education years were less likely to be heavy drinkers than white women even though they did not find racial differences in predicting heavy drinking. Moreover, black women with lower education who had lower income or were unemployed, and had unstable marriages showed a higher percentage of heavy drinkers, alcohol abuse and dependence than similar black women with higher education, income, jobs, and stable marriage relationships. Gray and Littlefield (2002) reviewed prior studies and reported that black women living in households with low family income, living in metropolitan areas, having no health insurance, being unemployed, being less educated, and never being married were more likely to initiate and continue alcohol use.

In addition to poor socioeconomic status, African American women who experienced traumatic events also had higher rates of problem drinking (Caetano et al., 2000; Jasinski et al., 2000). Caetano et al (2000) studied 555 white, 358 black, and 527 Hispanic couples in the U.S. to examine the relationship between intimate partner violence and drinking patterns. They studied both male-to-female partner violence and female-to-male partner violence. Both were higher among black couples, followed by Hispanic, and white couples. They found that nearly one-quarter of black women reported drinking during male-to-female partner violence incidents. This percentage was four times greater than the percentage among Hispanic women and two times greater than the percentage among white women. Moreover, over one-fifth of black women reported drinking during female-to-male partner violence, followed by white women and Hispanic women.

Being abused as a child also appears to increase heavy drinking among African American women. Jasinski, Williams, and Siegel (2000) studied 113 African-American women who experienced child abuse in their childhood (aged <12 years) to examine the association among characteristics of child sexual abuse, childhood physical abuse, lack of parental care, and heavy drinking in African-American women. They found that black women who experienced multiple types of sexual abuse were more likely to be heavy drinkers and women who experienced childhood physical abuse were also more likely to participate in binge drinking.

*Hispanic Women.* The positive relationship between Hispanic women's drinking and acculturation has been explained in many previous studies (Caetano, Ramisetty-Mikler, Wallish, McGrath, and Spence, 2008; Hanson, 1995; Mora, 2002; Rey, 1995). Acculturation leads to more drinking because highly acculturated immigrants adopt liberal norms and attitudes toward drinking and drunkenness, as well as positive expectancies about the effects of alcohol (Caetano et al., 2008). Through one review of prior research, Mora (2002) reported that Hispanic women are ethnically diverse, but women from Mexico women have the highest rates of heavy alcohol use and dependence compared to Cuban or Puerto Rican women. Compared to immigrant and second generation Hispanic women, there are fewer non-drinkers among third generation Hispanic women. Caetano et al. (2008) studied Hispanics in the Texas-Mexico border to examine the association between acculturation, drinking patterns, and heavy episodic drinking. The findings of the study showed that for women, the more acculturated women become to the U.S., the great the frequency of heavy episodic drinking as well as those identified as abusing or dependent on alcohol. In addition, being younger and having higher heavy episodic drinking during the past month increased the odds of having alcohol disorders.

*Asian American Women.* Asian women have not been considered as a unique ethnic group in studies of heavy drinking (Caetano, Clark, and Tam, 1998; Johnson and Nagoshi, 1989; Kitano and Louie, 2002). However, among Asian American women, differences in drinking levels emerge. For example, Chi et al. (1989) surveyed Chinese, Japanese, and Koreans to understand their drinking patterns and predictors of their drinking behaviors. They found that Japanese people showed the greatest portion of heavy drinking and Chinese people showed the lowest. They also reported that having peers who drink was the only significant factor of their drinking behavior. Moreover, Makimoto (1998) suggested that southeast Asians (e.g., Vietnamese) living in the U.S. appeared to be at the highest risk for heavy drinking because of their cultural preference toward alcohol and psychological problems due to their war histories and difficulties in adjusting to the American environment. In addition, economic status, educational attainment, degree of acculturation, and genetic and environmental factors (e.g., drinking norms and alcohol availability) influence drinking patterns among Asian Americans. Similar to Hispanic women, the level of acculturation also has been reported as a causal factor associated with Asian women's drinking (Kitano and Louie, 2002). For example, Asian American women's drinking patterns are similar to other immigrants as alcohol use tends to increase with acculturation.

*Native American Women.* Some studies reported that binge drinking is more common among Native American women than found in other racial/ethnic groups (Caetano et al., 2006; Timko, Sutkowi, Pavao, and Kimerling, 2008). Ward and Beck (1990) reviewed sociological theories to explain problem drinking behavior among Native Americans and Hispanics. They hypothesized that Native Americans were in a more favorable socioeconomic position and to have greater access to alcohol than Hispanic women who were new to the U.S. (Doshi and Jiles, 2006; Szlemko, Wood, and Thurman, 2006). Specifically, Doshi and Jiles (2006) studied American Indian/ Alaskan Native women to describe the prevalence of risky behaviors, including binge drinking. They found that women were more likely to binge drink if they were not married, had some post-high school education, had higher income, no health insurance coverage, had lower self-reported health status, and had difficulties seeing doctor due to cost. In addition, Szlemko et al (2006) found Native American women that were impoverished, had initiated alcohol use at an early age, and were more highly acculturated to the non-Native American values had higher levels of problem drinking.

## Adverse Experiences in Childhood Related to Women Drinking

Among adverse experiences in childhood, especially sexual abuse, has been shown to be a significant risk factor for women's alcohol use (Bulik, Prescott, and Kendler, 2001; Grayson and Nolen-Hoeksema, 2005; Koss et al., 2003; Pilowsky, Keyes, and Hasin, 2009; Timko et al., 2008; Vera, Alegria, Pattatucci-Aragon, and Pena, 2005). For example, Pilowsky, Keyes, and Hasin (2009) conducted a study of 43,093 adults age 18 and older. They examined the association between adverse childhood events (e.g., parental divorce, death of a biological parent, living with foster parents, living in an institution outside the home) that occurred in childhood (before age 18) and lifetime prevalence of alcohol dependence. They found that parental divorce was significantly associated with an increase in the odds of alcohol dependence. In addition, experiencing one or more adverse events in childhood was significantly associated with an increase in the likelihood of alcohol dependence. Other studies (Timko, Finney, and Moos, (2008) compared binge drinking women and non-binge drinking women to examine sociodemographics, physical and mental health, and adult and childhood adverse experiences associated with binge drinking. They found that those living with someone abusing substances, living with someone mentally ill, living with others victimized by violence, being emotionally abused, physically assaulted, and sexually assaulted significantly increased the odds of binge drinking. Shaw (2006) also found that lack of early maternal support was significantly associated with adult alcohol abuse.

Studies have shown that women who experience childhood abuse and neglect are much more likely to have problems during their lifetime with alcohol abuse and dependence. For example, Widom, Ireland, and Glynn (1995) found that having parent with drug or alcohol problems increases the likelihood of children having problems with alcoholism. Others have noted that compared to women who did not experience childhood sexual abuse, women with childhood sexual abuse history are more likely to use alcohol, to have alcohol dependence symptoms and problem drinking, to experience lifetime depressive episodes and anxiety than women with no child abuse history (Kendler et al., (2000). Others suggest that a history of childhood rape doubles the number of alcohol abuse symptoms (Epstein, Saunders, Kilpatrick, and Resnick, 1998; Miranda, Meyerson, Long, Marx, and Simpson, 2002).

Finally, Duncan et al. (1996) reported that a history of childhood physical assault was an important predictor of alcohol problems, such as driving while intoxicated, having alcohol-related accidents at home and while driving, more legal problems, workplace problems, and problems with family and friends. Thus, it appears that increased psychological distress predicts increased levels of alcohol misuse.

More specifically, some studies examine the interrelationship between childhood victimization within the family and development of women's alcohol problems. Studies have shown that women in alcoholism treatment programs experience higher rates of childhood victimization, significantly more severe violence by fathers and more childhood sexual abuse than did women in comparison groups (Miller and Downs, 1993; Miller, Downs, and Testa, 1993). Similarly, Miller et al (1993) also found that childhood sexual abuse and father-to-daughter violence were significant in predicting heavy drinking or alcohol problems in later adulthood.

## Adverse Experience in Adulthood Related to Women Drinking

Approximately 13% to 18% of American women have been the victim of rape in their adulthood and a majority of these rapes were committed by a spouse or intimate partner (Abbey, Zawacki, Buck, Clinton, and McAuslan, 2004). These traumatizing experiences have been clearly linked to alcohol abuse among women (Clum et al., 2002; Galvani, 2006; Kaysen et al., 2006; Kilpatrick, Acierno, Resnick, Saunders, and Best, 1997; Salomon et al., 2002; Ullman and Najdowski, 2009). For example, Kilpatrick et al. (1997) suggested that after an assault, the likelihood of alcohol abuse and drug use was significantly increased, even among women who with no previous substance use history. Intimate partner violence also has been reported as a risk factor of women's drinking (Salomon et al., 2002), with increased alcohol and illicit drug use following the assault.

Others (Clum et al., 2002) have found that alcohol use reduced the levels of perceived severity of the abuse, such as emotional and physical reactions to the assault. In addition, Ullman and Najdowski's (2009) study showed that among women who were re-victimized, they reported increased problem drinking. They noted that women who drink to cope, who experience negative social reactions in response to their assault disclosures, and who experience additional traumatic events also increase their level of drinking.

Relationship issues appear to be associated with women's alcohol use (Abbey et al., 1993; Covington, 2002; Covington and Surrey, 1997; Demers, Bisson, and Palluy, 1999; Leonard and Mudar, 2000; NIAAA, 2008; Olenick and Chalmers, 1991; Salomon et al., 2002; Skaff, Finney, and Moos, 1999). As women frequently initiate substance use in order to develop and maintain physical or psychological connections, women who have problems with their closest relationships tend to drink more than other women. These women often use substances to deal with problems in their relationship and may initiate use to try to change themselves to fit other's expectations. For example, Demers et al (1999) studied couples to assess how much the husband's drinking contributed to their wives level of drinking. They found that wives' drinking was positively related to their husband's drinking, both in terms of frequency and amount of binge drinking. Thus, male partners can introduce women to alcohol or other drugs and they often become suppliers when women became addicted (Salomon et al., 2002).

Peer relationships have also been shown to increase the risk for women's problem drinking (Abbey et al., 1993; Leonard and Mudar, 2000; Skaff et al., 1999). It appears that peer networks among women strongly influence alcohol consumption. Characterized by a higher level of alcohol involvement, peer influences are strongly associated with heavier drinking among both men and women (Skaff et al., 1999).

## Consequences of Risky Alcohol Use among Women

Women's alcohol abuse and alcoholism damage their health, safety, and general well-being. An enormous amount of research has shown high rates of alcohol-related health problems, such as liver disease, brain disease, cancer, heart disease, and sexually transmitted diseases (Kushnir, 1996; NIAAA, 2002, 2004; Rosa, Holleran, Rugh, and MacMaster, 2005). Moreover, a large number of studies have found that women who drink excessively are more likely to experience psychological difficulties such as depression and/or anxiety concurrently (Brady and Randall, 1999; DiNitto and Crisp, 2002; Nolen-Hoeksema, 2004). Many studies have emphasized the high likelihood of being victimized due to their own alcohol use and/or the drinking of men with whom they are associated. Studies include sexual assault, physical assault, domestic violence, and other violent crimes (Covington, 1998; Nolen-Hoeksema, 2004; Timko et al., 2008). Recently, research has highlighted the issue of alcohol use during the pregnancy. Women's alcohol consumption during their pregnancy can lead seriously harmful results for their babies which is called Fetal Alcohol Spectrum Disorder (Pagliaro and Pagliaro, 2000; Prescott, Neale, Corey, and Kendler, 1997; Schmidt et al., 1990).

## Women's Alcohol Use and Fetal Alcohol Spectrum Disorder (FASD)

Recently, research has emphasized the highly detrimental effects of alcohol use during pregnancy (Caetano et al., 2006; Centers for Disease Control and Prevention, 2002a, 2002b). The Centers for Disease Control and Prevention (CDC) (2002a) defines risky drinking for child-bearing age women as either 7 or more drinks per week or 5 or more drinks per occasion in the past 30 days. Alcohol is a toxic substance that is quickly transferred from the mother's to the baby's bloodstreamBecause all the organs of the fetus are forming, they are particularly vulnerable to toxic substances, especially during the first three months of pregnancy. In the best interests of the baby, a pregnant woman should avoid alcohol and all other toxic substances.

Despite warnings from the Surgeon General about the dangers of drinking while pregnant, the number of American women who drink alcohol while pregnant has not decreased during the past 15 years. Studies have shown that 10% of pregnant women use alcohol and approximately 2% engage in binge drinking or frequent use of alcohol (CDC, 2000a). The results further indicated that more than half of women who did not use birth control (and therefore might become pregnant) reported alcohol use and 12.4% reported binge drinking.

To date, researchers have not been able to determine the exact amount of alcohol that is "safe" for the development of the fetus. Some suggest that 3 or more drinks a day and daily or near-daily drinking greatly increases the risk for FASD (Barr and Streissguth, 2001). The risks of miscarriage, birth defects, growth retardation and mental disorders increase the more the mother drinks, and the more frequently she drinks. Even moderate, occasional drinking is a concern for pregnant women, but heavy drinking can gravely affect the fetus. A pregnant woman who frequently drinks heavily is more likely to give birth to a child with a specific condition known as fetal alcohol spectrum disorder, or FASD. Occasional heavy drinking also increases the risk of similar problems (DiNitto and McNeece, 2008; Pagliaro and Pagliaro, 2000).

FASD is one of the most severe outcomes of fetal alcohol exposure. Children with FASD have a number of problems such as growth retardation, mental disorders, an abnormally small head or other facial and skeletal abnormalities, malformations of the heart, and central nervous system disorders that last throughout their lifetime (Centers for Disease Control and Prevention, 2002b). Children who suffer from FASD are exposed to six times greater risk of suffering from Epilepsy and the probability of undergoing at least one seizure during their lifetime. Defects may be seen in the baby's heart, liver, and kidneys and he/she may develop vision and hearing problems as well. Children with fetal alcohol syndrome have difficulties with learning, attention, memory, and problem solving. Thus, there is a growing body of evidence that maternal drinking during pregnancy puts a child at greater risk for an even wider variety of neurologic and behavioral health problems than had been identified previously.

The prevalence of babies born with FASD range from 0.2 to 1.5 per 1,000 live births in the United States. When racial/ethnic groups are considered, certain groups show higher prevalence rates of FASD (Abel, 1995; Centers for Disease Control and Prevention, 2002b). For example, the prevalence of FASD among African American women aged 15 to 44 years of age is 2.29 per 1,000 births, while the rate among Caucasian women in this same age group is 0.26 per 1,000 births. American Indians/Alaska Natives have shown the highest rate of FASD (3.2 per 1,000 live births). Data also shows the relationship between women's socioeconomic status and the prevalence of FASD (Abel, 1995). Among low SES women whose income was $10,000 or less for a family of three, rates of FASD were 2.29 per 1,000 births. Among middle to high socioeconomic status women, prevalence of FASD was 0.26 per 1,000 births.

# CONCLUSION

This review of literature on women and alcohol use suggests that individual demographic characteristics, socioeconomic status, race/ethnicity, adverse experiences in childhood and adulthood, and interpersonal relationships are associated with the frequency and level of women's drinking. Especially among women of child-bearing age, the impact of alcohol consumption can have far-reaching and detrimental consequences. Alcohol use during pregnancy continues to be an important public health concern. Women's drinking can not only lead to serious harmful effects on their own health, but the impact of alcohol exposure on the unborn child may be highly damaging. Health care professionals must play an important role in educating women about this issue and should routinely ask all women who are pregnant or of childbearing age about their alcohol use, inform them of the risks of alcohol use while pregnant, and advise them not to consume alcohol while pregnant.

## REFERENCES


Abbey, A., Smith, M.J., and Scott, R.O. (1993). The relationship between reasons for drinking alcohol and alcohol consumption: An interactional approach. *Addictive Behaviors 18*, 659-670.

Abbey, A., Zawacki, T., Buck, P.O., Clinton, A.M., and McAuslan, P. (2004). Sexual assault and alcohol consumption: what do we know about their relationship and what types of research are still needed? *Agression and Violent Behavior, 9*, 271-303.

Abel, E.L. (1995). An Update on Incidence of FAS: FAS is not an equal opportunity birth defect. *Neurotoxicology and Teratology, 17*(4), 437-443.

Abma, J.C., and Mott, F.L. (1991). Substance use and prenatal care during pregnancy among young women. *Family Planning Perspectives, 23*(3), 117-122.

Brady, K.T., and Randall, C.L. (1999). Gender differences in substance use disorders. *Psychiatric Clinics of North America, 22*(2), 241-252.

Bulik, C.M., Prescott, C.A., and Kendler, K.S. (2001). Features of childhood sexual abuse and the development of psychiatric and substance use disorders. *The British Journal of Psychiatry, 179*(5), 444-449.

Caetano, R., Clark, C.L., and Tam, T. (1998). Alcohol consumption among racial/ethnic minorities: theory and research. *Alcohol Health and Research World, 22*(4), 233-238.

Caetano, R., Cunradi, C.B., Clark, C.L., and Schafer, J. (2000). Intimate partner violence and drinking patterns among white, black, and Hispanic couples in the U.S. *Journal of Substance Abuse, 11*(2), 123-138.

Caetano, R., and Kaskutas, L.A. (1995). Changes in drinking patterns among Whites, Blacks, and Hispanics, 1984-1992. *Journal of Studies on Alcohol 56*, 558-565.

Caetano, R., Ramisetty-Mikler, S., Floyd, L.R., and McGrath, C. (2006). The epidemiology of drinking among women of child-bearing age. *Alcoholism: Clinical and Experimental Research, 30*(6), 1023-1030.

Caetano, R., Ramisetty-Mikler, S., Wallish, L.S., McGrath, C., and Spence, R.T. (2008). Acculturation, drinking, and alcohol abuse and dependence among Hispanics in the Texas-Mexico border. *Alcoholism: Clinical and Experimental Research, 32*(2), 1-8.

Center for Disease Control and Prevention. (2009). Percent Distribution of current drinking status, drinking levels, and heavy drinking days by sex for persons 18 years of age and older: United States, NHIS, 1997-2008. from ftp://ftp.cdc.gov/pub/Health_Statistics/NCHS/Datasets/NHIS

Centers for Disease Control and Prevention. (2002a). Alcohol Use Among Women of Childbearing Age--United States, 1991-1999. *MMWR: Morbidity and Mortality Weekly Report, 51*(13), 273-276.

Centers for Disease Control and Prevention. (2002b). Fetal Alcohol Syndrome--Alaska, Arizona, Colorado, and New York, 1995-1997. *MMWR: Morbidity and Mortality Weekly Report, 51*(20), 433-434.

Chi, I., Lubben, J.E., and Kitano, H.H. (1989). Differences in drinking behavior among three Asian-American groups. *Journal of Studies on Alcohol, 50*(1), 15-23.

Clum, G.A., Nishith, P., and Calhoun, K.S. (2002). A preliminary investigation of alcohol use during trauma and peritraumatic reactions in female sexual assault victims. *Journal of Traumatic Stress, 15*(4), 321-328.

Covington, S. (1998). *The relational theory of women's psychological development: Implications for the criminal justice system*. Paper presented at the 50th Annual Meeting of the American Society of Criminology.

Covington, S. (2002). Helping women recover: Creating gender-responsive treatment. In S. L. A. Straussner and S. Brown (Eds.), *The Handbook of Addiction Treatment for Women*. San Francisco, CA: Josse-Bass.

Covington, S., and Surrey, J.L. (1997). The relational model of women's psychological development: Implications for substance abuse. In S. Wilsnack and R. Wilsnack (Eds.), *Gender and alcohol: Individual and social perspectives* (pp. 335-351). New Brunswick, NJ: Rutgers Center of Alcohol Studies.

Demers, A., Bisson, J., and Palluy, J. (1999). Wive's convergence with their husbands' alcohol use: Social conditions as mediators. *Journal of Studies on Alcohol, 60*, 368-377.

DiNitto, D.M., and Crisp, C. (2002). Addictions and women with major psychiatric disorders. In S. L. A. Straussner and S. Brown (Eds.), *The Handbook of Addiction Treatment for Women*. San Francisco, CA: Jossey-Bass.

DiNitto, D.M., and McNeece, C.A. (2008). Addictions and Social Work Practice. In D. M.DiNitto and C. A. McNeece (Eds.), *Social Work Issues and Opportunities: In a Challenging Profession*. Chicago, IL: Lyceum Books, INC.

Doshi, S.R., and Jiles, R. (2006). Health Behaviors among American Indian/Alaska Native women, 1998-2000 BRFSS. *Journal of Women's Health, 15*(8), 919-927.

Droomers, M., Schrijvers, C.T.M., Stronks, K., Mheen, D.v.d., and Mackenback, J.P. (1999). Educational differences in excessive alcohol consumption: The role of psychosocial and material stressors. *Preventive Medicine, 29*, 1-10.

Duncan, R.D., Saunders, B.E., Kilpatrick, D.G., Hanson, R.F., and Resnick, H.S. (1996). Childhood physical assault as a risk factor for PTSD, depression, and substance abuse: Findings from a national survey. *American Journal of Orthopsychiatry, 66*(3), 437-448.

Epstein, J.N., Saunders, B.E., Kilpatrick, D.G., and Resnick, H.S. (1998). PTSD as a mediator between childhood rape and alcohol use in adult women. *Child Abuse and Neglect, 22*(3), 223-234.

Galvani, S. (2006). Alcohol and domestic violence: Women's views. *Violence Against Women, 12*(7), 641-662.

Gomberg, E.S.L. (1994). Risk factors for drinking over a woman's life span. *Alcohol Health and Research World, 18*(3), 220.

Grant, B.F., Dawson, D.A., Stinson, F.S., Chou, S.P., Dufour, M.C., and Pickering, R.P. (2004). The 12-month prevalence and trends in DSM-IV alcohol abuse and dependence: United States, 1991-1992 and 2001-2002. *Drug Alcohol Depend, 74*(3), 223-234.

Gray, M., and Littlefield, M.B. (2002). Black women and addiction. In S. L. A. Straussner and S. Brown (Eds.), *The Handbookf of Addiction Treatment for Women*. San Francisco, CA: Jossey-Bass.

Grayson, C.E., and Nolen-Hoeksema, S. (2005). Motives to drink as mediators between childhood sexual assault and alcohol problems in adult women. *Journal of Traumatic Stress, 18*(2), 137-145.

Hanson, D.J. (1995). The United States of America. In D. B. Heath (Ed.), *International Handbook of Alcohol and Culture*. Westport, Conneticut: Greenwood Press.

Higgins, P.G., Clough, D.H., Frank, B., and Wallerstedt, C. (1995). Changes in health behaviors made by pregnant substance users. *The International Journal of the Addiction, 30*(10), 1323-1333.

Jasinski, J.L., Williams, L.M., and Siegel, J. (2000). Childhood physical and sexual abuse as risk factors for heavy drinking among African-American women: a prospective study. *Child Abuse and Neglect, 24*(8), 1061-1071.

Johnson, R.C., and Nagoshi, C.T. (1989). Asians, Asian-Americans and alcohol. *Journal of psychoactive drugs, 22*, 45-52.

Kaysen, D., Neighbors, C., Martell, J., Fossos, N., and Larimer, M.E. (2006). Incapacitated rape and alcohol use: A prospective analysis. *Addictive Behaviors, 31*, 1820-1832.

Kendler, K.S., Bulik, C.M., Silberg, J., Hettema, J.M., Myers, J., and Prescott, C.A. (2000). Childhood Sexual Abuse and Adult Psychiatric and Substance Use Disorders in Women: An Epidemiological and Cotwin Control Analysis. *Arch Gen Psychiatry, 57*(10), 953-959.

Kilpatrick, D.G., Acierno, R., Resnick, H.S., Saunders, B.E., and Best, C.L. (1997). A 2-year longitudinal analysis of the relationship between violent assault and substance use in women. *Journal of Consulting and Clinical Psychology, 65*(5), 834-847.

Kitano, K.J., and Louie, L.J. (2002). Asian and Pacific Islander women and addiction. In S. L. A. Straussner and S. Brown (Eds.), *The Handbook of Addiction Treatment for Women*. San Francisco, CA: Jossey-Bass.

Koss, M.P., Yuan, N.P., Dightman, D., Prince, R.J., Polacca, M., Sanderson, B., et al. (2003). Adverse childhood exposures and alcohol dependence among seven Native American tribes. *American Journal of Preventive Medicine, 25*(3), 238-244.

Kushnir, M. (1996). Men, women and alcohol: a distinctly unequal and dangerous relationship. *Journal of Insurance Medicine, 28*(1), 7-12.

Lantz, P.M., House, J.S., Lepkowski, J.M., Williams, D.R., Mero, R.P., and Chen, J. (1998). Socioeconomic factors, health behaviors, and mortality. *Journal of American Medical Association, 279*(21), 1703-1708.

Leonard, K.E., and Mudar, P.J. (2000). Alcohol use in the year before marriage: Alcohol expectancies and peer drinking as proximal influences on husband and wife alcohol involvement. *Alcoholism: Clinical and Experimental Research, 24*(11), 1666-1679.

Lillie-Blanton, M., MacKenzie, E., and Anthony, J.C. (1991). Black-white differences in alcohol use by women: Baltimore Survey findings. *Public Health Reports, 106*(2), 124-133.

Little, R.E., and Ervin, C.H. (1984). Alcohol use and reproduction. In S. Wilsnack and L. Beckman (Eds.), *Alcohol Problems in Women*. New York, NY: Guilford Press.

Lohr, M.J., Gillmore, M.R., Gilchrist, L.D., and Butler, S.S. (1992). Factors related to substance use by pregnant school-age adolescents. *Journal of Adolescent Health, 13*, 475-482.

Makimoto, K. (1998). Drinking patterns and drinking problems among Asian-Americans and Pacific Islanders. *Alcohol Health and Research World, 22*(4), 270-275.

Merrick, J.C. (1993). Maternal substance abuse during pregnancy: Policy implications in the United States. *The Journal of Legal Medicine, 14*, 57-71.

Miller, B.A., and Downs, W.r. (1993). The impact of family violence on the use of alcohol by women. *Alcohol Health and Research World, 17*(2), 137.

Miller, B.A., Downs, W.R., and Testa, M. (1993). interrelationships between victimization experiences and women's alcohol use. *Journal of Studies on Alcohol, Supplement*(11), 109-117.

Miranda, R., Meyerson, L.A., Long, P.J., Marx, B.P., and Simpson, S.M. (2002). Sexual assault and alcohol use: Exploring the self-medication hypothesis. *Violence and Victims, 17*(2), 205-217.

Mora, J. (2002). Latinas in cultural transition: Addiction, treatment, and recovery. In S. L. A. Straussner and S. Brown (Eds.), *The Handbook of Addiction Treatment for Women*. San Francisco, CA: Jossey-Bass.

Nakken, J.M. (2002). Addiction and women in the workplace. In S. L. A. Straussner and S. Brown (Eds.), *The Handbook of Addiction Treatment for Women*. San Francisco, CA: Jossey-Bass.

NIAAA. (2002). *Alcohol and Minorities: An update*: National Institute on Alcohol Abuse and Alcoholism.

NIAAA. (2004). *Alcohol- an important women's health issue*: NIAAA.

NIAAA. (2008). *Alcohol: A Women's Health Issue*. Retrieved. from. Nolen-Hoeksema, s. (2004). Gender differences in risk factors and consequences for alcohol use and problems. *Clinical Psychology Review, 24*, 981-1010.

Olenick, N.L., and Chalmers, D.K. (1991). Gender-specific drinking styles in alcoholics and nonalcoholics. *Journal of Studies on Alcohol, 52*(4), 325-330.

Pagliaro, A.M., and Pagliaro, L.A. (2000). *Substance Use Among Women: A Reference and Resource Guide*. Philadelphia, PA: Taylor and Francis

Pilowsky, D.J., Keyes, K.M., and Hasin, D.S. (2009). Adverse childhood events and lifetime alcohol dependence. *American Journal of Public Health, 99*(2), 258-263.

Prescott, C.A., Neale, M.C., Corey, L.A., and Kendler, K.S. (1997). Predictors of problem drinking and alcohol dependence in a population-based sample of female twins. *Journal of Studies on Alcohol, 58*, 167-181.

Rey, G.N. (1995). Mexico. In D. B. Heath (Ed.), *International Handbook on Alcohol and Culture*. Westport, Connecticut: Greenwood Press.

Rosa, M.R.D.L., Holleran, L.K., Rugh, D., and MacMaster, S.A. (2005). Substance abuse among U.S. Latinos: A review of the literature. In M. R. D. L. Rosa, L. K. Holleran and S. L. A. Straussner (Eds.), *Substance Abusing Latinos:Current Research on Epidemiology, Prevention, and Treatment* (pp. 1-20). Binghampton, NY: The Haworth Social Work Practice Press.

Salomon, A., Bassuk, S.S., and Huntington, N. (2002). The relationship between intimate partner violence and the use of additive substances in poor and homeless single mothers. *Violence Against Women, 8*(2), 785-815.

Schmidt, C., Klee, L., and Ames, G. (1990). Review and analysis of literature on indicators of women's drinking problems. *British Journal of Addiction, 85*(2), 179-192.

Shaw, B.A. (2006). Lack of emotional support from parents early in life and alcohol abuse later in life. *International Journal of Aging and Human Development, 63*(1), 49-72.

Skaff, M.M., Finney, J.W., and Moos, R.H. (1999). Gender differences in problem drinking and depression: different "Vulnerabilities?" *American Journal of Community Psychology, 27*(1), 25-54.

Szlemko, W.J., Wood, J.W., and Thurman, P.J. (2006). Native Americans and Alcohol: Past, present, and future. *The Journal of General Psychology, 133*(4), 435-451.

Timko, C., Sutkowi, A., Pavao, J., and Kimerling, R. (2008). Women's childhood and adult adverse experiences, mental health, and binge drinking: The California Women's Health Survey. *Substance Abuse Treatment, Prevention, and Policy, 3*(1), 15.

Ullman, S.E., and Najdowski, C.J. (2009). Revictimization as a moderator of psychosocial risk factors for problem drinking in female sexual assault survivors. *Journal of Studies on Alcohol and Drugs, 70*, 41-49.

Vera, M., Alegria, M., Pattatucci-Aragon, A.M., and Pena, M. (2005). Childhood sexual abuse and drug use among low-income urban Puerto Rican women. In M. R. D. L. Rosa, K. H. Lori and S. L. A. Straussner (Eds.), *Substance Abusing Lationos: Current Research on Epidemiology, Prevention, and Treatment* (pp. 45-68). Binghamton, NY: The Haworth Social Work Practice Press.

Ward, D.A., and Beck, W.L. (1990). Sociological theories and problem drinking behavior. In D. A. Ward (Ed.), *Alcoholism: Introduction to Theory and Treatment* (3rd ed.). Dubuque, Iowa: Kendall/Hunt Publishing Company.

Widom, C.S., Ireland, T., and Glynn, P.J. (1995). Alcohol abuse in abused and neglected children followed-up: Are they at increased risk? *Journal of Studies on Alcohol, 56*, 207-217.

Wilsnack, R.W., and Cheloha, R. (1987). Women's Roles and Problem Drinking across the Lifespan. *Social Problems, 34*(3), 231-248.

Wilsnack, S.C., Klassen, A.D., Schur, B.E., and Wilsnack, R.W. (1991). Predicting onset and chronicity of women's problem drinking: a five-year longitudinal analysis. *American Journal of Public Health, 81*(3), 305-318.

In: Pregnancy and Alcohol Consumption
Editor: Joshua D. Hoffman, pp. 331-346
ISBN 978-1-61761-122-3


*Chapter 14*

# ALCOHOL AND TIME TO PREGNANCY

***Audra L. Gollenberg[1], Maureen A. Cooney[1] and Courtney D. Lynch[2]***

1. Epidemiology Branch, Division of Epidemiology, Statistics and Prevention Research, Eunice Kennedy Shriver National Institute of Child Health and Human Development, National Institutes of Health, Department of Health and Human Services
2. The Ohio State University, School of Public Health, Departments of Epidemiology and Obstetrics and Gynecology, USA

## ABSTRACT

Secular trends showing a decrease in fertility across countries and an increase in the use and demand of infertility treatment in recent years have heightened the search for preventable contributors to impaired fecundity. There has been particular interest in the association between common exposures, such as alcohol intake, and reduced fecundability, given its global accessibility across socioeconomic gradients and thus, potential impact on markers of fecundity. An important marker of fecundity is time to pregnancy (TTP), measured as the at-risk time (in months or cycles) it takes a couple to achieve pregnancy. Sparse literature is available on the association between alcohol use and TTP and the existing studies have found conflicting results, largely from methodologic limitations and variability in study design. For example, some studies were based on large samples (>5,000) of participants, but collected alcohol information on only one partner, others used retrospective capture of both alcohol use and TTP information, a method which can be fraught with inaccuracies and bias. Several of the studies have observed a decreased fecundity for those consuming any alcohol as compared to unexposed individuals, yet still others have suggested a protective effect from certain types of alcoholic beverages. Moreover, other work has suggested that heavy drinking may contribute to the development of ovulatory disorders and thus, a difficulty in conceiving. It is important when reviewing the current state of the literature to take into consideration the different methodologies used in studying this association. Overall, the field requires more large, prospective cohort studies to elucidate the association between alcohol use by type and frequency and markers of fecundity using a couple-based approach before we can definitively inform couples regarding the risks and benefits of preconception alcohol use.

## INTRODUCTION

In 2002, the National Survey of Family Growth estimated that 7.3 million U.S. women ages 15-44 had sought infertility services at some point in their life [1]. Further, it was estimated that 11.8% of those women had an impaired ability to have children (i.e., impaired fecundity). Most of the women with an impaired ability to conceive (7.4%) reported taking longer than 12 months to become pregnant (i.e., the clinical definition of infertility) [2].

While some estimates show a decrease in the prevalence of infertility since 1982 this may be due in part to varying definitions as well as sparse national and international data on an outcome which has been poorly measured. Despite this difficulty conceiving remains an important public health problem [2]. Infertility treatment is expensive, often not fully covered by insurance, and treatment is associated with adverse health outcomes in resulting offspring [3]. This is particularly concerning in light of the recently recognized culture of impatience to conceive [4]. Couples wishing to become pregnant are often now very focused on achieving the optimal timing for sexual intercourse. Further, those who do not conceive right away are typically anxious to seek treatment.

While the advent of ovulation stimulating medication and assisted reproductive technologies (ART) has done much to help those experiencing difficulty conceiving, a primary prevention approach is clearly preferable both in terms of cost and health outcomes. Despite this, very few modifiable risk factors for infertility have been identified aside from smoking. The identification of such risk factors necessitates prospective investigation, as retrospective queries of women who have delivered suffer from selection bias (i.e., they are limited to women who eventually achieved pregnancy) and recall bias (i.e., women are often asked to recall their alcohol use many months or even years prior).

Alcohol consumption is a lifestyle factor that deserves attention. Recent estimates suggest that 41% of U.S. women are current regular drinkers (defined as >12 drinks in the last year) and an additional 17% are current infrequent drinkers (defined as ≤ 12 drinks in the last year [5]. Further, one of the most comprehensive studies to date to examine factors related to the probability of conception reported that only 17% of women reported no alcohol intake (reported on a weekly basis) while trying to become pregnant [6]. It should be noted, however, that this study took place in Denmark, where rates of alcohol consumption may be higher than in the United States. Given the high prevalence of alcohol use among women, even a small increase in fecundity impairment associated with alcohol consumption with trying to conceive would be important at the population level.

Alcohol is a known reproductive toxicant; it has been shown to have a direct impact on the hypothalamic-pituitary-gonadal axis [7]. Women who consume alcohol frequently or in large amounts have a higher prevalence of amenorrhea and menstrual disorders [8]. Heavy drinkers also have a higher incidence of miscarriage and other adverse pregnancy outcomes [9;10]. Although there have been several small studies examining the impact of male alcohol consumption on semen quality, there remains of dearth of information in this area [11;12].

This chapter reviews the state of the science on the relation between alcohol exposure and time to pregnancy (a common measure of fecundity impairment). We first review the retrospective observational studies that have been completed and then focus more thoroughly on the few prospective studies that have examined this issue. Finally, we discuss the public health significance of the weight of evidence to date and suggest future directions for research.

## RETROSPECTIVE DESIGNS

Until recently, most of what we knew about the influences on human fecundity came from retrospective epidemiologic studies. Retrospective studies of time to pregnancy (TTP) are defined by their recruitment of women (or couples) after they have become pregnant, ascertaining information about their waiting time to pregnancy and associated exposures upon entry into the study. This study design requires women to recall their past behaviors and their TTPs. Retrospective studies can be pregnancy based cohorts, where women are enrolled at some point during their pregnancy and asked to recall their TTPs or they can be constructed from a generalized population asking women to recall their reproductive history. Pregnancy cohorts offer the advantage that there is less time elapsed between recruitment and the time when she was trying to become pregnant, thus women may be able to remember TTP better than if they were asked to recall this years later after the pregnancy.

There are several limitations to retrospective studies which should be noted and a broad literature which discuss these in more detail [13-15]. As mentioned earlier, there is the potential for poor recall of TTP and any exposures when measured distantly from when they actually occurred and this could result in misclassification. It is possible that some of this misclassification could be differential if women who took longer or shorter times to become pregnant remembered their behaviors more or less accurately. It could also be argued that such misclassification, if it exists, would be non-differential, as the effects of these exposures, such as alcohol, on time to pregnancy are not well known. Another problem in retrospective measurement of lifestyle behaviors is that one has to rely on women remembering 'on average' what they consumed while trying to become pregnant. Therefore, any extremes might not be captured well in relation to the outcome. On the outcome side, recalled time to pregnancy has been demonstrated to be a reliable measure assessed via telephone and questionnaire over time [16-18] and at least one previous study has shown that TTP is valid if recalled over a short time period [19]. However, recently questions have been raised about the validity of long term recall of time to pregnancy [20].

Beyond the misclassification of both the exposure and the outcome in this type of study there are other concerns with a retrospective design to assess the effects of alcohol on TTP. By only including women who have a reported time to pregnancy, investigators will be limiting the study population to women who eventually got pregnant and thus eliminating any women who are infertile. This population could be captured, however, with the prospective design. Additionally, many women may consider that time to pregnancy would have to end in a live birth, thus pregnancies ending in miscarriage may not be included in such a sample.

Included in this review of retrospective studies of alcohol and fecundity are studies which employ a variety of study designs, but all of which include alcohol as a exposure and some measure of time to pregnancy defined most ideally as TTP, but often categorized by subfertility or infertility (TTP>12 months) as the outcome. This chapter does not address the association seen between alcohol and infertility as measured by medical diagnosis, although some study designs include women who utilized infertility services.

Most retrospective studies to date have reported no association between increased consumption of alcoholic beverages and time to pregnancy. However, it is important to consider both the study design and definitions of exposure and outcome while interpreting these results. Olsen and colleagues have the earliest reported null study of alcohol and time to pregnancy which was a case-control design [21]. In their study, cases were defined as women treated for infertility at a participating hospital and controls were women with a live birth from the same hospital during a similar time period (1977-1980). Questionnaires were used to assess use of alcohol while trying to conceive and intake was recorded in drinks per week. One drink was equivalent to one beer, one glass of wine, or one spirit. A similar study comparing 1818 infertile women and 2817 fertile women was conducted across multiple institutions in the U.S. and Canada [22]. In this case-control study, the authors ascertained alcohol use in consumption per week of wine (glasses/wk), beer (cans/wk), and liquor (oz/wk) and used logistic regression to estimate risk of infertility by alcohol consumption. No alteration of the odds ratio was found between groups. The case-control design and ensuing analysis (logistic regression) are not appropriate for the research question. Furthermore it is difficult to tell from this study whether the cases who had reported infertility were reporting their TTP from when they first started trying or when they first sought medical care.

In a different study of pregnant women, data on alcohol use and non-contracepting cycles were analyzed for 678 women with Cox proportional hazards [23]. No association was seen with an increase in consumption of alcoholic beverages and the fecundablity odds ratio. In a cross sectional study of 1909 women presenting for their first prenatal visit in Connecticut between 1980-82, no association was seen between self-reported consumption of alcohol while trying to become pregnant and TTP in a fecundability odds ratio model [24]. Curtis and colleagues published a study in 1997 on data from the Ontario Farm Family Health Study [25]. In this study, time to pregnancy was asked for each of the 2,607 planned pregnancies included. Questions about glasses per week of beer, wine, and liquor were asked of men and women for the time they were first married as well as during the year prior to the questionnaire and a time-weighted linear interpolation of these data were used to estimate the usual consumption for each interval of trying to conceive. Data were analyzed for both women and men using an analog of the Cox proportional hazards model and no associations were seen between alcohol and TTP. Yet another study of over 4000 women in multiple countries in Europe recruited both pregnant women and women from the general population who were defined as trying to become pregnant. In an analysis of alcohol (beer/wk, wine/wk/aperitifs/wk, and spirits/wk) while trying to become pregnant in both the male and female partners no effect of alcohol on time to pregnancy either categorized or examined continuously [26].

In the more recent retrospective studies, some associations between alcohol use and time to pregnancy have been observed [27-29]. In an analysis of data from the Danish National Birth Cohort, pregnant women (N=29,884) were asked to report how many glasses of wine, beer, or spirits they drank per week while trying to become pregnant. The outcome of TTP was categorized and subfecundity was defined as a TTP >12 months [28]. An association was observed (OR=1.3; 95%CI (1.0-1.7)) for subfecundity among parous women reporting >14 drinks per week while trying to become pregnant compared to women reporting between .5 and 2 drinks per week. When the whole population was considered, women who had no drinks compared to women who at least one drink had an increased odds for subfecundity (>12 months) as well (OR=1.5; 95%CI, 1.3- 1.6). This study suggested a shorter time to pregnancy among women who reported some alcohol intake versus none while women who had the highest alcohol compared to those who had a small intake had a longer time to pregnancy. Following up on their earlier work, Juhl and colleagues then looked at these data to see whether the type of alcoholic beverage consumed affected time to pregnancy [29]. In this analysis, they found that wine drinkers had a slightly shorter waiting time to pregnancy (fecundability odds ratios between 0.7 and 0.9, p<.05) than both non-wine drinkers and consumers of other alcoholic beverages. Finally in a recent study in the UK among 2112 pregnant women, a significantly longer TTP was observed if the male partner consumed >20 drinks per week (p<.001) compared to men who consumed no alcohol [27]. Moderate alcohol intake of either and both the male and female partner were not associated with time to pregnancy in this study.

Overall, the evidence from retrospective studies of alcohol and time to pregnancy are mixed. Many studies are not designed with this research question in mind and therefore the ascertainment of the exposure and the outcome are not uniformly well defined. It is important when considering this body of literature as a whole to take into consideration study design, the outcome measured, and how the exposure was ascertained. In summary, early retrospective studies have shown no effect of alcohol consumption (in either the male or female partner) to be associated with time to pregnancy, but more recent retrospective studies have shown suggestive effects that moderate alcohol consumption might decrease TTP, further emphasizing the need for prospective capture of both exposure and outcome.

## PROSPECTIVE DESIGNS

The strongest evidence of health effects is derived from studies employing the experimental design, in which groups of participants are randomized to receive a certain treatment/exposure and health endpoints are measured thereafter. However, this method is not an ethical option when studying the potentially harmful effects of toxins and/or certain lifestyle behaviors, thus investigators are left with observational study designs to answer pertinent questions regarding factors affecting fecundability. The prospective design involves recruiting couples preconceptionally and following them forward through time until pregnancy is achieved, or censoring if the study's end is reached first. The prospective design usually receives more weight than data collected through a retrospective design due to the investigator's ability to assign a temporal ordering between exposure(s) and outcome(s), minimize information bias in recalling past exposures, measure exposure(s) more accurately, and assess covariate information at multiple time points, as summarized by Buck et al. [30]. Alcohol use is typically assessed upon enrollment through questionnaire or interview and updated either monthly with additional questionnaires or daily through daily diaries in prospective TTP studies.

Prospective cohort studies with preconception enrollment have been described as expensive and difficult to conduct. However, empirical evidence suggests that such studies are feasible, even in the context of population-based sampling, and are often the only way to collect valid data on longitudinal and time-varying environmental, biological and lifestyle exposures that may affect both fecundity and fetal development [30]. In a comprehensive review, Buck et al. identified 15 studies that utilized the prospective pregnancy design with preconception enrollment. Recruitment and dropout rates varied widely by study depending on design, requirements, and recruitment strategies from 42 to 100% and 3 to 62%, respectively [30].

Prospective designs allow for the longitudinal capture of menses, sexual intercourse, lifestyle behaviors, environmental and biological factors, and cycle-based ascertainment of conception through biological measures, and do not rely on retrospective recall of TTP. Multiple types of selection bias may be avoided through the use of prospective studies, mostly due to issues inherent in this design. Whereas prospective studies of chronic diseases often require decades of follow-up, prospective pregnancy studies can be completed in a relatively short time period. Because prospective studies require recruitment of highly motivated individuals, it has been argued that they are not generalizable to all reproductive-aged women, and that retrospective studies have the advantage of being representative of the target population. As yet, there are no data to support this claim. Moreover, retrospective TTP studies are not representative of the referent population of all at-risk cycles because they systematically under-represent subfecund couples and over-represent fertile couples.

With regard to alcohol consumption, there have been four studies to date that have assessed the association between alcohol use and fecundability using a prospective cohort design [6;31-33]. Even within this domain of study design, there were differences in the methodologies employed and these factors will be discussed in light of the studies' results and interpretation.

The first prospective study seeking to answer the question of alcohol's effect on TTP was conducted from June 1987 to January 1989 by Florack et al. [32]. In this study, 259 female, Dutch workers aged 18-39 years and their partners were recruited and followed for up to 12 months of trying to conceive. Of the total eligible women contacted, the response rate was high at 85%. Alcohol use of both partners was assessed at baseline through a structured questionnaire and quantified as to the total number of alcoholic drinks per week [32]. The baseline questionnaire also collected information on caffeine intake, cigarette, pipe, or cigar smoking, occupational activity and exposures, and reproductive history. Throughout follow-up, participants tracked menstrual periods, occupational exposures, and changes in behavioral risk factors using a special calendar for a maximum of 12 months. If the expected date of menstruation was missed by >5 days, a first-morning urine sample was sent to the study laboratory for a pregnancy test using hCG measurement.

The authors analyzed the association between alcohol use and TTP using a discrete analog of the Cox proportional hazards model and estimating the fecundability odds ratio (FOR). After 1 year's participation in the study, 170 (65%) women had had at least one positive pregnancy test. The level of alcohol consumption of the female partner was not associated to fecundability (FOR= 1.1; 95% CI, 0.6-1.8 and FOR=1.2; 95% CI, 0.7-2.3) for women who consumed 5-10 drinks per week and ≥10 drinks per week, respectively, as compared to those who consumed <5 drinks per week at baseline. Among the partners, there was a small, positive relationship between alcohol consumption and fecundability (FOR=1.6; 95% CI, 1.0-2.4) for men who consumed ≥10 drinks per week as compared to those who consumed <5 drinks per week. The authors assessed a number of covariates as confounders (age, gravidity, previous spontaneous abortions, medical drug utilization, current chronic disease, educational level); however, none of the covariates altered the association between alcohol and fecundability.

Strengths of this study include prospective collection of TTP and of alcohol and covariate information on both partners. However, the authors appeared to rely on alcohol consumption at baseline as representative of participant use throughout follow-up, which may or may not hold true. In this manner, the authors were not able to allow alcohol use to vary from cycle to cycle in statistical models, thus altering the cycle-specific odds of conception. A second limitation acknowledged by the authors was the possibility of selection bias in their sample due to the likelihood that less fertile couples were more likely to enroll in their cohort and because they were more eager to participate. Indeed, the authors allowed participants to join the cohort even if they had been trying to conceive at baseline, and for some couples, this had been over a year. However, it was not clearly stated how TTP was categorized for couples who had initiated trying to conceive before study enrollment. Finally, this study did not collect information on frequency or timing of intercourse; therefore, it was not possible to determine the at-risk status of each cycle.

In the next two prospective studies, female alcohol use was associated with a reduced fecundability [6;33]. In the largest prospective study to date, Jensen et al. recruited 430 couples from 1992 to 1995 through a nationwide mailing of letters to trade union members in Denmark [6]. Eligible women were 20-35 years old, lived with a partner, had no children and had no previous reproductive experience and intended to discontinue contraception. An average participation rate of 16% was estimated. Couples were enrolled when they discontinued contraception and were followed for up to six menstrual cycles. At baseline, both partners completed a questionnaire on demographic, medical, reproductive, occupational, and lifestyle factors and the men provided a semen sample. Couples also completed a monthly questionnaire on changes in occupational exposures and lifestyle factors for the week before questionnaire completion (day 21), thus pertaining to days 14-21 in the cycle. For alcohol, caffeine and smoking intake, couples were asked to report on average intake as either daily or weekly consumption during the week prior to questionnaire completion. The total weekly alcohol intake was calculated by summing the intake of beer, wine and spirits. While trying to conceive, women completed daily diaries on vaginal bleeding and sexual intercourse. Cycles with no intercourse from day 11 to 20 were excluded from analyses as no couples who refrained from intercourse in that period became pregnant (47 cycles) [6].

TTP was defined as the number of cycles from the day couples discontinued contraception to pregnancy recognition. Couples who dropped out of the study before six follow-up cycles were censored at the cycle in which they stopped participation (n=22). Data were available on 423 couples with 1596 cycles, after excluding seven couples with azoospermia (absence of live spermatozoa in the semen) [6]. The association between alcohol intake and fecundability was analyzed through survival analysis techniques and the computation of the FOR.

Among women with a weekly average alcohol intake of <5 drinks, 179/280 (64%) conceived within six cycles compared with 75/136 (55%) of women with higher intake (Jensen). In adjusted analyses, there was a statistically significant trend of decreasing FOR with increasing alcohol intake (p=0.03). As compared to abstainers, the FORs for increasing weekly alcohol intake were the following: for 1-5 drinks, FOR=0.61; 95% CI, 0.40-0.93; for 6-10 drinks, FOR=0.55; 95% CI, 0.36-0.85; for 11-15 drinks, FOR=0.34; 95% CI, 0.22-0.52;

and >15 drinks, FOR=0.34; 95% CI, 0.11-1.07. These estimates were adjusted for cycle number, smoking in either partner, smoking exposure *in utero*, center of enrollment, diseases in female reproductive organs, women's body mass index, use of oral contraceptives before conception attempts, sperm concentration, and duration of menstrual cycle. For the male partners, there was no significant association between alcohol intake and conception probability. When the authors analyzed fecundability according to type of woman's alcohol intake (i.e. spirits, wine and beer), there was no significant association between alcohol intake and fecundability, though there was a suggestion of lower fecundability with higher alcohol intake.

Strengths of this study include prospective measurement of both exposure and outcome (i.e. alcohol intake and TTP), collection of lifestyle factors on both partners, and extensive adjustment of potential confounding factors. The authors were also able to eliminate couples with little or no chance of conceiving due to azoospermia. Limitations include a follow-up time period of only six cycles, when it is thought that a small proportion of normal and healthy couples may take up to 12 cycles to conceive. It is a strength that the authors collected alcohol information for each cycle of follow-up, but this information was restricted to the week prior to questionnaire completion. This method assumes that the most important exposure window for alcohol intake is during the menstrual week of days 14-21, when in reality this may not hold true. In addition, this method required a recall of alcohol intake over the past week, though this time period of recall was limited. Overall, Jensen et al. concluded that even modest amounts of alcohol intake by the female partner may increase TTP, whereas alcohol intake by the male partner had little effect on TTP.

In the next study published around the same time as that of Jensen et al., Hakim et al. recruited women employed at two semiconductor plants in Burlington, VT and East Fishkill, NY to participate in a prospective study of reproductive health from May 1989 to August 1991 (Hakim et al 1998). Eligibility required that women be of reproductive age, not using oral contraceptives or intrauterine devices, and not surgically sterilized. Participants completed a baseline questionnaire at enrollment and daily diaries on vaginal bleeding, unprotected sexual intercourse, and pregnancy symptoms throughout follow-up. Daily urine specimens were also collected by women throughout follow-up to detect hormonal changes indicative of ovulation and early pregnancy through hCG measurement. Urine specimens were stored in participants' home freezers and shipped to the study laboratory monthly. At baseline and monthly throughout follow-up, nurse coordinators interviewed women about their average daily consumption of mixed alcoholic drinks, beer, wine, cigarettes, coffee, tea and caffeinated soft drinks for the past month. Alcoholic drinks were categorized as 0 intake, up to 1 drink per week, 1-7 drinks per week, and >7 drinks per week.

The authors defined the unit of analysis as the number of menstrual cycles in which both ovulation and unprotected sexual intercourse occurred until the time of conception. The authors did not explicitly state how long women were followed to achieve pregnancy; however, women were given $100 for every 6 months of study involvement. Multivariable logistic regression models were used to compute the per cycle risk of conception and to estimate ORs and CIs while correcting for multiple cycles and conceptions per woman using the quasi-likelihood method. Age, race, education, pregnancy and fertility history, number of days of intercourse during a cycle, and smoking were considered as potential confounders.

**Table 1. Studies of Alcohol and Time to Pregnancy, 1983-2009**

| Year | 1st Author | Design | Population | Alcohol assessment | TTP assess-ment | Follow-up | Main results | Statistical Adjustments |
|---|---|---|---|---|---|---|---|---|
| Retrospective Studies | | | | | | | | |
| 1983 | Olsen | Retro-spective | n=5374 women (1069 infertility cases, 4305 live birth controls) | questionnaires/ drinks per week | recalled TTP | n/a | Alcohol not associated with subfecundity OR=0.9, (95% CI 0.7-1.1) | Case-control design; adjusted for smoking, OC use, age, residence, education, and parity |
| 1985 | Baird | Retro-spective | n=678 pregnant women | questionnaires/ drinks per week | recalled TTP | n/a | Alcohol use not associated with fecundability | None |
| 1993 | Joesoef | Retro-spective | n=4635 women (1818 infertile women and 2817 fertile women) | interviews/ drinks per week | recalled TTP | n/a | Alcohol use not associated with infertility OR=1.0, 95% CI 0.8-1.2 for the highest compared with no drinks per week | Case-control design; adjusted for smoking, maijuana use, cocaine use, BMI, education, age at menarche, gravidity, frequency of intercourse, and spontaenous abortions |
| 1993 | Hatch | Retro-spective | n=1909 pregnant women | interviews/ drinks per week | recalled TTP | n/a | Alcohol use not associated with fecundability | None |
| 1997 | Curtis | Retro-spective | n=2607 planned pregnancies; both male and female partners | questionnaires/ drinks per week | recalled TTP | n/a | Alcohol use not associated with fecundability women any vs. none: FOR=1.0, 95% CI 0.9-1.1; men any vs. none: FOR= 1.0 95% CI 0.9-1.1) | Adjusted for spouse's alcohol use, woman's age when trying to conceive, recent OC use, men's and women's smoking |
| 1997 | Olsen | Retro-spective | n=4035 pregnant women | questionnaires/ drinks per week | recalled TTP | n/a | Alcohol use not associated with fecundablity OR=1.3, 95% CI 0.8-2.1 for women in the highest intake vs. no intake; OR=1.3, 95% CI 0.9-1.7 for men in the highest versus no intake | Adjusted for female smoking, female age, OC use, coffee intake, and female working history; analyzed first pregnancies |

**Table 1. Studies of Alcohol and Time to Pregnancy, 1983-2009 (Continued)**

| Year | 1st Author | Design | Population | Alcohol assessment | TTP assess-ment | Follow-up | Main results | Statistical Adjustments |
|---|---|---|---|---|---|---|---|---|
| 2002 | Juhl | Retro-spective | n=39612 pregnant women | questionnaires/ drinks per week | recalled TTP | n/a | Alcohol use associated with shorter and longer TTP. Among parous women, >14 drinks per week vs. none: OR=1.3, 95% CI 1.0-1.7. Among all women, any intake vs. no intake: OR=1.2, 95% CI 1.1.-1.3. | Adjusted for age, parity, smoking, BMI |
| 2003 | Juhl | Retro-spective | n=29844 pregnant women | questionnaires/ drinks per week | recalled TTP | n/a | Alcohol use (wine use) is associated with a shorter TTP compared to women with no wine use. ORs 0.7-0.9 (p<.05) for varying amounts. Beer and spirits were not associated with fecundability. | Adjusted for age, parity, smoking, BMI, occupation, PID or abdominal issues |
| 2004 | Hassan | Retro-spective | n=2112 pregnant women | questionnaires/ drinks per week | recalled TTP | n/a | Alcohol use in the male partner associated with a subfecundity. Among men: drinking >20 drinks per week vs. none, OR=2.2, 95% CI 1.1-4.4 | Adjusted for women's age, weight, smoking, alcohol consumption, tea/coffee intake, drug abuse, parity, contraceptive use, menstrual pattern, men's age, men's smoking, drug abuse, coital frequencey and living standard |
| Prospective Studies | | | | | | | | |
| 1994 | Florack | Pro-spective | n=259 women and partners | Questionnaire at baseline; alcoholic drinks per week for current use | Diaries kept for men-strual periods; if missed >5 days, urine hCG test | 12 months | Alcohol use of women not associated with fecundability. For males, >10 drinks vs. <5, associated with a greater fecundability. FOR=1.6, 95% CI 1.0-2.4 | Confounders assessed but did not alter models |

| Year | 1st Author | Design | Population | Alcohol assessment | TTP assessment | Follow-up | Main results | Statistical Adjustments |
|---|---|---|---|---|---|---|---|---|
| 1998 | Jensen | Prospective | n=430 women and partners, 20-35 | Questionnaire at baseline; monthly questionnaire to update alcohol; alcohol use was the average for days 14-21 | Daily diaries on bleeding and inter-course | 6 cycles | Alcohol associated with decreased fecundability. 1-5 drinks vs. 0 drinks per week, FOR= 0.61, 95% CI 0.4-0.93; for >10 drinks vs. 0 drinks per week, FOR=0.34, 95% CI 0.22-0.52. Ptrend=0.03. | Adjusted for cycle number, smoking in both partners, smoking exposure in utero, reproductive organ diseases, BMI, OC use before conception, sperm concentration, and duration of menstrual cycle. |
| 1998 | Hakim | Prospective | n=124 women | At baseline and monthly, information on type and amount of alcohol intake | hCG assay for early pregnancy; hormones to test for ovulation in urine | Information not provided | Alcohol use is associated with a decreased fecundability. 13-90 g/week alcohol vs none: OR=0.4, 95% CI 0.21-0.77; >90g vs. none: non-significant but small sample. Caffeine and alcohol interaction observed. | Adjusted for age, frequency of sexual intercourse, caffeine intake, and restricted to nonsmokers. |
| 2009 | Buck Louis | Prospective | n=83 women | Daily diaries while trying to conceive; calculated drinks per cycle | Daily diaries and home hCG testing | 12 at-risk cycles | Alcohol use is associated with a decreased fecundability. For every increase in unit serving of alcohol consumed standardized to 28-day cycle: FOR=0.96, 95% CI 0.93-1.00 adjusted for confounders. | Adjusted for frequency of intercourse, PCBs, age, parity, serum lipids, and smoking |

TTP denotes time to pregnancy.
FOR denotes fecundability odds ratio, 95% CI denotes confidence interval.
OR denotes general odds ratio.
hCG denotes human chorionic gonadotropin testing for early pregnancy.
BMI denotes body mass index.
OC denotes oral contraceptives.
PID denotes pelvic inflammatory disease.
PCBs denote polychlorinated biphenyls.

After excluding 24 women who were anovular or did not report unprotected sexual intercourse, n=124 contributed at least one at-risk menstrual cycle to the analysis (total at-risk cycles = 678). Sixty-six (53.2%) women conceived 99 pregnancies throughout follow-up with a 14.6% conception rate per cycle. Because the authors observed a strong, negative effect of smoking on conception probability (smokers vs. nonsmokers: FOR=0.01; 95% CI, 0.0-0.19), the association between alcohol and fecundability was analyzed only among nonsmokers. The authors observed a statistically significant dose-response association between alcohol use and fecundability among nonsmokers: FOR=0.43; 95% CI, 0.25-0.76; FOR=0.40; 95% CI, 0.21-0.77, FOR=0.65; 95% CI, 0.20-2.15, respectively, for up to 1 drink/week, 1-7 drinks/week, and >7 drinks/week as compared to abstainers after adjustment for age, number of sexual intercourse occurrences per cycle, caffeine consumption. In addition, the authors conducted an interesting joint analysis of alcohol and caffeine consumption among nonsmoking women. The combination of alcohol and light caffeine appeared to further reduce the risk of conception among nonsmoking women. Women who consumed any alcohol and >100 mg of caffeine per day (~1 cup of coffee per day) had a significantly reduced risk of conception (FOR=0.26; 95% CI, 0.13-0.56) as compared to women who abstained from alcohol and consumed less than 100 mg caffeine per day.

Strengths of this study include repeated, prospective capture of alcohol use, ovulation, sexual intercourse, and conceptions including biomarkers of ovulation. However, updates on alcohol use were limited by participant recall over the previous month. The authors were also able to separate out the effects of smoking and alcohol with a stratified analysis among nonsmokers and to conduct an interesting joint analysis of the combined effects of caffeine and alcohol. Limitations include reliance on alcohol use captured retrospectively over the previous month, though this information was updated monthly, and the lack of information on partner use of alcohol and tobacco products. Nevertheless, the results from Hakim et al. appear to agree with that of the largest prospective study by Jensen et al. in that female alcohol use appears to decrease fecundability.

In the most recent prospective study of alcohol use and fecundability, Buck Louis et al. [31] recruited women aged 18-44 who were participants in the New York State Angler Cohort study who stated at enrollment that they were considering future pregnancies. Seventy-six percent (n=787) of women located in 1996-1997 were ineligible either due to age or not planning a future pregnancy. Of those eligible, n=113 (46%) reported they were planning a pregnancy in the next 6 months and were interested in participation. After excluding 14 women who were pregnant upon enrollment or before the baseline interview, 99 women enrolled in the study of which 83 women completed the daily diary cards for TTP calculation.

Study nurses conducted a baseline interview at the time of discontinuation of contraception to collect information about lifestyle and medical history. Participants were also instructed on the use of home pregnancy tests for use on the day menses was expected and one week later regardless of test result. Daily diaries were used throughout study follow-up of 12 at-risk cycles or until pregnancy was recognized, to capture menstruation, sexual intercourse, occasional use of birth control, cigarette smoking, alcohol and caffeine use, multivitamin use, and sport fish consumption.

Data were censored on the day following the participants' final outcome: the day following a first positive pregnancy test for women with live births, the day following a pregnancy loss, or the day following 12 cycles with at least one act of intercourse during the fertile window in the absence of pregnancy. TTP was defined as the number of menstrual cycles required for pregnancy as measured by a positive pregnancy test. For women who conceived prior to the first recorded menses and contributed 1-2 weeks of follow-up data, they were considered to have conceived at cycle 0. FORs were estimated with a discrete analog of the Cox model with time-varying covariates.

Of the 83 women with complete daily diaries, women who did not become pregnant reported consuming 15.4 (±14.6) alcoholic beverages per standardized menstrual cycle as compared to 9.2 (±10.8) beverages for those who did conceive ($p=0.05$). Alcohol consumption was associated with a significantly reduced FOR in the fully adjusted model (FOR=0.93; 95% CI, 0.93-0.99), after adjusting for polychlorinated biphenyls concentration, serum lipids, frequency of intercourse, age, parity, and cigarette usage.

This most recent study has several advantages including daily collection of alcohol use, sexual intercourse, and menstruation for 12 at-risk cycles making it likely the most accurate in terms of exposure collection and reporting. However, the sample size was limited at 83 women, thus it is the smallest study of the 4 prospective studies and did not have information on the male partners. Nevertheless, the study was powered to detect a statistically significant association between alcohol use and fecundability and the result agreed with 3 out of the 4 prospective studies to date.

Overall, 3 out of 5 prospective TTP studies found a negative association between alcohol use and fecundability suggesting that alcohol use may lengthen the time it takes to conceive. Of the 4 studies discussed here in detail, the one study that did not report this association [32] relied on baseline alcohol use as the measure of exposure throughout follow-up. The assumption that baseline alcohol use is representative of alcohol use while trying to conceive may have resulted in misclassification and a bias toward the null. In contrast, the other three studies that reported a negative association between alcohol use and fecundability updated participant alcohol use either monthly or daily throughout follow-up thus allowing alcohol use to vary by cycle. The second study to report no association between alcohol use and TTP analyzed this association in a prospective study primarily focused on caffeine consumption, though they provided little detail on the method of alcohol assessment, which limits interpretation [34]. In conclusion, the majority of prospective studies to date have reported that alcohol use by the female partner may increase TTP.

## Summary and Future Directions

While studies that have employed retrospective observational designs have yielded mixed results with regard to the association between alcohol use and fertility impairments, evidence from prospective studies is suggestive of an adverse impact of maternal alcohol consumption, even at low to moderate levels on impaired fecundity. In contrast, the evidence of an association between male alcohol consumption and increased waiting time to pregnancy is weak. As such, it is likely prudent to advise women who are planning a pregnancy to reduce or even discontinue alcohol use, especially if they are reporting a failure to conceive following several months of regular, well-timed intercourse.

Despite the numerous studies that have examined this issue over the years, there has yet to be a well-designed prospective study that collects enough detailed information on alcohol consumption to permit a thorough examination of the impact of various kinds of alcohol, frequency and timing of dose as well as interactions with other important covariates such as smoking, contraception use, and coital frequency. All of the prospective studies to date have examined the impact of alcohol use as a secondary analysis and therefore have been limited to the covariate information collected to fulfill the studies' primary aims. Furthermore, many prospective studies were still subject to misclassification of exposure due to recall bias, as several studies asked women to retrospectively recall their consumption over a period of a week or a month.

Detailed daily-level information that is recorded prospectively with self-report corroborated by a biomarker of exposure would be the "gold standard" method of alcohol intake assessment and would permit the necessary examination of type, timing and dose of alcohol in relation to the day-specific probabilities of conception. While retrospective studies are often logistically easier and less expensive to conduct, a prospective design is essential to this line of investigation. In order to have an accurate measure of the role that alcohol plays with regard to fecundity impairment studies must include all women who are attempting to conceive, including those who are later found to be infertile. A failure to include these women will result in a vast underestimate of the association between alcohol consumption and fecundity impairment. The issue of gravidity cannot be ignored. If, for instance, a woman who experiences an adverse outcome in her first pregnancy quits drinking alcohol as a precaution when she plans her second pregnancy, such behavior would result in a spurious association between abstinence from alcohol and adverse pregnancy outcomes (assuming the adverse outcome was due to some unrelated cause). As such, it is preferable to enroll nulligravid women in these studies whose fertility status is unknown.

In summary, the literature is suggestive of an adverse impact of alcohol use by women, even at mild or moderate levels, on the prevalence of fecundity impairments. While the effect of alcohol consumption on male fecundity remains unclear due to a lack of data; there remains the possibility of a joint effect of male and female alcohol consumption on waiting time to pregnancy. While a well-designed prospective study is required to elucidate the mechanisms and pathways of this association, available evidence is suggestive of an adverse impact of female alcohol consumption while trying to become pregnant. To this end clinicians should view alcohol as a modifiable lifestyle factor and encourage patients to alter their behavior if they are having trouble becoming pregnant, as this may be a low cost option for trying to maximize fecundity.

## References

[1] Chandra A, Martinez GM, Mosher WD, Abma JC, Jones J. Fertility, family planning, and reproductive health of U.S. women: data from the 2002 National Survey of Family Growth. *Vital Health Stat*. 23 2005;(25):1-160.

[2] Chandra A, Stephen EH. Impaired fecundity in the United States: 1982-1995. *Fam. Plann Perspect* 1998; 30(1):34-42.

[3] Jackson RA, Gibson KA, Wu YW, Croughan MS. Perinatal outcomes in singletons following in vitro fertilization: a meta-analysis. *Obstet. Gynecol.* 2004; 103(3):551-563.

[4] Leridon H. Sterility and subfecundity: from silence to impatience? *Popul. Engl. Sel.* 1992;35-54.

[5] Pleis JR, Lucas JW. Summary health statistics for U.S. adults: National Health Interview Survey, 2007. *Vital Health Stat*. 10 2009;(240):1-159.

[6] Jensen TK, Hjollund NH, Henriksen TB et al. Does moderate alcohol consumption affect fertility? Follow up study among couples planning first pregnancy. *BMJ* 1998; 317(7157):505-510.

[7] Gavaler JS, Van Thiel DH, Lester R. Ethanol: a gonadal toxin in the mature rat of both sexes. *Alcohol. Clin. Exp. Res*. 1980; 4(3):271-276.

[8] Becker U, Tonnesen H, Kaas-Claesson N, Gluud C. Menstrual disturbances and fertility in chronic alcoholic women. *Drug Alcohol Depend*. 1989; 24(1):75-82.

[9] Harlap S, Shiono PH. Alcohol, smoking, and incidence of spontaneous abortions in the first and second trimester. *Lancet* 1980; 2(8187):173-176.

[10] Hadi HA, Hill JA, Castillo RA. Alcohol and reproductive function: a review. *Obstet. Gynecol. Surv*. 1987; 42(2):69-74.

[11] Dunphy BC, Barratt CL, Cooke ID. Male alcohol consumption and fecundity in couples attending an infertility clinic. *Andrologia* 1991; 23(3):219-221.

[12] Parazzini F, Marchini M, Tozzi L, Mezzopane R, Fedele L. Risk factors for unexplained dyspermia in infertile men: a case-control study. *Arch. Androl*. 1993; 31(2):105-113.

[13] Baird DD, Weinberg CR, Rowland AS. Reporting errors in time-to-pregnancy data collected with a short questionnaire. Impact on power and estimation of fecundability ratios. *Am. J. Epidemiol*. 1991; 133(12):1282-1290.

[14] Joffe M. Feasibility of studying subfertility using retrospective self reports. *J. Epidemiol. Community Health* 1989; 43(3):268-274.

[15] Weinberg CR, Baird DD, Wilcox AJ. Sources of bias in studies of time to pregnancy. *Stat. Med*. 1994; 13(5-7):671-681.

[16] Joffe M, Villard L, Li Z, Plowman R, Vessey M. Long-term recall of time-to-pregnancy. *Fertil. Steril*. 1993; 60(1):99-104.

[17] Joffe M, Villard L, Zhimin L, Plowman R, Vessey M. A time to pregnancy questionnaire designed for long term recall: validity in Oxford, England. *J. Epidemiol. Community Health* 1995; 49:314-319.

[18] Joffe M, Key J, Best N, Keiding N, Scheike T, Jensen TK. Studying time to pregnancy by use of a retrospective design. *Am. J. Epidemiol*. 2005; 162(2):115-124.

[19] Zielhuis GA, Hulscher ME, Florack EI. Validity and reliability of a questionnaire on fecundability. *Int. J. Epidemiol*. 1992; 21(6):1151-1156.

[20] Cooney MA, Buck Louis GM, Sundaram R, McGuiness BM, Lynch CD. Validity of self-reported time to pregnancy. *Epidemiology* 2009; 20(1):56-59.

[21] Olsen J, Rachootin P, Schiodt AV, Damsbo N. Tobacco use, alcohol consumption and infertility. *Int. J. Epidemiol*. 1983; 12(2):179-184.

[22] Joesoef MR, Beral V, Aral SO, Rolfs RT, Cramer DW. Fertility and use of cigarettes, alcohol, marijuana, and cocaine. *Ann. Epidemiol*. 1993; 3(6):592-594.

[23] Baird DD, Wilcox AJ. Cigarette smoking associated with delayed conception. *JAMA* 1985; 253(20):2979-2983.

[24] Hatch EE, Bracken MB. Association of delayed conception with caffeine consumption. *Am. J. Epidemiol*. 1993; 138(12):1082-1092.

[25] Curtis KM, Savitz DA, Arbuckle TE. Effects of cigarette smoking, caffeine consumption, and alcohol intake on fecundability. *Am. J. Epidemiol.* 1997; 146(1):32-41.

[26] Olsen J, Bolumar F, Boldsen J, Bisanti L. Does moderate alcohol intake reduce fecundability? A European multicenter study on infertility and subfecundity. European Study Group on Infertility and Subfecundity. *Alcohol. Clin. Exp. Res.* 1997; 21(2):206-212.

[27] Hassan MA, Killick SR. Negative lifestyle is associated with a significant reduction in fecundity. *Fertil. Steril.* 2004; 81(2):384-392.

[28] Juhl M, Nyboe Andersen AM, Gronbaek M, Olsen J. Moderate alcohol consumption and waiting time to pregnancy. *Hum. Reprod.* 2001; 16(12):2705-2709.

[29] Juhl M, Olsen J, Andersen AM, Gronbaek M. Intake of wine, beer and spirits and waiting time to pregnancy. *Hum. Reprod.* 2003; 18(9):1967-1971.

[30] Buck GM, Lynch CD, Stanford JB et al. Prospective pregnancy study designs for assessing reproductive and developmental toxicants. *Environ. Health Perspect.* 2004; 112(1):79-86.

[31] Buck Louis GM, Dmochowski J, Lynch C, Kostyniak P, McGuinness BM, Vena JE. Polychlorinated biphenyl serum concentrations, lifestyle and time-to-pregnancy. *Hum. Reprod.* 2009; 24(2):451-458.

[32] Florack EI, Zielhuis GA, Rolland R. Cigarette smoking, alcohol consumption, and caffeine intake and fecundability. *Prev. Med.* 1994; 23(2):175-180.

[33] Hakim RB, Gray RH, Zacur H. Alcohol and caffeine consumption and decreased fertility. *Fertil. Steril.* 1998; 70(4):632-637.

[34] Wilcox A, Weinberg C, Baird D. Caffeinated beverages and decreased fertility. *Lancet* 1988; 2(8626-8627):1453-1456.

In: Pregnancy and Alcohol Consumption
Editor: Joshua D. Hoffman, pp. 347-357
ISBN 978-1-61761-122-3


*Chapter 15*

# BIOLOGICAL MARKERS OF EXPOSURE OF FOETUS TO ALCOHOL DURING PREGNANCY

***S. Lamy*** [1] ***and F. Thibaut*** [2*]
1. Centre de prévention de Normandie Renouvance, Rouen, France
2. University Hospital Ch Nicolle, INSERM U 614, Faculty of Medicine, Rouen, France

## ABSTRACT

The potential consequences of the increasing use of alcohol by pregnant women are a major public health concern. According to different studies, 20 to 89 % of women may drink alcohol during their pregnancy. Current research suggests that the consumption of seven or more standard drinks of alcohol (one standard drink = 13.6 grams of absolute alcohol) per week during pregnancy places the baby at risk of serious, lifelong developmental and cognitive disabilities. Maternal alcohol use during pregnancy may lead to fetal alcohol spectrum disorder (FASD). FASD is characterized by typical facial features, growth retardation, intellectual dysfunction and behavioral problems. The FASD is the first cause of developmental abnormalities known. Psychological and educational interventions may help women to reduce their alcohol intake during pregnancy. The National Institute of Drug Abuse (USA) reported that 75% of the infants exposed to alcohol or substance during pregnancy present medical problems as compared to only 27% of the nonexposed infants. The modalities of alcohol and substance use have changed during the last years and there is increasing evidence for polyconsumption (e.g. among cannabis users, 52.3% smoke tobacco and 32.4% use alcohol several times per week). The toxic effects of these substances during pregnancy may be increased by their combination. Alcohol and substance use prevalence (tobacco, cannabis, cocaine...) during pregnancy remains under estimated. Most of the published studies were based on the mother's interview. In most cases, the mother underreport the amount of alcohol used. Further studies measuring alcohol use in the mother's blood, hair or in the

* Correspondence: F. Thibaut, Psychiatry, CHU Ch. Nicolle, 1 rue de Germont, 76031 Rouen, France; email: Florence.Thibaut@chu-rouen.fr.

newborn's meconium are needed. In addition, a serious challenge in diagnosing FASD is the need for markers of alcohol use during pregnancy. Detecting patterns of maternal drinking that place fetuses at risk for fetal alcohol spectrum disorders (FASDs) is critical to diagnosis, treatment, and prevention but is challenging because information on antenatal drinking collected during pregnancy is often insufficient or lacking. Serum Gamma-glutamyltransferase (GGT), carbohydrate-deficient transferrin (CDT), and mean corpuscular volume of erythrocytes (MCV) appear to be the most efficient laboratory markers for detecting excessive alcohol consumption. Ethyl glucuronide (EtG) and ethyl sulfate (EtS) are also biomarkers of excessive alcohol use. They can be measured in the mother's blood, newborn's blood or meconium. Recently, fatty acid ethyl esters (FAEEs) measurements in meconium emerged as reliable, direct biological markers for establishing gestational ethanol exposure. We will review the available markers of alcohol use during pregnancy. Until now, when examining the association between prenatal alcohol exposure and fetal effects, epidemiological studies have ignored the timing and intensity of the exposure. New epidemiological study combining biological, pharmacological and mothers' interview approaches should permit a better evaluation of the consequences for the newborn and child exposed to alcohol during pregnancy as a function of intensity and timing of alcohol exposure.

## INTRODUCTION

All over the world, alcohol and substance consumption has dramatically increased during the past years. Alcohol use spans all socioeconomic classes, gender, race, education and cultural groups. In 2003, the World Health Organisation estimated that 140 million people throughout the world were suffering from alcohol dependence. The EMCDDA (European Monitoring Centre For Drugs And Drug Addiction) reported that the current situation of illicit drugs use in 2004 was the following in Europe: 65 million people have used at least once cannabis (20% of the population, 5% of them daily). Ten million people (3%) have used cocaine at least once. One million and 700,000 people are regular heroin users.

The potential consequences of the increasing use of alcohol and psychoactive substances during pregnancy are a major public health concern. The effects of various substances on foetus brain development may be reflective of both their inherent neurotoxicity and the patterns with which they are used (the age of foetus during exposure, the frequency and duration of exposure and the drug concentration). There is evidence for neurodevelopemental consequences of prenatal exposure to alcohol. The Syndrome of Fetal Alcoholisation (FAS) is the first cause of avoidable developmental abnormalities. The Fetal Alcohol Spectrum Disorder (FASD) is characterized by growth deficiencies, craniofacial dysmorphologies, and CNS damage. Prenatal exposure can cause intellectual disability, deficits in learning, attention, motor development and hyperactivity. The prevalence of FAS in typical, mixed-racial, and mixed-socioeconomic populations in the US is at least 2 to 7 per 1,000. Regarding all types of FAS disorders (FASD), the current prevalence of FASD in populations of young children may be as high as 2-5% in the US and Western European countries [23]. Generally speaking, these pregnancies are at high risk for both the mother and the foetus: more congenital malformations, premature births and/or hypotrophy are observed if the pregnant mother had been consuming alcohol. The National Institute of Drug Abuse (USA) reported that 75% of the infants exposed in utero to one or more drugs as compared to only 27% of the nonexposed infants, exhibited medical problems. Moreover, polyconsumption increases in the general population, consequently it is difficult to disentangle the consequences of the different drugs used during pregnancy on child development due to the potential interactions between these drugs. The consequences on child development will also depend on the time of drug use during pregnancy. A pregnant mother using alcohol will not necessarily give birth to a child with FAS, although there is no known safe level of alcohol consumption during pregnancy. Since the identification of the fetal alcohol syndrome in 1973, significant inroads have been made towards understanding the effects of alcohol on fetal development. Therefore, a high priority should be given to aims at reducing its prevalence through more effective diagnosis and early intervention. The need for objective methods for revealing alcohol abuse in its early phase has also been widely acknowledged. Unfortunately, the diagnosis of FAS and FADS is usually made after birth, when alcohol damage has become irreversible and permanent. Biological measurements can make a valuable contribution in assessing prenatal alcohol use and may help to prevent or at least to reduce the consequences of FAS syndrome. This review of the current literature was intended to summarize the data available on biological markers of alcohol excessive use during pregnancy.

## Epidemiology and Consequences of Alcohol Consumption during Pregnancy

Alcohol is a pharmacological depressant, blocking NMDA (N methyl D aspartate) receptor activity and increasing GABAergic activity, thereby decreasing cortical and subcortical activity. Alcohol can also disrupt growth factor receptor signalling by disrupting plasma membrane integrity. GABA receptors are present early in neuronal development, and can modulate progenitor cell proliferation, cell migration and neurite growth. Alcohol crosses the placental barrier during pregnancy and thus can have a severe impact on brain development [for review, 40].

Animal models of prenatal ethanol exposure have confirmed an increase in birth defects, including neurological dysfunction. Exposure during all gestational periods has dramatic teratogenic consequences [40]. There are reports of a decrease in spinal and cranial motor neuron production and size, neocortical and hippocampal dysgenesis, increased neuronal cell death, reduced or delayed neuronal migration and decreased myelination. In addition to direct antagonism of neurotransmitter receptors, receptor tyrosine kinase signalling is disrupted, leading to altered modulation of multiple histogenic events by neurotrophic factors. As well as alcohol's direct effects on the fetus, it also acts directly on the hypothalamic-pituitary-adrenal (HPA) axis of both the fetus and the mother [for review, 40].

Despite the international consensus recommending total abstinence during pregnancy, prenatal alcohol exposure remains a major public health issue. Alcohol use among women of childbearing age is prevalent in the United States, with approximately 1 in 25 pregnant women reporting binge drinking (5 or more drinks on any occasion) [12]. According to Alvik et al. [2], self-report is the best available method to obtain information about moderate alcohol consumption although alcohol consumption reported before and during pregnancy is often sensitive to response bias. Eighty-nine percent of the women were drinking alcohol before pregnancy and 23.5%, during pregnancy (after 7 weeks of pregnancy)[2].

De Chazeron and Llorca [9] using the AUDIT questionnaire (Alcohol Use Disorders Identification Test) reported that 52.2% of 837 French pregnant women indicated that they had consumed alcohol at least once during their pregnancy, and among those reporting abstinence, 54.5% had a positive AUDIT score. Of the pregnant women who consumed alcohol, 13.7% reported at least one binge drinking episode during pregnancy. Binge drinking was significantly more frequent than regular alcohol consumption during pregnancy (at least 1 drink more than 1 time per week). Nonindigenous west Australian women (n=4,839) were asked about alcohol consumption in each of the 4 time periods: the 3 months before pregnancy and each trimester of pregnancy; 79.8% reported drinking alcohol in the 3 months before pregnancy and 58.7% in at least 1 trimester during pregnancy [6]. The proportion of women consuming 1 to 2 drinks on a typical occasion did not change much during pregnancy, but the number of occasions declined. Although the proportion of women consuming more than 2 standard drinks on a typical occasion declined after the first trimester, 19% of women consumed this amount during at least one trimester of pregnancy and 4.3% of women consumed 5 or more standard drinks on a typical occasion during at least one trimester of pregnancy. In the first trimester of pregnancy, 14.8% of women drank outside the current Australian guidelines for alcohol consumption in pregnancy as compared to 10% in the second and third trimesters.

Using a questionnaire-based study, 151 postnatal Irish women were interviewed. Alcohol was consumed by 89% of women and 10% admitted binge drinking during pregnancy [25]. Only 44% of the study group was aware of the risk. Information on hazards of alcohol consumption during pregnancy in the general population seems necessary, especially in young women.

Maternal alcohol consumption during pregnancy places the fetus at risk for a number of neurological abnormalities and functional impairments. There are also many consequences of alcohol consumption during pregnancy on the future child development such as growth disorders [8]; learning or motor disorders [16], language disorders; attention deficit disorders [5, 21], memory disorders [37], executive dysfunctions [39]. The prevalence of depressive or anxiety disorders [16] may be increased in the child exposed to alcohol during pregnancy. Studying the relationship between alcohol consumption by the mother during pregnancy and the occurrence of FAS or FASD is very difficult using retrospective studies. According to the Fetal Alcohol Spectrum Disorder Advisory Workgroup recommandations, interviews of the mothers must be associated with biological measurements in order to reduce interview biases.

In spite of the heterogeneity of the methodologies reported in the existing literature (different types of interview, different biological measurements, psychiatric comorbidities, heterogeneity of economic status, etc), the prevalence of alcohol use increases in pregnant women, and in most cases, several substances are associated. The diagnosis of alcohol use disorders could be markedly improved by a more systematic use of specific questionnaires [38] such as the AUDIT [1, 14, 35], the Addiction Severity Index (ASI) [19, 24] or the CAGE questionnaire [10, 11] in association with laboratory tests, including serum gamma-glutamyltransferase (GGT), carbohydrate-deficient transferring (CDT), and mean corpuscular volume of erythrocytes (MCV). Recently, fatty acid ethyl esters (FAEEs) in meconium emerged as reliable, direct biological markers for establishing gestational ethanol exposure.

Among the minor nonoxidative products of ethanol metabolism, ethyl glucuronide (EtG) and ethyl sulfate (EtS) may also be measured.

## BIOLOGICAL MARKERS OF ALCOHOL CONSUMPTION

The diagnosis of FAS and FAD is usually made after birth, when alcohol damage has become irreversible and permanent. The clinical laboratory can make a valuable contribution in assessing prenatal alcohol use and may help to prevent this damage. Although none of the markers singularly has adequate sensitivity and specificity for screening, their diagnostic utility increases when measured as a panel. This is especially true in detecting alcohol use in pregnancy where the presence of several positive markers was correlated with the presence of alcohol-related fetal effects [7, 13].

Amniotic fluid, meconium, fetal hair, and maternal hair may provide a long historical record of prenatal exposure to alcohol or substances at different times of gestation: amniotic fluid for early pregnancy, meconium for the second and third trimester of gestation, fetal hair for the third trimester, and finally maternal hair for the whole period (hair growth is 1 cm/month). Placenta may also reveal the passage of a substance from the mother to the fetus. Cord blood and neonatal urine may be useful for determining acute exposure to alcohol in the period immediately previous to delivery.

Alcohol detection in maternal blood, oral fluid, urine and sweat reflects only acute consumption that occurred in the hours previous to collection and gives poor information concerning fetal exposure.

Different immunoassays were used as screening methods for alcohol testing in the above-reported matrices or as unique analytical investigation tools when chromatographic techniques coupled to mass spectrometry were not commonly available. However, in the last decade, both liquid and gas chromatography-mass spectrometric methodologies have been routinely applied after appropriate extraction of susbtances and their metabolites from these biological matrices [22].

Combining simultaneous analysis of maternal (hair, blood) and infant (cord blood, infant hair or meconium) matrices may increase the detection rate [31, 32, 33].

## GGT, MCV, CDT Measurements

Chronic ethanol consumption is known to induce a rise in serum Gamma-glutamyltransferase (GGT) which is currently the most widely used index of excessive ethanol intake (sensitivity: 15 to 85%; specificity: 80%). J. Hietala et al. [17] explored the relationship between ethanol consumption and GGT values in individuals with a wide variety of ethanol consumption and concluded that distinct effects of mild to moderate ethanol consumption on serum GGT levels should be considered in the clinical use of GGT measurement as a marker of ethanol abuse and liver status [17]. The International Federation of Clinical Chemistry's recommended methods for GGT measurements. Normal GGT levels were defined as GGT $\leq$ 28 U/L at a measurement temperature of 25°C.

CDT is a reliable marker of chronic or repeated alcohol abuse. It represents a group of isoforms of human transferrin (Tf), the main iron transport serum protein, which are deficient in sialic acid residues (asialo-, monosialo- and disialo-Tf) in comparison to the main isotransferrin which contains four sialic acid groups (tetrasialo-Tf). Among the different biomarkers of chronic alcohol abuse, CDT is worldwide recognized as the most reliable indicator [4]. It is at least as sensitive and more specific than GGT. In alcohol-dependent males abstinent for more than 4 days before the blood test, the following markers had low sensitivities (GGT: 33%; CDT: 14%; MCV: 42% respectively), whereas in those abstinent for less than 5 days, the markers had reasonably good sensitivities (GGT: 72%; CDT: 56%; MCV: 48% respectively). Half-life of plasma GGT, MCV and CDT are respectively of 4 weeks, 2-3 months and 14-16 days. Mean alcohol consumption in the 30 days prior to the blood test had a significant effect on CDT and GGT, but not on MCV. If a longer period of abstinence is suspected, MCV should also be measured. Normal MCV level is $\leq$ 95 fl. Using both CDT and GGT measurements, sensitivity can be enhanced to 90% [30]. Rink et al. [36] analyzed blood samples from alcohol-dependent patients ($n = 177$) as compared with a control group ($n = 181$). CDT, MCV, GGT were measured. None of the biomarkers reached sensitivity above 90% while all markers showed a good specificity. Combinations of different markers led to a significant increased sensitivity. Best sensitivity for men was achieved by using a combination of MCV, CDT, GGT (sensitivity: 98.6%, specificity: 86.4%). For women, similar results were yielded by combining MCV and CDT (sensitivity: 94.1%, specificity: 96%) [36].

## FAEE Measurements

Seven fatty acid ethyl esters (FAEEs): ethyl palmitate, ethyl palmitoleate, ethyl stearate, ethyl oleate, ethyl linoleate, ethyl linolenate, and ethyl arachidonate are products of nonoxidative ethanol metabolism. Meconium FAEE measurement is a novel biomarker of fetal ethanol exposure. FAEE was measured in 682 meconium specimens anonymously collected [15]. Meconium FAEE were extracted by liquid-liquid and solid-phase extraction and analyzed by gas chromatography with flame-ionization detection confirmed by gas chromatography with mass spectrometry. Seventeen of 682 meconium samples were positive (>2.0 nmol/g). FAEE analysis detected fivefold more ethanol-exposed pregnancies than standard postpartum questionnaires in this population (2.5% versus 0.5%). The FAEE concentrations of negative (95% CI: 0.38-0.49 nmol/g) versus positive (95% CI: 7.74-151.28 nmol/g) samples were distinct, further demonstrating the specificity of this biomarker in determining significant prenatal ethanol exposure. The FAEEs in meconium, particularly ethyl linoleate and ethyl AA, are biomarkers of high specificity for prenatal exposure to alcohol in newborns [31].

## EtG, EtS Measurements

New biomarkers such as ethyl glucuronide, ethyl sulfate are available but their routine use is yet limited.

Routinely used alcohol biomarkers can be influenced by age, gender and a variety of substances and non-alcohol-associated diseases and they do not fully cover the time axis for alcohol intake. Ethyl glucuronide (EtG) is a non-volatile, water-soluble, stable, direct metabolite of ethanol that can be detected in various body fluids, tissues and hair. Shortly after the consumption, even of small amounts of ethanol, EtG becomes positive. It can detect ethanol intake up to 80 hours after the complete elimination of alcohol from the body, covering a unique and important time spectrum for recent alcohol use. EtG seems to meet the need for a sensitive and specific marker to elucidate alcohol use not detected by standard testing [41, 42]. EtG is incorporated into the growing hair allowing retrospective investigation of chronic alcohol abuse [18]. A method for the sensitive and selective determination of EtG in hair has been developed using solid-phase extraction (SPE) and liquid chromatography-tandem mass spectrometry (LC-MS/MS). The detection of ethyl glucuronide and ethyl sulfate in meconium has also been investigated recently as an alternative to meconium FAEEs measurement and as an objective estimate of prenatal alcohol exposure, in addition to maternal self-reporting.

EtS, a direct ethanol metabolite, appears to offer potential as a biomarker for recent alcohol consumption. Although its window of assessment is similar to that of EtG, there are differences between the two markers in their pathways of synthesis and degradation. Morini et al. [26] reported the first study conducted to investigate the concentrations of EtG and EtS in meconium from newborns with or without intrauterine exposure to ethanol, defined by questionnaires and meconium FAEEs concentrations. FAEEs, EtG, and EtS were quantified in meconium by liquid chromatography tandem mass spectrometry. A positive cutoff of 2.0 nmol/g for EtG yielded the best sensitivity and specificity (100%) to discriminate for true prenatal exposure to ethanol. It was not possible to establish a proper cutoff for EtS because of the low number of positive samples in this study.

Meconium EtG can be proposed as an alternate biomarker for intrauterine alcohol exposure. In contrast to the 7 FAEEs, EtG represents only one measurement in meconium samples from newborns and a simple, low-cost, easy-to-perform immunoassay, which can be routinely applied in neonatology wards for the early diagnosis of prenatal exposure to ethanol.

In previous investigations, hair dosage of EtG and FAEEs were considered appropriate for the detection of excessive alcohol consumption [34, 43, 44].

Meconium appears so far as the best matrix in evaluating intrauterine exposure to ethanol, with EtG, and possibly EtS, as potentially good alternative biomarkers to FAEEs. However, the combined use of FAEE and EtG in meconium as markers for fetal alcohol exposure increases the accuracy of the interpretation and helps to avoid false positive and false-negative results [3, 26, 27, 28].

## Genetic Markers

Emerging biomarkers in alcoholism may also include in the future genetic markers for identifying individuals at risk for alcohol dependence or ethanol-induced damage in specific tissue. Much evidence coming from studies in humans and animals supports the hypothesis that alcohol addiction is a complex disease with both hereditary and environmental influences. Several rodent models show a high or low degree of alcohol preference, which provides a unique opportunity to approach the complexities underlying the genetic predisposition to alcohol abuse [29]. A few genes were also identified as candidate genes that may be involved in influencing alcohol consumption in the mice [29].

## Conclusion

Health problems created by excessive alcohol consumption had been rapidly increasing in the world. Fetal alcohol spectrum disorder (FASD) is the leading cause of non-genetic mental retardation. Moreover, the toxic effects of alcohol and substance use during pregnancy may be increased by their combination. We need to improve our knowledge of the prevalence of alcohol use during pregnancy and of its consequences on child development in order to target information for campaigns prevention and in order to implement specific mother and child medical care in high risk populations. The need for objective methods for revealing alcohol use during pregnancy has been widely acknowledged. Indeed, the retrospective detection of alcohol consumption during pregnancy is an important part of the diagnosis of fetal alcohol syndrome and fetal alcohol spectrum disorders. Using questionnaires, such as the ASI or the AUDIT, is cheap, easy, quick, noninvasive and has a relatively good sensitivity. However, questionnaires have been incomplete and it is necessary to concomitantly use biological measures to acurately evaluate the mother's alcohol consumption during pregnancy.

In the recent years, the evaluation of *in utero* exposure to alcohol abuse has been achieved by testing a combination of biological matrices of the newborn (eg, meconium, fetal hair, cord blood, serum cord blood, neonatal urine) and of the pregnant mother (eg, hair, blood, oral fluid, sweat, urine, breast milk), or of both (placenta, amniotic fluid). Overall, these matrices have the advantage of noninvasive collection (with the exception of amniotic fluid and neonatal urine) and of detection of exposure from different gestational periods. However, different factors may influence alcohol biomarkers such as duration of abstinence, age, gender, weight, concurrent medical illnesses (diabetis, liver cirrhosis, tumor, tuberculosis...), quantity of alcohol consumed, these confounding factors may increase the difficulty in establishing reliable sensitivity and specificity for these markers in the general population. Combining alcohol biomarkers such as GGT, MCV and CDT measurements may increase sensitivity. Detecting patterns of maternal drinking that place fetuses at risk for fetal alcohol spectrum disorders (FASDs) is critical to diagnosis, treatment, and prevention but is challenging because information on antenatal drinking collected during pregnancy is often insufficient or lacking. GGT, CDT, and MCV appear to be the most efficient laboratory markers for detecting excessive alcohol consumption in the pregnant mothers. Ethyl glucuronide (EtG) and ethyl sulfate (EtS) are also biomarkers of excessive alcohol use. These latter can be measured in the mother's blood, newborn's blood or meconium. Recently, fatty acid ethyl esters (FAEEs) measurements in meconium emerged as reliable, direct biological markers for establishing gestational ethanol exposure. These latter markers are also durably deposited in hair and in meconium (fifth month of pregnancy in total) and may also be measured in mothers or newborns'hair.

# REFERENCES


[1] Aalto M, Alho H, Halme JT et al. AUDIT and its abbreviated versions in detecting heavy and binge drinking in a general population survey. *Drug Alcohol Depend*, 2009, 103:25-9.

[2] Alvik A, Heyerdahl S, Haldorsen T et al. Alcohol use before and during pregnancy: a population-based study. *Acta Obstet. Gynecol*, Scand 2006, 85: 1292-8.

[3] Bakdash A, Burger P, Goecke TW et al. Quantification of fatty acid ethyl esters (FAEE) and ethyl glucuronide (EtG) in meconium from newborns for detection of alcohol abuse in a maternal health evaluation study. *Anal. Bioanal. Chem*, 2010, 396:2469-77.

[4] Bortolotti F, De Paoli G, Tagliaro F. Carbohydrate-deficient transferrin (CDT) as a marker of alcohol abuse: a critical review of the literature 2001-2005. *J. Chromatogr. B Analyt. Technol. Biomed. Life Sci,* 2006, 841:96-109.

[5] Coles CD, Platzman KA, Raskind-Hood CL et al. A comparison of children affected by prenatal alcohol exposure and attention deficit, hyperactivity disorder. *Alcohol. Clin. Exp. Res*, 1997, 21(1):150-61.

[6] Colvin L, Payne J, Kurinczuck JJ et al. Alcohol consumption during pregnancy in nonindigenous west Australian women. *Alcohol. Clin. Exp. Res,* 2007, 31:276-84.

[7] Cook JD. Biochemical markers of alcohol use in pregnant women. *Clin. Biochem*, 2003, 36:9-19.

[8] Day NL, Leech SL, Richardson GA et al. Prenatal alcohol exposure predicts continued deficits in offspring size at 14 years of age. *Alcohol. Clin. Exp. Res*, 2002, 99:283.

[9] De Chazeron I, Llorca PM, Venditelli F et al. Is pregnancy the time to change alcohol consumption habits in France? *Alcohol. Clin. Exp. Res*, 2008, 32:868-73.

[10] Dhalla S, Kopec JA. The CAGE questionnaire for alcohol misuse: a review of reliability and validity studies. *Clin. Invest. Med*, 2007, 30:33-41.

[11] Ewing T, John A. Detecting Alcoholism: The CAGE Questionnaire. *JAMA,* 1984, 252: 1905-7.

[12] Floyd DR, O'Connor MJ, Sokol RJ et al. Recognition and prevention of fetal alcohol syndrome. *Obstet Gynecol,* 2005, 106: 1059-64.

[13] Freeman WM, Salzberg AC, Gonzales SW et al. Classification of alcohol abuse by plasma protein biomarkers. *Biol. Psychiatry*, 2010, Mars 16, in press.

[14] Gache P, Michaud P, Landry U et al. The Alcohol Use Disorders Identification Test (AUDIT) as a screening tool for excessive drinking in primary care: reliability and validity of a French version. *Alcohol. Clin. Exp. Res*, 2005, 29:2001-7.

[15] Gareri J, Lynn H, Handley M et al. Prevalence of fetal ethanol exposure in a regional population-based sample by meconium analysis of fatty acid ethyl esters. *Ther. Drug Monit,* 2008, 30:239-45.

[16] Goldschmidt L, Richardson GA, Cornelius M et al. Prenatal marijuana and alcohol exposure and academic achievement at age 10. *Neurotoxicol. Teratol.* 2004, 26(4):521-32.

[17] Hietala J, Koivisto H, Anttila P et al. Comparison of the combined marker GGT-CDT and the conventional laboratory markers of alcohol abuse in heavy drinkers, moderate drinkers and abstainers. *Alcohol,* 2006, 41:528-33.

[18] Kharbouche H, Sporkert F, Staub C et al. Ethyl glucuronide: a biomarker of alcohol consumption. *Praxis,* 2009, 98:1299-306.

[19] Krenz S, Dieckmann S, Favrat B et al. French version of the Addiction Severity Index (5th edition): validity and reliability among swiss opiate-dependent patients. *Eur. Addict. Res,* 2004, 10:173-179.

[20] Lamy S, Thibaut F. Psychoactive substance use during pregnancy: a review. *Encéphale,* 2010, 36(1):33-8.

[21] Leech SL, Richardson GA, Goldschmidt L et al. Prenatal substance exposure: effects on attention and impulsivity of 6-year-olds. *Neurotoxicol. Teratol*, 1999, 21(2):109-18.

[22] Lozano J, Garcia-Algar O, Vall O et al. Biological matrices for the evaluation of in utero exposure to drugs of abuse. *Ther. Drug Monit,* 2007, 29:711-34.

[23] May PA, Gossage JP, Kalberg WO et al. Prevalence and epidemiologic characteristics of FASD from various research methods with an emphasis on recent in-school studies. *Dev. Disabil. Res. Rev*, 2009, 15:176-92.

[24] Mc Lellan AT, Kushner H, Metzger D et al. The Fifth Edition of the Addiction Severity Index. *J. Subst. Abuse Treat,* 1992, 9:199-213.

[25] Mc Millan H, Smaarani S, Walsh T et al. Smoking and alcohol in pregnancy. Survey in the immediate post-partum period. *Ir. Med. J,* 2006, 99:283.

[26] Morini L, Groppi A, Marchei E et al. Population baseline of meconium ethyl glucuronide and ethyl sulfate concentrations in newborns of nondrinking women in 2 mediterranean cohorts. *Ther. Drug Monit*, 2010 Mar 23 in press.

[27] Morini L, Marchei E, Vagnarelli F et al. Quantification of fatty acid ethyl esters (FAEE) and ethyl glucuronide (EtG) in meconium from newborns for detection of alcohol abuse in a maternal health evaluation study. *Anal. Bioanal. Chem*, 2010.

[28] Morini L, Marchei E, Vagnarelli F et al. Ethyl glucuronide and ethyl sulfate in meconium and hair-potential biomarkers of intrauterine exposure to ethanol. *Forensic. Sci. Int,* 2010, 196:74-7.

[29] Mulligan MK, Ponomarev I, Boehm SL et al. Alcohol trait and transcriptional genomic analysis of C57BL/6 substrains. *Genes Brain Behav*, 2008, 7:677-89.

[30] Niemelä O. Biomarkers in alcoholism. *Clin. Chim. Acta*, 2007, 377:39-49.

[31] Ostrea EM Jr., Brielawski DM, Posecion NC et al. Combined analysis of prenatal (maternal hair and blood) and neonatal (infant hair, cord blood and meconium) matrices to detect fetal exposure to environmental pesticides. *Environ. Res*, 2009, 109:116-22.

[32] Pichini S, Morini L, Marchei E et al. Ethylglucuronide and ethylsulfate in meconium to access gestational ethanol exposure: preliminary results in two Mediterranean cohorts. *Can. J. Clin. Pharmacol,* 2009, 16:370-5.

[33] Pichini S, Puig C, Zuccaro P et al. Assessment of exposure to opiates and cocaine during pregnancy in a Mediterranean city: preliminary results of the "Meconium Project". *Forensic. Sci. Int,* 2005, 153:59-65.

[34] Pragst F, Yegles M. Determination of fatty acid ethyl esters (FAEE) and ethyl glucuronide (EtG) in hair: a promising way for retrospective detection of alcohol abuse during pregnancy? *Ther. Drug Monit,* 2008, 30:255-63.

[35] Reinert DF, Allen JP. The alcohol use disorders identification test: an update of research findings. *Alcohol. Clin. Exp. Res*, 2007, 31:185-99.

[36] Rinck D, Freiling H, Freitag A et al. Combinations of carbohydrate-deficient transferrin, mean corpuscular erythrocyte volume, gamma-glutamyltransferase,

homocysteine and folate increase the significance of biological markers in alcohol dependent patients. *Drug Alcohol. Depend*, 2007, 89:60-5.

[37] Roebuck-Spencer TM, Mattson SN. Implicit strategy affects learning in children with heavy prenatal alcohol exposure. *Alcohol. Clin. Exp. Res*, 2004, 28:1424-31.

[38] Rubinsky AD, Kivlahan DR, Volk RJ et al. Estimating risk of alcohol dependence using alcohol screening scores. *Drug Alcohol. Depend*, 2010, 108:29-36.

[39] Schonfeld AM, Paley B, Frankel F et al. Executive functioning predicts social skills following prenatal alcohol exposure. *Child Neuropsychol*, 2006, 12:439-52.

[40] Thompson BL, Levitt P, Stanwood GD. Prenatal exposure to drugs: effects on brain development and implications for policy and education. *Nature Rev. Neurosci*, 2009, 40:303-312.

[41] Wurst FM, Metzger J. The ethanol conjugate ethyl glucuronide is a useful marker of recent alcohol consumption. *Alcohol. Clin. Exp. Res*, 2002, 26:1114-9.

[42] Wurst FM. Skipper GE. Weinmann W. Ethyl glucuronide--the direct ethanol metabolite on the threshold from science to routine use. *Addiction,* 2003, 98(S2):51-61.

[43] Yegles M, Labarthe A, Auwärter V et al. Comparison of ethyl glucuronide and fatty acid ethyl ester concentrations in hair of alcoholics, social drinkers and teetotallers. *Forensic. Sci. Int,* 2004, 145:167-73.

[44] Zimmermann CM, Jackson GP. Gas chromatography tandem mass spectrometry for biomarkers of alcohol abuse in human hair. *Ther. Drug Monit,* 2010, 32:216-23.

In: Pregnancy and Alcohol Consumption
Editor: Joshua D. Hoffman, pp. 359-364
ISBN 978-1-61761-122-3


*Chapter 16*

# ALCOHOL AND PREGNANCY: HISTORY, CURRENT SITUATION IN FRANCE AND DESCRIPTIVE STUDY OF THE DEVELOPMENT OF ADDICTIVE BEHAVIORS DURING PREGNANCY -

***M. Tanguy and S. Fanello***
Public Health University Department,
Teaching Hospital, Faculty of Medicine, Angers, France

## ABSTRACT

Alcohol consumption in France, a country with a strong wine tradition, is widely associated with conviviality, friendship and loyalty. However, excessive alcohol consumption is associated with well known adverse effects. During pregnancy, the problem is more severe. Binge drinking - a growing practice in France – and chronic consumption can cause disability to the unborn.

These damages are described as Foetal Alcohol Syndrome (FAS), Foetal Alcohol Effects (FAE) and Foetal Alcohol Spectrum Disorder (FASD). They can be avoided by informing women and encouraging abstinence from alcohol during pregnancy. Moreover, mothers who have an alcohol problem may find support and assistance. In France, mainly since 2002, public health policies have improved public information, prevention and management of disorders related to alcohol consumption during pregnancy. These measures need to be supported by careful training of all professionals providing health care to pregnant women.

---

Correspondence: M. Tanguy, Département de Santé Publique, UFR Médecine, 1 rue Haute de Reculée, 49933 Angers cedex 09, France; email: mtanguy@gmail.com.

## INTRODUCTION

In France, alcohol is the most widely spread psychoactive drug consumed by the adult population. A 2005 survey among people aged 12 to 75 years old showed that only 8.4% of them had never drunk in their lives [1]. It is the monthly or occasional consumption of alcohol that dominates according to 38.4% of respondents who say they have drunk less than once a week over the last twelve months. Furthermore, one third (32.7%) admitted to having drunk at least once a week, and 13.7% say they drink everyday.

Even if alcohol consumption is lower among women, it increases slowly over the years. The age of onset is now around 18-25 years, when fertility is at its peak. A general population survey carried out by the French National Institute of Prevention and Health Education (INPES) [2] showed that the daily drinkers were three times higher among men than women (20.3% vs. 7.3%, $p < 0.001$). However considering weekly consumption, the gap is smaller (21.7% vs. 11.8%, $p < 0.001$). Up to seven percent of women report an episode of binge drinking during the year (20% of women aged 20-25 years old) and 5% of women showed potential alcohol abuse.

## HISTORY OF FETAL ALCOHOL SYNDROME

Even though alcohol during pregnancy is a well identified risk since ancient times, it is difficult to warn against its consumption. The Old Testament relates the warning given by an angel to Samson's mother: "Behold, you shall conceive and bear a son; so then drink no wine or strong drink." - Judges 13:7

During the gin craze in England in 1725, a report from the Royal College of Physicians noted that "children born to mothers consuming gin are weak, feeble and distempered" [3]. The Royal College of Physicians asked for regulation of the production and sale of alcohol. A century later, in 1834, the House of Commons published a parliamentary report on the Effects of Drunkenness on the Nation, observing that children tend to be "born starved, shrivelled and imperfect in form" [4].

In 1899, Maurice Nicloux, a French biochemist, demonstrated that the alcohol consumed by pregnant women would be detected in foetal blood [5]. Around 1960, a French doctor, Paul Lemoine, noticed that hypotrophic babies present an unknown syndrome including severe and restricted intrauterine growth, hypotrophy, microcephaly, frequent cardiac and skeletal malformations especially associated with a facial dysmorphology and depressed nasal bridge. "The children looked as if they were siblings" he said [6]. He noticed that all these children had alcoholic mothers. In March 1964 to the Medico-surgical Society of Nantes Hospital a study of fifteen children: "Effects of maternal alcoholism in the offspring". In 1967, his report of abnormalities in 127 children of alcoholic mothers was published in *L'Ouest Médical* [7]. Although this study was initially viewed with scepticism, the Jellinek Prize was awarded in 1984 to Paul Lemoine for his work on alcoholism.

The Foetal Alcohol Syndrome (FAS) was named in 1973 by Drs. Kenneth Lyons Jones and David Weyhe Smith, two dysmorphologists. They identified a pattern of "craniofacial, limb, and cardiovascular defects associated with prenatal growth deficiency" in eight unrelated children of three ethnic groups, all born from alcoholics mothers. The study, publish in *The Lancet*: "Recognition of the Foetal Alcohol Syndrome in Early Infancy" had a significant impact [8]. Since then, a research unit on Alcohol and Drug Effects on the foetus was dedicated in Seattle to the prevention, intervention and treatment of the Foetal Alcohol Syndrome (FAS) and Foetal Alcohol Effects (FAE).

## CURRENT SITUATION IN FRANCE

The FAS incidence varies widely in the literature according to its definition, assessment methods and population studied. In France few studies have evaluated its incidence. A recent study in Reunion Island - a French overseas department – had estimated its incidence to 1.8 % of births. This is comparable to the results of a study in Clermont-Ferrand [9]. In the United States the incidence of FAS was estimated to 0.97% in 1995. The main factor associated with FAS was a low socio-economic level [10].

Despite evidence proving that alcohol consumption during pregnancy leads to FAS, there is still a controversy in France on the safety of occasional consumption. A recent multicenter survey of the 837 pregnant women indicated that more than half (52.2%) of them had consumed alcohol at least one time alcohol during their pregnancy and 13.7% reported a binge-drinking episode [9]. That makes a great difference with other countries like United States where only 12% of pregnant women report drinking alcohol [11]. In 2003, The French Society on Alcoholism (SFA) recommended abstinence as the best advice for pregnant women [12] The SFA also campaign for the training of perinatal professionals to the prevention and detection of FAS. The SFA recommended that the public be informed about the teratogenic effect of alcohol to the foetus at any dose. These recommendations were supported by French societies of paediatrics and obstetrics-gynaecology. The French National Academy of Medicine declared that alcohol consumption during pregnancy represents the major cause of non-genetically induced mental disabilities as well as child social inadaptability [13].

In 2004, the L3311-3 Article of the French Public Health Code was amended to include anti-alcohol information campaigns. There is a need to focus on FAS prevention in these campaigns as well as encourage pregnant women to abstain from alcohol. Information must also be given in colleges and high schools. The training of health professionals and medico-social sector should include information on the effects of alcohol on the foetus.

Since late 2004, the French Health Department and INPES have launched an annual campaign on the theme : "Zero alcohol during pregnancy." [14]. Since October 2007, all bottles of wine sold in France must display health warnings: "The consumption of alcoholic drinks during pregnancy, even in small amounts, can have severe consequences to health of your child". A picture depicting the silhouette of a pregnant woman drinking from a glass contained in a barred red circle must also appears.

From January to April 2006, a prospective, descriptive study was conducted by questionnaire among pregnant women attending a pre-natal consultation with a midwife, in a French Maternity situated in a Teaching Hospital (Centre Hospitalier Universitaire d'Angers) as well as in a Maternal and Child Health centre (PMI). 241 questionnaires were collected: 142 from the Maternity Hospital, 59 in the PMI and 40 in the liberal sector [15]. The cohort characteristics are shown in Table 1.

Smoking behaviour, psychosocial factors and environmental co-addiction (alcohol and illicit drugs such as cannabis, heroin and cocaine) were described and compared before and during pregnancy. A quarter of women smoked during their pregnancy with consumption exceeded ten cigarettes a day in 10% of cases. A third of women who reported smoking before pregnancy said they had ceased during the year. A French validated version - DETA questionnaire [16,17] - of the Mayfield's CAGE questionnaire to identifying alcoholism [18] was used. Subjects responding affirmatively to two or more questions were classified CAGE positive. The CAGE test had a sensitivity of 93% and a specificity of 76% for identification of alcohol dependence [19].

**Table 1. Social characteristics of pregnant women by visiting origins (size [%])**

| | PMI n = 59 | Maternity n = 142 | Liberal n = 40 |
|---|---|---|---|
| Single | 15 (25.4) | 7 (4.9) | 1(2.5) |
| Unwanted pregnancy | 11 (19.0) | 14 (9.9) | 0 |
| Abuse history | 13 (22.4) | 0. (9.2) | 1 (2.6) |
| Help of an Educator | 11 (19.0) | 3 (2.1) | 1 (2.6) |
| Withdraw from family | 11 (19.0) | 3 (2.1) | 1 (2.6) |
| Working | 16 (27.6) | 88 (62.0) | 30 (75.0) |
| Unemployed | 1 (17.2) | 22 (15.5) | 4 (10.0) |

**Table 2. Change of drinking habits during pregnancy by smoking status (size [%])**

| | Non smoker | Smoker | Total |
|---|---|---|---|
| Stop drinking | 43 (72.9) | 47 (59.5) | 90 (65.2) |
| Decrease consumption | 9 (15.3) | 22 (27.8) | 31 (22.5) |
| Not change | 7 (11.9) | 10 (12.7) | 17 (12.3) |

Two hundred and twenty of 241 women reported alcohol consumption before pregnancy, 137 completed the DETA questionnaire. Nine of them had an alcohol abuse. Seventeen claimed they had not changed their consumption during pregnancy. Ten of them drunk one to three glasses of alcohol every week. There was no significant difference between smokers and non smokers (Table 2). Forty-one women reported having used cannabis before pregnancy, six of them said that they continued during pregnancy, which was not the case of the five women who used heroin or cocaine before pregnancy.

This study shows that the majority of women who occasionally drink alcohol could cease if they were aware of its danger during pregnancy. However this fact must be tempered by the recurrence of addictions after pregnancy [20].

## CONCLUSION

Alcohol consumption among women is still a taboo question. It leads to shame and loss of self-confidence. Pregnant women must be helped by a large network of medical, social and educational workers trained to overcome this addiction. There are disparities between French regions in terms of assessment of this public health problem and its countermeasures. For example, there is a network for FASD Prevention and Care in regions like Reunion Island (REUNISAF). These structures aim at preventing damage to the offspring in families who already have a child with FASD. That must be developed nationwide.

Binge drinking is increasing in France even if it is not as widely reported as in neighbouring countries [21]. It can cause early pregnancy and damage to the developing brain of the unborn child. Prevention of adolescent alcohol abuse must be a priority.

Prevention tools, better public and health professional information for optimal care of high-risk women before, during and after pregnancy, should decrease the FAS incidence in the future.

## References


[1] Legleye S, Rosilio T, Nahon S. Alcoolisation, un phénomène complexe. In: Guilbert P, Gautier A, editors. Baromètre Santé 2005 : premiers résultats. St Denis: INPES; 2006,39-47.

[2] Beck F, Legleye S, Splika S, Briffault X, Gautier A, Lamboy B. Les niveaux d'usage des drogues en France en 2005, exploitation des données du Baromètre santé 2005. *Tendances* 2006; 48:6. Available from http://www.ofdt.fr/BDD/publications/docs/eftxfbm5.pdf

[3] Forbes R. Alcohol-related birth defects. *Public Health*. 1984; 98:238-241.

[4] Great Britain. Parliament. House of Commons. Select Committee on Inquiry into Drunkenness. Report form the Select Committee on Inquiry into Drunkenness.

[5] *Nicloux M. Sur le passage de l'alcool ingéré de la mère au fœtus. Canadien Royal Société de Biologie. 1899; 51:980.*

[6] Lemoine P. The history of alcoholic fetopathies. *J. FAS Int.* 2003; 1:e2.

[7] Lemoine P, Harousseau H, Borteyru JP, Menuet J. Les enfants de parents alcooliques: Anomalies observées. A propos de 127 cas [Children of alcoholic parents: Abnormalities observed in 127 cases]. *Ouest. Medical* 1968; 21:476-482.

[8] Jones KL, Smith DW. Recognition of the foetal alcohol syndrome in early infancy. *Lancet* 1973; 2:999–1001.

[9] de Chazeron I, Llorca PM, Ughetto S, Vendittelli F, Boussiron D, Sapin V, Coudore F, Lemery D. Is pregnancy the time to change alcohol consumption habits in France? *Alcohol Clin Exp Res.* 2008; 32:868-73.

[10] Seror E, Chapelon E, Bué M, Garnier-Lengliné H, Lebeaux-Legras C, Loudenot A, Lejeune C. Alcool et grossesse [Alcohol and pregnancy]. *Arch Pediatr.* 2009; 16:1364-1373.

[11] Floyd RL, Sidhu JS Monitoring prenatal alcohol exposure. *Am. J. Med. Genet C Semin. Med. Genet* 2004, 127:3-9

[12] Ades J, Balmes JL, Barrucand D, et al. Les conduites d'alcoolisation au cours de la grossesse. Recommandations de la Société française d'alcoologie. *Alcoologie et addictologie* 2003; 25:45S—104S

[13] Normand R.Consommation d'alcool, de tabac, ou de cannabis au cours de la grossesse. *Bull. Acad. Natle Med.*; 2004; 188: 519-521.

[14] Malet L, de Chazeron I, Llorca PM, Lemery D. Alcohol consumption during Pregnancy: an urge to increase prevention and screening. *Eur. J. Epidemiol.* 21: 787-788, 2006.

[15] Houdebine E, Guillaumin C, Rouquette A, Fanello S. Pregnant women and smoking: descriptive study and prognostic factors to stop smoking during pregnancy. *J. Gynecol. Obstet Biol. Reprod.*. 2009; 38:155-160.

[16] Rueff B. Dépistage des malades alcooliques par l'auto questionnaire DETA. Presse Med 1989; 18: 1654-1656.

[17] Huas D, Darne B, Rueff B, Lombrail P, Leblanc B. Malades alcooliques et consultations de médecine générale : prévalence et détection. *Rev. Prat. Med. Gen.* 1990; 8:45-49.

[18] Mayfield D, McLeod G, Hall P. The CAGE questionnaire: validation of a new alcoholism screening instrument. *Am. J. Psychiatry* 1974; 131:1121-1123.

[19] Bernadt MW, Mumford J, Taylor C, Smith B, Murray RM. Comparison of questionnaire and laboratory tests in the detection of excessive drinking and alcoholism. *Lancet* 1982; 1: 325-8.

[20] Fanello S, Moreau-Gout I, Cotinat JP, Descamps P. Critères de choix concernant l'alimentation du nouveau-né : une enquête auprès de 308 femmes [Decision-making criteria for feeding of newborns: a survey of 308 women] *Arch. Pediatr.*2003**, 10**:19–24

[21] Legleye S, Beck F, Spilka S, Nezet OL. Drogues à l'adolescence en 2005. Niveaux, contextes d'usage et évolutions à 17 ans en France – Résultats de la cinquième enquête nationale ESCAPAD [Drugs at adolescence in 2005. Levels, contexts of use and evolutions for seventeen-year-old] – Results from the national survey ESCAPAD 2005] Observatoire Français des Drogues et des Toxicomanies (OFDT); 2007.

# INDEX

## A

Abraham, 187, 239
absorption, 5, 10, 40, 45, 48, 52, 59, 85, 86
abuse, ix, x, 101, 120, 121, 127, 129, 130, 156, 157, 165, 168, 170, 171, 176, 195, 269, 271, 272, 315, 316, 317, 320, 321, 322, 328, 329, 340, 351, 352, 356
academic performance, xii, 281, 284
accessibility, xiii, 131, 256, 290, 331
acculturation, 319, 320
accuracy, 8, 267, 353
acetic acid, 74, 77
acetylcholinesterase, 131, 151
achievement test, 269
acidosis, 11, 82
acquired immunity, 44, 45
ACTH, 2, 36, 37
active site, 6, 179, 220
adaptation, 94, 150, 220, 309
adaptive functioning, 265, 268
Addiction Severity Index (ASI), 350
adenine, 30, 74
adenosine, 2, 29, 50
ADH, 2, 5, 6, 7, 8, 9, 10, 13, 14, 15, 16, 31, 47, 56, 147, 227, 228, 240
ADHD, 271, 276, 284, 293
adhesion, 3, 19, 21, 45, 48, 54, 65, 191, 205
adipose, 12
adipose tissue, 12
adjustment, 338, 342
adolescent drinking, 239
adolescents, 108, 122, 173, 267, 270, 276, 277, 278, 311, 328
ADP, 203
adrenaline, 37
adulthood, xiii, 38, 39, 48, 50, 51, 186, 268, 299, 322, 324
advantages, 238, 343
aetiology, 69, 80, 82, 85
affirming, 117
Africa, 258, 291
African American women, xiii, 315, 319, 320, 324
African Americans, 70
agencies, 120, 252, 255
aggregation, 78
aggression, 95, 131
agonist, 17, 21, 22, 208, 221, 243
alanine, 80
Alaska, 324, 326
Alaska Natives, 324
alcohol abuse, x, 39, 71, 81, 90, 91, 124, 130, 157, 160, 164, 165, 167, 169, 177, 178, 188, 190, 192, 195, 207, 251, 253, 256, 275, 317, 319, 321, 322, 323, 325, 326, 329, 349, 352, 353, 354, 355, 356, 357, 360, 362, 363
alcohol dependence, xiii, 70, 99, 130, 315, 317, 321, 327, 328, 348, 353, 357, 362
alcohol problems, 118, 126, 158, 191, 321, 322, 327
alcohol research, x, 225, 230
Alcohol Use Disorders Identification Test, 127, 157, 177, 350, 355
alcoholic liver disease, 34, 213, 219
alcoholics, xi, 12, 28, 31, 33, 34, 35, 36, 57, 62, 74, 246, 271, 279, 288, 328, 357, 360
alcoholism, xii, 51, 60, 63, 65, 71, 91, 151, 158, 170, 190, 253, 255, 277, 284, 299, 300, 301, 321, 322, 323, 353, 356, 360, 362, 364
alcohols, xi, 6, 83, 86, 91, 246, 253, 257
aldehydes, 6, 35, 55, 59, 147, 204, 218
alimentation, 364
allele, 241
alpha-tocopherol, 222
ALT, 184
alternative hypothesis, 14

alters, 23, 26, 34, 41, 45, 48, 49, 50, 51, 53, 58, 59, 65, 78, 95, 102, 131, 148, 150, 151, 182, 184, 186, 187, 192, 214, 242, 243, 265
alveolar macrophage, x, 175, 181, 184, 185, 187, 188, 189, 190, 191
alveoli, 16
amblyopia, 284
amenorrhea, 332
American Psychiatric Association, 316
amines, 11, 40
amino acids, 14, 33, 39, 42, 43, 58, 79, 80, 94, 101, 179, 202
amnion, 221
amniotic fluid, 14, 15, 26, 49, 72, 96, 351, 354
amplitude, 235
amplitudes, 15
amygdala, 22
anatomy, 49, 60, 132, 149, 237
anesthetics, 23
ANOVA, 135, 141, 142
ANS, 38
antagonism, 349
antibody, 34, 189
antidiuretic hormone, 2, 39
antigen, 45, 50
anti-inflammatory drugs, 80
antioxidant, x, 30, 46, 54, 56, 76, 79, 87, 89, 175, 179, 180, 181, 186, 188, 191, 192, 193, 199, 202, 210, 218, 222
anxiety, 55, 284, 295, 321, 323, 350
anxiety disorder, 55, 350
aorta, 146
apoptosis, 2, 12, 13, 23, 24, 27, 28, 29, 30, 32, 33, 44, 47, 51, 55, 58, 60, 62, 82, 94, 96, 100, 103, 120, 145, 146, 149, 180, 181, 182, 183, 185, 188, 191, 192, 193, 200, 202, 203, 204, 205, 206, 207, 210, 213, 215, 216, 218, 219, 220, 222, 240, 241
architecture, 205
aromatic compounds, 29
arousal, 216
arrest, 168
arrests, 33, 316
ARs, 77
arsenic, 84
arterial hypertension, 220
arteries, 82, 146, 197, 198, 209
arterioles, 39, 197, 236
artery, 24, 57, 101, 212, 244
ASI, 160, 354
Asian Americans, 320
aspartate, 3, 17, 18, 50, 208, 214, 219, 349
asphyxia, 209, 223
assault, 120, 322, 323, 325, 326, 327, 328, 329
assessment, 17, 118, 157, 159, 160, 161, 172, 183, 231, 247, 266, 267, 268, 269, 270, 271, 277, 339, 340, 341, 343, 344, 353, 361, 363
assessment tools, 172
astrocytes, 29, 212, 220, 222
asymmetry, 26
atherogenesis, 216
atherosclerosis, 214
atoms, 6, 83
ATP, 10, 30, 180, 204
atrium, 146
Attention Deficit Hyperactivity Disorder, 284
Attorney General, 276
authors, vii, 8, 29, 32, 73, 148, 158, 159, 160, 161, 163, 165, 198, 200, 201, 211, 231, 285, 291, 334, 336, 337, 338, 342
autism, 270
autoimmunity, 54
autonomy, 303, 309
autopsy, 191, 226, 229, 233
autosomal recessive, 85
axons, 19, 232, 236, 242

## B

BAC, 2, 10, 13, 15, 103, 236, 238
background, 70, 76, 167
bacteria, 185
bacterial infection, 44, 183, 185
bargaining, 272
barriers, 159, 167, 168, 171, 172
basal forebrain, 86, 90, 233
basal ganglia, 234, 236, 264, 278, 284
basal layer, 211
basement membrane, 213
BBB, 2, 10, 11, 28
beer, xi, 11, 16, 30, 107, 112, 118, 119, 227, 245, 247, 253, 257, 334, 337, 338, 346
behavioral change, 149, 266
behavioral disorders, 275
behavioral problems, xiv, 116, 347
behaviors, 108, 123, 124, 159, 162, 163, 268, 270, 295, 296, 319, 320, 321, 327, 333
beneficial effect, 11, 21, 200, 288
beta-carotene, 99
beverages, xi, xiii, 121, 124, 245, 246, 251, 252, 254, 257, 258, 289, 331, 334, 335, 343, 346
bias, xiii, 123, 248, 290, 292, 331, 332, 335, 336, 337, 343, 344, 345, 349
binge drinking, viii, 27, 41, 68, 69, 70, 91, 105, 107, 108, 109, 110, 114, 115, 116, 117, 119, 122, 123, 124, 126, 156, 162, 165, 176, 227, 246, 247, 250, 251, 289, 317, 320, 321, 322, 323, 329, 349, 350, 355, 360

bingeing, 265
bioavailability, 228
biochemistry, vii, 277
biological activity, 58, 79
biological consequences, 204
biological markers, vii, xiv, 47, 348, 349, 350, 354, 357
biological processes, 82, 89, 222
biological systems, 179
biomarkers, x, xiv, 10, 48, 58, 60, 175, 177, 178, 186, 342, 348, 352, 353, 354, 355, 356, 357
biomonitoring, 221
biosynthesis, 43, 77
biotin, 42, 80, 101
birth control, 157, 164, 165, 166, 167, 168, 324, 339, 342
birth rate, 164, 167
birth weight, 83, 97, 107, 161, 184, 192, 207, 230, 231, 283
births, 4, 70, 107, 115, 123, 130, 165, 166, 169, 171, 249, 324, 342, 348, 361
birthweight, 41
black women, xiii, 48, 315, 319, 320
Blacks, 325
blame, 272, 303
blastula, 139, 146
bleeding, 337, 338, 341
blepharoptosis, 284
blood clot, 136, 138
blood flow, 71, 78, 79, 80, 81, 83, 97, 103, 201, 202, 209, 212, 232, 233, 234, 235, 244
blood monocytes, 185
blood plasma, 12
blood pressure, 36, 50, 214
blood supply, 146
blood vessels, 90, 146, 209, 284
blood-brain barrier, 2, 10, 11, 26
bloodstream, 188, 227
BMI, 339, 340, 341
body fat, 13, 71
body fluid, 10, 12, 178, 353
body mass index, 47, 338, 341
body size, 208
body weight, 6, 10, 14, 30, 82, 230, 231, 234, 235, 236
bone, 20, 43, 56, 63, 145, 146, 184, 210, 284
bone marrow, 20, 184
bones, 43, 136, 144
brain abnormalities, 211, 213, 229, 286, 287
brain damage, ix, 103, 129, 130, 209, 226, 227, 228, 237, 238, 267, 268, 271, 272, 273
brain growth, 21, 65, 69, 74, 86, 95, 96, 196, 204, 229, 231, 232, 239, 240, 241, 286, 287
brain size, 208, 230, 231
brain stem, 50, 276
brain structure, 3, 24, 212, 230, 233, 237, 266
brainstem, 209, 232, 234, 235, 236, 264
breast feeding, xi, 245, 301
breast milk, 16, 354
breastfeeding, 16, 112
breathing, 79, 101
bronchoconstriction, 35
bronchodilator, 6
bronchopulmonary dysplasia, 183, 189
brothers, 300, 301, 304, 305
building blocks, 81
by-products, 180

## C

$Ca^{2+}$, 16, 18, 203
caffeine, 170, 336, 337, 341, 342, 343, 345, 346
calcium, 23, 26, 41, 43, 56, 198
campaigns, 156, 157, 253, 254, 257, 258, 259, 354, 361
cancer, 56, 62, 130, 223, 323
cannabis, xiv, 252, 260, 347, 348, 361, 362, 363
CAP, 20, 165, 166, 258
capillary, 192, 198, 214
carbohydrate, xiv, 2, 13, 16, 82, 177, 192, 348, 350, 356
carbohydrates, 5
carbon, 18, 33, 58, 198, 265
carbon dioxide, 58, 198
carbon monoxide, 18
carbonyl groups, 200
carcinogenesis, 35, 49
cardiac arrhythmia, 6
cardiac glycoside, 6
cardiac muscle, 10
cardiomyopathy, 130
cardiovascular system, 197
caregivers, 273, 274
carotene, 76
cartilage, 42, 134, 145, 146, 210
cartilaginous, 43, 150
caspases, 179, 204, 205, 206
catalytic activity, 6, 82, 209
catecholamines, 37
Caucasians, 6, 70, 291
causality, 308
cell culture, 13, 73, 76, 212, 214
cell cycle, 100
cell death, 7, 21, 27, 52, 54, 61, 69, 76, 83, 103, 120, 148, 152, 199, 203, 205, 207, 209, 211, 215, 216, 218, 222, 349
cell line, 27, 81, 97, 181, 184, 191, 199, 203, 219

cell lines, 199, 203
cell membranes, 45, 178
cell signaling, 45, 63
cell surface, 77, 185
cellular immunity, 44
central nervous system, xii, 2, 4, 12, 17, 18, 25, 26, 47, 59, 68, 92, 96, 136, 177, 188, 211, 213, 216, 217, 218, 258, 266, 267, 282, 299, 324
cerebellum, 18, 32, 49, 55, 180, 189, 207, 232, 234, 236, 238, 240, 241, 242, 243, 264, 265, 276, 284
cerebral blood flow, 242, 243
cerebral cortex, 25, 208, 211, 212, 233
cerebral palsy, 207
cerebrospinal fluid, 10
certificate, 107, 108
ceruloplasmin, 93
challenges, 171, 176, 269
character, 12, 26, 303
chemokines, 205
chemotaxis, 185
chicken, 79, 144
child abuse, viii, 106, 114, 120, 121, 124, 284, 320, 321
child benefit, 300
child development, 4, 36, 46, 349, 350, 354
child protection, 255
childhood, 101, 177, 267, 278, 282, 295, 310, 317, 320, 321, 322, 324, 325, 326, 327, 328, 329
childhood sexual abuse, 321, 322, 325
chlorine, 18, 201
cholesterol, 25, 44, 208, 253
chorion, 131, 132, 138, 221
chromatographic technique, 351
chromatography, 64, 133, 351, 352, 357
chronic diseases, 336
chronic drinking, 71
chronic hypoxia, 209
cigarette smoking, 89, 156, 289, 295, 342, 346
cimetidine, 228
circulation, 7, 9, 11, 12, 15, 16, 17, 28, 29, 30, 35, 36, 37, 39, 45, 72, 75, 81, 99, 132, 137, 138, 140, 141, 142, 143, 144, 145, 146, 147, 148, 150, 198, 201, 207, 208, 209, 220
cirrhosis, 130, 258, 301
citizenship, 252
classical conditioning, 223, 264, 279
classification, 247, 285, 287, 291
cleavage, 139, 206, 215
clients, 164, 165, 166, 271, 272, 279
clinical diagnosis, 70
clinical examination, 285, 290
clinical presentation, 264, 285, 288
clinical symptoms, 285
clinical trials, 162
closure, 73
CNN, 210
CNS, 2, 3, 7, 9, 17, 18, 19, 21, 22, 23, 24, 31, 38, 39, 42, 45, 56, 76, 145, 211, 212, 213, 217, 229, 264, 265, 268, 269, 270, 282, 283, 284, 285, 348
CO2, 5, 11, 12, 22
cocaine, xiv, 71, 119, 125, 170, 193, 228, 239, 240, 243, 339, 345, 347, 348, 356, 361, 362
coding, 35, 36, 46
coenzyme, 5, 10, 11, 14, 30
coffee, 338, 339, 340, 342
cognition, 23, 86, 90, 266, 268
cognitive abilities, 42, 217
cognitive deficit, 87, 96, 126
cognitive deficits, 87
cognitive development, 56
cognitive dysfunction, 226
cognitive flexibility, 271
cognitive function, 86, 106, 211, 229, 233, 268, 273
cognitive impairment, 87
cognitive performance, 268
cognitive process, 271
colleges, 361
collisions, 130
color, iv
coma, 13
combined effect, 244, 342
commissure, 233, 264
common symptoms, 39
communication, 152, 211, 220, 254, 257, 266, 268, 273
communication skills, 268
community, 98, 102, 127, 161, 162, 164, 165, 166, 167, 168, 172, 251, 267, 272, 274, 288, 298, 305
community service, 165, 166, 167
comorbidity, viii, 67, 267
compensation, 159
complement, 44, 256
complex interactions, 89, 271
complications, xii, 4, 30, 57, 183, 201, 207, 208, 255, 281, 283, 284, 288, 293
composition, 16, 23, 26, 28, 45, 48, 51, 72, 89, 307
compounds, vii, 1, 10, 11, 20, 36, 37, 83, 97, 178, 182, 201, 210
condensation, 44, 204, 206
conditioning, 158, 240, 276
conduct disorder, 270, 271
conference, 59, 256
confounders, 336, 338, 341
confounding variables, 267
congenital malformations, 9, 68, 103, 193, 223, 348
congestive heart failure, 6

conjugated dienes, 204
consent, 291, 292
consumption habits, xii, 281
consumption patterns, 248, 250, 288
consumption rates, 115, 250
content analysis, 257
contraceptives, 168, 338, 341
control group, 115, 160, 161, 162, 163, 164, 352
controlled research, 165
controlled trials, 159
coordination, 13, 164, 264, 268, 275, 276, 303
copper, 93, 223
coronary arteries, 223
corpus callosum, 19, 21, 49, 58, 227, 233, 236, 237, 239, 242, 243, 244, 264, 284
corpus luteum, 38
correlation, 34, 50, 81, 101, 178, 222, 230, 265
correlations, 229, 230, 296
cortex, 20, 22, 25, 48, 51, 62, 64, 78, 209, 212, 220, 233, 234, 236, 237, 241, 242, 243
cortical neurons, 20, 21, 22, 27, 32, 49, 58, 61, 188, 191
corticosteroids, 87
corticotropin, 37
cost, ix, 25, 50, 124, 130, 131, 155, 161, 169, 173, 252, 321, 332, 344, 353
cotyledon, 56, 97
counsel, 272
counseling, 122, 124, 127, 161, 162, 163, 164, 296
court proceedings, 272
covering, 249, 254, 353
cranial nerve, 239, 242
craving, 112
creatine, 3, 17, 50
crime, 272
criminal behavior, 272
criminal justice system, xi, 120, 263, 270, 274, 276, 326
critical analysis, 49
critical period, 47, 69, 85, 89, 95, 119, 138, 145, 156, 162, 184, 211, 226, 238, 265
Croatia, 281, 292, 298
CSF, 79, 190
cultural transition, 328
culture, 72, 73, 76, 99, 132, 219, 250, 332
curriculum, xii, 255, 282
cycles, xiii, 27, 166, 211, 331, 334, 336, 337, 338, 341, 342, 343
cyclooxygenase, 92
cystine, 2, 11, 190
cytochrome, 5, 7, 27, 32, 34, 55, 57, 62, 93, 97, 180, 187, 189, 199, 203, 215, 220, 221
cytokines, 3, 41, 78, 80, 84, 86, 87, 88, 90, 187, 205, 222
cytoplasm, 58, 74, 85, 197, 205
cytoskeleton, 20, 29, 38, 48, 206
cytotoxicity, 29, 44, 48, 79, 204, 215, 222, 223

## D

daily living, 268
damping, 12, 17, 24, 29
danger, xi, 246, 253, 308, 362
data collection, 124, 247, 248
data processing, 284
decomposition, 11, 203
defects, ix, x, 36, 43, 49, 65, 68, 73, 74, 75, 76, 77, 79, 80, 82, 83, 85, 86, 87, 88, 94, 96, 98, 115, 116, 119, 124, 125, 129, 130, 131, 134, 144, 149, 195, 196, 198, 207, 212, 226, 246, 264, 265, 283, 284, 324, 349, 360, 363
defence, 30, 89, 199, 201
deficiencies, xii, 9, 19, 39, 40, 46, 86, 184, 267, 283, 299, 309, 348
deficiency, viii, xii, 17, 23, 29, 33, 39, 40, 41, 42, 43, 45, 54, 56, 57, 67, 72, 75, 76, 77, 78, 82, 83, 84, 85, 87, 88, 90, 93, 94, 95, 96, 97, 98, 100, 184, 189, 211, 267, 281, 360
deficit, 266, 271, 275, 286, 287, 350, 355
deformation, 19, 152
degradation, 29, 30, 74, 78, 79, 205, 241, 353
delinquent behavior, 271
demographic characteristics, 160, 317, 324
demyelination, 204
denial, 117, 118, 124, 309
Denmark, 332, 337
deoxyribonucleic acid, 2
Department of Health and Human Services, 116, 125, 126, 127, 173, 331
Department of Justice, 272, 276
dependent variable, 231, 237, 238
dephosphorylation, 19, 65
deposition, 33, 34
deposits, 213
depression, 55, 85, 171, 284, 323, 326, 329
deprivation, 82, 91, 100, 318
detection, x, 63, 126, 172, 175, 186, 191, 192, 219, 247, 285, 290, 291, 297, 351, 352, 353, 354, 355, 356, 361, 364
detention, 106
deterrence, 273
detoxification, 8, 9, 10, 53, 77, 164, 179, 180, 181, 182, 183, 300
developing brain, 21, 22, 23, 25, 50, 55, 208, 211, 227, 265, 363
developmental disorder, vii, 1, 290

developmental process, viii, 42, 67, 69, 197
deviation, 268
diabetes, 30, 130, 198, 199, 267
diagnostic criteria, 266, 285, 286, 287, 288
diagnostic parameters, 285
diastolic blood pressure, 222
diet, 15, 33, 46, 71, 82, 85, 86, 87, 88, 93
dietary intake, 28, 31
differential diagnosis, 266, 269, 287
diffusion, 16, 241, 244, 259
dioxin, 219
direct observation, 131
directives, 285
disability, xiv, 106, 117, 120, 264, 274, 283, 348, 359
disadvantages, 238
disorder, viii, ix, xi, xiv, 40, 63, 94, 100, 105, 106, 121, 124, 125, 129, 130, 149, 150, 152, 172, 192, 212, 216, 217, 225, 226, 241, 264, 266, 268, 270, 271, 272, 275, 278, 284, 290, 294, 295, 296, 297, 324, 347, 354, 355
displacement, 210, 264, 265
disposition, 47
dissociation, 205
distress, 316
disturbances, 32, 59, 69, 345
diversity, 4, 247
dizygotic, 198
DNA, ix, 2, 7, 27, 29, 32, 35, 46, 49, 59, 72, 81, 93, 129, 138, 139, 140, 142, 143, 150, 179, 180, 181, 182, 188, 199, 202, 204, 205, 206, 212, 215, 219, 220, 222, 265
DNA damage, 32, 181, 188, 204, 212, 215
DNA repair, 204
docosahexaenoic acid, 24, 26, 42, 48, 56, 57, 81
doctors, 113, 117, 307
dogs, 244
domestic violence, 168, 323, 326
donors, 11, 65
dopamine, 2, 18, 23, 37
dopaminergic, 19, 23, 52
dorsal aorta, 131, 151
dosage, 200, 353
drinking pattern, 68, 70, 227, 229, 243, 247, 248, 265, 293, 319, 320, 325
drinking patterns, 68, 70, 243, 247, 248, 293, 319, 320, 325
drinking styles, 328
drinking water, 81, 182
Drosophila, 130
drug abuse, 268, 283, 284, 340
drug action, 93
drug interaction, 228, 243
drug testing, 120
drug treatment, 121, 166, 167
drugs, 71, 97, 103, 111, 112, 113, 114, 118, 119, 120, 124, 149, 165, 166, 170, 171, 198, 227, 228, 237, 241, 265, 272, 296, 323, 348, 356, 357, 361
dynamics, 72, 75
dyslexia, 276
dysplasia, 21

## E

economic status, vii, 67, 71, 118, 160, 320, 350
ectoderm, 197, 210
ectopic pregnancy, 123
edema, 131, 207
Education, 109, 110, 127, 254, 276, 360
educational attainment, 117, 320
educational background, 289
efficiency, 6, 27, 187, 228
eicosapentaenoic acid, 28, 50
electron, 3, 179, 180, 181, 199, 202, 221
electrons, 40, 76, 181, 203
elementary school, 292
eligibility criteria, 167
embryogenesis, ix, 77, 102, 103, 129, 131, 132, 134, 138, 142, 144, 145, 146, 147, 150, 152, 197, 211, 222
embryonic stem cells, 217
emotion, 233
emotional disorder, 106
employment, 166, 167, 270, 289, 305, 306, 308, 312, 317
employment status, 289
encoding, 70, 180, 210, 228
encouragement, 112, 121, 124
endocrine, 57, 186, 198
endoderm, 197
endothelial cells, 20, 24, 78, 92, 100, 203, 205, 207, 216, 243
endothelial dysfunction, 201
endothelium, 198, 207, 216
endotoxemia, 192
endotoxins, 83
England, 345, 360
enrollment, 161, 165, 166, 335, 337, 338, 342
environmental conditions, 120
environmental factors, 68, 70, 201, 246, 282, 320
environmental influences, 269, 353
enzymatic activity, 6, 7, 8, 10, 31, 32, 179, 180, 203
enzymes, 6, 10, 11, 22, 27, 31, 32, 34, 35, 36, 37, 43, 46, 51, 70, 77, 80, 82, 84, 147, 179, 181, 188, 189, 200, 201, 202, 206, 216, 227, 228
EPA, 2, 28
epidemic, 249, 278

epidemiologic studies, 333
epidemiology, 98, 102, 170, 173, 279, 293, 297, 298, 325
epidermis, 93
epinephrine, 37, 59
epithelia, 190
epithelial cells, 187
epithelium, 211
equilibrium, 31
erythrocytes, xiv, 34, 146, 348, 350
essential fatty acids, 45
ester, 198, 219, 357
estrogen, 10, 37, 39, 198
ethanol metabolism, 33, 61, 95, 100, 147, 180, 190, 351, 352
ethical issues, 127
ethnic diversity, 228
ethnic groups, xii, 7, 70, 228, 281, 297, 319, 320, 324, 360
ethnicity, 70, 108, 117, 315, 317, 319, 324
ethyl alcohol, 63, 228
etiology, 54, 207
event-related potential, 295
exaggeration, 100
excitability, 25, 49, 208
excitation, 22, 208
excitotoxicity, 31, 208, 209, 219
exclusion, 35, 302, 310
excretion, 13, 17, 30, 43, 45
execution, 4, 205, 206, 233, 264, 295, 303
executive function, 265, 266, 268, 271, 273, 284
executive functioning, 265, 266, 268, 271, 284
experimental condition, 89, 204
experimental design, 146, 163, 335
experts, xii, 124, 263
external influences, 237
external validity, 163
externalizing behavior, ix, 155

## F

facial asymmetry, 144
FAD, 351
false positive, 353
family history, 258, 269
family income, 319
family life, 300, 301
family members, 106, 258, 269, 284
family planning, 163, 164, 167, 168, 344
family support, ix, 155
family violence, 328
fatty acids, vii, 1, 6, 7, 10, 12, 13, 24, 26, 27, 28, 29, 32, 42, 45, 54, 74, 80, 100, 178, 179
fears, 123, 301
febrile seizure, 295
feedback, 272
feelings, 158
femur, 230
fermentation, 11
fertility, xiii, 238, 331, 338, 343, 344, 345, 346, 360
fertilization, 40, 132, 134, 196, 344
fetal abnormalities, 68, 83, 92
fetal development, vii, x, 1, 4, 7, 9, 20, 31, 33, 41, 43, 62, 68, 69, 71, 72, 82, 86, 90, 93, 196, 197, 199, 200, 213, 226, 243, 288, 336, 349
fetal growth, x, 53, 54, 63, 79, 80, 82, 90, 94, 97, 170, 195, 197, 201, 205, 219, 220, 240, 277
fetal growth retardation, 53, 94
fetal nutrition, 94
fiber, 132, 232
fibers, 19, 213
fibroblast growth factor, 146, 212
Finland, 1
fish, 131, 132, 133, 143, 149, 150, 151, 342
fluid, 15, 18, 45, 181, 197, 351, 354
fluid balance, 18
folate, vii, 1, 17, 33, 43, 46, 49, 54, 57, 81, 357
folic acid, 59, 81, 90, 94, 97, 99, 191, 200, 215
folklore, 16
follicle, 2, 38
follicle stimulating hormone, 2, 38
Ford, 189, 190
forebrain, 65, 73, 208, 210, 211, 232, 233, 236, 241
formaldehyde, 6, 62
formula, 74, 237
fragments, 56
France, vi, xi, xiv, xv, 144, 245, 246, 247, 248, 249, 250, 252, 253, 254, 256, 258, 259, 261, 289, 296, 299, 300, 347, 355, 359, 360, 361, 363, 364
fraternal twins, 76
free radicals, 30, 75, 93, 147, 197, 199, 201, 210, 211
frequencies, 36, 228, 249
friendship, xiv, 359
frontal cortex, 239
frontal lobe, 236
fructose, 11, 14
functional changes, 213
funding, 118, 166
fusion, 205, 206, 214

## G

gastroenteritis, 284
gastrointestinal tract, 5
gastrulation, 97, 102, 197, 210, 211, 222, 242
gel, 141
gender differences, 10

gene expression, 42, 60, 62, 76, 100, 103, 131, 146, 150, 151, 208, 210, 211, 212, 232, 234, 236, 237, 241
gene mapping, 151
general intelligence, 265
general practitioner, xii, 169, 263
genes, 24, 36, 42, 45, 46, 62, 70, 76, 84, 90, 94, 98, 99, 131, 150, 180, 205, 207, 210, 211, 212, 228, 354
genetic disease, 131
genetic factors, x, 46, 53, 70, 71, 94, 189, 195, 294
genetic marker, 353
genetic syndromes, 276
genetics, 89, 150, 239, 271, 272
genome, 132
genotype, 54
genre, 259, 260
Georgia, 175
germ layer, 197
gestation, xi, 6, 8, 9, 11, 14, 15, 19, 20, 23, 25, 28, 31, 32, 36, 37, 38, 40, 42, 43, 44, 45, 61, 64, 69, 71, 72, 73, 75, 77, 82, 83, 86, 89, 92, 97, 98, 176, 184, 185, 192, 196, 197, 200, 202, 204, 207, 208, 210, 211, 216, 223, 225, 227, 229, 230, 231, 243, 292,351
gestational age, 7, 28, 31, 39, 115, 208, 223, 266, 267
gestational diabetes, 267
gland, 16
glasses, xi, 245, 249, 250, 251, 258, 334, 362
glia, 211, 213, 220
glial cells, 208, 217, 220, 221
glucose, 14, 58, 79, 80, 81, 101, 200, 202, 207, 212
glutamate, 2, 17, 18, 19, 22, 38, 59, 208, 235, 239
glutamic acid, 22
glutathione, x, 2, 3, 7, 31, 33, 49, 53, 61, 62, 65, 76, 175, 180, 181, 182, 185, 186, 189, 192, 199, 200, 202, 214, 217, 221
glycine, 19, 52
glycoproteins, 38
gray matter, 218
Great Britain, 363
Greece, 263, 306
growth factor, 3, 20, 43, 53, 62, 209, 210, 211, 212, 349
growth hormone, 43, 64, 222
growth rate, 43
growth spurt, 23, 229, 239
guardian, 300, 302, 305
guidance, 20, 21, 54, 165
guidelines, 170, 216, 239, 266, 285, 296, 350
Guinea, 187, 188, 189, 214

## H

hair, xiv, 178, 188, 191, 192, 193, 347, 351, 353, 354, 356, 357
half-life, 78, 85, 178
harmful effects, viii, 26, 105, 198, 212, 256, 325, 335
harmonization, 266
hazards, 10, 334, 336, 350
HE, 98, 151, 152, 217, 294, 295, 297, 298
headache, 36
health care professionals, 255
health education, 246
health effects, 4, 335
health insurance, 306, 319, 321
health problems, xiii, 130, 159, 300, 315, 323, 324
health services, 168
health status, 125, 130, 321
hearing loss, 284
heart disease, 130, 323
heart rate, 131, 146
heartburn, 228
heat shock protein, 96, 131
heavy drinking, vii, xiii, 4, 34, 67, 162, 172, 317, 318, 319, 320, 322, 324, 325, 327, 331
height, 266, 267, 283
hematopoietic stem cells, 20, 33, 53, 59
heme, 18, 27
hemisphere, 233
hemoglobin, 34, 192
hemorrhage, 48
hepatocytes, 27, 29, 34, 48, 55, 74, 87, 199, 200, 214
hepatomegaly, 213
heroin, 71, 119, 348, 361, 362
heterogeneity, 32, 182, 268, 350
high blood pressure, 78
high fat, 5, 33
high school, 114, 122, 156, 321, 361
higher education, xii, 281, 289, 319
high-risk populations, xii, 281
hippocampus, 18, 19, 26, 55, 78, 86, 91, 180, 189, 207, 209, 233, 234, 235, 236, 242, 264, 265, 284
Hispanic population, 115
Hispanics, 320, 321, 325
histidine, 7, 33, 80
histone, 265
homeostasis, viii, 18, 31, 43, 61, 67, 83, 84, 85, 86, 88, 182, 186, 205
homework, 302
homicide, 120
homocysteine, 357
hormonal control, 16
hospitalization, 158, 178, 189

HPA axis, 36, 39
human brain, 19, 23, 187, 230
human chorionic gonadotropin, 3, 38, 198, 341
human condition, 131, 144, 238
human development, 58, 196
human subjects, 226
humoral immunity, 44, 184
Hunter, 97, 151, 184, 189
husband, 120, 300, 305, 322, 327
hybrid, 33
hydrocephalus, 21
hydrogen, 74, 76, 180, 199, 201, 202, 203, 204
hydrogen peroxide, 74, 76, 180, 199, 201, 202, 203
hydrolases, 11
hydronephrosis, 284
hydroperoxides, 222
hydroxide, 203
hydroxyl, 76, 179, 180, 199, 201, 202
hygiene, 309
hyoid, 134
hyperactivity, xi, 50, 263, 266, 270, 271, 275, 348, 355
hypersensitivity, 94
hypertelorism, 267, 284
hypertension, 78, 130, 207, 214, 253
hyperuricemia, 30
hypoplasia, 21, 100, 131, 212, 267, 283, 284, 285
hypothalamus, 19, 36, 37, 38, 49
hypothesis, x, 20, 24, 37, 50, 147, 195, 219, 328, 353
hypoxia, x, 23, 25, 27, 48, 71, 76, 79, 80, 82, 99, 195, 196, 198, 199, 201, 207, 208, 209, 213, 215, 234, 242

## I

ICAM, 3, 45
ideal, xii, 263
identical twins, 70, 76
IFN, 48
illegal drug use, 121
image, 135, 253
image analysis, 135
immune function, x, 65, 82, 175, 176, 185, 193
immune response, 28, 34, 42, 44, 45, 54, 88, 184, 185
immune system, 12, 29, 34, 40, 44, 45, 46, 53, 184, 186
immunity, 28, 41, 44, 45, 55, 184, 185, 186, 214
immunization, 183, 191
immunoglobulin, 3, 34, 41, 44, 45, 46
immunoglobulins, 34, 44, 46
immunohistochemistry, 214
immunoreactivity, 59
immunosuppression, 186
impacts, xii, 30, 47, 263
impairments, xi, 41, 63, 69, 70, 81, 83, 85, 102, 263, 270, 271, 277, 282, 284, 288, 293, 343, 344, 350, 270, 271, 356
in utero, vii, x, xiii, 1, 17, 22, 24, 25, 27, 28, 31, 38, 43, 45, 47, 69, 72, 100, 175, 176, 177, 178, 179, 182, 183, 184, 185, 186, 187, 190, 191, 192, 198, 207, 230, 259, 267, 299, 310, 338, 341, 348, 354, 356
in vivo, 4, 6, 10, 11, 12, 13, 17, 20, 21, 23, 24, 26, 28, 29, 32, 33, 34, 35, 38, 39, 40, 43, 47, 49, 50, 51, 55, 60, 65, 72, 75, 76, 93, 94, 95, 185, 188, 202, 209, 213, 217, 222, 223, 241
incarceration, xii, 123, 168, 263, 269, 274
incidence, xiii, 4, 40, 69, 70, 71, 73, 79, 82, 83, 84, 90, 130, 148, 163, 164, 183, 186, 187, 230, 247, 252, 297, 310, 315, 318, 332, 345, 361, 363
inclusion, 249, 290
independence, 270
Indians, 149, 172, 324
indirect effect, 23, 38, 209
indirect measure, 78
induction, 9, 18, 34, 41, 84, 85, 86, 87, 88, 89, 93, 142, 145, 181, 182, 188, 191, 198, 203, 206
infancy, 61, 96, 126, 150, 190, 218, 241, 260, 277, 284, 296, 363
infant care, 254
infants, viii, xi, xiv, 11, 47, 49, 53, 70, 86, 92, 103, 105, 107, 115, 120, 127, 164, 166, 167, 176, 177, 178, 183, 189, 191, 192, 226, 229, 230, 245, 246, 247, 253, 255, 265, 347, 348
infarction, 81, 209, 215
infertility, xiii, 331, 332, 333, 334, 339, 345, 346
inflammation, 49, 50, 74, 86, 87, 95, 98, 187, 188, 203, 204, 215, 284
inflammatory cells, 184
inflammatory disease, 49, 204
inflammatory mediators, viii, 67, 75, 79, 86
informed consent, 291, 292
ingest, 201
ingestion, 9, 11, 16, 34, 36, 74, 86, 101, 144, 181, 185, 187, 190, 196
inherited disorder, 85
inhibition, 8, 9, 10, 22, 23, 27, 30, 38, 42, 45, 53, 54, 63, 72, 77, 79, 93, 94, 136, 147, 202, 208, 210, 212, 215, 220, 222, 241, 268, 271, 295
inhibitor, 2, 9, 27, 32, 37, 65, 75, 78, 79, 100, 102, 181, 265
initiation, 76, 79, 120, 179, 206
innate immunity, 44, 46, 185, 188, 190
insight, viii, 67, 68, 106, 124, 238
insulin, 3, 43, 53, 209, 212
integration, 19, 20, 21, 29, 46, 106, 232, 233

intellectual disabilities, 276
intelligence, xiii, 106, 268, 271, 273, 299, 303, 308
intelligence quotient, xiii, 299, 303
intelligence tests, 271
intensive care unit, 188
interest groups, 253
interface, 198, 222
interference, vii, 1, 9, 34, 43, 80
interneuron, 54
interneurons, 20, 21, 51
interpersonal relations, 324
interpersonal relationships, 324
intervention, 4, 68, 89, 95, 120, 122, 127, 157, 159, 160, 161, 162, 163, 164, 166, 167, 169, 170, 171, 172, 223, 296, 311, 349, 361
intervention strategies, 68, 89, 168
intestinal tract, 18
intestine, 48, 86, 184, 203
intimate partner violence, 319, 328
intoxication, 100, 204, 316
intrauterine growth retardation, 39, 101, 196, 215
ion channels, 23, 25, 50, 198, 208
ionization, 352
ions, 3, 41
IQ scores, 69, 265
Ireland, 258, 289, 321, 329
iron, 27, 33, 64, 79, 219, 300, 352
iron transport, 352
irritability, 308
ischemia, 27, 76, 202, 207, 209, 215
isozymes, 49, 227, 228
Israel, 296
Italy, 289, 298

J

Japan, 258
job satisfaction, 318

K

$K^+$, 18
keratin, 215
kidney, 6, 8, 10, 34, 41, 86, 283, 284
kidneys, 83, 258, 283, 284, 324
kindergarten, 291
kindergarten children, 291
kinetic constants, 8
kinetic studies, 217
kinetics, 8, 13, 14, 15, 60, 99, 227, 240
knots, 205
Korea, 258

L

labeling, 156, 157
labile zinc, 103
laboratory tests, 285, 350, 364
lack of control, 307
lack of opportunities, 269
lactate level, 62
lactation, 3, 16, 18, 22, 36, 45, 46, 48, 51, 52, 53, 59, 60, 82, 95, 215, 219
lactic acid, 30, 201
language development, 270
later life, 55, 208
Latinos, 328
law enforcement, 120, 275
lawyers, xii, 263, 270, 272
learning, xi, xii, 18, 24, 68, 82, 231, 233, 263, 264, 265, 270, 271, 272, 275, 276, 277, 278, 279, 281, 284, 293, 302, 304, 324, 348, 350, 357
learning difficulties, 293
learning disabilities, xi, xii, 263, 264, 270, 272, 277, 281
legislation, xi, 114, 121, 245, 246, 251, 252
leisure, 270, 305, 306, 307
leisure time, 270
leptin, 38, 39, 55
lesions, 35, 199, 203
leucine, 80
level of education, 258
life expectancy, xi, 245
lifestyle behaviors, 333, 335, 336
lifestyle changes, 160
lifetime, ix, 10, 12, 13, 107, 155, 160, 169, 321, 324, 328
ligand, 18, 20, 23, 27, 50, 83, 151, 180, 183, 206
limitations, xiii, 231, 331, 333
lipid metabolism, 7, 26, 42, 62, 82
lipid peroxidation, 2, 7, 33, 34, 35, 46, 51, 56, 58, 79, 179, 180, 181, 182, 200, 203, 204, 212, 221, 222
lipids, 3, 7, 26, 47, 49, 54, 59, 75, 178, 199, 202, 204, 341, 343
lipolysis, 11
lipoproteins, 204
liposomes, 204
liquid chromatography, 353
liver, 6, 7, 8, 9, 10, 11, 12, 14, 15, 16, 27, 28, 31, 32, 33, 34, 35, 37, 41, 43, 49, 53, 54, 57, 58, 59, 60, 61, 64, 74, 78, 81, 83, 84, 85, 86, 87, 88, 89, 90, 98, 102, 178, 180, 181, 184, 187, 188, 192, 199, 200, 213, 214, 220, 221, 222, 227, 228, 239, 258,323, 324, 351, 354
liver cancer, 258
liver cirrhosis, 64, 258, 354

liver damage, 59
liver disease, 11, 34, 57, 323
living environment, 275
localization, 23, 54, 58, 64
locus, 235, 242
longitudinal study, 52
low risk, viii, 106
loyalty, xiv, 359
lumen, 85
lung disease, 183, 184, 188, 191
luteinizing hormone, 3, 38, 52, 55
lymphocytes, 44, 183, 184, 193
lymphoid, 184, 205
lymphoid tissue, 184
lysine, 7, 11, 33, 34, 80

## M

machinery, 30
macrocytosis, 60
macromolecules, 138, 147, 179
macrophages, 8, 44, 45, 74, 182, 184, 187, 191, 201, 203, 206, 223
magazines, 254
major depressive disorder, 156
majority, 21, 73, 78, 106, 117, 119, 120, 124, 138, 145, 146, 156, 161, 162, 165, 168, 176, 177, 212, 229, 251, 255, 256, 265, 290, 291, 322, 343, 362
malabsorption, 85
malnutrition, 94, 95, 196, 202, 217, 255
mammal, 16
mammalian brain, 17, 212
mammalian tissues, 11, 12
management, ix, xv, 156, 164, 165, 171, 172, 293, 308, 359
mandates, 121
marijuana, 119, 125, 170, 345, 355
marital status, xiii, 108, 289, 315, 317, 318
markers, xiii, xiv, 13, 30, 31, 32, 63, 145, 177, 182, 187, 190, 191, 192, 205, 331, 348, 351, 352, 353, 354, 355
mass spectrometry, 351, 352, 353, 357
MAST, 158
mast cells, 60
maternal care, 61
maternal smoking, 54, 95
maternal support, 321
mathematics, 302
matrix, 203, 353
maxilla, 267
meconium, xiv, 12, 29, 178, 187, 191, 198, 214, 215, 348, 350, 351, 352, 353, 354, 355, 356
media, xi, 245, 251, 252, 296
Medicaid, 108, 109, 110
medical care, 121, 334, 354
medication, 300, 328, 332
Mediterranean, 356
medulla, 37
megakaryocyte, 60
membrane permeability, 204
membranes, 20, 26, 46, 75, 81, 152, 179, 181, 204
memory, 18, 23, 41, 63, 83, 86, 90, 95, 102, 106, 233, 248, 265, 266, 268, 271, 272, 273, 293, 303, 306, 309, 324, 350
meningitis, 183, 300
menstruation, 336, 342, 343
mental development, 164
mental disorder, 173, 272, 324
mental health, 156, 168, 284, 321, 329
mental illness, 271, 274, 295
mental retardation, vii, ix, x, xii, 99, 130, 155, 177, 195, 196, 265, 268, 299, 354
mesencephalon, 145
mesoderm, 152, 197, 210
messages, viii, 106, 254, 255, 257, 259, 307
messenger RNA, 152
meta-analysis, 344
metabolic pathways, 5, 29, 47
metabolism, viii, x, 2, 6, 10, 12, 13, 28, 30, 43, 46, 51, 54, 56, 57, 59, 63, 65, 67, 70, 71, 72, 73, 74, 76, 77, 79, 83, 87, 89, 90, 91, 92, 93, 97, 98, 99, 102, 145, 178, 180, 182, 195, 198, 227, 228, 239, 265
metabolites, vii, x, 1, 10, 13, 19, 23, 25, 26, 31, 35, 36, 42, 45, 46, 57, 73, 77, 79, 103, 182, 187, 196, 198, 204, 208, 214, 265, 282, 351
metabolizing, ix, 10, 36, 46, 129, 152, 189, 227
metals, 41, 80
methodology, 114, 291
methylation, 150, 232, 265
Mexico, 320, 325, 328
mice, 10, 19, 20, 28, 32, 37, 41, 49, 51, 55, 57, 59, 70, 72, 73, 74, 75, 76, 78, 79, 81, 83, 84, 85, 86, 88, 92, 93, 94, 95, 100, 102, 103, 150, 210, 211, 216, 222, 354
Michigan Alcoholism Screening Test, 158, 177
microcephaly, 46, 73, 74, 75, 95, 144, 145, 211, 231, 264, 360
microheterogeneity, 48
microscope, 134, 135, 146, 213
microsomes, 34
microstructure, 229, 241, 295
middle class, 71
migration, 19, 20, 21, 22, 29, 55, 61, 62, 136, 145, 148, 152, 204, 210, 211, 218, 219, 222, 264, 349
minorities, 325
minority groups, 183

miscarriage, 282, 324, 332, 333
misconceptions, 259
misunderstanding, 273, 274
mitochondria, 10, 27, 179, 180, 199, 201, 203, 204, 215, 217, 222
mitochondrial damage, 200
moderating factors, 318
modern society, 106
modification, 35, 40, 43, 100, 199
modules, 256
molecular biology, 50
molecular oxygen, 180, 199
molecular weight, 22, 31, 83
molecules, 20, 35, 40, 45, 81, 146, 179, 191, 205, 207, 212, 220
monitoring, 120
morbidity, vii, 67, 68, 87, 89, 183
morphogenesis, 9, 42, 132, 147, 149, 220, 277, 286, 287
morphological abnormalities, 21, 83
morphology, 37, 56, 73, 132, 134, 210, 214, 232, 278, 294
morphometric, 278
mortality rate, 13, 161, 282
morula, 196
motivation, 17, 160, 302, 306
motor behavior, 264
motor skills, 106, 265, 268
MRI, 17, 229, 232, 233, 275
mRNA, ix, 6, 8, 9, 32, 44, 63, 77, 95, 129, 131, 141, 142, 144, 147, 149, 152, 180, 181, 216, 240
multidimensional, 244
multiplication, 302, 307
muscles, 146
musculoskeletal system, 197
music, 309
mutant, 10, 32, 41, 220
mutation, 77, 99
myelin, 74, 204, 222
myopathy, 34


## N


$Na^+$, 18
NaCl, 134
NAD, 14, 74, 76, 220
NADH, 14, 30, 76
nanometers, 44
National Institutes of Health, 175, 225, 331
National Survey, 114, 332, 344
Native Americans, 70, 321, 329
natural killer cell, 45, 193
necrosis, 12, 29, 47, 102, 202, 203, 204, 209, 214, 215
negative outcomes, 274
neglect, 114, 120, 269, 271, 316, 321
neocortex, 20, 22, 86, 221, 222
neonates, 16, 23, 28, 29, 36, 41, 46, 120, 188, 192, 209, 215
nerve, 223, 283
nerve growth factor, 223
nervous system, xiii, 19, 26, 46, 56, 95, 98, 197, 204, 208, 218, 299
Netherlands, 1, 258
neural development, vii, 1, 19, 227
neural network, 19
neuroactive peptides, 18
neurobiology, 275
neuroblasts, 25
neurodegeneration, 24, 28, 51, 59, 96, 204, 218
neurodegenerative disorders, 27
neuroendocrine system, 36
neurogenesis, 25, 132, 150, 211, 241, 242
neuronal apoptosis, 23, 24, 26, 47, 52, 56, 65
neuronal cells, 18, 20, 21, 25, 26, 28, 38
neurons, 12, 19, 20, 21, 23, 24, 25, 28, 29, 31, 32, 37, 41, 47, 48, 50, 58, 62, 86, 120, 188, 203, 211, 212, 216, 217, 220, 222, 233, 237, 238, 241
neuroprotection, 222
neuropsychology, 278
neurotoxicity, 99, 218, 221, 348
neurotransmitter, 2, 17, 18, 21, 23, 25, 37, 45, 46, 349
neurotrophic factors, 240, 241, 244, 349
neutrophils, 203
New Zealand, 289
nicotinamide, 74
nicotine, 60, 221
nitric oxide, 3, 11, 26, 30, 37, 51, 52, 60, 61, 63, 65, 70, 76, 90, 91, 201, 202, 212, 214, 215, 216, 219, 220, 221, 222
nitric oxide synthase, 3, 63, 65, 70, 76, 91, 201, 212, 214, 216, 219, 221
nitrogen, 40, 199, 203, 220
nitrogen dioxide, 203
NMDA receptors, 17, 19, 58
nonsmokers, 341, 342
norepinephrine, 37
normal development, 17, 25, 117, 138, 147, 150
North America, ix, 130, 155, 156, 162, 173, 325
notochord, 131, 136, 145
Nrf2, 188, 193
NSAIDs, 79
nuclear receptors, 9, 77
nuclei, 196, 206, 232, 234, 235, 240, 242
nucleic acid, 35, 82, 138, 199
nucleotides, 202

nucleus, 18, 19, 50, 58, 180, 205, 206, 233, 235, 242
nursery school, 302
nurses, 342
nursing, 61, 258
nutrient transfer, 81
nutrients, 41, 71, 80, 83, 89, 147, 198, 201, 206, 209
nutrition, 58, 71, 88, 89, 92, 95, 97, 229, 265

## O

offenders, 274, 276
olfaction, 233, 243
oligomers, 52
oocyte, 196
opiates, 248, 356
opportunities, 131, 222, 223, 252
optic nerve, 131, 264
oral health, 151
organ, 9, 30, 36, 40, 42, 72, 82, 119, 181, 186, 190, 197, 198, 204, 205, 211, 221, 228, 341
organelles, 85
organism, 153, 199
organizing, 304
oscillations, 48
ossification, 43, 63, 84
overlap, 269
overproduction, 61
ovulation, 3, 38, 332, 338, 341, 342
oxidation, 3, 5, 6, 7, 8, 9, 11, 13, 14, 26, 32, 35, 53, 54, 74, 76, 77, 79, 93, 179, 182
oxidation products, 26
oxidative damage, 199, 200, 202
oxidative reaction, 203
oxidative stress, viii, x, 24, 27, 30, 31, 32, 33, 42, 46, 51, 55, 57, 60, 61, 62, 64, 67, 70, 72, 74, 75, 79, 96, 100, 145, 147, 149, 179, 180, 181, 182, 188, 190, 195, 196, 198, 199, 200, 201, 202, 207, 213, 215, 216, 218, 219, 220, 221
oxygen, x, 30, 32, 41, 51, 74, 76, 80, 180, 196, 197, 198, 199, 201, 203, 206, 207, 217, 218, 221, 241
oxygen consumption, 180, 201, 203

## P

p53, 41, 202, 219
Pacific, 70, 327, 328
Pacific Islanders, 328
pain, 300, 304
paints, 255
palate, 83, 267
palivizumab, 183, 186
pancreas, 12, 83, 86, 178, 200
parallel, 199, 238, 253
parameter, 13, 14
parity, 229, 339, 340, 341, 343
Parliament, 363
patent ductus arteriosus, 183, 212
pathogenesis, 70, 78, 101, 181, 207, 209
pathogens, 185
pathology, 51, 63, 201, 208, 209, 220, 310
pathophysiology, 48, 184, 187, 191, 215
pathways, vii, 1, 4, 5, 7, 9, 10, 12, 13, 19, 21, 33, 40, 42, 46, 54, 59, 61, 68, 71, 74, 98, 178, 197, 203, 204, 209, 214, 223, 227, 240, 344, 353
pattern recognition, 44
PCR, 141, 142, 144, 147
peer influence, 323
pelvic inflammatory disease, 341
peptides, 62
percentile, 266, 267, 268, 286, 287
performance, 16, 122, 240, 243, 268, 277, 286, 287, 316
perfusion, 29, 36, 42, 61, 80, 82, 207, 208
perinatal, 37, 51, 56, 87, 99, 168, 189, 207, 218, 249, 256, 282, 283, 361
peripheral blood, 10, 34, 47
peripheral blood mononuclear cell, 47
peripheral nervous system, 3, 18, 25
permeability, 3, 27, 55, 81
permit, xiv, 343, 344, 348
peroxidation, 34, 54, 78, 179, 199, 200, 204
peroxide, 76, 200, 203
peroxynitrite, 12, 30, 55, 58, 202, 203, 204, 205, 215, 216, 217, 220, 221, 222, 223
personality characteristics, 279
pesticides, 356
PGE, 39, 42, 79, 90
pH, 33, 201
phagocytosis, 182, 185, 191, 204
pharmacokinetics, 74, 242, 243
phenotype, 4, 69, 88, 125, 150, 215, 264, 267, 275, 279, 288, 296
philtrum, 144, 177, 210, 266, 267, 269, 283, 284, 285, 286, 287, 288
phosphatidylserine, 3, 26, 47, 206, 220
phosphocreatine, 50
phospholipids, 64, 100
phosphorus, 81
phosphorylation, 19, 21, 23, 24, 52, 65, 179, 205, 236, 237, 241
photomicrographs, 134, 135, 136
physical abuse, 320
physical education, 303
physical features, 191, 229, 267, 278
physicochemical properties, 34
physiology, 13, 30, 31, 38, 39, 51, 52, 60, 63, 90, 102, 187

pigs, 7, 22, 72
pilot study, 161, 164, 165, 171, 241
pitch, 307
pituitary gland, 36, 264
placenta, 7, 8, 10, 12, 17, 25, 28, 29, 36, 37, 42, 46, 49, 54, 62, 64, 71, 72, 75, 80, 81, 83, 89, 90, 92, 94, 95, 96, 97, 99, 100, 101, 180, 181, 197, 198, 201, 204, 205, 207, 208, 209, 213, 214, 216, 217, 218, 220, 221, 223, 255, 354
placental abruption, 41, 57
placental barrier, 28, 38, 42, 44, 46, 197, 209, 349
planning, 4, 43, 116, 163, 268, 271, 288, 290, 293, 296, 305, 342, 343, 345
plants, 338
plasma levels, 9, 28, 30, 36, 38, 40, 208
plasma membrane, 24, 26, 29, 44, 204, 206, 220, 349
plasma proteins, 200
plasticity, 95
platelet aggregation, 78
platelets, 12
plausibility, 97
plea bargaining, 272
pneumonia, 183, 185, 284
polarity, 146
police, 272, 308
political party, 252
polling, 254
polymerization, 203, 216
polymorphism, 6, 64, 76, 182
polymorphisms, 70, 102, 180, 182, 244
polyunsaturated fat, 3, 7, 26, 27, 49, 53, 54, 62, 63, 78, 81, 181, 204
polyunsaturated fatty acids, 3, 7, 26, 27, 49, 53, 62, 63, 78, 81, 204
pools, 181, 182, 183
Portugal, 247
positive feedback, 27
positive relationship, 320, 336
post traumatic stress disorder, 156
poverty, 271
precursor cells, 145
preeclampsia, 30, 54, 62, 78, 102, 198, 199, 201, 206, 213, 216, 219, 220, 222
prefrontal cortex, 54
premature infant, 37, 176, 189, 218
prematurity, 178, 183, 186, 191, 192
preterm delivery, 37, 187, 205, 207
preterm infants, 187, 216
prevention, ix, xii, xiv, xv, 116, 122, 124, 156, 157, 162, 163, 164, 165, 168, 169, 171, 172, 173, 186, 188, 189, 191, 196, 215, 250, 252, 254, 256, 257, 258, 260, 266, 277, 279, 281, 288, 293, 296, 297, 332, 348, 354, 355, 359, 361, 364
primary function, 85, 87
primary school, 257, 294, 303
primate, 92, 94, 229, 232
probability, 158, 181, 324, 332, 338, 342
probation officers, 270
problem behavior, 271
problem behaviors, 271
problem drinkers, 126, 318
problem drinking, 157, 162, 318, 319, 321, 322, 323, 328, 329
problem solving, 324
producers, 11, 246, 252, 258
productivity, ix, 155
progesterone, 25, 198, 208, 216
prognosis, 40
programming, vii, 1, 4, 36, 37, 38, 39, 40, 55, 56, 59, 60, 64, 65, 89, 186, 193
pro-inflammatory, 58, 184, 185
project, 20, 108, 149, 163, 232
prolactin, 16, 36, 202, 217, 222
proliferation, 19, 20, 24, 25, 28, 33, 43, 44, 52, 59, 60, 64, 73, 82, 146, 180, 183, 205, 211, 229, 349
promoter, 78, 87, 150
prophylaxis, 187, 222
prostacyclins, 81
prostaglandins, viii, 67, 72, 78, 81, 92, 97
proteases, 179, 204, 205, 206, 220
protective factors, 288
protective mechanisms, 33
protein oxidation, 179, 182, 214
protein structure, 6
protein synthesis, 72, 74
proteins, 7, 19, 20, 21, 23, 31, 33, 34, 36, 40, 42, 44, 45, 46, 75, 77, 82, 85, 86, 96, 98, 131, 143, 179, 180, 182, 198, 199, 200, 202, 203, 205, 206, 209, 240, 241, 244
proteinuria, 207
psychiatric disorders, 268, 276, 326
psychiatric hospitals, xiii, 299
psychiatric illness, 156
psychoactive drug, 327, 360
psychological assessments, 273
psychological connections, 322
psychological development, 326
psychological distress, 322
psychological problems, 320
psychology, 276
psychosocial factors, 361
psychotropic drugs, 295
PTSD, 326
puberty, 4, 284
public awareness, 122, 178, 256
public domain, 118

public health, x, xiv, xv, 106, 156, 169, 195, 196, 252, 324, 332, 333, 347, 348, 349, 359, 363
pulmonary hypertension, 47, 59
pumps, 18
purines, 29, 43
pyramidal cells, 233, 235
pyrimidine, 29

## R

race, 70, 108, 117, 118, 315, 317, 319, 324, 338, 348
racial differences, 319
radical formation, 71, 222
radical reactions, 204
radicals, 27, 43, 74, 76, 179, 180, 199, 201, 204, 215, 217
radio, 254, 284
rape, 321, 322, 326, 327
reactions, 40, 44, 76, 80, 179, 199, 201, 206, 265, 322, 326
reactive oxygen, 24, 30, 46, 57, 73, 74, 75, 76, 79, 83, 87, 89, 93, 147, 176, 179, 198, 199, 214, 220, 222, 241
reactivity, 6, 7, 10, 32, 35, 40, 46, 54, 202, 219, 236
reading, 303, 313
reality, xii, 4, 252, 299, 309, 338
reasoning, xii, 106, 266, 271, 273, 281, 302
recall, 24, 36, 46, 113, 248, 271, 273, 332, 333, 336, 338, 342, 344, 345
recalling, 335
receptors, 9, 17, 18, 19, 22, 23, 30, 38, 44, 45, 50, 53, 55, 57, 75, 76, 77, 147, 179, 183, 204, 208, 210, 212, 219, 223, 349
recognition, 22, 52, 54, 63, 86, 93, 102, 156, 160, 170, 172, 196, 198, 217, 231, 240, 259, 274, 275, 288, 297, 316, 337
recommendations, iv, 43, 117, 127, 167, 186, 191, 252, 255, 285, 361
reconciliation, 274
recruiting, 335
recurrence, 362
recycling, 43, 203, 254
red blood cells, 13
redistribution, 60, 75, 86, 180, 220
regression, viii, 25, 105, 108, 334, 338
regression analysis, viii, 105, 108
regression model, 338
rehabilitation, 273, 284, 300
rehabilitation program, 300
reinforcement, 200, 288
relational theory, 326
relatives, 158
relaxation, 11, 78, 257
relevance, vii, 1, 6, 9, 22, 23, 27, 28, 30, 32, 33, 37, 40, 41, 43, 65, 73, 79, 92, 201, 213, 217, 218, 285
reliability, 177, 271, 300, 345, 355, 356
religion, 117
religious beliefs, 113, 117
repair, 35, 87, 89, 201, 204, 208, 222
repetitions, 137, 140
replication, 167
reproduction, 38, 50, 82, 92, 95, 220, 238, 259, 260, 327
reproductive age, 106, 119, 157, 228, 289, 338
reproductive organs, 338
reproductive toxicant, 332
requirements, 28, 40, 43, 82, 120, 160, 258, 270, 336
residues, 7, 11, 33, 34, 179, 202, 203, 221, 352
resistance, 42, 82, 187, 197, 209, 241, 247, 305
resources, 159
respect, 46, 144, 253, 267, 306
respiration, 5, 11, 14, 74, 180, 182, 202
respiratory distress syndrome, 185
respiratory syncytial virus, 183, 186, 189, 191
responsiveness, 53
retardation, ix, x, xii, xiv, 4, 21, 40, 46, 68, 73, 75, 85, 91, 129, 130, 147, 177, 195, 196, 200, 211, 226, 264, 267, 281, 282, 283, 284, 285, 286, 287, 324, 347
reticulum, 27, 216
retina, 197
retinol, 6, 8, 9, 54, 76, 77, 89, 93, 95
retirement, 310
ribonucleic acid, 3
rights, iv, xii, 120, 263, 272
risk factors, x, xii, 71, 89, 90, 98, 102, 151, 225, 227, 229, 253, 281, 288, 289, 290, 293, 318, 327, 328, 329, 332, 336
RNA, ix, 3, 29, 72, 81, 129, 131, 138, 139, 140, 141, 142, 143, 145, 147
rodents, 14, 35, 81, 82, 83, 86, 204
room temperature, 11, 139
rural areas, 292
rural population, 291
Russia, 258

## S

saliva, 63
saturated fat, 26
scavengers, 202, 210
schizophrenia, 90, 91, 99, 100
school performance, xii, 281, 282
school reports, 303, 312
scoliosis, 284
screening, ix, 42, 95, 117, 118, 124, 126, 127, 151, 156, 157, 158, 159, 160, 163, 164, 167, 169, 172,

187, 188, 192, 198, 239, 247, 260, 266, 270, 275, 288, 290, 291, 296, 297, 351, 355, 357, 364
sebum, 178
second generation, 320
secondary education, 257
secretion, 34, 55, 56
seizure, 284, 295, 324
selectivity, 241
selenium, 76, 191
self-confidence, 305, 362
self-discipline, 47
self-regulation, 277
self-reports, 269
semen, 332, 337
semiconductor, 338
sensitivity, 13, 25, 38, 43, 51, 55, 58, 62, 65, 70, 118, 158, 177, 178, 182, 200, 207, 288, 303, 351, 352, 353, 354, 362
sensitization, 37, 38
sensorimotor gating, 91
sentencing, 273, 274
sepsis, x, 175, 183, 184, 187, 188, 192, 193, 202
septum, 236
serotonin, 2, 12, 18, 19, 23, 45, 51, 65
serum, 25, 28, 30, 34, 47, 51, 53, 63, 77, 97, 213, 341, 343, 346, 350, 351, 352, 354
service provider, 167
SES, 71, 319, 324
severe stress, 88
sex, 10, 27, 37, 39, 48, 64, 325
sex differences, 10, 64
sex hormones, 10, 37, 39
sexual abuse, 168, 304, 320, 321, 322, 327, 329
sexual behavior, 271
sexual behaviour, 39, 284
sexually transmitted diseases, 323
shame, 123, 362
sheep, 43, 53, 72, 185, 190, 216, 223, 229, 232, 238, 242, 243, 244
shock, 150, 257
shortage, 210
short-term memory, 87, 102
shrinkage, 206
sialic acid, 352
sibling, 294
siblings, 164, 284, 295, 360
side effects, 114
signal transduction, 17, 18, 21, 23, 47, 179, 183, 199, 203, 212, 223, 244
signaling pathway, 20, 23, 24, 43, 146, 232
signalling, 50, 54, 55, 56, 62, 63, 72, 76, 77, 78, 98, 201, 205, 207, 211, 212, 222, 349
signals, 37, 38, 61, 202
signs, 106, 121, 200, 206, 226, 266, 285
sister chromatid exchange, 35
skeletal muscle, 6, 10, 34
skeleton, 93, 132, 133, 134, 136, 150
small intestine, 83, 228
smoking, 71, 90, 99, 114, 119, 241, 254, 289, 295, 297, 332, 336, 337, 338, 339, 340, 341, 342, 344, 345, 346, 362, 364
smooth muscle, 78, 223
smooth muscle cells, 223
sociability, 246
social activities, 233
social behavior, 131
social change, 292
social consequences, xii, 158, 281
social desirability, 123, 158, 248
social events, 161
social integration, 171
social network, 168
social problems, xiii, 299, 315
social responsibility, 270
social roles, 318
social services, ix, 121, 155, 268, 301
social situations, 161
social skills, 106, 233, 266, 278, 357
social standing, 117
social stigmatization, 123
social workers, 269, 300, 304
socialization, 268
societal cost, ix, 156
socioeconomic status, xii, 70, 156, 265, 281, 289, 317, 318, 319, 324
sodium, 203
South Africa, 71, 98, 99, 102, 258, 277, 291, 297, 298
South Dakota, 120
South Korea, 258
space, 108, 181, 185, 197, 209, 301
Spain, 258
spatial learning, 86
spatial memory, 102, 308
specialists, 253
species, 5, 11, 24, 30, 36, 46, 73, 74, 76, 79, 83, 87, 89, 131, 145, 147, 176, 179, 198, 199, 201, 203, 214, 218, 220, 222, 229, 232, 238, 241
spectroscopy, 18
speech, xii, 106, 281, 284, 303
sperm, 196, 338, 341
spinal cord, 131
spontaneous abortion, 68, 205, 294, 336, 345
spontaneous recovery, 163
standard deviation, 266, 267, 268
standardization, 186

State Department, 127
state laws, 119
state legislatures, 120
statistics, 125, 248, 317, 345
stem cells, 25, 223
steroids, 10, 23, 25, 37, 59, 61, 208, 209, 217, 221
stigma, 117, 119, 158, 168, 178
stigmatized, 304, 306
stillbirth, 41, 123, 282
stimulus, 17, 38, 220
stoichiometry, 33
stomach, 5, 12, 63
strabismus, 284
strategy, 145, 164, 271, 278, 357
strategy use, 271
stressors, 79, 182, 208, 318, 326
striatum, 236, 241
stroma, 203, 209
structural changes, 81
structural defects, 287
structuring, 304
stupor, 13
styrene, 93
subcutaneous injection, 85
substance abuse, 88, 121, 160, 167, 168, 171, 173, 256, 272, 276, 326, 328
substance use, xiv, 121, 172, 188, 248, 256, 271, 272, 274, 316, 322, 325, 327, 328, 347, 354, 356
substrates, 6, 9, 203
supervision, 274, 301, 304, 312
suppression, 27, 45, 50, 79, 101, 182
Supreme Court, 121
surface area, 211, 264
surfactant, 185, 187, 190, 192, 193
surfactant proteins, 185
surveillance, 107, 115, 120, 149, 186, 259, 290
survey, viii, 105, 107, 108, 114, 115, 119, 120, 122, 123, 124, 156, 170, 241, 248, 249, 250, 256, 257, 289, 296, 326, 355, 360, 361, 364
survey design, 249
survival, 13, 24, 40, 87, 99, 102, 146, 198, 206, 211, 212, 308, 337
survivors, 329
susceptibility, vii, xi, 4, 7, 35, 43, 44, 46, 67, 70, 76, 94, 95, 189, 191, 201, 216, 217, 232, 263, 265, 270, 294
suspensions, 316
sweat, 13, 351, 354
Switzerland, 258
symptoms, 25, 31, 36, 89, 207, 300, 301, 316, 321, 338
synaptic plasticity, 21
syncytium, 197, 205
syndrome, ix, x, xi, xii, 53, 90, 94, 98, 100, 101, 102, 129, 130, 144, 148, 151, 152, 195, 196, 207, 213, 222, 239, 245, 246, 259, 263, 264, 266, 267, 269, 275, 276, 278, 279, 281, 282, 283, 284, 285, 287, 293, 295, 296, 297, 298, 299, 300, 301, 303, 305, 306, 308, 309, 310, 311, 316, 349, 360, 363
synthesis, 18, 26, 28, 37, 41, 45, 47, 51, 72, 77, 78, 79, 92, 93, 99, 100, 147, 181, 208, 223, 353

## T

T cell, 56, 184, 185
T regulatory cells, 184
tactics, 309
target behavior, 163
target population, 336
T-cell receptor, 45
teens, 108, 122
teeth, 210
telencephalon, 22
temperature, 33, 35, 139, 351
tension, 197, 217, 308
tensions, 308
teratogen, 56, 88, 91, 97, 99, 119, 151, 226, 232
teratology, 82, 149, 152, 212, 226, 232, 278
terminals, 11, 23, 51
territory, 249, 252
testing, 119, 121, 341, 351, 353, 354
testosterone, 10, 25, 37, 38, 39, 57, 64
tetralogy, 284
thalamus, 64, 232, 235, 242
therapeutic intervention, x, 175, 186
therapeutics, 58
therapy, 191, 218
thermodynamics, 190
thromboxanes, 81, 92
thymus, 184, 188
thyroid, 3, 20, 38, 39, 42, 52, 53, 59, 64
thyroid stimulating hormone, 38
time periods, 350
tissue, 6, 7, 9, 10, 12, 22, 25, 27, 28, 30, 34, 42, 46, 60, 79, 90, 150, 178, 180, 181, 182, 184, 201, 210, 221, 228, 230, 234, 353
Title V, 122
TLR, 3, 44, 45, 74
TLR4, 63
TNF, 3, 34, 41, 84, 87, 206, 207, 221
TNF-α, 3, 34, 41, 84, 207, 221
tobacco, vii, xiv, 67, 71, 119, 149, 159, 249, 252, 253, 254, 255, 342, 347
tobacco smoking, vii, 67
toxic effect, xiv, 4, 46, 130, 209, 347, 354
toxic side effect, 46
toxic substances, 323

toxicity, 7, 12, 13, 17, 29, 33, 34, 35, 44, 46, 64, 70, 74, 91, 92, 93, 97, 99, 102, 145, 146, 147, 151, 179, 182, 211, 212, 214, 219, 220, 228, 282
toxicology, 119, 131, 149, 191, 221
toxin, 130, 345
trace elements, 76, 88
trade union, 337
traditions, 291
training, ix, xv, 155, 159, 166, 167, 255, 256, 259, 275, 288, 303, 305, 312, 359, 361
training programs, 166
trajectory, 117
transaminases, 213
transcription, 24, 63, 82, 84, 179, 205, 210
transcription factors, 63, 84, 179, 210
transcripts, 52
transduction, 180
transference, x, 195, 196
transferrin, xiv, 2, 13, 192, 348, 352, 355, 356
transforming growth factor, 24, 50, 59, 61
translation, 187
translocation, 180
transmission, 11, 18, 23, 37, 49, 56, 99, 233
transport, x, 3, 28, 41, 42, 51, 53, 54, 56, 72, 80, 81, 82, 83, 85, 93, 94, 95, 101, 151, 180, 196, 198, 199, 201, 202, 221, 241
transportation, 308
trauma, 326
traumatic brain injury, 216
traumatic events, 319, 322
trial, 120, 122, 127, 160, 163, 169, 170, 171, 273, 274
tricarboxylic acid, 5, 11
tricarboxylic acid cycle, 11
triggers, 3, 64, 205, 210
triglycerides, 28, 62, 100
triiodothyronine, 3, 38, 39
trisomy, 288
TSH, 3, 38
tubal ligation, 164
tuberculosis, 354
tumor, 3, 64, 206, 219, 223, 354
tumor necrosis factor, 3, 64, 206, 219, 223
tumours, 9
turnover, 8, 205
twins, 70, 101, 328
type 1 diabetes, 61
tyrosine, 19, 21, 40, 52, 65, 203, 218, 349
Tyrosine, 220

## U

UK, 247, 258, 335
ultrasound, 230, 239, 241
umbilical cord, 28, 29, 48, 51, 81, 120
underlying mechanisms, 41
undernutrition, 71
uniform, 208, 212
urban population, xii, 281, 289
urethane, 84, 93
uric acid, 29, 47, 53, 65
urinary tract, 40
urine, 12, 39, 79, 307, 336, 338, 340, 341, 351, 354
US Department of Health and Human Services, 239, 242
uterus, 40, 97, 196

## V

variations, 6, 9, 19, 35, 46, 49, 107, 115, 181, 182, 248, 250, 265, 292
vascular cell adhesion molecule, 3
vascular system, 197
vasculature, 82, 202, 203
vasoactive intestinal peptide, 3, 20, 238
vasoconstriction, 42, 62, 78, 82, 90
vasodilation, 12
vasodilator, 42, 53, 78
vasopressin, 2, 39, 48
VCAM, 3, 45
vein, 146, 198
velo-cardio-facial syndrome, 288
ventilation, 23
ventricle, 146
ventricular septal defect, 212, 284
verbal fluency, 271
Verbal IQ, 271
vertebrae, 78
vertebrates, 21, 136, 146, 149
vessels, 48, 81, 136, 138, 209, 283
victimization, xi, 263, 270, 274, 322, 328
victims, xiii, 299, 326
violence, 271, 300, 301, 308, 319, 321, 322, 325
violent behaviour, 284
violent crime, 323
viral infection, 88, 185
virus infection, 187, 191
vision, 82, 302, 307, 324
visual system, 148
visualization, 218
vitamin A, 9, 50, 51, 92, 98, 210
vitamin B6, 42, 101
vitamin C, 60, 99, 200, 221
vitamin E, 76, 99, 181, 192, 200
vitamins, 80, 97, 200, 222
vocabulary, 303, 307, 313

vulnerability, 55, 58, 68, 69, 71, 94, 96, 149, 186, 191, 204, 211, 212, 220, 231, 237, 238, 240, 241, 242, 243, 265, 272

## W

wealth, 46, 232
websites, 252, 255, 258
weight gain, 16
welfare, 114, 120, 121, 123, 165
Western Cape Province, 98, 291, 297
Western Europe, 348
white blood cells, 12, 29, 35
white matter, 56, 207, 218, 236, 242, 244
wild type, 10, 57, 76, 84, 87
windows, 22, 42, 69, 151, 232, 234, 236, 238, 240
withdrawal, 316
witnesses, 270
workers, 292, 336, 362
working memory, 83, 271
workplace, 322, 328
World Health Organisation, 348

## Y

yolk, 75, 89, 133, 138, 143, 147
young women, 124, 325, 350

## Z

zinc, vii, viii, 1, 6, 45, 46, 49, 53, 55, 56, 60, 63, 67, 74, 83, 84, 85, 87, 89, 90, 91, 92, 93, 94, 95, 96, 97, 98, 100, 102, 202, 223
zygote, 196